RESEARCH METHODS IN HEALTH

Dedication

For my daughters,
Zoe Sanipreeya Rice and Emma Inturatana Rice

RESEARCH METHODS

IN HEALTH

FOUNDATIONS FOR
EVIDENCE-BASED PRACTICE

THIRD EDITION

Edited by **Pranee Liamputtong**

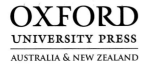

OXFORD
UNIVERSITY PRESS
AUSTRALIA & NEW ZEALAND

OXFORD
UNIVERSITY PRESS

Oxford University Press is a department of the University of Oxford.

It furthers the University's objective of excellence in research, scholarship, and education by publishing worldwide. Oxford is a registered trademark of Oxford University Press in the UK and in certain other countries.

Published in Australia by
Oxford University Press
253 Normanby Road, South Melbourne, Victoria 3205, Australia

© Pranee Liamputtong 2017

The moral rights of the author have been asserted.

First edition published 2010

Second edition published 2013

Third edition published 2017

National Library of Australia Cataloguing-in-Publication entry

Title: Research methods in health: foundations for evidence-based practice / PraneeLiamputtong (editor).

Edition: 3rd edition

ISBN 9780190304300 (paperback)

Notes: Includes bibliographical references and index.

Subjects: Health–Research–Methodology.
Medical sciences–Research–Methodology.
Evidence-based medicine.
Research–Methodology.

Other Creators/Contributors:
Liamputtong, Pranee, 1955-, editor.

Dewey Number: 610.7

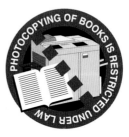

Edited by Adrienne de Kretser, Righting Writing
Text design by Ana Cosma
Cover image from Getty/jpgfactory
Typeset by Newgen KnowledgeWorks Pvt. Ltd., Chennai, India
Proofread by Philip Bryan
Indexed by Frances Paterson
Printed by Shek Wah Tong in Hong Kong

BRIEF CONTENTS

PART I METHODS AND PRINCIPLES 1

PART II QUALITATIVE APPROACHES AND PRACTICES 65

PART III QUANTITATIVE APPROACHES AND PRACTICES 191

PART IV EVIDENCE-BASED PRACTICE AND SYSTEMATIC REVIEWS 291

PART V **MIXED METHODS RESEARCH** 359

PART VI **MAKING SENSE OF AND PRESENTING DATA**.................419

EXPANDED CONTENTS

PART I METHODS AND PRINCIPLES... 1

1 The Science of Words and the Science of Numbers 3

PRANEE LIAMPUTTONG

2 Getting Started: Designing and Planning a Research Project 29

PRANEE LIAMPUTTONG AND VIRGINIA SCHMIED

3 What is Ethical Research?...49

PAUL RAMCHARAN

PART II QUALITATIVE APPROACHES AND PRACTICES 65

4 The In-depth Interviewing Method in Health 67

TANYA SERRY AND PRANEE LIAMPUTTONG

FIGURES

FIGURES AND TABLES

TABLES

PREFACE

In 2011, Norman Denzin (2011, p. 645) contended that 'like an elephant in the living room the evidence-based model is an intruder whose presence can no longer be ignored'. This is even more true in 2017. Globally, evidence-based practice (EBP) has become a major preoccupation of researchers and practitioners in health care. EBP lends itself neatly to the practice of some health practitioners, particularly those who rely on interventions in their practice. No doubt EBP is very useful for certain health researchers and practitioners, but it overemphasises certain kinds of research and undervalues or ignores other kinds that can contribute greatly to health practices. Politically, this has prompted many researchers to suggest that EBP is developed to privilege certain health researchers, practitioners and health practices. The main debate is the question of what type of evidence we need in health care practice. Of course not all evidence can be gathered from the approach advocated by EBP, and this is when we need to carry out research to find appropriate evidence that will be suitable for our practice and our clients. This is the precise reason for this book to be born.

In this book I bring together contributors who write about research methods that readers can adopt to find their evidence. I include both qualitative and quantitative approaches, as we need to select the method that is appropriate for the questions we ask. I also include chapters on the mixed methods research design so that readers can see that there are times when we need to consider both approaches in finding evidence we need. The volume also introduces ways in which we can make sense of the research data we have collected and instructions on how to write up the data in a more meaningful way.

In this third edition, I introduce a new chapter (Chapter 2) on designing and planning a research project that students and researchers will find useful. This is the result of demand from readers who wished to see such a chapter included in the book. In any piece of research, ethical issues are crucial. How do we carry out research without harming our research participants? In our preoccupation with finding evidence, we may forget that there is another party that we must acknowledge, and we must design our research carefully so that they will not be harmed. Chapter 3 deals with this important matter. Also, researchers and practitioners have to find appropriate methods or approaches when dealing with disadvantaged groups, such as indigenous populations. How to work with marginalised people in our research endeavour is dealt with in Chapter 22.

Part IV of this text comprises chapters dedicated to EBP and systematic review. As mentioned above, EBP has become a norm in most health care areas. Chapters in this Part will point to this. A systematic review of hard evidence is recognised as the best way for EBP. A new chapter on metasynthesis of qualitative evidence was included in the second edition of this book and it has proved to be very useful for researchers who wish to make qualitative evidence more convincing. Metasynthesis has been seen as a way for qualitative research to be included in EBP. Cheryl Beck (2009) said this clearly in the title of her piece on EBP and qualitative research: *Metasynthesis: A Goldmine for Evidence-based Practice*. I believe the inclusion of this chapter in the second edition was useful for many readers and practitioners who wish to find evidence based on qualitative inquiry.

In most textbooks on qualitative and quantitative research, the quantitative approach is treated first. To me this implies that qualitative research takes second place and confirms the common perception that it is a 'soft' science. In putting qualitative research first, I am arguing that this approach is as legitimate as the quantitative one in the academic and practical worlds.

As in any good textbook, a Glossary is included at the end of this book. It should be noted that many of the entries in this Glossary are contested in the literature in terms of definition and use. Readers may find that some of the definitions that I use in this book are different from others, but they represent what writers refer to in their chapters. The margin notes are an abbreviated version of the relevant Glossary entry.

This book is intended as a foundation for EBP in health. It is written mainly for undergraduate students. Each chapter includes concrete or real examples. Each chapter also contains 'Tutorial exercises' at the end, and most contain 'Stop and think' boxes throughout, which will give students practice in using research to generate evidence. The volume also includes examples of research practices in each chapter. I believe these will provide students and readers with concrete examples that can be adopted as evidence in health care. Each chapter also provides further reading lists and websites that will allow students to delve deeper into the methods and issues. Although the book is intended for undergraduates, it has been very useful for postgraduate students and novice researchers who need to make themselves more familiar with different types of research and the processes involved.

I wish to express my gratitude to many people who helped to make this book possible. First, I would like to express my thanks to the contributors, many of whom worked hard to deliver their chapters within the time-frame that I set. I would like to thank the two reviewers who provided useful comments. I thank Debra James and Melpo Christofi of Oxford University Press in Melbourne who believed in this book and helped to bring it to birth; I greatly appreciate their assistance. Last, I thank my two children, Zoe Sanipreeya Rice and Emma Inturatana Rice, who understand the busy life of an academic mother.

Two chapters in this book reproduce sections that have been published in journals.

In Chapter 17, Table 17.1 is reproduced from Iles & Davidson (2006), Evidence based practice: A survey of physiotherapists' current practice, in *Physiotherapy Research International*, with permission from Wiley-Blackwell. In Chapter 27, an example from the journal *Sexual Health* (see Rawson & Liamputtong 2009) is used with permission from CSIRO Publishing. The link to this issue of *Sexual Health* is <www.publish.csiro.au/nid/166/issue/5048.htm>. An example from *Archives of Physical Medicine and Rehabilitation* (see Shields *et al.* 2008b) is used here with permission from Elsevier Science.

Pranee Liamputtong

Sydney, April 2016

GUIDED TOUR

- A list of **Abbreviations** at the beginning of the book provides a quick reference to help you with unfamiliar acronyms.

ABBREVIATIONS

ACCHO	Aboriginal community controlled health organisation
ACL	anterior cruciate ligament
AHW	Aboriginal health worker
AMS	Aboriginal Medical Service
ANOVA	analysis of variance
CAQDAS	computer-assisted qualitative data analysis software
CDM	clinical data-mining
CEBM	Centre for Evidence-Based Medicine
CONSORT	Consolidated Standards of Reporting Trial
CPG	clinical practice guideline
CPR	collaborative participatory research
CTT	classical test theory
EBM	evidence-based medicine
EBP	evidence-based practice

- Each chapter opens with **Chapter objectives** that are clearly defined to focus your learning on the main points of the text.

Chapter objectives

In this chapter you will learn:

- about evidence and evidence-based practice
- about different research designs in health
- the nature of qualitative and quantitative approaches
- the usefulness of mixed methods
- about rigour, reliability and validity in research
- about sampling issues

- **Key terms** highlight important concepts that will be addressed in the chapter.

Key terms

Bias	Ontology
Constructivism	Phenomenology
Convenience sampling	Positivism
Data saturation	Pragmatism
Effectiveness/efficacy	Probability sampling method
Epistemology	Purposive sampling
Ethnography	Qualitative research
Evidence	Quantitative research
Evidence-based practice	Reliability
Knowledge	Research participant
Knowledge acquisition	Rigour
Metasynthesis	Systematic review
Mixed methods	Validity
Non-probability sampling	Variable

- **Key terms**, with their definitions, are placed in the **margin notes** throughout the text to provide concise explanations of the main concepts and aid your understanding as you read.

Introduction

Knowledge is essential to human survival. Over the course of history, there have been many ways of knowing, from divine revelation to tradition and the authority of elders. By the beginning of the seventeenth century, people began to rely on a different way of knowing—the research method (Grinnell *et al.* 2011a, p. 16).

Knowledge: An accepted body of facts or ideas acquired through the use of the senses or reason, or through research methods.

According to Grinnell and colleagues (2014a, p. 8), **knowledge** is 'an accepted body of facts or ideas which is acquired through the use of the senses or reason'. In the old days, we used to believe that the Earth was flat. Our belief came about through those who were in 'authority', who told us so, or because people in our society had always believed that the world was flat. Now we know that the Earth is spherical because scientists have travelled into space to observe it from this perspective. However, Grinnell and colleagues argue that the most efficient way of 'knowing something' (**knowledge acquisition**) is through research findings, which have been gathered through the use of research methods.

Knowledge acquisition: The most efficient way of 'knowing something' is through research findings, which have been gathered through the use of research methods.

What has knowledge got to do with evidence and evidence-based practice? I contend that it is through our knowledge that evidence can be generated. This evidence can then be used for our practice. Without knowledge, there will not be evidence that we can use. But how can we find knowledge? For scientists and health practitioners, the answer is through research and research methods (Neutens 2014). According to Grinnell and colleagues (2014a, p. 17),

---

- **Stop and think** questions appear at regular intervals, inviting you to critically reflect and consider your own responses to important issues discussed throughout the chapter.

STOP AND THINK

- Considering what has been discussed above, what is your opinion regarding evidence and evidence-based health care?
- Should all EBP be based on an RCT or quantitative research approach only? Why?
- What type of evidence would you need in your own profession? With colleagues who have a different professional background from you, discuss what evidence would be more appropriate for your work and your prospective clients.

- **Research in practice** boxes introduce the reader to practical cases and examples that demonstrate how research can be applied in clinical practice.

RESEARCH IN PRACTICE

A PRACTICAL CONSIDERATION IN THE CHOICE OF RESEARCH APPROACH

Emma is a podiatrist and owns her practice. Through her work, she has treated many competitive athletes who come to her because of their foot injuries. This is particularly so around the time of major competitive events like the Commonwealth and Olympic Games. She does not know the real prevalence of the injuries in her city, so she cannot say exactly what would be the rate of injuries; she only knows that she has treated many athletes. She would like to know about this as she needs to prepare her practice in terms of the number of podiatrists that she needs to employ and the purchase of essential equipment. Emma has also noticed that some athletes do not follow her advice about how to avoid or prevent foot injuries, or adhere to this non-compliance. Hence, this is the beginning of her research endeavour.

From reading literature on sports injuries, Emma realises that there are different ways in which she can find her answers. If she wants to ascertain the prevalence of foot injuries among competitive athletes, she would need to use a quantitative approach, as this would allow her to determine the number of such injuries in her city. However, if she wants to understand why the athletes do not follow her advice or adhere to her treatment plans, she must talk to them and allow them to tell her stories, as this will provide her with in-depth understanding of their issues, which may help her to develop treatment plans that better cater for their personal needs. So, Emma has choices as to how she can obtain evidence that can inform her work.

- Clearly presented **Tables** and **Figures** encourage analysis of relevant data by presenting facts in a format that assists comprehension.

TABLE 1.1   Comparison of qualitative and quantitative approaches

QUALITATIVE APPROACH	QUANTITATIVE APPROACH
Words	Numbers
Participants' points of view	Researcher's point of view
Meaning	Behaviour
Contextual understanding	Generalisation
Rich, deep data	Hard, reliable data
Unstructured	Structured
Process	Static
Micro	Macro
Natural settings	Artificial settings
Theory emergent	Theory testing
Researcher close	Researcher distant

FIGURE 1.1   Hierarchy of evidence

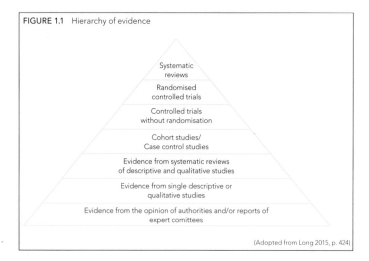

Systematic
reviews

Randomised
controlled trials

Controlled trials
without randomisation

Cohort studies/
Case control studies

Evidence from systematic reviews
of descriptive and qualitative studies

Evidence from single descriptive or
qualitative studies

Evidence from the opinion of authorities and/or reports of
expert comittees

(Adopted from Long 2015, p. 424)

- Each chapter ends with a **Summary** that draws together important ideas. To reinforce what has been covered, these link back to chapter opening objectives.

Summary

Neither quantitative nor qualitative methodology is in any ultimate sense superior to the other. The two approaches exist along a continuum on which neither pole is more 'scientific' or more suited to … knowledge development. (Williams *et al.* 2014, p. 94).

In this chapter, I have introduced the concept of evidence and evidence-based practice in health. I have argued that in many situations and for many health issues, researchers and practitioners need to find the 'best' evidence, and this may require us to carry out a research study to find our answers. I have provided readers with firm foundations for carrying out research in health. I have suggested that researchers should not favour one method over another based on their own preferences. Rather, we need to carefully consider the research questions to which we wish to find answers.

- **Practice exercises** consolidate your understanding of a particular concept covered within the chapter. They are appropriate for use in class-based discussions.

Practice exercises

1 You have been asked by your superior to find the 'best' evidence that can be used to develop culturally sensitive maternal and child health services for Indigenous Australians. How would you find this 'best' evidence? Discuss various types of evidence that you could obtain.

2 There has been a good deal of discussion in your local area about young people, who are seen as likely to engage in risky health-related behaviour such as smoking heavily, driving very fast, and not paying attention to their diet. You want to understand why young people tend to take such health risks. Which research approach (qualitative or quantitative) is likely to give you greater in-depth understanding of their lives, the meaning they attach to risk-taking behaviour and their lived experiences of risk? Discuss.

- **Further reading** and annotated **Websites** advise you of relevant works in the subject and allow you to conduct additional reading and learning that will be of interest.

Further reading

Alvesson, M. & Sandberg, J. (2013). *Constructing research questions: doing interesting research.* London: Sage.

Bryman, A. (2016). *Social research methods*, 5th edn. Oxford: Oxford University Press.

Dingwall, R. & McDonnell, M.B. (2015). *The Sage handbook of research management.* London: Sage.

Fawcett, B. & Pockett, R. (2015). *Turning ideas into research: theory, design & practice.* London: Sage.

Websites

https://www.youtube.com/watch?v=GYywR7SA03E

Dr Michael Quinn Patton talks about designing and planning a research project to find knowledge.

https://www.youtube.com/watch?v=LWLYCYeCFak

This video discusses how to develop a research question.

- A consolidated **Glossary** is located at the end of the book to provide quick reference to all the key terms listed throughout the text.

GLOSSARY

Allocation bias
A type of selection bias that occurs when the process of allocating participants to groups leads to differences in the baseline characteristics of those groups.

Allocation concealment
The randomised allocation sequence being concealed from investigators who are involved in recruiting participants.

Alternating treatment design
Two or three treatments of interest are provided in rapid succession and in an alternating format, within a session, in a session-by-session format or in a day-by-day format. The results are graphed together to clearly show the difference in rate and stability of learning in each treatment condition.

associations between exposure and outcome factors.

Anonymity
Refers to a person being unknown to the researcher and hence to anyone else. Further, if the person took part in a public health survey their confidentiality was maintained.

Ascertainment bias
Occurs when the results or conclusions of the trial are distorted by the knowledge of which intervention each participant is receiving.

Assessment bias
Occurs if an investigator's assessment of a participant lacks objectivity. Subjective outcome measures are prone to exaggerate the effect of the intervention.

ABOUT THIS BOOK

This book contains twenty-seven chapters and is divided into six parts. Part I contains three introductory chapters. The first, by Pranee Liamputtong, introduces issues relevant to evidence and evidence-based practice. It suggests that evidence can be obtained from different sources. It argues that the hierarchical system used in the EBP model privileges certain research methods and that not all evidence can be found in EBP. It follows with discussion on several salient points in carrying out research in the health sciences. These include the selection of the method appropriate to the questions for which researchers wish to find evidence. When asking qualitative and/or quantitative questions, researchers need to ensure that the method is selected appropriately. Each approach will provide different types of evidence and we should not assume that one approach can provide the best or all the evidence we need. Different ontological and epistemological positions adopted by qualitative and quantitative approaches are introduced in this chapter. Issues of rigour, validity and reliability within both approaches are crucial for good research; these are included in this chapter. The last section is dedicated to sampling issues.

Chapter 2 is a new chapter in this edition. Pranee Liamputtong and Virginia Schmied introduce salient issues that researchers must consider in designing and planning for their research. The chapter commences with discussions about what we need to think when designing our research project. Regardless of the nature of research enquiry, research is a cyclical process. The chapter includes the research process that researchers tend to follow. In this section, the authors point out subtle differences between qualitative and quantitative research. In any research project, research questions are essential. Often, our research questions derive from research problems. These are discussed in this chapter. In planning a research project, a literature review offers researchers many benefits. The chapter discusses why we need to conduct a literature review and where we can find the literature. The last section of the chapter focuses on a research proposal and its structure. This is important for all research projects, as the research proposal will dictate the direction and success of our research project.

In Chapter 3, Paul Ramcharan outlines the emergence of the largely unregulated social research ethical frameworks and, by contrast, those associated with health and medical research that arose from the Helsinki Declaration. The convergence of the two discourses in the past decade is described and explained. This is supplemented by a consideration of the Australian NHMRC National Statement on Ethical Conduct in Human Research and the position of both the National Office for Research Ethics Committees and the Research Ethics Framework of the Economic and Social Research Council in the UK. The nature and principles of contemporary ethical frameworks are described and case studies are provided to highlight issues around anonymity/confidentiality, privacy, informed consent, dependence and vulnerability, data storage and potential conflicts of interest. Readers are given additional examples through which they might work using ethical principles and the seminal concepts of beneficence, non-maleficence, discomfort and justice. In these case studies, students are asked to work as researchers or together as a Human Research Ethics Committee (HREC) to come to a decision about the balance of risk and benefit in each case study. Remaining issues around ethical regulation are described. These include the extent to which regulation is paternalistic, difficulties in maintaining independence of decision-making from conflicts of interest, contradictions between the need for clearly established protocols for decision-making versus research with emergent designs, issues around vulnerable groups, and the importance of ethics as process.

Part II commences with Chapter 4 on the in-depth interviewing method in health, by Tanya Serry and Pranee Liamputtong. They argue that, among qualitative research methods, the in-depth interviewing method is the most commonly employed by qualitative researchers. Conversation, it is argued, is a fundamental means of interaction between individuals in society. Through conversation, people have an opportunity to know others, learn about their feelings and experiences, and the world in which they live. The authors suggest that interviewing is a way of collecting empirical data about the social world of individuals by inviting them to talk about their lives in depth. In an interview conversation, the researcher asks questions then listens to what people say about their dreams, fears and hopes. The researcher hears about the interviewees' perspectives in their own words, and learns about their family and social life and work. Most people, including researchers, will say they know about the in-depth interview method, or they have heard about it, and that it is not difficult to ask questions and talk to people. But, as the authors suggest in this chapter, undertaking a good in-depth interview requires a lot more than knowing how to ask questions and talk to people. There are many things to consider and there are techniques that can be used to elicit detailed and accurate information from the research participants. The authors provide practical steps for in-depth interviews and case studies from their research in speech pathology and public health.

Chapter 5 is about the focus group method in health and nursing. Patricia Davidson, Elizabeth Halcomb and Leila Gholizadeh argue that focus groups are a useful strategy for obtaining the collective perspective of a group of individuals with common characteristics; they are also useful for studying issues and concerns about a topic that is not well known. Focus groups are particularly valuable in obtaining the views and perspectives of underrepresented and marginalised individuals, and can be tailored to address contextual factors and concerns. Commonly, focus groups consist of five to fifteen people who share their opinions and experiences about a particular issue with the guidance of a moderator. Focus groups can also promote interaction and encourage deliberation of crucial issues by stimulating group discussion. In health research, this method can be informative in exploring issues as well as providing an evaluation technique. This chapter discusses pragmatic issues in conducting focus groups and proposes strategies to ensure methodological rigour.

In Chapter 6, Priscilla Ennals and Linsey Howie write about narrative enquiry in occupational therapy. They contend that the numerous methodologies comprising qualitative research can be confusing to the uninitiated health professional. Narrative enquiry is a research method used more recently in health science research to examine clients' thoughts and experiences of illness, interventions, rehabilitation and recovery, and service provision. In illuminating experience from a consumer's perspective, narrative enquiry enlarges our understanding of phenomena and engages participants in the research process. However, the potential for narrative research to inform health practice through the retrospective telling of events or experiences relevant to specific professions is not fully appreciated. The aim of this chapter is to provide a detailed account of narrative enquiry and the processes involved in the design and conduct of narrative studies that seek to establish the meaning of human experiences conveyed through stories. This chapter gives an outline of the method, its origins and uses in other disciplines, and an overview of the place of narrative within qualitative research. A clear account of sampling procedures, participant recruitment and engagement, data collection and analysis, with reference to key authors in this area of research, is presented using a step-by-step approach to demystify poorly understood aspects of this method.

Jon Willis and Karen Anderson discuss the use of ethnography in health research, in Chapter 7. They suggest that ethnography focuses on describing and understanding the practices and beliefs of groups of people within the context of the shared cultures that structure and give meaning to their actions and interactions. From the health perspective, ethnography provides unique insights into the ways that patients understand illness and the struggle for health, the social contexts in which health practitioners are trained, the ways in which we organise and validate health-related actions, whether as consumers or practitioners, and how societies privilege particular models of health and illness while dismissing others. In this chapter, the authors explore the origins of ethnography in early twentieth-century anthropological practice, and chart its development as a methodological paradigm. Using examples, they demonstrate the array of tools and approaches that ethnographic methodology now encompasses in a range of social and health science disciplines. They explore in particular the influence of the Chicago School and the symbolic interactionists on the application of ecological principles in the ethnography of urban societies, as well as the impact of postmodernism, and the insights offered by cultural theory to our understanding of the circulation of health-related information, meanings and rationalities within complex social networks. Finally, they examine recent examples of ethnography in the area of health, including focused ethnography, institutional ethnography and ethno-nursing.

Chapter 8, by Pauline Wong, Pranee Liamputtong and Helen Rawson, is about using grounded theory in health research. The authors point out that qualitative methods have been used in health professions such as nursing for many years to describe, interpret and better understand the perspectives of clients, families and nurses. Grounded theory is a qualitative method that allows researchers to explore and explain social processes, structures and interactions. The focus for grounded theory research is on discovering the main concern of people in the situation, the processes that are at work for these people, and how these processes are maintained or limited. For example, health professionals and nurses could explore the goal-setting process from the client's perspective, in order to better understand how to negotiate this process with clients and provide client-centred care. There are several approaches to grounded theory, but each includes a core set of methods that researchers apply in order to develop an explanatory framework for the situation. The aim of this chapter is to introduce the grounded theory method, including the main techniques that distinguish it from other methods. The chapter begins with a brief description of the history of grounded theory, and a consideration of different modes or approaches. It then describes the steps to be taken in a grounded theory study, including theoretical sampling, constant comparison for analysis, and development of theory. An example of some of these steps is given using the authors' research. Potential uses of the method for understanding social processes and interactions in nursing, including examples of published research in the field, are also provided.

Christine Carpenter, in Chapter 9, discusses phenomenology as a methodological approach to rehabilitation research. She contends that the aim of phenomenological research is to understand the lived experience of a phenomenon, for example spinal cord injury or physiotherapy services in the home, from the individual's perspective, and to examine the meanings they give to that experience. The choice of a particular method reflects the type of question being asked; the method in turn contributes to a coherent and rigorous qualitative study design that includes data collection methods, participant recruitment, data analysis and the role of the researcher. These design features are discussed and illustrated by drawing on research examples relevant to rehabilitation practice and physical therapy. In order to listen actively and genuinely to research participants' perspectives, researchers are required to reflect upon, and make explicit, their own understandings and beliefs about the phenomenon being studied, and this is examined in this chapter. Christine suggests that health care practitioners are required to be accountable in terms of the evidence supporting the clinical decisions they make on behalf of patients or clients. EBP, as originally conceived, privileged a hierarchy of evidence derived primarily from experimental research. Practitioners recognised that this narrow definition of 'best' evidence did not reflect the complex issues involved in living with a chronic condition or disability, or of the model of patient-focused or client-centred and interdisciplinary approaches characteristic of rehabilitation practice. Qualitative research can make a significant contribution to the generation of evidence to support clinical reasoning and practice. This contribution is also discussed using examples of phenomenological research relevant to rehabilitation.

Chapter 10, by David Nilsson, presents the use of clinical data-mining as practice-based evidence for social workers. David argues that clinical data-mining involves the use and analysis of available clinical information for research purposes. It is a form of practice-based research that is carried out by practitioners and is designed to inform and address practice issues. It is essentially a specific form of secondary data analysis. It has been used by social work practitioners and other health professionals in a range of research studies. The chapter begins by defining this method, provides a context for its use, compares it to other research methods, and outlines its advantages and drawbacks for social work practitioners. The process involved in clinical data-mining is then outlined, followed by a case study using David's study of psychosocial problems faced by 'frequent flyers' in a paediatric diabetes unit in a children's hospital. As well as outlining the methodology and findings of the study, they provide a reflective account of David's experience of using clinical data-mining in this example.

Part III is dedicated to quantitative research methods and comprises five chapters. In Chapter 11, Christine Imms and Susan Greaves argue that health clinicians use tools frequently in clinical practice and during research. We use the data obtained to support practice, understand the condition of the client, determine intervention choices and measure change. We must know how and for what purpose these tools were developed, so we can choose the right measure for our intended use. Understanding the psychometric properties of the tools we use is critical to knowing how much trust we can place in the findings. Christine and Susan point out that research studies that do this—that is, investigate the properties of clinical measurement tools—seek to evaluate aspects of validity and reliability. Validity studies aim to demonstrate that a measurement tool actually measures what it intended. Reliability studies evaluate the ability of the tool to measure consistently. Often, preliminary validity and reliability studies are conducted during development of a measurement tool, but as validity and reliability are not 'all or none' constructs, evidence about a tool's reliability and validity must be built over time. This requires the clinician to have the knowledge to be a critical consumer of validity and reliability studies. This chapter provides a basic framework to enable clinicians to become critical consumers of measurement studies. Readers are introduced to two theories of measurement development—classical test theory and item response theory—and are helped to understand the range of research studies required to develop a valid and reliable measure. They learn to critically appraise the research methods used to validate a clinical measurement tool and interpret reliability statistics. Reading this research critically will enable the clinician to determine the relative validity and reliability of the measurement tools they require in daily practice and, as a result, assist their selection of optimum tools for use with clients.

Miranda Rose's Chapter 12 is about single-subject experimental designs (SSEDs) in the health sciences. This chapter covers salient issues relevant to SSEDs. It defines SSEDs, describes their history and the need for them, and contextualises them within the broader research design schema to highlight the phases and stages of research activity they are best suited to. The chapter describes the types of SSEDs commonly used in health science research. It discusses the statistical and visual analysis techniques commonly used in SSEDs, outlines their limitations, highlights current controversies in their implementation and analysis, and suggests possible future directions for their development. A practical case study and reflective account regarding the use of the method is provided. It also describes the use of a published SSED in the investigation of treatment efficacy for aphasic word retrieval impairments. The strengths and limitations of the design and analysis methods are discussed. Last, alternative designs and the decision-making process in selecting a SSED are described.

Chapter 13, by Margot Schofield and Christine Forrester-Knauss, introduces surveys and questionnaires in health research. Surveys are a very common descriptive research method. They are particularly useful for collecting data about research phenomena that are not directly observable. This chapter provides an overview of the types of surveys used in health research, such as cross-sectional and longitudinal surveys, and describes how these relate to study aims and design. A variety of methods of administering surveys is described, including paper and pencil surveys, online surveys and interviewer-administered surveys (face-to-face, telephone and internet formats). The relative advantages and disadvantages of the different methods are explored, such as cost, time, facilities and the personnel required. The chapter also outlines key issues in survey design such as determining the topics to be covered, the use of standardised scales (advantages and disadvantages), how to design questions and response options, how to sequence questions, the use of screening questions, the design of questions on sensitive topics, avoiding bias, and consideration of closed versus open-ended responses. Issues about the validity and reliability of survey responses are addressed and methods for checking validity and reliability outlined. Examples of both cross-sectional and longitudinal survey design are provided.

In Chapter 14, Melissa Graham writes about epidemiology in health research. She argues that epidemiology is concerned with the study of the distribution and determinants of health states in populations. Epidemiology can help us to determine the extent of ill health or disease in the community, identify the cause of ill health and the risk factors for disease, understand the natural history and prognosis of ill health, investigate disease outbreaks or epidemics, evaluate existing and new preventive and therapeutic programs and services, and provide the foundation for developing public policy and regulation. Essentially, this means that epidemiology can provide the answers to questions asked in the health sector, such as: How much disease is there? Who gets it? Where are most people affected? When did they have it? What happens over time? More important is how we as health professionals apply this to prevent and control health problems. This chapter aims to introduce readers to the underlying principles of observational descriptive and analytical epidemiology, drawing on examples from contemporary practice. It also introduces readers to sources of existing epidemiological data and discusses practical applications to help answer questions of person, place and time. A case study that draws on existing data is presented.

Chapter 15, by Karl B. Landorf, introduces clinical trials in health. Karl suggests that clinical trials that evaluate the effectiveness of interventions or treatments are abundant in the health sciences. It is essential that such evaluations ensure that the effects detected are directly attributable to the intervention being investigated and not to other extraneous causes. However, not all clinical trials provide the framework to achieve this. If poorly executed, they may provide invalid results, due to inherent bias or poor methodology. Often such trials—non-randomised or uncontrolled trials ('the bad' or 'the ugly')—overestimate the effectiveness of an intervention. Fortunately, there are methods to overcome this. For some time now, the randomised controlled trial has been considered the 'gold standard' when evaluating the efficacy or effectiveness of an intervention. There are two key features to a randomised controlled trial, which in its simplest form includes (1) comparison of a group that receives an intervention with one that does not, and (2) random allocation into those groups. The main aim of using randomised trials is to ensure, as much as possible, that the characteristics of the participants (people who receive the interventions) at the beginning of the trial are similar across groups. Nevertheless, some randomised trials fail to adhere to good design principles. If appropriate randomisation is not adequately carried out, bias or systematic unwanted effects will be present. This bias will ultimately affect the accuracy of the results of the trial, generally leading to an overestimation of the effectiveness of the intervention being evaluated. Accordingly, all trials are not created equal. Certain clinical trial designs provide more accurate results than others. Randomised controlled trials are considered the gold standard, however, if there is not enough attention to detail, results from even these trials can be biased or contain errors. To minimise such errors, appropriate methods (e.g. allocation concealment and blinding) and planning (e.g. prospective sample size calculations and statistical analysis) are essential. Clinical trials should also be registered before commencement with a recognised trial register and the results reported, using the recommendations outlined in the CONSORT statement. By being aware of such matters, clinicians and researchers will assist in improving the quality of clinical trials, thus encouraging a higher standard.

Part IV is about EBP and systematic review. It has four chapters. First, in Chapter 16, Deirdre Fetherstonhaugh, Rhonda Nay and Margaret Winbolt discuss evidence-based health care. They point out that basing practice on the best available evidence is now an expectation in health care. Nevertheless, finding and translating the evidence into practice poses significant challenges for health professionals. This chapter introduces readers to evidence-based concepts in health care, provides a potted history of its development and outlines methods used to locate and appraise the evidence. As most practitioners will be more involved in using the evidence than in primary research or research appraisal, the main focus of the chapter is on translating evidence into everyday practice. There are numerous known barriers to changing practice and these are outlined, along with strategies that can be used to overcome them. A case study reporting the trials, failures and successes of translating evidence into practice, with relevant activities, assist readers to learn by doing. The chapter adopts a person-centred and interdisciplinary care approach.

Megan Davidson and Ross Iles, in Chapter 17, introduce EBP in therapeutic health care. They point out that EBP is defined as the use of best research evidence, along with clinical expertise, available resources and patient's preferences to determine the optimal assessment, treatment or management option in a specific situation. The skills to be acquired for the evidence-based practitioner centre on the use of 'best research evidence'. The five-step EBP approach of Sackett is a widely used framework. Step 1 is to recognise a knowledge gap and formulate an answerable clinical question. The type of question—whether it relates to therapy effectiveness, prognosis, diagnosis or human experiences—dictates the type of research design that is best able to answer the question. In Step 2, the evidence-based practitioner searches for the available research that is best able to answer the clinical question. Important resources for this step include sources of pre-appraised evidence such as clinical practice guidelines and systematic reviews. Databases such as the Cochrane Library, Clinical Evidence and PEDro (the Physiotherapy Evidence Database) are of most value, followed by abstracting databases such as Medline and Cinahl. In Step 3, the practitioner critically evaluates the research evidence against accepted quality criteria in order to determine how much influence the research evidence will have when considering Step 4. Step 4 is the integration of the research evidence with the other aspects of EBP (expertise, resources, patient preferences) that results in a practical clinical outcome. The final step, Step 5, is to reflect on Steps 1–4, seeking to improve one's effectiveness and efficiency as an evidence-based practitioner. In this chapter, Megan and Ross demonstrate, using an example of a therapy question and a diagnosis question, how the evidence-based physiotherapy practitioner might undertake the five-step process. They also present published surveys of physiotherapy practice that demonstrate that many practitioners do not have sufficient skills to undertake the five steps, and the implications of this for patients and clients of physiotherapists.

In Chapter 18, Terese Bondas, Elisabeth Hall and Anita Wikberg describe and discuss metasynthesis, i.e. research on previous qualitative studies in a field of interest that refers to both the analytic processes and the novel interpretation that is created. They argue that metasynthesis research in health science research can make a difference in the life of people that it may concern, and that the findings of metasynthesis studies may further the disciplinary development. Metasynthesis is compared to other review types such as integrative reviews, systematic reviews, meta-analysis and secondary analysis, but is the type of review that aggregates and synthesises qualitative findings only. The main features of metasynthesis development are described from meta-ethnography by Noblit and Hare (1988), to be continued with metastudy including meta-data analysis, meta-method analysis and meta-theory analysis to create a metasynthesis by Paterson and colleagues (2001), and further with metasummary to qualitative research synthesis by Sandelowski and Barroso (2007). Noblit and Hare's meta-ethnography and Sandelowski and Barroso's qualitative research synthesis study are exemplified with research by the authors. The reader is guided along the phases: getting started (conceiving the synthesis, deciding what is relevant to the initial interest), deciding the target of the study, reading the studies (appraising included reports, determining how studies are related), targeted comparison, translating the studies into one another, forming the qualitative metasynthesis and finally expressing and presenting the metasynthesis. The authors argue that the most important validity question is whether the metasynthesis study enlarges human science knowledge for the benefit of patients and their families.

Nora Shields discusses how to conduct the systematic reviews often used in EBP, in Chapter 19. A systematic review is a comprehensive identification and synthesis of all relevant studies on a review question. It is conducted according to an explicit and reproducible method to minimise the risk of reviewer bias. Systematic reviews help health professionals cope with large volumes of literature by summarising it and providing more reliable evidence, which can aid clinical decision-making. They are also used by researchers to identify gaps and strengths in the current literature, assisting research design. Nora argues that the method of conducting a systematic review should be transparent, easily replicated and scientifically rigorous. This chapter sets out a six-step process for completing a systematic review, including how to set an answerable clinical question, search for relevant information, decide what should be included and excluded, assess the quality of the included studies, extract relevant data, synthesise the findings of your review and consider the relevance of your review to your clinical practice. The PICO method is recommended to assist with Steps 1–3. Throughout the chapter, emphasis is placed on practical advice for students regarding decision-making and where to look for further information. Nora also suggests that, despite the advantages of systematic reviews, this method is not infallible. Areas of potential problems, such as sensitivity and specificity of the search strategy, validity of the quality assessment procedure, publication bias, data pooling and interpretation, are discussed, so that care can be taken to avoid some of the pitfalls inherent in this research method.

In Part V, chapters relevant to mixed methods research are included. Chapter 20 presents the writing of Carol Grbich on integrated methods in health research. Carol contends that the nature of allied health with its multidisciplinary focus provides the best environment for a mix of methodological approaches in research. These enable the practitioner to give a wider overview of the setting or situation before going deeper into the reasons why, the experience of and the explanation of particular behaviours. This chapter attempts to clarify the range of mixes in methodological approaches that the health professional may find useful. In particular, parallel methods and the sequencing of methods are discussed, together with indications of how these might be used within a range of methodological approaches such as ethnography, narratives, case studies and grounded theory. Multiple data sets can then be put together in a variety of ways to enhance the impact of such approaches.

In Chapter 21, Ann Taket introduces the use of mixed methods in health research. She suggests that the term 'mixed methods' can be understood in different ways. First of all, it can refer to different kinds of methods being used within a single study—often it is used to refer to mixing qualitative and quantitative methods—but it can also refer to mixing different kinds of qualitative method within a study. Second, it may refer to mixing that occurs at different stages in the research process; for example in data collection, in data analysis or indeed in both these stages. Third, we need to consider different modes or ways of mixing methods within a single study. Sometimes a research study is divided into a number of stages, carried out sequentially, so we may have a qualitative stage followed by a quantitative stage or vice versa; for example, a qualitative component (focus groups) may be used to help define and pilot a structured survey instrument. Sometimes the mixing is parallel—a qualitative component in a study runs alongside a quantitative one, without interaction, answering different research questions. Or the mixing may be a blend—two (or more) interacting strands, answering the same research question(s). Ann then considers the different potential reasons for mixing different types of qualitative method: promoting choice and empowerment for research participants, enabling participation, accessing different research participants, and triangulation. She also discusses some of the issues involved in using mixed methods in health research, illustrated with examples taken from her own research. The chapter ends with a discussion of some of the challenges (or fears) expressed about mixed methods.

Collaborative participatory research with disadvantaged communities is presented by Anke van der Sterren, Peter Waples-Crowe and Priscilla Pyett in Chapter 22. In recent years, the overwhelming evidence of the links between social factors and health inequalities has led to increasing calls for collaborative and partnership approaches to health research with disadvantaged and marginalised groups. Participatory action research (PAR) has a long tradition in developing countries and has been used in health research with many disadvantaged communities. In PAR, community members participate in research to bring about changes that will improve their circumstances. PAR involves a cycle of observe, reflect, plan, act, observe and so on. It is often used by consumer and advocacy groups or by practitioners carrying out evaluation of their programs. Academic research, on the other hand, because of the way it is funded, rarely includes sufficient time or financial resources to carry out the actions required of a PAR project. Collaborative participatory research (CPR) is a term used to describe a more practical approach to partnerships between academics or practitioners and the community groups they are researching. In CPR, participation by community members may vary from cooperating with and supporting the research team, through various levels of collaboration to full engagement as co-researchers. There is no doubt that CPR is more time-consuming than more conventional research methods. But it is also well established that CPR can increase the validity and improve the relevance of the research to the communities involved. This in turn increases the uptake of findings and the likelihood of results being of benefit to the communities. This chapter describes collaborative and participatory research methods for health research, focusing on research with Indigenous communities. It also discusses the ethical, methodological and practical challenges associated with CPR. The case study describes a collaborative project conducted with an urban Indigenous community organisation. The project was carried out in three phases: research, resource development, and training and dissemination.

Part VI is concerned with how to make sense of data and how to present it. In Chapter 23, Pranee Liamputtong and Tanya Serry discuss how to make sense of qualitative data. Once data have been collected, researchers need to organise the data in a more meaningful way. This is what qualitative researchers refer to as data analysis. Qualitative research has several ways of making sense of the data. The simplest and most common are content analysis and thematic analysis. The procedures for these data analysis methods are given in this chapter.

Chapter 24, by Tanya Serry and Pranee Liamputtong, introduces computer-assisted qualitative data analysis (CAQDAS). They argue that in this postmodern world, computers have extensively impacted on our lives and, not surprisingly, this is the case when we do research. For qualitative research, as in other fields of research, the use of computers has gained increasing prominence in both data collection and data analysis. Computer-assisted qualitative data analysis software or CAQDAS refers to a specifically designed program that can take over a substantial amount of the manual labour involved in analysing data. In this chapter, Tanya and Pranee briefly discuss some of the key functions available via CAQDAS. They describe how they have adopted CAQDAS in their own research and times when they have decided not to use it. However, they do not present a step-by-step approach to using CAQDAS, nor do they promote any one CAQDAS program over another. There is no 'industry leader' in regards to CAQDAS options. At the end of the chapter, they provide a list of CAQDAS options for readers to explore.

In Chapter 25, Jane Pierson writes about data analysis in quantitative research. This chapter covers essential matters in analysing quantitative data: the place and purpose of quantitative data analysis in health research, selection of data analysis procedures, procedures for examining association and relationships between two or more variables (chi-square, bi-variate correlation, and multiple regression), and procedures for examining differences between two or more measures of central tendency (t tests and non-parametric equivalents, ANOVAs and non-parametric equivalents, factorial ANOVAS, and post hoc tests).

Paul O'Halloran, in Chapter 26, tells us how to read and make sense of statistical data. He contends that reading and interpreting statistical data, whether it is original data from a computer package or data from a journal article, can be a considerable challenge to students and practitioners alike. Many people become overwhelmed by a mass of figures and are unclear about what specific pieces of information will aid their interpretation of the data. This can be a problem because, with the adoption of EBP, the ability to interpret statistical data is an important skill for all health care professionals. The aim of this chapter is to give readers the background information and tools that will enable them to pinpoint the critical figures and issues when reading and interpreting statistical data. This is done by examining core issues related to interpreting statistical data within a health context. That is, a practical case study involving data that are pertinent to health professionals is used to illustrate key issues. Topics examined in the chapter include key issues when interpreting descriptive statistics (e.g. strengths and limitations of descriptive statistics and how to interpret means, standard deviations and confidence intervals), key issues when interpreting inferential statistics (e.g. how to interpret findings that are statistically significant and how to interpret findings that are *not* statistically significant), statistical versus clinical significance (e.g. amount of change, complete elimination of symptoms, and similarity with normative samples at the end of an intervention), and common errors when interpreting statistical data (e.g. overinterpretation of data).

The last chapter, Chapter 27, is about how to present our end product in qualitative and quantitative data and how to evaluate qualitative and quantitative published materials to assess the strength of evidence. Pranee Liamputtong, Nora Shields and Annemarie Gallichio point out that once researchers have conducted a piece of research, it is essential to put the information down on paper: we need to write about it. We need to write in order to disseminate our research findings so that other people can read and make use of them, whether for improving current health and welfare practices or using them as the basis for developing new research projects. In many cases, this not only completes the project but is also the best way to disseminate the findings to wider audiences. In this chapter, the authors discuss some of the characteristics of qualitative and quantitative writing. They outline the styles of research report commonly used to disseminate findings drawn from both qualitative and quantitative research projects. There are a number of techniques to observe when writing good qualitative and quantitative research papers, and these are included in this chapter. The new part of this chapter focuses on how readers can evaluate qualitative and quantitative published materials which will be valuable to many students and researchers.

ABOUT THE EDITOR

Pranee Liamputtong is Professor of Public Health at the School of Science and Health, Western Sydney University, Australia. Previously, she held a position of Personal Chair in Public Health at the School of Public Health, La Trobe University, Australia. Pranee has also taught in the School of Sociology and Anthropology and worked as a public health research fellow at the Centre for the Study of Mothers' and Children's Health, La Trobe University. Pranee's particular interests include issues related to cultural and social influences on childbearing, childrearing, motherhood, infant feeding practices, and reproductive and sexual health. Her current research includes HIV/AIDS, breast cancer and sexuality.

Pranee has published several books and a large number of papers in these areas. These include *Maternity and Reproductive Health in Asian Societies* (with Lenore Manderson, Harwood Academic Press, 1996); *Asian Mothers, Western Birth* (Ausmed Publications, 1999); *Living in a New Country: Understanding Migrants' Health* (Ausmed Publications, 1999); *Hmong Women and Reproduction* (Bergin & Garvey, 2000); *Coming of Age in South and Southeast Asia: Youth, Courtship and Sexuality* (with Lenore Manderson, Curzon Press, 2002); *Health, Social Change and Communities* (with Heather Gardner, Oxford University Press, 2003). Her more recent books include *Reproduction, Childbearing and Motherhood: A Cross-Cultural Perspective* (Nova Science Publishers, 2007); *Childrearing and Infant Care Issues: A Cross-Cultural Perspective* (Nova Science Publishers, 2007); *The Journey of Becoming a Mother amongst Thai Women in Northern Thailand* (Lexington Books, 2007); *Population, Community, & Health Promotion* (with Sansnee Jirojwong, Oxford University Press, 2008); *Infant Feeding Practices: A Cross-Cultural Perspective* (Springer, New York, 2011); *Motherhood and Postnatal Depression: Narratives of Women and their Partners* (with Carolyn Westall, Springer, Dordrecht, The Netherlands, 2011); *Health, Illness and Well-Being: Perspectives and Social Determinants* (with Rebecca Fanany and Glenda Verrinder, Oxford University Press, 2012), *Contemporary Socio-Cultural and Political Perspectives in Thailand* (Springer, 2014); *Public Health: Local and Global Perspectives* (Cambridge University Press, 2016).

Pranee is a general editor of a book series, *HIV/AIDS and Cross-Cultural Research*. The series is being published by Springer in the Netherlands. Her two new books in the series were published by Springer in 2013. These were *Stigma, Discrimination and Living with HIV/AIDS* and *Women, Motherhood and Living with HIV/AIDS*. The third one in the series is *Children, Young People and Living with HIV/AIDS: A Cross-Cultural Perspective*, published in 2016. Pranee and her colleague in Thailand are in the final process of writing a book on antiretroviral drugs and Thai women living with HIV/AIDS, for Springer (to be published in 2017).

Pranee has also written and edited a number of research method books. Her first research method book was *Qualitative Research Methods: A Health Focus* (with Douglas Ezzy, Oxford University Press, 1999); the second edition of the book was titled *Qualitative Research Methods* (2005); the third edition was published in 2009. Pranee has also published a book on doing qualitative research online: *Health Research in Cyberspace: Methodological, Practical and Personal Issues* (Nova Science Publishers, 2006). Her new books include *Researching the Vulnerable: A Guide to Sensitive Research Methods* (Sage, 2007); *Undertaking Sensitive Research: Managing Boundaries, Emotions and Risk* (with Virginia Dickson-Swift and Erica James, Cambridge University Press, 2008); *Knowing Differently: Arts-Based and Collaborative Research Methods* (with Jean Rumbold, Nova Science Publishers, 2008); *Doing Cross-Cultural Research: Ethical and Methodological Issues* (Springer, 2008), *Performing Qualitative Cross-Cultural Research* (Cambridge University Press, 2010); *Research Methods in Health: Foundations for Evidence-Based Practice* (Oxford University Press, 2010, 2013); *Focus Group Methodology: Principles and Practice* (Sage, 2011); and *Using Participatory Qualitative Research Methodologies in Health* (with Gina Higginbottom, Sage, 2015). She is now editing a series of research methods in health and social sciences for Springer.

ABOUT THE CONTRIBUTORS

Karen Anderson is a Lecturer in public health at La Trobe University, Melbourne. She has recently completed a major ethnographic study of the way health promotion principles are deployed in the training and practice of Australian nurses.

Terese Bondas is a Professor of Nursing Science at the Faculty of Professional Studies, Nord University (previously University of Nordland), Norway, and Adjunct Professor (Methods of Health Research), University of Eastern Finland. Terese initialised and led the interdisciplinary research network 'Childbearing in the European countries: a qualitative research network' (BFiN) and an interdisciplinary Nordic research network in health care leadership (NiV). She is involved in research that develops the Caritative Leadership theory that she has created, and several international research projects in the research areas of caring, childbearing, and development of qualitative methods.

Christine Carpenter was educated as a physical therapist in Liverpool, England, and attained her graduate degrees in Educational Studies at the University of British Columbia, Canada. Before becoming an educator and researcher, she worked as a physical therapist for over twenty years in rehabilitation settings, primarily with people who had sustained spinal cord injury. Her current research initiatives are focused on the long-term experience and quality of life issues involved in living with a disability or chronic condition. She has co-written three books on qualitative research and evidence-based practice for occupational and physical therapists.

Megan Davidson is Adjunct Associate Professor in the School of Allied Health at La Trobe University, Melbourne. She has over twenty years' experience in curriculum design and teaching in evidence-based practice for physiotherapy and other health sciences students. Her education research interests are in the areas of interprofessional education, the assessment of clinical performance, and evidence-based practice. As a Director of the independent consulting group Health Workforce Consulting, she undertakes project work primarily for professional organisations and universities.

Patricia Davidson is Dean of the School of Nursing at Johns Hopkins University, USA, and a professor in the Faculty of Health at the University of Technology Sydney (UTS). Formerly, she was Professor and Director of the Cardiovascular and Chronic Care Centre in Faculty of Health at UTS. Patricia is the Counsel General of the International Council on Women's Health Issues. Her current research activities include models of delivering chronic care, development and evaluation of guidelines for palliative care of patients with heart failure, Indigenous health, novel models of care in heart failure management, perspectives of cultural diversity in heart disease, prevention and management of heart disease in women. She is particularly interested in methods of research that engage vulnerable and marginalised communities.

Priscilla Ennals is a Lecturer in occupational therapy and researcher within the Living with Disability Research Centre at La Trobe University, Melbourne. Her current research interests include mental health and occupational participation, how mental health and ill health impact what people do, and how what people do impacts their mental health and well-being. Her recently completed PhD used a grounded theory method to explore the experience of studying at university for students with mental ill health.

Deirdre Fetherstonhaugh is the Director of the Australian Centre for Evidence-Based Aged Care at La Trobe University, Melbourne. Her research focuses on the translation and implementation of research evidence into practice, the ethical implications of clinical practice, decision-making in dementia, sexuality and dementia, clinical risk in residential aged care, and the reality of person-centred care.

Christine Forrester-Knauss is a Research Fellow in the Department of Developmental Psychology, University of Bern and at the Swiss Tropical and Public Health Institute in Basel, Switzerland. She completed her PhD in the area of body dissatisfaction in adolescents at the University of Bern. Christine has worked on several research projects in Switzerland and Australia, including gender and health, body image and eating disorders, and evaluation of psychotherapy.

Annemarie Gallichio (formerly Nevill) is a Lecturer with the School of Health and Social Development at Deakin University, Melbourne. She lectures in the area of social health, health promotion and health sciences, and is an experienced online educator. Annemarie is a critical feminist ethnographer, and her main research interest focuses on how older female genocide survivors living in diaspora are able to heal. Using decolonial epistemology, she is also interested in the roles of culture, indigeneity and tradition, including religion and spirituality, in the health of diasporic populations. She has co-edited a book on social exclusion and health.

Leila Gholizadeh is a Lecturer at the University of Technology, Sydney. She completed her Master's degree at Tabriz University of Medical Sciences in 1999 and her PhD at the University of Western Sydney in 2009. She is interested in mixed method research and used that methodology in her PhD project to study the relationship between perceived and estimated absolute risk of cardiovascular disease in Middle Eastern women.

Melissa Graham is a Senior Lecturer in epidemiology and health research methods at Deakin University, Melbourne. Her area of interest is women's reproductive health, specifically the role of reproductive health in social exclusion, the impact of hysterectomy on health and well-being, the determinants of reproductive health, and the experience of and impact of childlessness on health.

Carol Grbich is an Emeritus Professor in the School of Medicine at Flinders University, Adelaide. She is author of several texts on qualitative research approaches, including *Qualitative Research in Health: An Introduction* (Prentice Hall, 2004) *New Approaches to Social Research* (Sage, 2004) and *Qualitative Data Analysis* (Sage, 2007, 2013). She is the foundation editor of the *International Journal of Multiple Research Approaches*.

Susan Greaves is Senior Occupational Therapist (Neurodevelopment) at the Royal Children's Hospital in Melbourne and recently completed her doctorate at La Trobe University. Her PhD research project concerned the development of a bimanual outcome measure for young infants with hemiplegic cerebral palsy. She has published three peer-reviewed journal articles and co-authored three book chapters.

Elizabeth Halcomb is Professor of Primary Health Care Nursing at the University of Wollongong, School of Nursing and Midwifery. Her research interests include general practice nursing, chronic disease, healthy ageing and the nursing workforce. She has experience in a range of research methods, including focus groups, systematic reviews, mixed methods and survey research. She is co-editor of the text *Mixed methods research for nursing and the health sciences* (Wiley-Blackwell, 2009), and the editor of *Nurse Researcher.*

Elisabeth O.C. Hall is Professor Emerita in Clinical Nursing and connected to the Department of Nursing Science, School of Public Health, Aarhus University, Aarhus, Denmark. Elisabeth was born in Sweden where she became a registered nurse and nurse teacher, and she earned her Master's and PhD degrees in nursing science from Aarhus University. Elisabeth's area of interest is caring and family nursing when a premature or small child is critically ill; her teaching and supervising has concerned nursing theories, qualitative research methods and own research. She has published extensively in these areas.

Linsey Howie is an Adjunct Associate Professor in the Department of Occupational Therapy in the School of Allied Health, La Trobe University, Melbourne. She has a keen interest in qualitative research methodologies including grounded theory and phenomenology, and has supervised Honours and higher degree students using narrative enquiry. Linsey is a former Head of School of Occupational Therapy and Deputy Dean in the Faculty of Health Sciences at La Trobe University.

Ross Iles is a Senior Lecturer and Advanced Research Coordinator in the Department of Physiotherapy at Monash University and a Research Fellow at the Institute for Safety, Compensation and Recovery Research (ISCRR) in Melbourne. His interest in physiotherapists' use of evidence-based practice formed the basis of his Honours thesis and he has taught research-related subjects to physiotherapy students at La Trobe and Monash universities. He has completed the postgraduate Diploma of Work Disability Prevention at the University of Sherbrooke, Canada, and he has published multiple papers in peer-reviewed journals.

Christine Imms' research encompasses intervention effectiveness and outcome measurement for children. She is the Professor of Occupational Therapy and member of the National Centre for Clinical Outcomes Research at The Australian Catholic University and an Honorary Research Affiliate at the Royal Children's Hospital and Murdoch Children's Research Institute in Melbourne, and the CanChild Centre for Childhood Disability Research, Ontario, Canada.

Karl B. Landorf is an Associate Professor and Research Coordinator at La Trobe University, Melbourne. He is also Group Leader of the Foot and Ankle Research Group in the Lower Extremity and Gait Studies program at La Trobe University and Research Fellow in the Allied Health Department of Melbourne Health. His research interests include musculoskeletal disorders of the foot and ankle, health outcome assessment and clinical trial methodology.

Rhonda Nay is Emeritus Professor at La Trobe University, Melbourne. She was previously Professor of Interdisciplinary Aged Care at La Trobe University, Director of the Victorian and Tasmanian Dementia Training Studies Centre, and Director of the Institute for Social Participation. Her research focused on dementia and translating research into practice.

David Nilsson is a Senior Lecturer in the joint faculty of Health, Education and Social Care at Kingston University and St George's University of London. His practice experience was largely in the field of hospital social work and he has conducted a number of research studies on health social work.

Paul O'Halloran is a health psychologist and a Senior Lecturer, who has been lecturing in research methods at La Trobe University, Melbourne, at undergraduate and postgraduate level for more than ten years. Paul is an active researcher in areas such as chronic illness conditions and mood and physical activity.

Jane Pierson is a Lecturer in the School of Psychology and Public Health at La Trobe University, Melbourne. Jane has a substantial history of involvement in health research and evaluation in Australia and the UK. The bulk has been in neuropsychology and gerontology, with extensive experience in the analysis of quantitative data and data from mixed method studies. Jane also has wide experience, in Australia and the UK, in educating undergraduate and postgraduate students, and health professionals, in quantitative research methods and related data analysis procedures.

Priscilla Pyett has over twenty years' experience as a sociologist and health researcher working with collaborative methodologies. She has worked extensively with Aboriginal community controlled health organisations and with many other marginalised groups.

Paul Ramcharan is Senior Lecturer in Disability Studies at RMIT University, Melbourne. Paul has nearly twenty years' experience in the field and, between 2001 and 2006, was coordinator of a research initiative designed to support the implementation of Valuing People (2001), a national policy focused on people with intellectual disabilities.

Helen Rawson is a Research Fellow in the School of Nursing and Midwifery, Deakin University, Geelong, Australia, and in the Centre for Nursing Research–Deakin University and Monash Health Partnership, Melbourne, Australia. Her research focus is the delivery of evidence-based quality care for older people across all health settings, and incorporates both qualitative and quantitative research methods.

Miranda Rose is a Principal Research Fellow in the Discipline of Speech Pathology in the School of Allied Health at La Trobe University, Melbourne, and an Australian Research Council Future Fellow. Her doctoral studies included single-subject experimental designs to investigate the efficacy of speech pathology treatments for aphasia. Miranda currently runs funded research projects investigating innovative treatments for aphasia, community support programs for living with chronic aphasia, and the gesture and multimodality communication skills of people with aphasia.

Virginia Schmied is Professor of Midwifery and Director of Research in the School of Nursing and Midwifery, University of Western Sydney, and holds a Visiting Professorship at the University of Central Lancashire in the UK. She is a leading Australian researcher in midwifery and child and family health. Her program of scholarship, teaching and research is grounded in social science theory and methods and focuses on transition to motherhood, breastfeeding and infant feeding decisions, perinatal mental health, postnatal care and strengthening universal health services for families and children. Virginia has been successful in competitive grants, has published over 170 refereed journal articles, book chapters and published reports, and regularly presents at national and international conferences. Her research has been translated into policy and practice, for example through the development of teaching resources for consumers and health professionals.

Margot Schofield was Professor of Counselling and Psychotherapy in the School of Psychology and Public Health at La Trobe University, Melbourne. She has extensive experience in the design of both cross-sectional and longitudinal surveys, and has been a founding investigator on the Australian Longitudinal Study of Women's Health. Her current research focuses on the development of psychotherapists and counsellors, process and outcome evaluation of counselling and clinical supervision, art-based approaches in mental health recovery, couples counselling and family mediation, women's health, and the use of internet surveys.

Tanya Serry is a speech pathologist, Lecturer and researcher at La Trobe University, Melbourne. Her PhD used an interpretative phenomenological approach to examine theoretical premises and current practices across various stakeholders in order to develop an integrated understanding of processes in place for supporting young schoolchildren who have reading difficulty. Tanya has published a number of scholarly articles and various book chapters, and has assisted with editing the *Australian Communication Quarterly* and the *International Journal of Speech-Language Pathology* for a number of years.

Nora Shields is Professor of Clinical and Community Practice in the School of Allied Health at La Trobe University, Melbourne. She teaches postgraduate students the process of how to conduct a systematic review. Her publications include fourteen high-quality systematic reviews.

Ann Taket is Professor of Health and Social Exclusion and Director of the Centre for Health through Action on Social Exclusion at Deakin University, Melbourne. She has over twenty years' experience in public health-related research. She has particular interests in participatory methods, the use of mixed methods, research with marginalised or disadvantaged groups, and the prevention of violence and abuse.

Anke van der Sterren works at the Alcohol Tobacco and Other Drug Association as a Researcher and Project Officer. She has worked as a researcher in a number of Aboriginal and Torres Strait Islander health contexts, including at the Centre for Excellence in Indigenous Tobacco Control at the University of Melbourne.

Peter Waples-Crowe is a Koori with over twenty-five years' experience working in Aboriginal health. He was formerly a Team Leader at the Victorian Aboriginal Community Controlled Health Organisation.

Anita Wikberg is a Senior Lecturer in Health Care at Novia University of Applied Sciences, Finland. She is a registered nurse and midwife and has worked and lived in Finland, Sweden, Zambia, Lesotho, Nepal and Vietnam. She has anMNSc (caring science) from Abo Akademi University in Finland and has obtained her PhD in Caring sciences.

Jon Willis is an anthropologist and social epidemiologist who has conducted ethnographic research in Singapore and South Africa and in a range of Indigenous communities in Australia. He is best known for his work on the sexual and health cultures of the Pitjantjatjara people of Australia's Western Desert. Jon is an Associate Professor and Research Director of the Poche Centre for Indigenous Health at the University of Queensland, Brisbane.

Margaret Winbolt is a Senior Research Fellow in the Australian Centre for Evidence-Based Aged Care at La Trobe University, Melbourne. Margaret is a registered nurse and has over thirty years' experience and knowledge of the care of people with dementia, and the needs of people with dementia and their carers.

Pauline Wong is a Lecturer in the School of Nursing and Midwifery at La Trobe University, Melbourne. Currently, she teaches in the undergraduate Bachelor of Nursing degree. Pauline's PhD thesis used a grounded theoretical framework to portray the families' journey of heightened emotional vulnerability, regaining control and resilience when a relative is admitted unexpectedly to an Australian ICU. The recommendations can be used by health care professionals to inform clinical practice that is inclusive of families and critically ill patients.

ABBREVIATIONS

ACCHO	Aboriginal community controlled health organisation
ACL	anterior cruciate ligament
AHW	Aboriginal health worker
AMS	Aboriginal Medical Service
ANOVA	analysis of variance
CAQDAS	computer-assisted qualitative data analysis software
CDM	clinical data-mining
CEBM	Centre for Evidence-Based Medicine
CONSORT	Consolidated Standards of Reporting Trial
CPG	clinical practice guideline
CPR	collaborative participatory research
CTT	classical test theory
EBM	evidence-based medicine
EBP	evidence-based practice
GP	general practitioner
HREC	Human Research Ethics Committee
ICC	intraclass correlation coefficients
IRT	item response theory
LOA	limits of agreement
MANOVA	multivariate analysis of variance
MOU	memorandum of understanding
NHMRC	National Health and Medical Research Council
PAR	participatory action research
PBR	practice-based research
PEDro	Physiotherapy Evidence Database
PICO	Population, Intervention or Indicator, Comparator or Control, Outcome
PRR	prevalence rate ratio
RBP	research-based practice
RCT	randomised controlled trial
SDD	smallest detectable difference

SDT	Self-Discovery Tapestry
SEM	standard error of measurement
SPSS	Statistical Package for the Social Sciences
SSED	single-subject experimental design

ACKNOWLEDGMENTS

The author and the publisher wish to thank the following copyright holders for reproduction of their material.

British Sociological Association for 'Criteria for the evaluation of qualitative research papers', Blaxter, *Medical Sociology News*, 22(1), 68–71, 1996. Reproduced with permission from the British Sociological Association © The British Sociological Association www.britsoc.co.uk; **CSIRO publishing** for 'Influence of traditional Vietnamese culture on the utilisation of mainstream health services for sexual health issues by second-generation Vietnamese Australian young women', Rawson, H. & Liamputtong, P., *Sexual Health*, 6, 75-81, 2009; **Elsevier** for 'Effects of a Community-Based Progressive Resistance Training Program on Muscle Performance and Physical Function in Adults With Down Syndrome: A Randomized Controlled Trial', Shields, N., Taylor, N. & Dodd, K.J., *Archives of Physical Medicine and Rehabilitation*, 89, 1215–20, 2008/'Testing the reliability and efficiency of the pilot Mixed Methods Appraisal Tool (MMAT) for systematic mixed studies review', Pace et al, *International Journal of Nursing Studies*, pp51–52, 20012/*Evidence-based medicine: How to practice and teach EBM*, Sackett et al, Copyright Elsevier, 1997; **Sage Publications**, *An Introduction to Qualitative Research*, 3ed, Uwe Flick, 2006; **Solutions for Public Health (SPH)** for 'Critical Appraisal Skills Programme' 2007.

Every effort has been made to trace the original source of copyright material contained in this book. The publisher will be pleased to hear from copyright holders to rectify any errors or omissions.

METHODS AND PRINCIPLES

1

The Science of Words and the Science of Numbers

PRANEE LIAMPUTTONG

Chapter objectives

In this chapter you will learn:

- about evidence and evidence-based practice
- about different research designs in health
- the nature of qualitative and quantitative approaches
- the usefulness of mixed methods
- about rigour, reliability and validity in research
- about sampling issues

Key terms

Bias

Constructivism

Convenience sampling

Data saturation

Effectiveness/efficacy

Epistemology

Ethnography

Evidence

Evidence-based practice

Knowledge

Knowledge acquisition

Metasynthesis

Mixed methods

Non-probability sampling

Ontology

Phenomenology

Positivism

Pragmatism

Probability sampling method

Purposive sampling

Qualitative research

Quantitative research

Reliability

Research participant

Rigour

Systematic review

Validity

Variable

Introduction

Knowledge is essential to human survival. Over the course of history, there have been many ways of knowing, from divine revelation to tradition and the authority of elders. By the beginning of the seventeenth century, people began to rely on a different way of knowing—the research method (Grinnell *et al.* 2011a, p. 16).

Knowledge: An accepted body of facts or ideas acquired through the use of the senses or reason, or through research methods.

According to Grinnell and colleagues (2014a, p. 8), **knowledge** is 'an accepted body of facts or ideas which is acquired through the use of the senses or reason'. In the old days, we used to believe that the Earth was flat. Our belief came about through those who were in 'authority', who told us so, or because people in our society had always believed that the world was flat. Now we know that the Earth is spherical because scientists have travelled into space to observe it from this perspective. However, Grinnell and colleagues argue that the most efficient way of 'knowing something' **(knowledge acquisition)** is through research findings, which have been gathered through the use of research methods.

Knowledge acquisition: The most efficient way of 'knowing something' is through research findings, which have been gathered through the use of research methods.

What has knowledge got to do with evidence and evidence-based practice? I contend that it is through our knowledge that evidence can be generated. This evidence can then be used for our practice. Without knowledge, there will not be evidence that we can use. But how can we find knowledge? For scientists and health practitioners, the answer is through research and research methods (Neutens 2014). According to Grinnell and colleagues (2014a, p. 17), the research method of knowing comprises two 'complementary research approaches': the qualitative approach and the quantitative approach. Qualitative research relies on 'qualitative and descriptive methods of data collection'. Data are presented in the form of words, and sometimes as diagrams or drawings, but not as numbers (Patton 2015). The quantitative approach, on the other hand, 'relies on quantification in collecting and analyzing data and uses statistical analyses' (Patton 2015). Data obtained in a quantitative study are presented in the form of numbers, not in the form of words, as is the case for the qualitative approach. These two approaches will be discussed later in this chapter.

Evidence and evidence-based practice

It is our belief that you must know the basics of research methodology to even begin to use the concept of evidence-based practice effectively (Grinnell & Unrau 2008, p. v).

This quotation expresses the main reason why this book has been written. Thus it is intended to provide the foundations for evidence-based practice (EBP) in health. As I have suggested, evidence can be derived from knowledge and knowledge can be obtained through research.

Evidence: Evidence in the context of EBP is what results from a systematic review and appraisal of all available literature relevant to a carefully designed question and protocol.

Evidence, according to Manuel and colleagues (2014, p. 186), is 'information' that can be used to support and guide practices, programs and policies in health and social care in order to enhance the health and well-being of individuals, families and communities. For example, you might be interested in depression among young people and in the most effective way to assess their risk for suicide and to prevent it. Types of evidence that you may be interested in may include:

- perceptions and experiences of depression and suicide among young people
- factors that are related to the onset of depression in young people
- risk factors and protective factors that are relevant to depression and suicide among young people
- evidence-based methods that can be used to carry out an appropriate assessment of suicide risk
- strategies or interventions that can be used in practice
- prevention programs and policies that can have a positive impact on these health and social problems.

As you can see, there are several types of evidence that you can use to find answers to the questions about the health issue in which you are interested. Now it has to be asked: which type is the 'best' evidence that you can use, and how do you obtain this evidence? This depends on the questions you ask. It has been debated among researchers and practitioners whether there is a universal way to judge which evidence is the best (Altheide & Johnson 2011). Researchers and practitioners come from different disciplines and surely will have different perspectives on the types of evidence they see as useful or not useful for their research purposes and professional practices (Altheide & Johnson 2011; Manuel *et al.* 2014; Liamputtong 2016). What is seen as the best evidence for some researchers and practitioners may not be seen as such by others. It is at this point that I wish to bring up the issue of EBP.

Fundamentally, **evidence-based practice** in the area of health care refers to:

> the process that includes finding empirical evidence regarding the effectiveness and/or efficacy of various treatment options and then determining the relevance of those options to specific client(s). This information is then considered critically, when developing the final treatment plan for the client or clients (Mullen *et al.* 2014, p. 204; see also Chapters 15, 16, 17, 18).

One approach for evaluating evidence within the model of EBP is through a hierarchical ranking system (Manuel *et al.* 2014, p. 194; see Chapter 17). Within this system, evidence is evaluated according to the research design that was used to generate it. For instance, when evaluating a health care intervention, a well-designed experiment, specifically a randomised controlled trial (RCT) or, better, the systematic review of a number of RCTs, is perceived as the gold standard (Evans 2003; Aoun & Kristjanson 2005; Packer 2011; Liamputtong 2016; see Chapters 15, 16, 17).

However, the hierarchical ranking system may ignore some of the limitations of RCTs, and neglect observational studies (Aoun & Kristjanson 2005; Packer 2011; Manuel *et al.* 2014; Long 2015). For instance, confidence in the RCT is based on knowing that the research was correctly undertaken (see Chapter 15) but, more often than not, published research using RCTs presents conflicting findings (see Chapter 15). Some researchers argue that a hierarchical approach is

Evidence-based practice: A process that requires the practitioner to find empirical evidence about the effectiveness or efficacy of different treatment options and to determine the relevance of that evidence to a particular client's situation.

FIGURE 1.1   Hierarchy of evidence

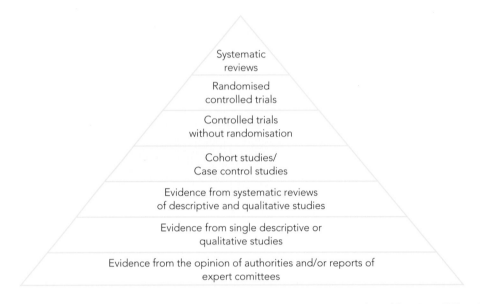

(Adopted from Long 2015, p. 424)

Effectiveness/ efficacy: A measure used to determine whether the treatment or intervention has an intended or expected outcome. In medicine, however, it refers to the ability of a treatment or intervention to reproduce a desired outcome under ideal circumstances.

Ethnography: A research method that focuses on the scientific study of the lived culture of groups of people, used to discover and describe individual social and cultural groups.

based solely on seeing whether the intervention works as intended, or on the measurement of the **efficacy** of intervention 'with little attention to the appropriateness and feasibility of the interventions in the real practice world' (Manuel *et al.* 2014, p. 193). More importantly, as Packer (2011, p. 37, original emphasis) argued, 'the gold standard also prevents researchers from studying, let alone questioning, the forms of life in which people find themselves and in which things are found. People are *not* in fact independently existing entities. We exist together, in *shared* forms of life.'

More importantly, within this hierarchical system, qualitative evidence is often placed at the bottom of the hierarchy (Grypdonck 2006; Savage 2006; Manuel *et al.* 2014; Long 2015; Liamputtong 2016). In this model, the contribution to EBP of findings from qualitative research is undervalued, and at worst discounted (Gibson & Martin 2003; Aoun & Kristjanson 2005; Grypdonck 2006; Denzin 2009, 2011; Altheide & Johnson 2011; Liamputtong 2016). Qualitative research, despite its increasing contributions to the evidence base of health and social care, is still underrepresented in some health care areas that place a high value on evidence from the hierarchical system (Johnson & Waterfield 2004; Long 2015; Liamputtong 2016). This is in part, as Gibson and Martin (2003, p. 353) suggest, due to 'mistaken attempts to evaluate qualitative studies according to the evidence-based hierarchy, where the status of qualitative research is not acknowledged'. Many qualitative researchers argue that this is flawed, as qualitative studies also employ rigorous methods of data collection and analysis (Johnson & Waterfield 2004; Annells 2005; Hammersley 2005; Denzin 2009, 2011; Houser 2015; Liamputtong 2016). Savage (2006, p. 383), for example, argues that **ethnography,** one of the qualitative research methods, is essentially useful due to 'the attention that it gives to context and its synthesis of findings from different methods'. More importantly, ethnography provides 'a holistic way of exploring the relationship between the different kinds of evidence that underpin clinical practice' (see also Altheide & Johnson 2011; see Chapter 7). Similarly, Houser (2015, p. 400) contends that phenomenological research offers means for finding evidence of nursing practices which 'support and enhance the ways patients respond to the challenges in their health care'. **Phenomenology** is valuable as it allows us to understand 'the ways in which patients react and respond to both everyday experiences and unique events' (see also Chapter 9).

It is argued that the hierarchical model of evidence is only one way of organising different types of evidence. It is important for health researchers and practitioners to know this, so that they can evaluate the quality of evidence that can be found with respect to a specific health issue (Schmidt & Brown 2015a; Liamputtong 2016). And no doubt it can be very useful for some health practices, for example in therapeutic science (e.g. see Chapters 15, 17). However, Manuel and colleagues (2014, p. 194) believe that 'the decision on what evidence to use should be placed in context with your research study'. Researchers and practitioners need to consider the relevance and feasibility of evidence and whether the evidence accords with the values and preferences of the clients (Houser 2015). And this is what I advocate in this chapter: that we need to consider different types of evidence and that this evidence can be derived from the findings of different types of research (see also Chapter 2). This book will give readers an understanding of the different methods that researchers and practitioners can use or draw on in producing evidence: qualitative methods (see Part II), quantitative methods (see Part III), mixed methods (see Chapters 20, 21) and collaborative approaches (see Chapter 22).

It is worth noting that EBP has emerged from the long-standing commitment among health practitioners to social research and science. But there has been a significant change in how research and practice are related. In the past, according to Mullen and colleagues (2014), research and practice were seen as separate activities and/or as the roles of two different professions. Research was undertaken by researchers to add to the knowledge base, which was eventually drawn upon by practitioners to provide evidence on which to base their practice. Now these differences are blurred, and research and practice are often combined. In EBP, many of the practice questions largely resemble the essential parts of research questions: 'We search for evidence—especially research evidence—to answer our practice questions using established research criteria when the evidence comes from research studies, and we collect data on the processes and outcomes of our interventions' (p. 214).

In EBP, practitioners need to be clear about what is known and not known about any health problem or health practice that will be 'best' for their clients (Mullen *et al.* 2014; Schmidt & Brown 2015a). But all too often, we know little about the particular health problems of some population groups, or about treatment options that are not empirically based (Liamputtong 2016). Although there is research evidence that practitioners may find in existing literature, Mullen and colleagues (2014) argue that there are still many health issues that remain unknown to us. Currently, EBP does not apply to many of the health issues of certain population groups, for example certain ethnic minorities and indigenous groups, recent immigrants and

Phenomenology:
A methodological approach that seeks to understand, describe and interpret human behaviour and the meaning that individuals make of their experiences.

refugees, gays and lesbians, rural communities, and people with uncommon or particularly challenging health problems. In her analysis of the impact of evidence-based medicine (EBM) on vulnerable or disadvantaged groups, Rogers (2004, p. 141) points out that EBM 'turns our attention away from social and cultural factors that influence health and focuses on a narrow biomedical and individualistic model of health. Those with the greatest burden of ill health are left disenfranchised, as there is little research that is relevant to them, there is poor access to treatments, and attention is diverted away from activities that might have a much greater impact on their health.' It is clear that there is a need for more research with different groups of people as part of the EBP process. Also, much of the EBP focus, in terms of both research and application, has been centred on a subset of health issues. Research is needed in other fields, in both health issues and practices.

More importantly, depending on the research or practice question, practitioners may need evidence other than that which relates to the efficacy of interventions, to inform their practice (Aoun & Kristjanson 2005; Manuel *et al.* 2014; Houser 2015; Liamputtong 2016). Evidence that we use in EBP cannot and should not be based solely on the findings of RCTs. Rather, it should be derived from many sources (Hawker *et al.* 2002; Shaw 2011; Houser 2015; Liamputtong 2016). Some health topics or issues are not appropriate for an RCT (Aoun & Kristjanson 2005; Schmidt & Brown 2015a). Fahy (2008, p. 2), for example, contends that most maternity care practices will never be found by RCTs. However, evidence for practice in midwifery is needed so that midwives will be able to help women 'to make the best decisions for themselves by taking the best available evidence into account'. She also suggests that 'a more expansive definition of evidence and evidence-based practice' is needed. Additionally, there are many ethical concerns regarding RCTs (see Chapter 3). For instance, you may be interested in knowing about the meaning and interpretation of body weight because there have been higher rates of diabetes or anorexia nervosa in your city, or you may need to know about the understanding of homelessness among poor families and how they deal with it, because you have noticed that there are increasing numbers of homeless young people in poorer areas of your city. The 'best' evidence for these issues will not be generated by RCTs but by qualitative research. These scenarios illustrate situations where you need to look for other types of evidence.

Therefore, if there is no available evidence that you can find from systematic reviews or from other sources such as the relevant literature, evidence can be obtained by gaining knowledge through your own research. As Shaw (2011, p. 20) contends, '"valid scientific knowledge" can take many forms'. In this book, I argue that evidence can be generated by both qualitative and quantitative research (see also Beck 2009; Schmidt & Brown 2015a; Chapter 2). No doubt, most health care providers will trust the so-called 'hard' evidence obtained through quantitative approaches such as surveys with closed-ended questions, clinical measurements and RCTs (see chapters in Part III). As I have pointed out, the quantitative approach is seen as being empirical science and as being more systematic than qualitative research, so the findings of this approach are regarded as more reliable. But I argue that evidence derived from the qualitative approach can help you to understand the issue and to use the findings in your practice. Qualitative research provides evidence that you may not be able to obtain from quantitative research or from a **systematic review** of quantitative research (Patton 2015; Olsen *et al.* 2016). Seeley and colleagues (2008), for example, point out that the quantitative part of their research, which involved more than 2000 participants, failed to provide a good understanding of some of their findings regarding the impact of HIV and AIDS on families. It was only through the life histories of 24 families that they were able to explain these findings in a more meaningful way. Their study clearly points to the importance of qualitative evidence in health care and practice. Indeed, many researchers have argued that 'qualitative research findings have much to offer evidence-based practice' (Hawker *et al.* 2002, p. 1285; see also Grypdonck 2006; Jack 2006; Daly *et al.* 2007; Meadows-Oliver 2009; Houser 2015; Olsen *et al.* 2016; Chapters 9, 18). As Sandelowski (2004, p. 1382) puts it, 'Qualitative research is the best thing to be happening to evidence-based practice'.

Within the emergence of EBP in health care, Grypdonck (2006, p. 1379) contends that qualitative research contributes greatly to the appropriateness of care. She argues that health practitioners need to have a good understanding of:

> what it means to be ill, to live with an illness, to be subject to physical limitations, to see one's intellectual capacities gradually diminish, or to be healed again, to rise from [near] death after a bone marrow transplant, leaving one's sick life behind, to meet people who take care of you in a way that makes you feel really understood and really cared for.

Practitioners may not obtain knowledge from existing literature in order to address these crucial issues of health and illness. Such knowledge can only be gained through the integration of research into their daily work (see Chapter 9, for example). Surely, by gaining a better understanding of the lived experience of patients and clients, health practitioners will be able to provide more sensitive and appropriate care.

I argue here that qualitative enquiry is an essential means of eliciting evidence from diverse individuals, population groups and contexts. In clinical encounters, Knight and Mattick (2006, p. 1084) say this clearly: 'The inclusion of qualitative research within EBM brings closer the link between individual patients' perspectives and "scientific" perspectives'. Long (2015, p. 423) contends that we should not underestimate the contributions of qualitative research because data from qualitative enquiry can offer the perspective of the consumers/patients, which is a crucial part of EBP in health care. The findings from qualitative research can be used to 'enhance evidence-based practice' by integrating the values and preferences of consumers/patients into the guides for health care practice (Houser 2015, p. 34). Houser (2015, p. 388) also suggests that qualitative research is especially valuable in EBP as it allows us to identify the needs, motives and preferences of the patients. Qualitative research is 'helpful in describing the acceptability of an intervention. Interventions that require lifestyle adjustment, attitude changes, or behavioural alterations are particularly well suited to qualitative studies'. Although practitioners must use 'scientific evidence' in their evidence-based health care, they must also 'see a social or human problem through the eyes of the patient' (see also Streubert & Carpenter 2011). Indeed, qualitative enquiry not only offers an in-depth understanding

Systematic review:
A comprehensive identification and synthesis of the available literature on a specified topic. In a systematic review, literature is treated like data.

about patients but also 'adds another dimension to quantitative evidence: one based on the human experience' (Houser 2015, p. 389).

In relation to interventions in health care, qualitative research can contribute to many things (Audrey 2011; Young *et al.* 2012; Houser 2015):

- it allows health care providers to pinpoint the needs of people that they serve
- it helps health care providers to develop interventions which are more acceptable to their patients
- it helps health care providers to enhance the understanding of the effect of an intervention from the patients' perspectives within their own social/cultural contexts
- it gives health care providers a more accurate understanding of the reasons for attrition, cessation of treatment, or lack of adherence to a treatment protocol.

However, there is still a sense of distrust of qualitative research. This is mainly due to a perception that qualitative enquiry is unable to produce useful and valid findings (Hammersley 2008; Torrance 2008, 2011; Houser 2015), a perception that stems largely from insufficient understanding of the philosophical framework for qualitative work, which has its focus on meaning and experience, the social construction of reality, and the relationship between the researched and the researcher (Patton 2015).

Recently, however, we have witnessed an attempt to synthesise qualitative findings in a form of metasynthesis because the synthesis provides 'stronger credibility' than individual studies can offer within EBP (Thorne 2009, p. 571; Houser 2015). **Metasynthesis,** according to Zuzelo (2012, p. 500), 'offers a mechanism to help establish qualitative research as a viable source of evidence for EBP'. With the acceptance of metasynthesis of qualitative research in EBP, 'the pursuit of "what works" in evidence-based practice can be enhanced by examining "what is at work" when individuals and communities experience interventions and report these experiences in their own words' (Padgett 2012, p. 193; see also Chapter 18).

Metasynthesis: A generic term that represents the collection of approaches of qualitative research on previous qualitative studies in a field of interest.

STOP AND THINK

- Considering what has been discussed above, what is your opinion regarding evidence and evidence-based health care?
- Should all EBP be based on an RCT or quantitative research approach only? Why?
- What type of evidence would you need in your own profession? With colleagues who have a different professional background from you, discuss what evidence would be more appropriate for your work and your prospective clients.

Research designs: which one?

Designs are built about the questions we ask. Then, understanding, insight, and knowledge emerge from inquiry into the questions we ask. That means determining what data to collect and what cases to study (Patton 2015, p. 254).

Before selecting a research design, you must think carefully about your research questions (see also Chapter 2). What are the questions or health issues to which we need or wish to find answers? Researchers need to consider carefully whether qualitative or quantitative research or mixed-method research is best suited to addressing the research problem (Patton 2015). Once you have thought this through, you will be able to select a research design that will be appropriate for the questions you ask. For example, if you wish to understand why some young women smoke and you want to learn from them about their perceptions of smoking, gender issues and societal pressure, their needs and concerns about smoking and their body, or if you want to really understand why many working-class men will not stop smoking, can you find your answers by conducting an RCT or a case control study? Will these methods allow you to find applicable answers? On the other hand, if you wish to find out how many young women smoke, or the prevalence of diabetes among young children in your local area, can these questions be addressed by the use of a qualitative approach? Before you can answer these questions, you will need to understand what each approach can offer you and what it cannot (its limitations) (Houser 2015; Patton 2015). Hence, a good understanding of research methods is essential.

Often, we hear students and novice researchers make comments like 'I want to do a qualitative research study because I am not very good with numbers', or 'I want to use quantitative research because I am not interested in qualitative research' or, worse, 'I do not want to use qualitative research because I don't like it – too many flowery words and not objective enough'. I would suggest that this is not a good way of selecting your approach. You need to find out which approach is the best way to find answers to your research questions (or to find evidence for practice), and this can be either a qualitative or a quantitative approach. If you cannot find your complete answers (or evidence) using either of these approaches alone, you may need to go further and to use a mixed-methods design.

The choice of a research design or 'strategy of inquiry' (Denzin & Lincoln 2011) must be 'tailored to' the specific research question being investigated (Bryman 2016, p. 36). If researchers are interested in how individuals within a specific social group perceive health and illness, a qualitative approach, which allows us to examine how individuals interpret their social world, will be the most appropriate research strategy to use. Also, if researchers are interested in a topic that we know little about, a more exploratory position is preferable. This is when a qualitative approach will serve our needs better because such approaches are typically associated with the generation of new findings rather than the testing of existing theory (see chapters in Part I). On the other hand, if researchers are interested in finding out about the causes of a health problem, or its prevalence (e.g. the rate of diabetes in Australia), a quantitative approach will provide more appropriate answers (Fawcett & Pockett 2015; see Chapters 2, 13, 14).

Another salient issue relevant to the choice of research design is related to the nature of the topic and the characteristics of the individuals or groups being researched (Patton 2015). For instance, if you need to engage with hard-to-reach individuals or groups, for example those engaged in illicit activities such as violence, drug use and dealing, or those living with stigmatised illnesses such as mental health problems and HIV/AIDS, or with indigenous people, it is unlikely that a quantitative approach would allow you to gain the necessary rapport or the confidence of the participants. These are some of the reasons that most researchers in these areas have adopted a qualitative approach as their research strategy (see Liamputtong 2007, 2013, 2016; see Chapters 2, 21 in this volume).

RESEARCH IN PRACTICE

A PRACTICAL CONSIDERATION IN THE CHOICE OF RESEARCH APPROACH

Emma is a podiatrist and owns her practice. Through her work, she has treated many competitive athletes who come to her because of their foot injuries. This is particularly so around the time of major competitive events like the Commonwealth and Olympic Games. She does not know the real prevalence of the injuries in her city, so she cannot say exactly what would be the rate of injuries; she only knows that she has treated many athletes. She would like to know about this as she needs to prepare her practice in terms of the number of podiatrists that she needs to employ and the purchase of essential equipment. Emma has also noticed that some athletes do not follow her advice about how to avoid or prevent foot injuries, or adhere to her treatments, despite the fact that she has followed the recommendations from a systematic review which showed that the advice that she has given and the treatments she has adopted are 'the best' options. This has really puzzled her. She wants to know the reasons for this non-compliance. Hence, this is the beginning of her research endeavour.

From reading literature on sports injuries, Emma realises that there are different ways in which she can find her answers. If she wants to ascertain the prevalence of foot injuries among competitive athletes, she would need to use a quantitative approach, as this would allow her to determine the number of such injuries in her city. However, if she wants to understand why the athletes do not follow her advice or adhere to her treatment plans, she must talk to them and allow them to tell her their stories, as this will provide her with in-depth understanding of their issues, which may help her to develop treatment plans that better cater for their personal needs. So, Emma has choices as to how she can obtain evidence that can inform her work.

If you were Emma, how would you go about doing your research in order to find the evidence that you need? How would you design your research if you were a public health practitioner, a nurse or a social worker? Discuss your choice of research design.

Ontology and epistemology

Ontology refers to the question of whether or not there is a single objective reality.

In any research undertaking, it is crucial that researchers examine the ontological and epistemological positions that underlie the way in which research is undertaken. **Ontology** refers to the question of whether or not there is a single objective reality (Denzin & Lincoln

2005; Lincoln *et al.* 2011; Creswell 2013; see Chapter 20). Here 'reality' refers to the existence of what is real in the natural or social worlds. If we adopt the ontological standpoint of objective reality, we must take a position of objective detachment and ensure that the research process is free from bias. Researchers who adopt this position would argue that reality can be accurately captured (Grbich 2013). These researchers will adopt a quantitative approach for their research.

Other researchers would reject the position of objective reality. They would argue that it is impossible to carry out research in a detached way, that if we wish to understand the realities and experiences of other people, we must acknowledge our own subjectivities, which include our own beliefs, values and emotions, in the process of carrying out research. These researchers will make use of a qualitative approach for their research.

Epistemology is concerned with the nature of knowledge and how knowledge is obtained. It is 'the science of knowing' or 'systems of knowledge' (Babbie 2016, p. 6). It begs 'the question of what is (or should be) regarded as acceptable knowledge in a discipline'. A central concern is 'the question of whether the social world can and should be studied according to the same principles, procedures, and ethos as the natural sciences' (Bryman 2016, p. 27). There are five major epistemological paradigms that can be used to explain the nature of knowledge (Guba & Lincoln 1994, 2008; Lincoln *et al.* 2011). These paradigms give different understandings of what reality is in the natural and social worlds, and how we come to know that reality. In this chapter I shall focus on the two paradigms on which qualitative and quantitative approaches are respectively based: constructivism and positivism. A more detailed discussion of research paradigms can be found in Denzin and Lincoln (2005), Willis (2007), Dickson-Swift *et al.* (2008a) and Lincoln *et al.* (2011). See also Chapter 20.

> **Epistemology** is concerned with the nature of knowledge and how knowledge is obtained.

Constructivism suggests that 'reality' is socially constructed. It is also referred to as interpretivism (Patton 2015; Bryman 2016). Constructivist researchers believe that there are multiple truths which are individually constructed (Guba & Lincoln 1994, 2008; Lincoln *et al.* 2011; Grbich 2013; Creswell 2014). Reality is seen as being shaped by social factors such as class, gender, race, ethnicity, culture and age (Grbich 2013). To constructivist researchers, reality is not firmly rooted in nature, but is a product of our own making. Thus, it is possible that many different views of reality exist and that they are all legitimate (Houser 2015). One of the central beliefs of researchers working within this paradigm is that research is a very subjective process, due to the active involvement of the researcher in the construction and conduct of the research (Grbich 2013; Creswell 2014). Constructivist researchers also argue that 'reality is defined by the research participants' interpretations of their own realities' (Williams *et al.* 2014, p. 80; Houser 2015). Research situated within this paradigm, as Grbich (2013, p. 8) points out, focuses on 'exploration of the way people interpret and make sense of their experiences in the worlds in which they live, and how the contexts of events and situations and the placement of these within wider social environments have impacted on constructed understanding'.

> **Constructivism:** An epistemology that suggests that 'reality' is socially constructed. Constructivist researchers believe that there are multiple truths, individually constructed, and that reality is a product of our own making.

According to Bryman (2016, p. 26), constructivist researchers hold 'a view that the subject matter of the social sciences—people and their institutions—is fundamentally different from that of the natural sciences'. When the social world is studied, it 'requires a different logic of research procedure, one that reflects the distinctiveness of humans as against the natural order' (p. 26). Within this constructivist paradigm, researchers are required to 'grasp the subjective meaning of social action' (p. 26). This necessitates the use of research methods that would allow people to articulate the meanings of their social realities, and this requires the use of a qualitative approach.

In contrast, **positivism** is underpinned by the ontological belief that there is an objective reality that can be accessed (Guba & Lincoln 1994; Willis 2007; Lincoln *et al.* 2011; Grbich 2013). This is often referred to as 'naïve realism' (Dickson-Swift *et al.* 2008a). Positivism is also known as naturalism, logical empiricism, and behaviouralism. Based on positivism, the world is seen as 'something available for study in a more or less unchanging form' (Houser 2015, p. 33). Positivism views reality as being independent of our experiences of it, and being accessible through careful thinking, and observing and recording of our experiences (Moses & Knutsen 2007; Patton 2015; Bryman 2016). The aim of positivist enquiry is to explain, predict or control that reality (Houser 2015). Positivist scientific enquiry attempts to 'make unbiased observations of the natural and social world' (Houser 2015, p. 33). One of the central ideas of research approaches based on a positivist paradigm is the generation and testing of hypotheses through scientific means (Bryman 2016).

According to Grinnell and colleagues (2014b), positivism strives toward measurability, objectivity, reducing uncertainty, duplication, and the use of standardised procedures. Knowledge generated through this paradigm is based on 'objective measurements' of the real world, and not on the 'opinions, beliefs, or past experiences' of individuals. Positivism argues that research must be as 'objective' as possible; the things that are being studied must not be affected by the researcher (Houser 2015). Positivist researchers attempt to undertake research in such a way that their studies can be duplicated by others. Further, 'a true-to-the-bone positivist researcher' will use only well-accepted standardised procedures. Research is regarded as credible only when others accept its findings, and before those others accept them they must be satisfied that the study is 'conducted according to accepted scientific standardized procedures' (Grinnell *et al.* 2014b, p. 62).

Differences in ontology and epistemology lead to different data collection methods (Williams *et al.* 2014). Objective reality can be explored through the data collection method of standardised observation, which is the practice commonly employed in research that uses a quantitative approach. However, it is not possible to establish subjective reality through standardised measurement and observation. The only way to find out about the subjective reality of our research participants is to ask them about it, and the answer will come back in words, not in numbers. This is the hallmark of the qualitative approach.

In summary, constructivism influences qualitative research, whereas positivism dominates quantitative research (Willis 2007; Patton 2015; Babbie 2016). If researchers wish to examine the subjective nature of phenomena, and the multiple realities of those involved in the research, a constructivist paradigm is essential, and of course this necessitates the use of a qualitative approach. If researchers want to investigate the objective nature of phenomena, a positivistic paradigm is crucial, and hence a quantitative approach is indicated (Williams *et al.* 2014).

Positivism views reality as being independent of our experiences of it, and being accessible through careful thinking, and observing and recording of our experiences.

It is important to point out here that traditional research methods and designs are heavily influenced by scientific positivism, since it is seen as 'the crowning achievement of Western civilization' (Denzin & Lincoln 2008, p. 8). But many constructivist researchers reject the use of positivist assumptions and methods. Positivist methods, for some researchers, are just one way of 'telling stories about societies or social worlds'. These methods may not be better or worse than any other methods, but they 'tell different kinds of stories'. Other constructivist researchers, however, believe that the criteria used in positivist science are 'irrelevant to their work'. They argue that 'such criteria reproduce only a certain kind of science, a science that silences too many voices' (Denzin & Lincoln 2005, p. 12).

In this chapter I wish to introduce a third paradigm: **pragmatism**. This paradigm has become increasingly popular among health researchers from a variety of disciplines (Creswell 2014; Patton 2015). Pragmatists argue that reality exists not only as natural and physical realities, but also as psychological and social realities, which include subjective experience and thought, language and culture. Knowledge, according to pragmatists, is both constructed and based on the reality of the world in which we live and which we experience. As such, pragmatists advocate that researchers should employ a combination of methods that work best for answering their research questions (Biesta 2010; Cresswell 2015; Curry & Nunez-Smith 2015). Moses and Knutsen (2007) contend that this paradigm offers a 'fully fledged metaphysical position', which combines the most attractive characteristics of constructivism and positivism. Pragmatism, for mixed-methods researchers, 'opens the door to multiple methods, different worldviews, and different assumptions as well as different forms of data collection and analysis' (Creswell 2014, p. 11; see also Chapter 20).

> **Pragmatism** argues that reality exists not only as natural and physical realities, but also as psychological and social realities, which include subjective experience and thought, language and culture.

The major push for the methodological pluralism that underlies pragmatism is the belief that knowledge can be generated from diverse theories and sources, and in many ways through different research methods. Hence we must embrace methodological diversity in our research. Methodological pluralism encourages objectives-driven research instead of methods-driven research. As I have indicated above, the reason for this is that certain methods, regardless of their ontological and epistemological positions, may be more suitable for some questions than for others. In order to understand complex social phenomena, methodological pluralism is crucial.

Qualitative and quantitative approaches: a comparison

Qualitative research is recognised as 'the word science' (Denzin 2008, p. 321). It relies heavily on words or stories that people tell us, as researchers (Liamputtong 2013; Creswell 2014; Patton 2015). Qualitative research is research that has its focus on the social world instead of the world of nature. Fundamentally, researching social life differs from researching natural phenomena. In the social world, we deal with the subjective experiences of human beings, and our 'understanding of reality can change over time and in different social contexts' (Dew

> **Qualitative research:** Research strategies that emphasise words rather than numbers in data collection and analysis. The focus of qualitative research is on the generation of theories.

2007, p. 434). This sets qualitative enquiry apart from researching the natural world, which can be treated as 'objects or things'. The term qualitative, according to Denzin and Lincoln (2011, p. 8), emphasises 'the qualities of entities' as well as the 'processes and meanings that are not experimentally examined or measured in terms of quantity, amount, intensity, or frequency'. Qualitative research is based on inductive reasoning; reasoning which 'moves from the particular to the general'. Inductive reasoning will allow researchers to adopt particular understandings and develop a general conceptual understanding about the issue they examine (Schmidt & Brown 2015a, p. 17; Babbie 2016, p. 23). Researchers use qualitative research to address questions that are associated with the 'hows and whys' of people's actions which are more difficult to articulate through the use of quantitative methods, and when they need to examine phenomena that they know little about or when they attempt to generate theory (Mauk 2015, p. 229). In qualitative research, we use 'words to provide evidence' (Mauk 2015, p. 229).

Quantitative research, on the other hand, is known as the science of numbers. It is also referred to as positivist science. Quantitative research is based on deductive reasoning; reasoning which mobilises from 'the general to the particular' (Schmidt & Brown 2015a, p. 17; Babbie 2016, p. 24). For quantitative researchers, the need to be objective and structured is crucial, as quantitative research attempts to measure things and avoid any **bias** that could influence the findings (Houser 2015; Babbie 2016; Bryman 2016). Quantitative research can produce evidence which 'describe a phenomenon, explain relationships and differences among **variables**, predict relationships and differences among variables, or determine causality' (Peters 2015, p. 175).

Qualitative research is more flexible and fluid in its approach than quantitative research. This has led some researchers to see it as less worthwhile because it is not governed by clear rules (Patton 2015). Quantitative researchers have argued that the interpretive nature of qualitative research makes it 'soft' science, lacking in reliability and validity, and of little value in contributing to scientific knowledge (Hammersley 2008; Denzin 2008; Torrance 2008; Denzin & Lincoln 2011). But the interpretive and flexible approach is necessary because the focus of qualitative research is on meaning and interpretation (Liamputtong 2007, 2013; Patton 2015). Essentially, qualitative research aims to 'capture lived experiences of the social world and the meanings people give these experiences from their own perspective' (Corti & Thompson 2004, p. 327).

Because of its flexibility and fluidity, qualitative research is more suited to understanding the meanings, interpretations and subjective experiences of individuals (Lincoln *et al.* 2011; Houser 2015; Patton 2015; Babbie 2016). In particular, as suggested earlier, qualitative enquiry allows the researchers to hear the voices of those who are marginalised in society (Liamputtong 2007, 2013). The in-depth nature of qualitative methods allows the participants to express their feelings and experiences in their own words.

While quantitative research has always been the dominant research approach in the health sciences, in the past decade or so qualitative research has been gradually accepted as a crucial component in increasing our understanding of health (Neutens 2014; Houser 2015). In many areas of health, researchers have argued about the value of interpretive data. In public health in particular, the 'new public health' recognises the need to 'describe' and 'understand' people (Padgett 2012). For example, Baum (2015) argues for the need for qualitative methods, since they provide great understanding about the complexities of human behaviour and their health issues. In a nutshell, qualitative research is crucial for dealing with the complexity of public health issues that we face globally (Liamputtong 2016). This is reflected in Part II of this book.

Bryman (2016, pp. 401) provides some contrasts between qualitative and quantitative research approaches, which are presented in Table 1.1.

TABLE 1.1 Comparison of qualitative and quantitative approaches

QUALITATIVE APPROACH	QUANTITATIVE APPROACH
Words	Numbers
Participants' points of view	Researcher's point of view
Meaning	Behaviour
Contextual understanding	Generalisation
Rich, deep data	Hard, reliable data
Unstructured	Structured
Process	Static
Micro	Macro
Natural settings	Artificial settings
Theory emergent	Theory testing
Researcher close	Researcher distant

RESISTANCE TO PARTICIPATING IN FALLS PREVENTION EXERCISE

Zoe is a physiotherapist who works in a community health care centre which looks after old people from the local area. She has noticed that there are many old people who recently experienced falls, particularly people from ethnic communities. To prevent future falls, these people come to exercise programs conducted by physiotherapists at the centre, but despite many instructions about doing further exercise at home to prevent falls they seem not to adhere to the recommended exercises. There is no available evidence that Zoe can draw on to improve the situation, and she decides to conduct some research to find the answers that might give her a greater understanding of these old people. She carries out her research using in-depth interviewing, one of the most common methods in qualitative research.

Her study reveals that although preventing further falls is considered important, many old people do not believe that falls are preventable or are unsure about it. Most older people can suggest strategies to prevent falls, including being careful and taking

RESEARCH IN PRACTICE

it slowly. However, few describe evidence-based approaches such as exercise or medication reviews as strategies to prevent falls. Most old people think that physiotherapy and exercise are beneficial in improving physical function, mobility, strength and balance. Zoe finds that family, the client–clinician relationship and personal experience affect their decision-making and exercise participation.

From her study, Zoe recommends a clear explanation of the role of exercise in preventing falls; she says that when engaging this group of older people it is important that clinicians understand the personal motivating and de-motivating factors for such exercise.

Adapted from Lam (2012).

Mixed methods

> In some ways, the differences between quantitative and qualitative methods involve trade-offs between breadth and depth … Qualitative methods typically produce a wealth of detailed data about a much smaller number of people and cases (Patton 2015, p. 257).

Mixed methods:
A research design that combines methods from qualitative and quantitative research approaches within a single study.

How then do we combine the depth and the breadth? **Mixed methods** research offers a way of doing this. In some situations, we find that neither a qualitative nor a quantitative approach alone can provide enough information for us to use, so a combination of the two is required (Feilzer 2010; Creswell & Plano Clark 2011; Flyvbjerg 2011; Cresswell 2014, 2015; Curry & Nunez-Smith 2015; Bryman 2016). This is referred to as a mixed methods research design. According to Curry and Nunez-Smith (2015), quantitative approaches have been the dominant means for conducting research in health sciences. However, many contemporary issues in health and social care are difficult, and often impossible, to investigate using quantitative methods alone. Flyvbjerg (2011, p. 313) contends that 'research is problem-driven and not methodology-driven, meaning that those methods are employed that for a given problematic best help answer the research questions at hand'. We may find that the combination of both research approaches will provide the best evidence that we need.

Mixed methods research has been termed 'the third methodological movement' (Tashakkori & Teddlie 2010 p. 5) because it is the movement that follows the development of quantitative and qualitative research (Creswell & Plano Clark 2014). It has also been referred to as 'multiple ways of seeing and hearing' (Greene 2007, p. 20). These multiple ways of seeing and hearing are what we witness in our everyday life (Creswell & Plano Clark 2014). Therefore, using mixed methods would allow us to find strong evidence that we need in our EBPs.

According to Bryman (2016, p. 34), although qualitative and quantitative approaches have different ontologies, epistemologies and research strategies, 'the distinction is not a hard-and-fast one'. He contends that research which has 'the broad characteristics of one research strategy may also have a characteristic of the other'. Thus within one research project, the two can be combined (Teddlie & Tashakkori 2011; Edmonds & Kennedy 2012; Spicer 2012). Bryman (2016, p. 635) also suggests that this strategy 'would seem to allow the various strengths to be capitalized upon and the weaknesses offset somewhat'.

The term 'mixed methods research' should not be confused with the combination of methods from within one research approach (Creswell 2015; Bryman 2016). For example, the combined use of in-depth interviews and focus groups is not mixed methods research, because both these methods belong to the qualitative approach. Similarly, the use of both a questionnaire (with closed-ended questions) and an RCT is not mixed methods research because both methods come from the quantitative approach. Only research that employs both qualitative and quantitative methods, such as using focus groups and a questionnaire, is classed as mixed methods research. As suggested by Curry and Nunez-Smith (2015, p. 4), mixed methods research underscores 'the interplay of qualitative and quantitative methods in a single research study'. Some researchers, however, may use the term to refer to the combination of different methods from one approach (see Chapter 21).

There are different ways in which researchers can combine the methods. Hammersley (1996) proposes three approaches: triangulation, facilitation and complementarity. Triangulation refers to the use of qualitative research to confirm the findings from quantitative research, or vice versa. In facilitation, one research approach is used in order to facilitate research using the other approach. When the two approaches are used so that different aspects of an investigation can be articulated, this is referred to as complementarity. You may like to read Teddlie and Tashakkori (2011), Cresswell (2015), Curry and Nunez-Smith (2015) and Bryman (2016) who provide useful ways of combining qualitative and quantitative research in a mixed methods design. See also Chapters 20 and 21.

STOP AND THINK

You have been asked to find some evidence for the provision of paediatric health care and the effectiveness of falls prevention to families from culturally and linguistically diverse backgrounds (CALD). You have to develop a research project which will allow you to find appropriate evidence for your workplace.

- Which research design might provide the best evidence for you?
- If you think the first research area (the provision of paediatric health care) should be carried out using a qualitative approach, can you use quantitative research to find evidence too? If you agree, how would you explain the option?
- Can these two evidences be found using a mixed methods approach? What would this approach offer you?

Research rigour: trustworthiness and reliability/validity

Both qualitative and quantitative research approaches have criteria that can be used to evaluate the **rigour** (authenticity/credibility/strength) of the research. Within the qualitative approach, we use the term 'trustworthiness', which refers to the quality of qualitative

Rigour: Rigorous research is trustworthy and can be relied on by other researchers.

enquiry (Liamputtong 2013; see also Chapters 4, 8). A trustworthy research is a research in which researchers have 'drawn the correct conclusions about the meaning of an event or phenomemon' (Houser 2015, p. 146). In health research and practice, trustworthiness means that 'the findings must be authentic enough to allow practitioners to act upon them with confidence' (Raines 2011, p. 497). In quantitative research, the concepts of reliability and validity are used (Dougherty 2015; Babbie 2016). 'Reliability' refers to 'the stability of findings' and validity represents 'the truthfulness of findings' (Carpenter & Suto 2008, p. 148). **Reliability** is 'the consistency and trustworthiness of research findings' (Kvale 2007, p. 22). Often, it is considered in relation to 'whether a particular technique, applied repeatedly to the same object, yields the same result each time' (Babbie 2016, p. 146). **Validity** bears upon measurement and is 'concerned with the integrity of the conclusions that are generated from a piece of research' (Bryman 2016, p. 41). Validity 'refers to the extent to which an empirical measure adequately reflects the real meaning of the concept under consideration' (Babbie 2016, p. 148). The most commonly used validity concepts are internal and external validity. Internal validity is related to 'the issue of whether a method investigates what it purports to investigate' (Kvale 2007, p. 22), while external validity relates to 'whether the results of a study can be generalized beyond the specific research context' (Bryman 2016, p. 42). See also Chapters 11, 13, 15, 16, 17.

The attainment of validity in quantitative research is based on strict observance of the rules and standards of the approach. Thus it follows that attempting to apply those rules to qualitative research becomes problematic. Angen (2000, p. 379) contends that when qualitative research is judged by the validity criteria used in the quantitative approach, it may be seen as 'being too subjective, lacking in rigour, and/or being unscientific'. As a consequence, qualitative research may be denied legitimacy.

The concepts of validity and reliability are seen as incompatible with the ontological and epistemological foundations of qualitative research (Carpenter & Suto 2008, p. 148; Liamputtong 2013; Patton 2015). Since qualitative research is descriptive and unique to a specific historical, social and cultural context (Johnson & Waterfield 2004), it cannot be repeated in order to establish reliability. Qualitative researchers hold the view that reality is socially constructed by an individual and, while this socially constructed reality cannot be measured, it can be interpreted. For qualitative research, understanding cannot be separated from context. Hence qualitative data cannot be 'tested for validity' using the same rules and standards, which are based on 'assumptions of objective reality and positivist neutrality' (Johnson & Waterfield 2004, pp. 122–3; see also Angen 2000).

Qualitative researchers have, however, developed some criteria that can be used to judge the trustworthiness of their research. Here I refer to the work of Lincoln and Guba (1985, 1989), who propose four criteria that many qualitative researchers have adopted; these can be used 'as a translation of the more traditional terms associated with quantitative research' (Carpenter & Suto 2008, p. 149). Hence credibility equates to internal validity, and transferability to external validity, dependability to reliability, and confirmability to

---

Reliability: The extent to which a measurement instrument is dependable, stable and consistent when repeated under identical conditions.

Validity: The degree to which a scale measures what it is supposed to measure.

objectivity (see also Padgett 2008; Raines 2011; Liamputtong 2013; Patton 2015; Creswell 2014; Bryman 2016).

Credibility 'refers to the truth or believability of findings' (Mauk 2015, p. 236). It relates to the questions 'Can these findings be regarded as truthful?' (Raines 2011, p. 455) or 'How believable are the findings?' (Bryman 2016, p. 44). It scrutinises the matter of 'fit' between what the participants say and the representation of those viewpoints by the researchers (Padgett 2008). Credibility asks whether 'the explanation fits the description and whether the description is credible' (Tobin & Begley 2004, p. 391).

Transferability (or applicability) relates to 'whether findings from one study can be transferred to a similar context; application of findings to a different situation' (Mauk 2015, p. 236). It begs the questions of 'To what degree can the study findings be *generalised* or applied to other individuals or groups, contexts, or settings?' or 'Do the findings apply to other contexts?' (Bryman 2016, p. 44). It attempts to establish the 'generalisability of inquiry' (Tobin & Begley 2004, p. 392). Transferability pertains to 'the degree to which qualitative findings inform and facilitate insights within contexts other than that in which the research was conducted' (Carpenter & Suto 2008, pp. 149–50; see also Padgett 2008).

Dependability raises questions about whether the research findings 'fit' the data that have been collected (Carpenter & Suto 2008), or 'are the findings likely to apply at other times' (Bryman 2016, p. 44). Dependability 'addresses the consistency or congruency of the results' (Raines 2011, p. 456). It is gained through an auditing process, which requires the researchers to ensure that 'the process of research is logical, traceable and clearly documented' (Tobin & Begley 2004, p. 392).

Confirmability asks if the researcher has 'allowed his or her values to intrude to a high degree' (Bryman 2016, p. 44). It attempts to show that the findings, and the interpretations of the findings, do not derive from the imagination of the researchers but are clearly linked to the data. Confirmability is 'the degree to which findings are determined by the respondents and conditions of the inquiry and not by the biases, motivations, interests or perspectives of the inquirer' (Lincoln & Guba 1985, p. 290).

Table 1.2 compares rigour criteria employed in qualitative research with those used in quantitative research.

TABLE 1.2 Rigour criteria employed in qualitative and quantitative research

QUALITATIVE RESEARCH	QUANTITATIVE RESEARCH
Credibility	Internal validity
Transferability	External validity
Dependability	Reliability
Confirmability	Objectivity

Source: Carpenter & Suto (2008, p. 149).

Sampling issues

Here I discuss two salient issues in relation to sampling: sampling methods and sample size.

Sampling methods

Issues in sampling methods centre around whether the sample is based on a probability or a non-probability method. **Probability sampling methods** are methods in which 'the probability of an element being selected is known in advance' (Schutt 2014, p. 298). In research involving people, an element means a **research participant**. Within these methods, elements are randomly selected and hence there should be no systematic bias, as 'nothing but chance determines which elements are included in the sample' (Schutt 2014, p. 298). It means that 'every element in the accessible population has an equal chance of being selected for inclusion in the study' (White 2015, p. 300; see also Seale 2012b; Houser 2015; Patton 2015; Babbie 2016). Because of this characteristic, probability sample methods are important in quantitative research where, in most cases, the intent is to generalise the findings for the sample to the population from which the sample was taken (see also Chapters 11–15, 25, 26). The four most common methods for drawing random samples are simple random sampling, systematic random sampling, stratified random sampling, and cluster random sampling (Seale 2012b; Schutt 2014; Houser 2015).

In **non-probability sampling** methods, on the other hand, the likelihood of a potential research participant being selected is not known in advance (Seale 2012b; Schutt 2014; Babbie 2016). Additionally, random selection procedures commonly employed in probability sampling are not used in non-probability sampling methods. The latter do not provide representative samples for the populations from which they are drawn, so the findings cannot be generalised to a larger group of people (White 2015). However, these methods are useful for research questions that do not need to involve large populations, and particularly for qualitative research projects (Johnson & Waterfield 2004; Seale 2012b; Schutt 2014; Patton 2015; Babbie 2016).

Qualitative researchers therefore usually rely on non-probability sampling methods. Since qualitative research is concerned with in-depth understanding of the issue or issues under examination, it relies heavily on individuals who are able to provide information-rich accounts of their experiences. It usually involves a small number of individuals. Morse (2007, p. 530, original emphasis) contends that 'qualitative researchers sample for *meaning*, rather than frequency. We are not interested in how much, or how many, but in *what*'. Qualitative research aims to examine a 'process' or the 'meanings' that people give to their own social situations. It does not require a generalisation of the findings, as in positivist science (Hesse-Biber & Leavy 2011; Houser 2015). Qualitative research also relies heavily on purposive sampling strategies (Hesse-Biber & Leavy 2011; Liamputtong 2013; Houser 2015; Patton 2015; Bryman 2016). **Purposive sampling** is a deliberate selection of specific individuals, events or settings because of the crucial information they can provide, which cannot be obtained as adequately through other channels (Patton 2015; White 2015; Babbie 2016). For example, in research that is concerned with how cancer patients cope with pain, purposive sampling will require

---

Probability sampling method: The probability of a participant being selected is known in advance. The intent is to generalise the findings for the sample to the population from which it was taken.

Research participant: A person who agrees to take part in the study on equal terms.

Non-probability sampling: The probability of a potential research participant being selected is not known in advance. The findings cannot be generalised to a larger group of people.

Purposive sampling looks for cases that will be able to provide rich or in-depth information about the issue being examined, not a representative sample as in quantitative research.

the researcher to find participants who have pain, instead of randomly selecting any cancer patients from an oncologist's patient list (Padgett 2008). The powers of purposive sampling techniques, Patton (2015, p. 264, original emphasis) suggests, 'lie in selecting *information-rich cases* for study in depth'. Information-rich cases are individuals or events or settings from which researchers can learn extensively about issues they wish to examine (Houser 2015).

Another sampling method commonly adopted in qualitative research is **convenience sampling**. It is also known as accidental sampling (Houser 2015). This method allows researchers to find individuals who are conveniently available and willing to participate in a study (Patton 2015; White 2015). Convenience sampling is crucial when it is difficult to find individuals who meet some specified criteria such as age, gender, ethnicity or social class. This may happen more often in research that requires the conduct of fieldwork, such as ethnography. Researchers need to find key informants who are able to provide in-depth information on the research issues and site. Often, researchers make decisions on the basis of 'who is available, who has some specialized knowledge of the setting, and who is willing to serve in that role' (Hesse-Biber & Leavy 2011, p. 46; see also Liamputtong 2013; Bryman 2016).

> Convenience **sampling** allows researchers to find individuals who are conveniently available and willing to participate in a study.

Sample size

The question of sample size is considered differently in qualitative and quantitative approaches. A crucial point in qualitative research is selecting the research participants meaningfully and strategically, instead of attempting to make statistical comparisons or to 'create a representative sample' (Carpenter & Suto 2008, p. 80; see also Patton 2015). Hence the important question is whether the sample provides data that will allow the research questions or aims to be thoroughly addressed (Mason 2002; Houser 2015). The focus of decisions about sample size in qualitative research is on flexibility and depth. A fundamental concern of qualitative research is quality, not quantity. Qualitative researchers do not intend to maximise the breadth of their research (Padgett 2008; Liamputtong 2013; Patton 2015).

In qualitative research, no set formula is rigidly used to determine the sample size, as is the case for quantitative research (Morse 1998; Patton 2015). The sampling process is flexible and, at the commencement of the research, the number of participants to be recruited is not definitely known. However, **data saturation**, a concept associated with grounded theory, is used by qualitative researchers as a way of justifying the number of research participants, and this is established during the data collection process (Houser 2015). Saturation is considered to have occurred when little or no new data are being generated (Padgett 2008; Liamputtong 2013; White 2015). The sample is adequate when 'the emerging themes have been efficiently and effectively saturated with optimal quality data' (Carpenter & Suto 2008, p. 152), and when 'sufficient data to account for all aspects of the phenomenon have been obtained' (Morse *et al.* 2002, p. 12).

> **Data saturation** occurs when little or no new data are being generated and new data fit into the categories already developed.

In quantitative research, sample sizes tend to be larger than those of qualitative research. Researchers have more confidence about generalising their results if they have larger samples. Often, during the planning stage of their research, quantitative researchers attempt to determine how large a sample they must have in order to achieve their purposes. As Schutt

(2014, p. 311) points out, quantitative researchers must 'consider the degree of confidence desired, the homogeneity of the population, the complexity of the analysis they plan, and the expected strength of the relationships they will measure'. Generally, quantitative researchers can use the following criteria when considering their sample size (Schutt 2014; Houser 2015):

- the larger the sample size, the less the sampling error
- samples of more diverse populations need to be larger than samples of more homogeneous populations
- if only a few variables are to be examined, a smaller sample will suffice, but if a more complex analysis involving sample subgroups is required, then a larger sample will be needed
- if the researchers wish to test hypotheses, and expect very strong effects, they will need a smaller sample size to find these effects, but if they expect smaller effects, a larger sample is required.

Sample size can be estimated by using existing tables (Peat 2001), or calculated using relevant formulae (Friedman *et al.* 1998; Seale 2012b). Ideally, more precise estimation of the necessary sample size should be carried out by the use of the statistical power analysis method (Seale 2012b; Polit & Beck 2014; Houser 2015). A power analysis refers to a statistical method that is 'used to determine the acceptable sample size to detect the true effect or difference in the outcome variable' (White 2015, p. 310). This analysis allows 'a good advance estimate of the strength of the hypothesized relationship in the population' (Schutt 2014, p. 311; Polit & Beck 2014). However, it is a complicated analysis and it may require researchers to work with a statistician to determine the size of their research sample.

**RESEARCH
IN PRACTICE**

OBTAINING EVIDENCE FROM WOMEN LIVING WITH HIV/AIDS IN THAILAND

I would like to give readers a reflective practice example from my own research that I conducted collaboratively with colleagues from two universities in Thailand (see Liamputtong et al. 2009, 2012).

Thai women are now experiencing a high prevalence of HIV and AIDS. In this study, we examined the women's perspectives on community attitudes towards women currently living with HIV/AIDS. We also looked at strategies employed by women in order to deal with any stigma and discrimination they might feel or experience in their communities. Last, we examined the reasons that women had for participating in drug/vaccine trials.

A qualitative method was adopted in this study because it enabled us to examine the interpretations and meanings of HIV/AIDS within the women's perspectives. The strength of using such a method is that it has a holistic focus, which allows for flexibility and also allows the participants to raise issues and topics that may not have been included by the researcher.

A purposive sampling technique was adopted for this research; that is, only Thai women who had HIV/AIDS and who were participating, or had participated, in HIV clinical trials, and female drug users who had been participating in vaccine trials, were approached to participate. Due to the sensitivity of this research, we would approach the women and invite them to take part, with caution. For the same reason, we relied on snowball sampling; that is, our participants suggested others who were interested in participating. We also enlisted the assistance of leaders of two HIV and AIDS support groups to access the women in this study.

We used a number of in-depth interviews and some participant observations to collect data with twenty-six Thai women. We interviewed the women in places that they selected. Most often, the interviews were done in a café or in a shopping mall. Since the women wished to preserve their confidentiality and identities as HIV persons, they did not wish us to interview them in their own homes.

Interviews were conducted in the Thai language to allow the women to articulate about their lived experiences and to allow us to maintain the subtlety and any hidden meanings in their narratives. Before the study began, ethical approval was obtained from the Faculty of Health Sciences Human Ethics Committee, La Trobe University, Melbourne, and from the Ethics Committee at Chulalongkorn University, Thailand. We also sought consent from each woman in the study. Each interview took between one and two hours. Each participant was given 200 Thai baht as compensation for the time spent in participating in the study.

With permission from the participants, we audio-recorded the interviews. The tapes were then transcribed in Thai, for data analysis. The in-depth data were analysed using a thematic analysis. All transcripts were coded, and emerging themes were subsequently identified and presented in the results section of the report on the research.

As you can see, there are many issues we need to consider in carrying out a piece of research: not only which approach and which method to use, but who will be our research participants, how we will find them and how many we need for our project. Also, ethical issues requiring consideration need to be identified, we need to consider how we will make sense of the data we have collected, and how we will present these data and their analysis. All these matters are covered in this book.

Summary

Neither quantitative nor qualitative methodology is in any ultimate sense superior to the other. The two approaches exist along a continuum on which neither pole is more 'scientific' or more suited to … knowledge development. (Williams *et al.* 2014, p. 94).

In this chapter, I have introduced the concept of evidence and evidence-based practice in health. I have argued that in many situations and for many health issues, researchers and practitioners need to find the 'best' evidence, and this may require us to carry out a research study to find our answers. I have provided readers with firm foundations for carrying out research in health. I have suggested that researchers should not favour one method over another based on their own preferences. Rather, we need to carefully consider the research questions to which we wish to find answers.

Qualitative and quantitative research approaches, as Williams and colleagues (2014, p. 93) contend, 'each have their special uses'. Rather than asking which approach is best, it would be more appropriate for us to ask 'under what conditions each approach is better than the other in order to answer a particular research question' (Williams *et al.* 2014, p. 93). This is what I have advocated in this chapter.

In summary, I argue that knowledge is essential in the era of EBP in health care. Without knowledge, evidence cannot be generated. Without 'appropriate' evidence, our practice may not be applicable or suitable to those who health care providers/practitioners need to serve.

Practice exercises

1   You have been asked by your superior to find the 'best' evidence that can be used to develop culturally sensitive maternal and child health services for Indigenous Australians. How would you find this 'best' evidence? Discuss various types of evidence that you could obtain.

2   There has been a good deal of discussion in your local area about young people, who are seen as likely to engage in risky health-related behaviour such as smoking heavily, driving very fast, and not paying attention to their diet. You want to understand why young people tend to take such health risks. Which research approach (qualitative or quantitative) is likely to give you greater in-depth understanding of their lives, the meaning they attach to risk-taking behaviour and their lived experiences of risk? Discuss.

3   You want to ascertain the prevalence of risk-taking behaviour among young people in your city. What approach will provide you with an estimate of this prevalence, and how will you go about doing the research? Discuss.

4   As you need to design a research study that will provide the best answers that you can find, what important issues do you need to consider? Write a short account of your proposed research, taking into account salient issues that have been discussed in this chapter.

Further reading

Aoun, S.M. & Kristjanson, L.J. (2005). Evidence in palliative care research: how should it be gathered? *Medical Journal of Australia*, 183(5), 264–6.

Curry, L. & Nunez-Smith, M. (2015). *Mixed methods in health sciences research*. Thousand Oaks, CA: Sage.

Denzin, N.K. (2009). The elephant in the living room: or extending the conversation about the politics of evidence. *Qualitative Research*, 9(2), 139–60.

Flemming, K. (2010). The use of morphine to treat cancer-related pain: a synthesis of quantitative and qualitative research. *Journal of Pain and Symptom Management*, 39, 139–54.

Gibson, B.E. & Martin, D.K. (2003). Qualitative research and evidence-based physiotherapy practice. *Physiotherapy*, 89, 350–8.

Grypdonck, M.H.F. (2006). Qualitative health research in the era of evidence-based practice. *Qualitative Health Research*, 16(10), 1371–85.

Hammell, K.W. & Carpenter, C. (2004). *Qualitative research in evidence-based rehabilitation*. Edinburgh: Churchill Livingstone.

Hawker, S., Payne, S., Kerr, C., Hardey, M. & Powell, J. (2002). Appraising the evidence: reviewing disparate data systematically. *Qualitative Health Research*, 12(9), 1284–99.

Johnson, R. & Waterfield, J. (2004). Making words count: the value of qualitative research. *Physiotherapy Research International*, 9(3), 121–31.

Liamputtong, P. (2013). *Qualitative research methods*, 4th edn. Melbourne: Oxford University Press.

Mullen, E.J., Bellamy, J.L. & Bledsoe, S.E. (2014). Evidence-based practice. In R.M. Grinnell & Y.A. Unrau (eds), *Social work research and evaluation: foundations of evidence-based practice*, 10th edn. New York: Oxford University Press, 200–17.

Olsen, K., Young, R.A. & Schultz, I.Z. (2015). *Handbook of qualitative health research for evidence-based practice*. New York: Springer.

Patton, M.Q. (2015). *Qualitative research and evaluation methods*, 4th edn. Thousand Oaks, CA: Sage.

Spicer, N. (2012). Combining qualitative and quantitative methods. In C. Seale (ed.), *Researching society and culture*, 3rd edn. London: Sage, 479–93.

Websites

http://libguides.library.curtin.edu.au/c.php?g=202374&p=1332674

> Critical appraisal is an integral process in evidence-based practice. This website contains several critical appraisal tools that researchers can use to make informed decisions about the quality of research evidence.

http://methods.cochrane.org/qi/

> This website is about the Cochrane Qualitative and Implementation Methods Group. It provides useful information about the use of qualitative research synthesis in evidence-based practice.

www.womenandhealthcarereform.ca/

> This website provides useful discussions on evidence and women's health care. It argues that 'because women are not all the same, changes to the health care system may variously affect the health, well-being and work of particular groups of women. This means that when evidence is used by decision-makers in the development and implementation of health care reforms, women need to question what is being counted as evidence, whose perspective and experience is being counted, if the differing contexts of women's lives are being considered, and which women's needs are being included and excluded.'

http://en.wikipedia.org/wiki/Evidence-based_medicine

This website provides a good discussion on EBP and its limitations.

www.gla.ac.uk/media/media_48396_en.pdf

This website contains a set of slides on the contribution of the qualitative approach to EBP, which will be useful for the many readers who are sceptical about the value of qualitative research.

www.conted.ox.ac.uk/courses/details.php?id=48

This is the website of Oxford University's MSc in Evidence-Based Health Care program. It is part of the Oxford International Programme in Evidence-Based Health Care. It is offered as a part-time course consisting of six taught modules and a dissertation. The course provides extensive coverage of the role of research methods, including both qualitative and quantitative approaches, in providing the information needed for EBP.

www.climatecrisis.net/an-inconvenienttruth.php

www.takepart.com/an-inconvenient-truth/film

This is the website of the award-winning documentary on global warming entitled *The Inconvenient Truth*. It features Al Gore, the former US Vice President and Nobel Prize winner, who discussed his personal journey relating to the changing climate and global warming as well as the statistical trends. This document is a good example of a mixed methods research. It combines both qualitative and quantitative information to tell a single story.

2

Getting Started: Designing and Planning a Research Project

PRANEE LIAMPUTTONG AND VIRGINIA SCHMIED

Chapter objectives

In this chapter, you will learn about:

- what we need to consider in designing a research project
- the research process
- research questions and research problems
- the importance of literature review and where we can find literature
- the essence of a research proposal and its structure

Key terms

Boolean operator

Literature review

Narrative review

Research

Research design

Research problem

Research process

Research proposal

Research question

Introduction

> The best research starts with two words: 'I wonder'. A sense of curiosity is all that is needed to begin the research process. Observations about a problem become questions, and these questions lead to … research' (Houser 2015, p. 77).

As we suggested in Chapter 1, knowledge can be obtained through many means. According to Cohen and Manion (2000), there are three main ways of knowing: experience, reasoning and research. Often, we generate new knowledge through research (Fawcett & Pockett 2015). Scientific research, Schmidt and Brown (2015a, p. 7) contend, is perceived to 'yield the best source of evidence'. In an attempt to provide evidence-based health care, research is undertaken so that knowledge which addresses the practice concern is generated (Grove *et al.* 2013). In this chapter, we will discuss the research process—how we design and plan for a research project in order to obtain knowledge that can be used as evidence in our practice. We will first discuss salient issues regarding how to design a research project that can assist us to find evidence that we need in our practice. We will then take you through the research process, the importance of research questions, and the literature review. Last, we will discuss the essence of a research proposal and the common structure that researchers tend to construct when planning for their research project.

Designing research

In the health sciences, **research** is a 'planned and systematic activity' (Schmidt & Brown 2015a, p. 14) that results in the construction of new knowledge which can be used to provide answers to some health problems or as evidence for health care practice (Polit & Beck 2011).

In conducting any piece of research, **we** must carefully consider our research design. The term **research design** signifies several issues. First, it refers to the type of research enquiry. As discussed in Chapter 1, there are different types of research design. At a basic level, we can categorise the research design into three major designs: qualitative, quantitative and mixed method research. Each research design serves different purposes and leads to different data collection methods and findings (Fawcett & Pockett 2015). All forms of research design, however, aim to find evidence that we can use for our evidence-based practice (EBP) (Houser 2015). We need to ensure that the research design will be appropriate to the research questions of our study.

A research design also refers to 'an outline of the study' (Houser 2015, p. 131). It is a 'formalised plan' that we prepare before conducting our research (Gabriel 2013, p. 359). This is a research proposal and we will discuss this later in this chapter. At a macro level, research design signifies the research's 'overall approach' situated within the type of knowledge that we seek and the questions that need to be answered (Houser 2015, p. 131). This level of research design was covered in Chapter 1, in the Ontology and Epistemology section. At a micro level, design refers to the 'research design' of the study. In qualitative research, the design details

Research: A planned activity that results in the construction of new knowledge which can be used to provide answers to some health problems or as evidence for health care practice.

Research design: The type of research enquiry as well as an outline of the study.

the planned approach that researchers use for gathering data. This includes our beliefs about the nature of knowledge to be generated. The planned approach also includes criteria for selecting research participants, strategies for data collection, and data analysis. In quantitative studies, the design describes how the participants will be selected and put into groups. It also includes information about a measurement strategy and a plan for data analysis. Some types of quantitative research include discussion on how the intervention will be done (Houser 2015; see also Chapter 1).

Importantly, in designing a research project, we need to carefully address the nature of the research questions that we will examine. We must select a particular research design that is appropriate to the nature of research questions that we wish to examine (Parfrey & Ravani 2009; Houser 2015; Bryman 2016). For example, a research question which focuses on the effectiveness of an intervention will need a quantitative approach that will lead to an 'objectively measured outcome' (Houser 2015, p. 36). However, research questions that emphasise the acceptability of an intervention will necessitate the use of a qualitative approach. The new intervention may be effective, but the consumers may find it unpleasant and burdensome. This may have an impact on their compliance. To find out these issues, we must ask the consumers about their lived experiences, needs and preferences. This is when we need to employ qualitative enquiry in our research (Liamputtong 2013; Houser 2015).

Additionally, in designing a research project, we must consider the purpose of the study. A research design that serves the purpose of the study must be selected. We need to ask if our research aims to be an exploratory study or a confirmatory study. Exploratory studies 'explore and describe a given phenomenon' (Houser 2015, p. 135). Often, exploratory research projects employ qualitative or mixed methods, but some quantitative research can also be an exploratory study if measurement is used, such as research projects that use survey methods. Survey methods are often adopted in exploratory research projects. Confirmatory research includes research that examines relationships between variables. This type of research is used to statistically test the relationships among variables. Bias must be minimised (see Chapter 1). Careful definition of the variables and concepts of interest is crucial so they can be appropriately measured and analysed (Houser 2015; Bryman 2016). Thus, most quantitative research falls within the parameters of confirmatory research.

The research process

The term 'research' means 'to search again' (Schmidt & Brown 2015a, p. 14). However, the search needs to be purposeful and choreographed according to the research questions that we intend to examine. The planned activity that we construct for our research project is referred to as the '**research process**' (Neutens 2014, p. 7).

A research process is cyclical and comprises several stages. Commonly, it commences with determining a research problem by identifying a gap in knowledge about health. The literature is then reviewed to ascertain key knowledge about the issue and to establish relevant evidence.

Research process:
A planned activity that researchers use to construct their research project, choreographed according to the research questions that they intend to examine.

An appropriate research design which is suitable for the philosophical assumption, the nature of the question, and the overall aim of the researcher is then determined. A sampling strategy is decided upon. It details both how research participants will be recruited (and designated into groups if appropriate), and how many participants will be included in the study. Ethical issues must be addressed prior to data collection. Data are then collected and analysed using the most appropriate data collection methods and analytic techniques. The findings are disseminated to the appropriate audiences. In EBP, the findings are used to enhance practice. Often, the adoption of the research findings is recommended through particular protocols for practice in health care (Houser 2015). This process is presented in Figure 2.1.

FIGURE 2.1   The cyclical stages of a research project

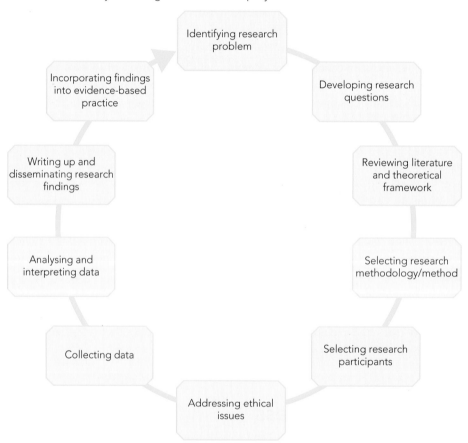

The cyclical research process described above holds true for both qualitative and quantitative research. However, there are slight differences in some of the stages. Quantitative research usually commences with identifying problems and developing relevant research questions. Variables which will be examined or tested are determined. Relevant literature is reviewed and an appropriate research design is selected. Appropriate measurement tools and research samples are chosen. Once all these have been designed, data collection and analysis follow. When data have been analysed, the study findings are disseminated to appropriate audiences as well as incorporated into EBP (Grinnell *et al.* 2014b). For most quantitative research, decisions are usually firmly made before the commencement of data collection. Only in some emergent research topics is the research plan adapted during the study.

However, the research cycle of qualitative research takes a slightly different approach. This form also commences with problem identification and addressing the research questions on which researchers seek to find evidence. A literature review is conducted to find gaps in existing knowledge. However, researchers normally identify research participants who will provide knowledge appropriate to their research questions prior to the selection of research methods. This is crucial, as researchers need to select research methods that are appropriate to their research participants. Once research methods are decided, data collection will follow. After data analysis is done, the findings are disseminated to appropriate audiences and incorporated into EBP. In qualitative research, the processes from identifying the problem, selecting research participants and methods, to data analysis and interpretations are intermingled. It is not a one-way process, as in most quantitative research; rather it is a two-way process (Williams *et al.* 2014). The design of qualitative research is, as Houser (2015, p. 32) points out, 'a fluid process, one that may be considered a work in progress until the final plan is complete'.

Research problems and research questions

In designing and planning for research, it is crucial that we consider our research problems and establish research questions from the beginning. Conceptually, a **research question** is 'a question that provides an explicit statement of what it is the researcher wants to know about' (Bryman 2016, p. 7). Often, research questions are framed as questions to which we hope to find answers through our research (Houser 2015).

Research questions are crucial in the research process since they push us to think carefully about the area of interest on which we need to seek knowledge (Bryman 2016). Well-founded research questions will allow researchers to generate new knowledge that can significantly contribute to evidence-based health care practice (Natalier 2013). According to Bryman (2016), research questions will guide our literature review, assist us to select the appropriate research design, indicate what data should be collected and who should be selected as research participants, and offer ideas for data analysis. Research questions also provide readers with 'a clearer sense of what the research is about' (Bryman 2016, p. 9). Hence, the research question is the pivotal component of the research process—it will keep us focused (Natalier 2013).

Research questions are generally derived from **research problems**. Here, the research problem is 'an area of concern when there is a gap in knowledge that requires a solution that can be described, explained, or predicted' in order to improve health care practice (Adams 2015, p. 72). This knowledge gap, or what is not known about the issue,

Research question:
A question that a researcher intends to answer through conducting the proposed research.

Research problem: An area of concern about which little is known and which needs an answer in order to improve health care practice. Often, it determines the complexity of the research project.

determines the complexity of the research needed to produce important knowledge in health (Creswell 2014).

Research problems can be generated from a number of sources. They can derive from our personal experiences, health and social issues, clinical practice observations, theoretical frameworks, research reports, research priorities, professional literature, and consumer/patient feedbacks (Sandberg & Alvesson 2011; Alvesson & Sandberg 2013; Houser 2015). A research problem can be determined by asking questions such as the following:

- What role does health inequality play in morbidity rates among ethnic minority groups?
- What factors predispose women to breast cancer?
- What are the needs of stroke survivors?
- Why has adolescent obesity increased so rapidly in the past ten years?
- What contributes to the high incidence of postnatal depression among women in rural areas?
- What is the mental health impact of being a Muslim woman/person living in Australia today?

These types of questions could assist us to identify an important research problem for our study (Grove *et al.* 2013, p. 75).

RESEARCH IN PRACTICE

Below, we provide examples of research questions from two studies.

In their research on social support among women living with breast cancer in Thailand, Suwankhong and Liamputtong (2016) contend that little is known about social support among breast cancer survivors in southern Thailand's rural community. There are few quantitative studies that shed light on social support among this group (Anusasananun *et al.* 2013; Lueboonthavatchai 2007). In their study, Suwankhong and Liamputtong wish to examine social support among women living with breast cancer in southern Thailand. They argue that it is important for nurses and health care providers to understand how these vulnerable women deal with the challenges resulting from breast cancer.

This understanding can help health care providers, including nurses, create ways that can help to enhance the women's quality of life. The research questions of their study included: What are their coping resources? How do these sources operate after the diagnosis of breast cancer? Do these support sources provide a way of coping with the distress of living with breast cancer?

Social, emotional and mental health problems, such as depression, domestic violence, drug and/or alcohol abuse and lack of social support, in women in pregnancy and following birth are recognised as a major public health issue and are associated with poor outcomes for women and their children. To identify women who are experiencing, or are likely to experience, social and emotional problems, many health services are implementing routine psychosocial assessment in pregnancy and after birth. Very little is known about how women respond to or experience psychosocial assessment, particularly on their first antenatal visit, or how midwives and/or child health nurses conduct these assessments. Rollans and colleagues (2013) wanted to describe the process and impact of the psychosocial assessment undertaken by midwives in the antenatal booking visit and by child and family health nurses (CFHN) in the postnatal universal home visit. In particular, they wanted to capture the dynamics of the interaction between women and professionals during psychosocial assessment, describing the actions of midwives and nurses, the reactions of the women and their subsequent engagement in ongoing services. The research questions included: What approach (actions and interactions) do midwives and CFHN take to psychosocial assessment and to engaging women and families in services? How do women react to psychosocial assessment, particularly in disclosing sensitive and intimate information to midwives and CFHN? What psychosocial services and support are available, offered to and accessed by women during the perinatal period?

STOP AND THINK

Fawcett and Pockett (2015, p. 8) suggest that research questions 'flow from the generation of good ideas. In turn, good ideas flow from moments of inspiration, from detailed work in specific areas, from big-picture scenarios and from making links and connections'.

You are asked to come up with some research questions on which you can find evidence in your discipline.

- Based on Fawcett and Pockett's points, what would be your 'good ideas' that can lead to research questions?
- How will you go about developing these research questions? Discuss.

Literature review

Once you have developed your research questions, you need to review relevant literature. A **literature review** constitutes a crucial part of every research project (Ridley 2012; Bryman 2016). A literature review refers to 'an organised written presentation' of what researchers will find when they review the literature (Grove *et al.* 2013, p. 97). It pulls together existing publications on a particular issue and offers pertinent research findings.

Why do a literature review?

The literature review provides a critical analysis of what is known and what is not known, and shapes the groundwork for research which would lead to evidence-based practice in health care (Houser 2015). The literature review can summarise the body of knowledge on a specific issue, and point to a paucity of knowledge on the subject. In a nutshell, the literature review is the first step that allows us to appraise the importance of our research question and a possible research design for our study (Houser 2015).

Literature review: A written presentation resulting from reviewing literature. It provides a critical analysis of what is known and what is not known, and shapes the groundwork for research which would lead to EBP in health care.

Once we have decided on a research topic, we need to conduct a literature review for a number of reasons. In reviewing the literature, we can determine, appraise and theorise a body of knowledge which is related to the topic that we wish to examine. This will not only establish a background for the study but also offers a justification for investigating a specific research question. The purpose of a literature review is 'to justify the proposal in terms of a gap in existing knowledge' (Jones 2013, p. 42). According to Bryman (2016, p. 94), a literature review offers researchers many advantages. It allows us to know:

- what is already known about the issue
- what concepts and theories have been adopted
- what research design and methods have been utilised
- whether there are any unanswered questions and/or controversies about the issue
- who are the key contributors to research on the topic
- how the literature links with your research questions/topics.

Within the health sciences, the literature review may refer to the systematic review of literature that we conduct to evaluate existing knowledge on the efficacy of an intervention, for example, the evidence base for the preferred treatment of back pain or foot injuries. This will not be the focus of this section. Readers can find information about this in Chapters 18, 19, 20 in this volume.

Our aim here is to discuss the literature review as used in planning a research project. This type of review is known as the **narrative review** and is a commonly adopted form in most research projects (Bryman 2016). Narrative review will illustrate how ideas, conceptual frameworks and methodologies have been established within a specific health issue. In the narrative review, we critique existing research by evaluating, scrutinising and integrating it and place it within the context of our research (Jones 2013; Bryman 2016). Often, when we conduct a narrative review, we compare and contrast the findings from different studies. In this approach, we are not too concerned about different research designs, methods or research settings (Mileham 2015).

In conducting a literature review, we are not expected to list all the published work (Grove *et al.* 2013). Most literature reviews synthesise the literature, place it into a progression of relevant issues, often from general ideas to specific issues, and summarise the literature by suggesting the central themes (Creswell 2014). The literature review may be done in a few ways. Cooper (2010) suggests four types of literature review. These are the review that integrates what previous researchers have done and suggested, reviews that critique existing literature, reviews that create links among relevant topics, and reviews that identify the fundamental issues in the areas (Creswell 2014; Bryman 2016).

Where do we find literature?

Most researchers search through scholarly literature, which includes peer-reviewed articles in scholarly journals, monographs, books, research reports, conference proceedings, internet sites, theses and dissertations, government reports, and practice guidelines (Natalier 2013;

Narrative review: Illustrates how ideas, conceptual frameworks, and methodologies have been established within a specific health issue. Researchers critique existing research by evaluating, scrutinising and integrating it within the context of their research.

Houser 2015). At the simplest level, we may be able to locate some relevant literature by looking at the references cited in published journal articles, books, monographs and reports. This will allow us to identify some keywords which would help to define the boundaries of our research project. This in turn will assist us to search relevant literature through electronic databases (Houser 2015; Bryman 2016).

Most scholarly literature can be found through electronic databases (Ridley 2012; Bryman 2016), although books, dissertations, individual journals and websites may not be included in major databases (Houser 2015). Electronic databases differ in subject (e.g. nursing versus biomedical), content type (e.g. full text versus bibliographic records), search interface (the search engine), and indexing (e.g. free-text or text-word searching versus subject headings) (Houser 2015). Most academic libraries have access to computer databases, both commercial and those in the public domain. These databases offer an accessible entry point to a large number of journals, conference papers, and other materials on numerous different research topics (Creswell 2014; Bryman 2016).

TABLE 2.1   Major bibliographic databases

DATABASE	DESCRIPTION
MEDLINE	The National Library of Medicine's (NLM) premier bibliographic database. It includes the fields of medicine, nursing, veterinary medicine, dentistry, the preclinical sciences and the health care system
CINAHL (Cumulative Index to Nursing and Allied Health Literature)	This database covers comprehensive records of nursing journals in the English language as well as journal titles from seventeen allied health disciplines. It also includes books, book chapters, dissertations, patient education documents, audio-visual materials, and software
MEDLINEplus	The NLM's website for private and up-to-date consumer health information
PsysINFO	The database provides summaries of serial literature in psychology and relevant disciplines from around the world
National Library of Medicine	This database covers updated weekly journal citations
BIOETHICSLINE	It includes citations to journal articles that cover the ethical, legal, and public policy issues of biomedical and health care research. The database also contains citations to monographs, chapters in monographs, court decision, bills, laws, newspaper articles, audio-visual materials and unpublished documents from many areas, including the health sciences, religion, philosophy and law

(continued)

TABLE 2.1   Major bibliographic databases (*continued*)

DATABASE	DESCRIPTION
Social Work Abstracts	It covers over 35,000 citations from social work and other related journals on issues like homelessness, child and family welfare, ageing, substance abuse, HIV/AIDS, legislation, and community organisation. It spans from 1977 to the present
HAPI (Health and Psychosocial Instruments)	The database indicates evaluation and measurement and instruments found in the health and psychosocial literature (e.g. checklists, tests and questionnaires). It does not include copies of the instruments
Health Management Information Consortium	The database contains health systems and services, public health, health administration and management, health policy, occupational and environmental health, and clinical medicine
International Bibliography of Social Sciences	The database includes literature from several social science areas including anthropology, sociology, health, politics and economics
Applied Social Sciences Index and Abstract	It covers health, psychology, sociology, social services, politics, race relations, economics, and education

A free database that is valuable for research is Google Scholar. Google Scholar offers a means of extensively searching for literature across many sources, including peer-reviewed articles, books, abstracts, theses, and full papers from academic publishers, universities, professional societies, and other authoritative organisations (Creswell 2014). Unless the published article is in an open access journal, however, you will require library access to get the paper.

For a comprehensive literature search, several databases might be used. Reference librarians tend to be very knowledgeable about which database to use for your research project, the terms and keywords that you should use for the search, and how to build a search strategy. Work with them when you have decided which health issue/topic you will examine.

Often, the **Boolean operators** 'and', 'or', and 'not' are used to build the search strategy. Boolean operators refer to terms which determine the relationship between two or more search words. These three basic terms can be linked to expand or condense the search. The 'and' operator will narrow down the search while the 'or' operator will expand the search. The 'not' operator will ensure that records with the specified word are not included (Grove *et al.* 2013; Jones 2013). For example, typing the keywords 'refugee' and 'migrant' will yield records of publications which are relevant to both refugees and migrants; 'refugee' or 'migrant' will result in records of publications which encompass either refugee or migrants; 'refugee' not 'migrant' will provide records which incorporate only refugees but not migrants.

Boolean operator: A term that determines the relationship between two or more search words in searching through electronic databases. There are three basic terms: 'and', 'or', and 'not'. These three terms can be linked to expand or condense the search.

Here, we provide an example from a literature review of the study on social support and breast cancer conducted by Suwankhong and Liamputtong (2016).

Women living with breast cancer face many changes in their lives and encounter numerous traumatic experiences (Fernandes *et al.* 2014; Sprung *et al.* 2011). They have to deal with the traumatic physical and psychological experiences of the diagnosis of breast cancer and treatment which disrupt their daily lives and often lead to a poor quality of life (Holland & Holahan 2003; Liamputtong & Suwankhong 2015). It has been demonstrated that women who are diagnosed with breast cancer are susceptible to many emotional debilities, including anxiety, fear of dying, depression, and negative and suicidal thoughts (Sprung *et al.* 2011; Taleghani *et al.* 2006). The long, and often traumatic, processes of breast cancer treatment have also affected the emotional and physical well-being of many women (Liamputtong & Suwankhong 2015; Fernandes *et al.* 2014).

It has been theorised that social support plays a crucial role in the health and well-being of people with serious illnesses (Ell *et al.* 1992; Uchino 2006). Individuals who have no social support may have a poorer quality of life, especially those who are ill. Social support assists individuals who confront crises to cope with and manage their difficult lives better (Ell *et al.* 1992; Holland & Holahan 2003; Kavitha & Jayan 2014). Social support enhances human functioning and hence improves their quality of life.

Social support has been an essential means of reducing distress among people living with breast cancer (Kavitha & Jayan 2014; Dumrongthanapakorn & Liamputtong 2015). Many studies have confirmed that social support plays a vital role in promoting psychological health outcomes among individuals living with breast cancer (Kavitha & Jayan 2014;

Uchino 2006; Yoo *et al.* 2010). Social support is linked with better health and quality of life for people living with breast cancer (Yoo *et al.* 2010). Specifically, social support helps to decrease the stress associated with the diagnosis of breast cancer among the women, improves their emotional well-being, and produces positive changes in their lives (Holland & Holahan 2003). In contrast, women who have insufficient social support have a higher risk of psychosocial distress and depression, as well as of the progression of their cancer (Drageset *et al.* 2012).

According to Bloom *et al.* (2001), there are two distinct concepts of social support that most researchers have agreed upon. First is structural support, which refers to 'the network of relationships' between individuals and others including relatives, friends, neighbours, and so on (p. 1513). The second aspect of social support is functional support, which includes tangible assistance, emotional support and the availability of information (Mbekenga *et al.* 2011). Tangible or instrumental support refers to the specific assistance that others provide to the individual, such as financial assistance, performing household chores, childcare, or transport to medical appointments. Emotional support includes messages which signify that the individual is cared for, loved, and valued. It has been suggested that the perception of the availability of tangible and emotional support is more critical than its actual occurrence (Drageset *et al.* 2012). Informational support means the provision of knowledge that is relevant to the situation that the individual is encountering (Bloom *et al.* 2001).

According to Cohen *et al.* (2000), each type of support has its own function but they play integrative

RESEARCH IN PRACTICE

roles in meeting the needs of individuals. Different social support can be obtained from different sources, and may become essential at different stages and trajectories of the person's illness.

Landmark *et al.* (2002) point to some typical sources of support: family members, close friends, peers and health care professionals. These offer different levels of social support.

STOP AND THINK

You are asked to write a literature review as part of an assignment in your research method subject.

- What important things do you need to do to ensure that your literature search is comprehensive?
- How would you go about doing this?

Research proposal: an essential part of the research plan

Once the research design and process have been decided, it is essential to construct a research proposal. This will provide a more concrete plan about your research project.

What is a research proposal?

Research proposal:
A formal written document which provides full details of the research that the person intends to conduct.

A **research proposal** is 'a document which is the product of a process of planning and designing' (Punch 2016, p. 12). It is the result of synchronising all important components of the research design into a written plan, a formal document which provides full details of the research that you intend to conduct. Hence, it is a substantial document which justifies and outlines the proposed research project (Harper 2007). The written document must be submitted to an institution or funding body and an ethics committee for approval prior to undertaking a research project (Natalier 2013; Neutens 2014).

Punch (2016, p. 2) suggests a '4 Ps' view of the proposal: Phase, Process, Product, Plan. The research proposal is a phase of the whole research process; it is the phase that initiates the research, and thus a very important first step. A research proposal is developed through a process of planning and designing the research and this proposal guides the execution of the research. This includes placing it in context and connecting it to relevant literature. The finished proposal is a product which sets out the proposed plan for the research to be carried out.

Research proposals have always been an important part of conducting research. A proposal sets out the exact nature of the issue to be examined, a detailed description of the procedures and methods to be employed, and a time-frame to keep the process on schedule (Kelly 2012; Babbie 2014; Bryman 2016). A research proposal gives readers a preview of why your study will be conducted and how it will be undertaken (Babbie 2014). Writing a research proposal is therefore essential before undertaking a piece of research.

Research proposal and its structure

A research proposal must be able to persuade readers that your research is crucial, well-planned and will offer important outcomes (Harper 2007; Endacott 2008; Punch 2016). Bryman (2016, p. 85) suggests that, in writing up a research proposal, we need to consider several salient issues.

- What are your research questions?
- What are your research objectives?
- Why are these objectives worthy of research?
- What does the literature say about your research questions and objectives?
- What methodology/methods will you use to generate the data that can answer your research questions?
- Why is this methodology/method suitable to your research questions?
- Who will be your research participants and how will you find them?
- What data analysis method will you employ to analyse the data?
- What possible ethical issues may arise?
- What is your time-line?

  Most research proposals will contain the following sections:

- significance of the proposed project
- background and rationale
- research questions
- hypotheses/suppositions
- objectives
- theoretical framework
- research design (methodology and methods for data collection and analysis)
- time-frame.

Significance of the proposed project

What is the value of your proposed research project? Why do you have to conduct this research? This has to be said clearly and convincingly in the proposal. This section of the proposal is essential if we want to convince others that what we propose is of value and worthy of being researched. The best way to do this is to show how the findings might be applied to health care services or how they might enable the development of other kinds of research that have been previously impossible (Rossman & Rallis 2012; Locke *et al.* 2013).

Background and rationale

The section on background and rationale indicates the importance and urgency of the project. The emphasis here is typically on relevant previous research (Punch 2016). This means you have to include some relevant literature and then point to the gap in knowledge. This section also emphasises the situation and factors that prompted you to develop the proposed project.

Research questions

Research questions make explicit statements about the problem or issue you want an answer to (Bryman 2016; see earlier). They emerge from the background and rationale of the proposed research, and are the immediate objectives that are addressed in the proposal. The answer to the research questions therefore helps to fulfil the purpose and objectives of the research. As discussed earlier, research questions give direction for a research project (Parfrey & Ravani 2009; Kelly 2012; Bryman 2016). In one project there may be several research questions, depending on its scope. It is very important to state in this section, as clearly as possible, what the proposed research will look for.

Hypothesis/supposition

Most quantitative research specifies some hypotheses which can be used to test the relationships of variables that we wish to examine in the research project. This is particularly so for experimental research, for example, using a randomised control design or survey research that is based on a cross-sectional design (Bryman 2016; see also Part III). However, due to its ontological and epistemological foundations, a hypothesis is not applicable to most qualitative research (see Chapter 1). But some qualitative researchers include a supposition in their research. Similar to hypotheses, suppositions contain statements about the relationship between two or more variables. But they are not subject to testable assertions, as in quantitative research. Suppositions seek information for clarification, not for verification. Suppositions are usually written as declarations and without the predictive statements of a hypothesis. For example, 'Lack of social support may contribute to the emotional burden of women living with breast cancer', 'Poor living conditions would lead to negative health outcomes among homeless youth', 'Religious beliefs may act as a buffer against stress among people from poor backgrounds'.

Research objectives

Research objectives are specific statements that clearly outline what our proposed project will achieve. The research objectives should be stated as clearly as possible, in terms of what results the proposed project is expected to accomplish, not how those results will be attained.

Important questions to be answered in the objectives section include what you are planning to do (what will be done, with whom, why and where) and what you will achieve by carrying out the proposed project.

Theoretical framework

We need to include a theoretical framework that situates the health issue that we examine in the research. Theories interrelate with individual findings and allow greater generalisation (Willis *et al.* 2009; Rossman & Rallis 2012; Anfara & Mertz 2014). There are many theories that we can adopt, such as critical theory, social support theory, the health belief model, health promotion framework, transcultural nursing and so on (Anfara & Mertz 2014). We must select a theory to suit our proposed research, and set the problem explicitly within the chosen framework. This will allow readers to see what main variables will be considered, what the relationships are between the variables, and how information about them comes together to answer the research question of the proposal.

In quantitative research, theories are used to develop hypotheses and the data are collected to test the theory (Bryman 2016). In qualitative research, theories are used to explain the findings. This will help to strengthen the conceptual knowledge that we develop from qualitative findings (Liamputtong 2013). Regardless, it is essential to discuss the theoretical framework in detail in the proposal, particularly when the theory and concepts used may not be well known among reviewers who are outside the science discipline (Punch 2016).

Research designs (methodology)

There are several points that require special attention within this section. At a basic level, we need to plan the design to fit our available time, energy, facilities and money. The research design must also correspond with the availability of data from participants. One important consideration is the extent to which it is desirable or possible to impose upon the persons who will form the pool of research participants, and therefore the data that we will obtain. The important thing to consider here is the suitability of the research design that we propose to find answers to our research questions (see above).

There are several subsections that can be included in a research design section: research methodology, research methods, study setting, research participants and data analysis.

The research methodology is one of the most important parts of the research design. Here, we refer to the methodological frameworks that researchers adopt to suit their research questions. Within this section, we should discuss the ontological and epistemological foundation on which our research questions are based (see Chapter 1). This will strengthen the foundation of our research and allow readers to understand why we have selected the qualitative, quantitative or mixed methods approach for our research project.

In qualitative research, there are a number of methodological frameworks from which researchers can choose. These include phenomenology, ethnography, symbolic interactionism, hermeneutics, feminism and postmodernism (see Creswell 2013; Liamputtong 2013, 2016).

We need to select a methodological framework that matches the research questions and aims of our research proposal.

We also need to discuss reasons for selecting the particular method/s for the proposed research. There is a diverse range of data collection methods and the approach selected will be determined by the research methodology as well as what is appropriate for the study sample. In qualitative research, interviews and focus groups are a very common method of data collection when we are trying to understand a person's experience of a phenomenon. In quantitative research, methods such as surveys using validated instruments as well as collection of physical measures such as blood pressure, hormone levels etc. are more common.

The proposal needs to illustrate that the method is appropriate, adequate and feasible (Rossman & Rallis 2012; see Chapter 1 and section above on research design). For example, if we need to discover and understand in great depth the experience of living with disability, then in-depth interviewing, life history or ethnography may be chosen as a method. If we want to see the prevalence of domestic violence or diabetes in our local areas, quantitative research such as epidemiology would be more appropriate. The proposal must clearly and precisely describe the method to be used in order to achieve the proposal's objectives (see Parts II and III).

The proposal needs to specify the research participants, and their social demographics should be described as precisely as possible. The proposal should also state where and how the participants will be selected. Usually, some sampling frameworks will be cited (see Chapter 1). In qualitative research, it is not always feasible to clearly determine the number of people to be included in the sample. Sample size may be guided by saturation or other non-numerical criteria (see Chapter 1 for sampling techniques). Thus, in some qualitative research proposals, we may not specify the size of the samples to be recruited. If the number is given, evidence to justify the sample size is essential (Liamputtong 2013; Corbin & Strauss 2015).

Data analysis should be discussed in detail in the research design section (Kelly 2012). For qualitative research, it is usually not enough just to state that the data will be analysed using a particular method, as many readers may not be familiar with that data analysis method. Qualitative research proposals need to provide some details about the analysis process so that the reviewers can clearly see how we intend to manage the data, and what analytic techniques will be employed (Bazeley 2013; see Chapters 23, 24, 25).

Time-frame

Most research projects take a considerable time to complete (Kelly 2012; Bryman 2016). Even a small pilot project may take twelve months, and almost every proposal submitted to major funding agencies asks for at least two or three years funding. A time-frame is essential for several reasons (Locke *et al.* 2013). First, it keeps us on schedule throughout a long period of research. It allows us to justify the need for that period of funding, particularly if we show that every month is filled with what has to be done to complete the project. A well-planned time-frame will help reviewers to understand the nature of the proposed project, and this in turn can prevent possible criticism from reviewers that the project cannot be completed in the time proposed.

Here, due to space limits, we show the research design from a project regarding disclosure/non-disclosure among HIV-positive women in Thailand, conducted by Liamputtong and Haritavorn (see Liamputtong & Haritavorn 2016). Note that this proposal is also discussed in Chapter 1.

Research design (methodology)

In this study, a qualitative approach is adopted because qualitative researchers accept that, to understand people's behaviour, we must attempt to understand the meanings and interpretations that people give to their behaviour (Cresswell 2014; Bryman 2016). This approach is particularly useful when we have little knowledge of the participants and their world views (Padgett 2012; Liamputtong 2013). Because we aim to understand the lived experiences of women living with HIV/AIDS, descriptive phenomenology is adopted as our methodological framework. Descriptive phenomenology allows us to understand the issues under study from the experiences of those who have lived through them (Carpenter 2013). Hence, this permits us to examine the experiences of HIV-positive women and how they dealt with HIV/AIDS. Within the phenomenological framework, the in-depth interviewing method is usually adopted by qualitative researchers. In this study, in-depth interviews will be conducted with a number of Thai women who live with HIV/AIDS.

Purposive sampling technique (Patton 2015) will be adopted; only Thai women living with HIV/AIDs who are mothers will be approached to participate in the study. The participants will be recruited through advertising on bulletin boards at hospitals where drug trials have been undertaken and personal contacts made by the Thai co-researchers, who have carried out a number of HIV/AIDS research projects with Thai women. In conducting research related to HIV/AIDS, the recruitment process needs to be highly sensitive to the needs of the participants. The sensitivity of this research will guide our decisions about how we would approach the women and invite them to take part in this research. We will directly contact potential participants ourselves only after being introduced by our network or gatekeepers. Because of the sensitive nature of this study, we will also rely on snowball sampling techniques; that is, our previous participants will suggest others who are interested in participating. We will enlist the assistance of leaders of two HIV/AIDS support groups to access the women in this study. We will also take part in the activities of the groups as part of the methodology of our study.

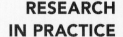

RESEARCH IN PRACTICE

The number of participants will be determined by a theoretical sampling technique, which is to stop recruiting when little new data emerge; this signifies data saturation (Liamputtong 2013; Patton 2015).

Interviews will be conducted by both authors in the Thai language to maintain as much as possible the subtlety, and any hidden meanings, of the participants' statements (Liamputtong 2010). Interviews will be conducted at a place where the women feel most comfortable. For this study, we will use the following questions to prompt the women to talk with us: (1) Do you tell anyone about your HIV/AIDS? (2) Please tell us about your reasons for disclosure/non-disclosure. (3) Who do you tell as a first person? (4) In your own experience, what are the consequences of your disclosure? These questions will be followed by other prompted questions to allow the women to articulate more about the issues.

Prior to the commencement of the study, ethical approval will be obtained from the Human Ethics Committee of La Trobe University, Melbourne, and Chulalongkorn University, Thailand. Before making an appointment for interviews, the participants' consent to participate in the study will be sought. After a full explanation of the study, the length of interviewing time and the scope of questions, the participants will be asked to sign a consent form, which will be kept in a locked filing cabinet to protect the confidentiality of the participants. Each interview will take between one and two hours. Individual participants will be paid 200 Thai baht as a compensation for their time in taking part in this study. This incentive is necessary for sensitive research because it is a way to show that research participants are respected for their time and knowledge.

With permission from the participants, interviews will be audio-recorded. The tapes will then be transcribed verbatim in Thai for data analysis.

The transcripts will not contain the real name of our participants; we will invent a fictitious name for each woman. The in-depth data will be analysed using a thematic analysis (Braun & Clarke 2006; Bazeley 2013; Clark & Braun 2013). This method of data analysis aims to identify, analyse and report patterns or themes within the data. Initially, we will perform open coding where codes will first be developed and named. Then, axial coding will be applied, which will be used to develop the final themes within the data. This will be done by reorganising the codes that we have developed from the data during open coding in new ways by making connections between categories and subcategories. This will result in themes, and they will be used to explain the lived experiences of the participants in the study.

Summary

In this chapter, we have introduced issues relating to research design and the research process.

We have suggested that the research design should be focused on answering the research questions with credibility. We need to decide what type of knowledge we need to generate, which will allow us to make decisions about the research method that is appropriate to our research questions. When this has been decided on, we need to write a research plan, i.e. a research proposal. This proposal must be developed at the beginning as it forms a written plan for us to follow.

In conducting a piece of research, we need to remember that the research process can be messy, and it may not proceed as we have written or planned in the research proposal. This is rather common. Bryman (2016, p. 13) warns us that 'research is often a lot less smooth than the accounts of the research process you read in books … In fact, research is full of false starts, blind alleys, mistakes, and enforced changes to research plans'. Bear this in mind when planning for and designing your research project.

Practice exercises

1 Through your personal and professional experiences, you notice that children in your local area seem to be inactive in their daily life. You do not know exactly what contributes to their inactive life but you would like to do something about it. What will you do to fulfil this need?

2 You are asked to conduct a piece of research in order to find evidence regarding support for mental health issues among homeless young people. How will you go about designing this project? Discuss salient issues that need to be considered.

3 You need to write a research proposal on work-related injuries in your local area. What issues do you need to consider and how will you go about writing the proposal?

Further reading

Alvesson, M. & Sandberg, J. (2013). *Constructing research questions: doing interesting research*. London: Sage.

Bryman, A. (2016). *Social research methods*, 5th edn. Oxford: Oxford University Press.

Dingwall, R. & McDonnell, M.B. (2015). *The Sage handbook of research management*. London: Sage.

Fawcett, B. & Pockett, R. (2015). *Turning ideas into research: theory, design & practice*. London: Sage.

Harper, P.J. (2007). Writing research proposals: five rules. *HIV Nursing*, 8(2), 15–17.

Locke, L.F., Spirduso, W. & Silverman, S.J. (2013). *Proposals that work: a guide for planning dissertations and grant proposals*, 6th edn. Thousand Oaks, CA: Sage.

Natalier, K. (2013). Research design. In M. Walter (ed.), *Social research methods*, 3rd edn. Melbourne: Oxford University Press, pp. 25–49.

Parfrey, P. & Ravani, P. (2009). On framing the research question and choosing the appropriate research design. *Methods in Molecular Biology*, 473, 1–17.

Punch, K.F. (2016). *Developing effective research proposals*, 3rd edn. London: Sage.

Ridley, D. (2012). *The literature review: a step-by-step guide for students*, 2nd edn. London: Sage.

Rossman, G.B. & Rallis, S.F. (2012). *Learning in the field: an introduction to qualitative research*, 3rd edn. Thousand Oaks, CA: Sage.

Sandberg, J. & Alvesson, M. (2011). Ways of constructing research questions: gap spotting or problematization? *Organization*, 18(1), 23–44.

Websites

https://www.youtube.com/watch?v=GYywR7SA03E

> Dr Michael Quinn Patton talks about designing and planning a research project to find knowledge.

https://www.youtube.com/watch?v=LWLYCYeCFak

> This video discusses how to develop a research question.

https://www.lib.ncsu.edu/tutorials/litreview/

> This website, created by North Carolina State University Library, is about literature reviews for graduate students. It provides useful tips about conducting a literature review and includes the following questions: What is a literature review? What purpose does it serve in research? What should you expect when writing one?

www.sp2.upenn.edu/app/uploads/2014/08/DSW-Literature-Review-Powerpoint.pdf

> This website contains slides that discuss literature review.

www.studygs.net/proposal.htm

> This US-based website suggests how to write a research proposal.

http://www2.le.ac.uk/offices/ld/resources/writing/writing-resources/planning-dissertation

> This website is very useful for students to start planning their research projects. The contents are relevant to what is in this chapter.

3

What is Ethical Research?

PAUL RAMCHARAN

Chapter objectives

In this chapter you will learn:

- basic principles of research ethics as they relate to health and social care research
- about developments and changes to ethical regulation since Helsinki (1964)
- how contemporary human research ethics committees operate
- how to critically appraise ethical regulation and key topics of continuing debate
- how to support readers to apply their learning in their review of other studies and in constructing their own research ethically

Key terms

Anonymity

Confidentiality

Deontological ethics

Ethical principles

Human research ethics
    committee

Informed consent

Research ethics

Research participant

Sensitive topics

Theme

Utilitarian

Virtue ethics

Vulnerable people

Introduction

All human interaction produces a relationship between the people involved. These relationships can be passing or long-term; they can be affective or business-like; they can be warm or distanced; they can be pleasurable or not, as the case might be. Like all forms of human interaction, research undertaken on human research subjects or in which human subjects are participants raises questions about what motivates a person to enter into an interaction, how a person should comport themselves, and how a person's interaction affects the other(s) involved. Researchers in health and social care research rely on members of the public who choose to accept invitations to be involved in research. As such, it is in the interests of researchers to carry out their research in a way that supports this outcome (Israel 2015; Tollich 2015). But how do researchers accomplish this? What are the rules of conduct for such relationships? And how can we be sure that researchers are acting in a moral or ethical way? This area of research is often referred to as **research ethics**, the subject matter of this chapter.

Research ethics: Finding the balance between the risks associated with a research project and its benefits.

STOP AND THINK

Consider why you see the following as questionable. What does this tell you about your own values?

- Living prisoners are given by the king to a medical practitioner for research using vivisection, i.e. surgery while alive (reported of Herophilus, 335–280 BCE).
- In 1796 a doctor, Edward Jenner, injects a young boy with material from cowpox blisters on a sufferer of the disease, in order to examine the effects. He later does the same on many more research subjects.

These and other examples are reported on the following website: <http://en.wikipedia.org/wiki/Human_experimentation#History>.

Are your values the same as other people's? Would you expect them to feel the same way? If they are common values, should they be seen as a criterion of good and ethical research?

There are many more recent examples. Under Nazi experimentation 400,000 people were subjected to varying means of sterilisation as a means of ensuring that feeble genes could not damage the national gene pool; experiments were conducted on 1500 pairs of twins, of which only 200 survived; thousands were subjected to freezing experiments to establish how best to protect Nazi troops on the front line. Between 1932 and 1972, a total of 399 poor African Americans were denied treatment for syphilis despite penicillin having been found to be a cure in 1947. The Tuskegee Syphilis study, as it was called, resulted in the death of some study patients, the passing on of syphilis to others, as well as suffering discomfort unnecessarily (see Liamputtong 2010, 2013).

The power relationships in these examples are worth noting: researchers gained power by royal decree and, in Jenner's case, by government plaudit and public funding. In situations of sanctioned coercion or in working with vulnerable or ill-informed subjects, it is easier for researchers to exert their will over the research 'subject'—a term that has long been rejected in favour of 'participant'. A '**research participant**' refers to a person who agrees to take part in the study, on equal terms. Equality of power in the research relationship therefore requires the freedom, that is, autonomy and will, to choose to take part in a study whose nature is well understood by the prospective participants.

Given the experiences of the Second World War, in 1948 principles of medical research were established at Nuremberg, and in 1964 the World Medical Association extended and formalised the Nuremberg principles in the Helsinki Declaration, a declaration considered to the present day to be the seminal work on which ethical regulation is based.

> Research participant:
> A person who agrees to take part in the study, on equal terms.

STOP AND THINK

- Is it enough to have principles for doing research ethically, that researchers follow by choice? Or should there be regulation, where what researchers do or intend to do is scrutinised, permission is granted or withheld, and sanctions can be applied?
- If you think there should be regulation, then who should have the power to say whether a piece of research is ethical and can go ahead?

The Helsinki Declaration, part of which will be considered later, was written originally for medical research, and much social research did not come under its regulatory aegis until fairly recently. Consider the following two case studies.

MALPRACTICE IN ETHNOGRAPHIC RESEARCH

Covert observation of homosexual acts

A researcher acted as a 'Watch Queen', warning men participating in homosexual acts in public lavatories if a member of the public was approaching. The researcher conducted fifty interviews there and then. However, where this was not possible, the researcher copied the men's car registration numbers and traced their home addresses. He later disguised himself and undertook a 'health survey' with fifty more participants, part of which covered homosexuality (Humphreys 1975).

Fake electric shocks test participants' ethics

A researcher recruited research participants and paid them a small sum to take part in an experiment which they were told was about memory and learning in different conditions. The participant was introduced to a 'learner' (an actor) and an 'experimenter' (the researcher). The experimenter told the participant that the learner would have to memorise word pairs and that when they got one wrong a shock would be administered by the participant (no shock was actually administered, but the participant did not know this). The participant was given a small shock to indicate the 'learner's' experience. The participant was told they would have to raise the shock intensity 15 volts for each incorrect answer. The 'learner' cried

RESEARCH IN PRACTICE

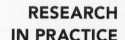

>>

out each time a 'shock' was administered, more loudly as the voltage increased. If the participant wanted to stop taking part, the researcher used successive prompts: please continue; the experiment requires that you continue; it is absolutely essential that you continue; you have no other choice; you must go on (Milgram 1974).

In small groups, consider these case studies. Have the researchers done anything wrong? Why? Report your group's view and discuss whether there are any differences in your opinions. Have your views on whether or not to regulate research changed through your discussions?

Converging principles in medical, health and social care research?

Up to the 1980s, within social research, there remained considerable debate around the probity of covert or disguised research (see e.g. Erikson 1967; Douglas 1976; Denzin 1982). Bulmer (1982) contends that the covert research debate lays bare some of the key principles on which contemporary research ethics is based: to the end of this section, therefore, key ethical principles will be italicised (or bolded if they are Glossary entries). For example, some would argue that Humphreys' (1975) covert study of homosexuality did not allow **informed consent**, that is, that people from whom data was collected understood the research and agreed to participate on the basis of this understanding; the research approach used both *disguise* and *deception* and involved an invasion of *privacy* with records linking car registration and home addresses.

Informed consent: Before data collection, participants are informed of the aims and methods of the research and asked for their consent.

Anonymity: A person is unknown to the researcher and hence to anyone else.

Confidentiality: Concealing the true identity of participants to protect them from any negative consequences, particularly those marginalised and stigmatised in society.

Humphreys points out that although he used deception and invaded people's privacy, at no time was the anonymity of the person breached. The term **anonymity** refers to a person being unknown to the researcher and hence to anyone else. Furthermore, where the person took part in the public health survey their confidentiality was maintained. **Confidentiality** differs from anonymity in that the researcher knows the person's identity and further things about them but does not divulge this identity or acts, circumstances or places that might lead to identification in any way at any time. Humphreys argues that his study *benefited* a population that was deeply misunderstood, that was persecuted for its sexuality and most certainly for its public expression. In short, Humphreys' argument was that the *risks* of the research were outweighed by the research *benefits*. This central issue is one that will be revisited shortly.

Milgram's experiment has similar issues of deception and confidentiality (of people 'willing to administer shocks' to strangers!). Three further principles emerge from this study. The first is that if a person is paid to become involved in a piece of research, they are more likely to do what they are told or to give answers or views they expect will be those the researcher wishes to hear. This is methodologically as well as ethically unsound. Such payment could be seen as an *inducement* if it covers more than expenses or token appreciation (Grady 2001). Second, the researcher exerted undue pressure for compliance; the participant did not actively consent and did not have *equal power* to that of the researcher. Third, many of the participants showed signs of stress and distress at what they were doing; they showed *discomfort* and may well have been harmed by their experience.

Unifying concepts for these principles have been widely attributed to the work of Beauchamp and Childress (2001) in their *Principles of Biomedical Ethics*, first published in 1979. The authors argue for four key **ethical principles**: *respecting autonomy*—the person making an informed decision about being involved; *beneficence*—the obligation to provide benefits not necessarily to the participant, but certainly to the 'public good'; *non-maleficence*—avoiding bad intention or the causing of harm or discomfort disproportionate to the benefits of the research; and *justice*—the concept that benefits, risks and costs are equitably distributed. These ideas appear widely in contemporary regulatory research ethics frameworks (see Israel 2015; Bryman 2016).

Ethical principles: There are four principles that researchers must adhere to in their research: respecting autonomy, beneficence, non-maleficence and justice.

Understanding and applying the principles of ethical research

Even where the principles of research ethics have been shared (Lacey 1998), the organisational response has varied across countries and in relation to health, as opposed to social or behaviourally focused research. For example, in the USA, institutional review boards (set up after the Belmont Report 1979) have gradually extended from medical and behavioural studies to cover social and social care research. In contrast, in the UK the regulation of social care research remains a hot topic for debate (Dominelli & Holloway 2008), with a Social Care Research Ethics Committee housed at the Social Care Institute of Excellence, a quasi-government organisation set up in 2008.

In Australia, the Medical Council's *Statement on human experimentation* was issued in 1966 in direct response to the Helsinki Declaration, followed by a subcommittee recommendation in 1976 in Supplementary Note 1 to make it a requirement for all proposed research involving human subjects to be examined by an institutional ethics committee. By 1985, no human research without permission from the appropriate committee could be accorded public funding. Before that, research in social sciences such as psychology, sociology and anthropology was guided by statements from their Australian Associations. The National Health and Medical Research Council (NHMRC), established in 1992, issued its *National statement on ethical conduct in research involving humans* (NHMRC 1999b), and updated it in the *National statement on ethical conduct in human research* (2007). In what follows, the regulatory framework is considered in relation to some of the key ethical principles outlined above.

The membership of a **human research ethics committee** (HREC) can be a decisive factor in that the committee needs to have knowledge of and expertise in the merit and standards that apply across research paradigms and groups, to make fair and just decisions and to do

Human research ethics committee: A group of people that includes researchers, health and social care professionals, a lawyer, lay members, and a balance of men and women.

so with due process (De Vries *et al.* 2004; Edwards *et al.* 2004; Bryman 2016). The NHMRC guidelines (2007) recommend an ethics committee makeup that includes researchers, health and social care professionals, a lawyer, lay members, and someone with a pastoral role in the community. They also indicate the need to have a balance of men and women as well as people who are regularly present and those who are co-opted for specialist expertise.

Below is a summary of key requirements for research ethics committees and the key issues in their decision-making.

Generic requirements

When submitting an application to an HREC, the researcher will be required to submit a research proposal. In this regard, the 2008 Helsinki Declaration says:

> Article 12 'Medical research involving human subjects must conform to generally accepted scientific principles.'

> Article 14 'The design and performance of each research study involving human subjects must be clearly described in a research protocol. The protocol should contain a statement of the ethical considerations involved.'

The reason for this is that 'a poorly designed study is by definition unethical' (Lynoe *et al.* 1999, p. 152) since it cannot produce the benefits claimed. Any risk would be too great when set against a study that has no benefit. The protocol is likely to require some review of literature, a statement of the study's aims, the numbers in the sample and means of recruitment, the approach to analysis, and research tools such as questionnaires being used alongside consideration of the ethical issues. However, there are some criticisms of Lynoe's dictum.

STOP AND THINK

Is there anything ethically questionable about the following research? A new drug for cancer is being tested. The researchers have proposed a double-blind randomised controlled trial (see Chapter 15). This means that, before analysis of results, neither the researcher nor the participants knows which are given the new drug and which receive a placebo.

In this example, a sacrifice of methodological rigour is important because it would be wrong to ask people to forgo a life-saving treatment and 'intolerable' if they did not know whether they were in the experimental or placebo group (Kent 1996). Not all well-designed projects are ethical, however, simply because they are well designed,.

A second criticism is that qualitative studies and their research relationships can be complex (De Laine 2000; Guillemin & Gillam 2004; Tollich 2015). Moreover, an emergent research design means that the researcher is initially less clear on samples and sample size and has to alter the approach to data collection to test emergent theories. Action research, which is increasingly used in the health and social care fields, requires reorientation of the research as it proceeds (Khanlou & Peter 2004; Higginbottom & Liamputtong 2015). There are also issues of proportionality. The latter argument is that, judged against the invasiveness and potential threats to the physical integrity of the body in much medical research, health and social research produces far less risk. It is far more efficient to use a lighter touch than to subject all research to the same degree of scrutiny, to satisfy the surveillance needs of an audit culture (Strathern 2000). Moreover, that a committee has the right to judge whether a person can respond suggests a degree of paternalism that infringes autonomy and the individual's right to choose.

In stating the four principles listed above, the most recent NHMRC guidelines (2007) implicitly recognise a broad base of research approaches. Further, the guidelines on qualitative research adapt the Helsinki Declaration emphasis on 'generally accepted scientific principles' and 'scientific protocols' to, among other things, emphasise the applicability of findings and not the capacity for generalisation (para 3.1.4), and rigour being judged not on sample size (para 3.1.6) or validity and reliability as in quantitative approaches (para 3.18) but on 'quality and credibility of data collection and analysis' (para 3.18). See also Chapter 1.

STOP AND THINK

- What are the four key ethical principles outlined by Beauchamp and Childress (2001) and why are these important?
- Did ethical regulation emerge so as to control what researchers do; to protect those who are involved as participants or subjects in research; to bring to bear commonly held values and beliefs as they relate to research relationships?
- Who regulates research ethics, and why do researchers comply?

Read the Preamble of the *National statement on ethical conduct in human research* (2007): <www.nhmrc.gov.au/guidelines-publications/e72>.

Beneficence/non-maleficence

The UK has long had an electronic ethics application form, and in Australia the National Ethics Application Form was introduced in early 2009. What, in addition to the research proposal, will the health researcher need to do to complete the forms? Earlier, it was argued that at all times the benefits of research must outweigh its risks, and this is a central idea on which HREC members seek to base their judgment.

Lists of risks are given in Table 3.1. These are not exhaustive: in their deliberations HREC members will also consider the seriousness of the risk, its probability of occurrence, and strategies to minimise the risk and address any risk that remains (see NHMRC 2007, pp. 15–18).

As well as the actual process of carrying out research, harm can be produced by the way in which data is collected, stored and published. Data collection for web surveys, for example, should be undertaken using methods in which identities cannot be accessed; transcript data should de-identify the participants and be stored in locked filing cabinets and on password-protected computers. In publication, major problems can

TABLE 3.1   Thinking about potential ethical risks in a research project

POTENTIAL RISKS	
Health	Injury to body (e.g. through invasive medical procedure); using healthy volunteers for experiment (e.g. sleep deprivation and mechanical manipulation study); side effects (e.g. of a new drug); discomfort or inconvenience (e.g. of procedure from lengthy sessions, interviews or focus groups); placebo and delay of treatment; indirect risk (e.g. on public transport as a result of a procedure)
Psychological	Stress (e.g. of procedure or of memories and thoughts); emotional (memories, procedure or effect on relationships); identity (e.g. a person's self-ascription of deviance, vulnerability, powerlessness); distress (e.g. as a result of the approach taken to data collection or its inconvenience); worry over effects of participating (e.g. of a service provider who knows a person who has taken part); arrangements for withdrawal from the study
To the community	Disproportionate impacts on marginalised groups or in sensitive areas; economic, political and social effects of working with some groups (e.g. from minority ethnic or religious communities, indigenous groups, those seeking asylum, those socio-economically disadvantaged, those who are disenfranchised and those without a voice)

emerge regarding the identity of participants even if names are not used. For example, stating the participant's gender and the city location of a facility (the only one in that city) that provides a service for very few clients may, given additional information on the participant's history, inadvertently give away their identity. There needs to be sensitivity towards maintaining confidentiality and anonymity, for example by using pseudonyms, making sure quotations are not attributed, or using composite stories, that is, combining the views of several participants to describe a recurrent **theme** or theory (see Dickson-Swift *et al.* 2008a; Liamputtong 2010, 2013).

Theme: A grouping of data emerging from the research, to which the researcher gives a name.

If there are substantial risks, what are the benefits against which these should be offset? Table 3.2 lists some of the benefits against which risks can be offset.

Given the complexity of research, there are a number of other key issues that are considered below, with a focus on completing HREC application forms.

TABLE 3.2　Some potential benefits accruing from a research study

BENEFITS	
To knowledge	Knowledge may have direct application (utility) or it may be for 'enlightenment'; it may be personal in terms of increase in skills, insight or understanding
To the participant	Taking part, hope, a chance to reconsider life, identity and relationships may benefit; public service (i.e. giving back by contributing); the direct change to services, life outcome; identity (e.g. chance to reformulate their identity by taking part); new technology and interventions; learning resources
To the public good	Public knowledge of an issue; practitioner resources and knowledge; contributing to the community's ability to address problems of health or disadvantage, to deliver economic benefits, or to challenge injustice and promote equality

STOP AND THINK

Discuss the ethics of the following scenarios.

A part-time doctoral student also runs a counselling service in which she has developed a new method of working with clients. The student has submitted an application to the HREC to evaluate this new method of counselling. Participants are receiving treatment free as long as they agree to complete a questionnaire and a battery of health measures every two weeks, and undergo an interview at the end. The cost of the eight sessions would ordinarily be $720.

In a study of quality of life and health outcomes among people with intellectual disabilities, a participant is unable to answer some questions about the health professionals with whom he has had contact. With the participant's permission, a staff member has joined the discussion but remains seated for the rest of the interview in which the participant is evaluating the service he receives.

Autonomy

In the first scenario, there is a potential conflict of interest as it is in the interests of the student to produce results that promote her own counselling approach. The 'payment' (i.e. non-presentation of a bill) at the end of the therapy sessions may mean that participants carry on with sessions even if these create discomfort. Especially where it is the researcher who administers the questionnaires or conducts the final interview, participants may not feel free to give their real views. In the second scenario, the professional service received by the client might not be honestly reported because of the presence of one of the providers.

Another aspect of autonomy is the prospective participant's understanding of the research, in making a decision about whether to participate. As well as the research proposal, the applicant is required to produce a plain language statement that outlines the details of the study in language that is intelligible to participants. This should inform the potential participant of the project's title and aim, the investigators involved, the funding source, rights as a participant (including the right to withdraw, to have identifiable data withdrawn, to have questions answered), what is expected, the risks and relevant safeguards, the benefits of the research, and to whom complaints or questions should be directed. Similar information should be included in a letter or frontispiece to postal questionnaires or as a series of boxes that have to be clicked before completion of web-based surveys. This approach assumes that return of a questionnaire or submission via the web implies consent to participate.

The plain language statement mentioned above is submitted with the HREC application along with a consent form signed by the participant (and, in some circumstances, by their guardian or advocate) and witnessed by the researcher. These should be kept in a locked filing cabinet. Consent forms usually have statements or tick boxes in which the participant says they have read the plain language statement, understand confidentiality and anonymity issues for the study, recognise that they have the right to withdraw from the study at any time without consequence, and understand that the researcher commits to keeping the data secure.

Issues around consent and autonomy

Are there exceptions?

STOP AND THINK

Discuss whether consent is necessary in the following case studies.

- A study was undertaken to assess the impact of HIV status on outcomes of intensive care treatment and to assess whether HIV patients should be prioritised for non-HIV intensive care treatment. The participants were not told they were being tested for HIV and no staff were informed about the person's HIV status (see Bhagwanjee *et al.* 1997a).
- Although questions later arose around his 'interviews' and methods (Fleck & Muller 1997), a Nazi concentration camp inmate collects data which, when he is released, form the basis of a book on the psychology of living in extreme conditions (Bettelheim 1943).

In defence of their HIV study, Bhagwanjee and associates (1997a) point out that an HREC had given consent for their study, they could not have gained consent on admission, and no staff were informed of any person's HIV status. The study was undertaken in Natal, South Africa, where they report that: 'By the end of 1992 over 300 000 people were infected … If the worst case scenario materialises, by 2010 it is estimated that 28–52% of all deaths will be related to HIV infection' (1997b, p. 1082). The HREC held that the study was of national importance and sufficiently in the *public interest* to waive the right to consent in this case, though this position was by no means universally accepted (e.g. Kale 1997).

Had Bettelheim made known his data collection and study intentions, it is probable that he would not have survived the concentration camp. In such situations, is the study's benefit great enough to warrant disguise and deception? As recently pointed out by Liamputtong (2007, p. 138), 'sensitive researchers need to think carefully about what method will be best for them to use to work with vulnerable individuals and groups and the moral and ethical issues that go with the method'. This raises wider issues in relation to working with sensitive topics and with vulnerable groups, as discussed below.

Sensitive topics and vulnerable groups

Lee and Renzetti (1993) define **sensitive topics** as those that may touch deep emotions (e.g. death or dying, eating disorders, sexual abuse), areas that may be culturally taboo for research (e.g. religion or homosexuality in some cultures), areas in which the research threatens powerful interests (e.g. the arms trade or large corporations) or areas of deviance (e.g. drug-taking cultures or places in which there is or may be illegal activity). Awareness of the likely effects of participation is important in this respect, alongside the research method being adopted and the strategy for withdrawal. For example, interviews may be one-off or they may require more time and more visits. If the interview takes place on one occasion, the researcher needs to have a view on whether the sensitivity of the interview may lead to an emotional reaction at a later date (see Liamputtong 2007; Dickson-Swift *et al.* 2008a).

> **Sensitive topics:** Those that may cause emotional upset or pose physical or emotional risks for research participants.

Where the interview is held over several meetings, other ethical issues arise because of the different level of rapport and emotional involvement involved (Minichiello *et al.* 2008; Morris 2015; see Chapter 4). A one-off consent sheet hardly suffices; it is important to establish 'consent as a process' (Cutcliffe & Ramcharan 2002; Royal College of Nursing Research Society 2005; Wiles *et al.* 2005). The closeness of the relationship may lead to a delusion of alliance (Stacey 1988) or to new issues about gauging how much trust exists within the research relationship (McDonald *et al.* 2008). Researchers need to be careful not to exert subtle pressure and to ensure that the relationship does not become too intrusive (Stalker 1998). And, given the relationship that develops, the researcher needs to manage an exit strategy that does the least harm (Booth 1999).

In considering such issues, HREC members tend to perceive such issues of vulnerability in terms of the level of risk. This is a third area of contention in much HREC decision-making, as outlined below.

Risk and vulnerability

Some **vulnerable people** may find it difficult to understand the language and concepts of research, and therefore informed consent sheets or plain language statements will be beyond them (Liamputtong 2007, 2010). The irony for much health and social care research is that social justice, that is, the requirement that all people are treated fairly and equally, means a disproportionate interest in such groups (Bryman 2016). It is also inconceivable that such

> **Vulnerable people:** Individuals who are marginalised or discriminated against because of their class, ethnicity, gender, age, illness, disability or sexual preference.

research should be suspended, for it would be unethical to stop potentially useful research on the grounds of difficulty in understanding. There have been a number of responses to this issue.

In the past, some organisations have sought to organise in-house ethics procedures for the 'best interests' of 'their' clients, meaning that researchers have to submit ethics applications to more than one HREC. Iacono (2006) reports that one HREC in Australia empowered the Office of the Public Advocate to assess the capacity of potential participants to consent to 'subjecting vulnerable people to a substantial number of probing questions, thus multiplying the effects any research might subsequently have had' (Ramcharan 2006, p. 183). Thankfully, the present Australian NHMRC guidelines propose a responsibility to 'adopt a review process that eliminates unnecessary duplication of ethical review' (NHMRC 2007, Section 5.3.1, p. 87), but the institution still has a responsibility to 'identify any local circumstances … and provide for their management' (Section 5.3.3a, p. 87).

In the UK, the latter point has been formalised into a research governance framework (Department of Health 2005a). This means that researchers have had to apply to the institutions in which the research is taking place, which again involves committees. As well as the resulting delays, there are issues about the independence of local services to make such decisions. The Helsinki Declaration understandably specified that decision-making should remain independent of the researcher and sponsor, to avoid conflicts of interest: it is conceivable that some organisations might use their power to prevent challenging or unwanted research by claiming, for example, that their clients are overresearched or would be unable to participate meaningfully.

A second approach is that HRECs identify levels of risk for each application. One of the criteria for risk relates to 'vulnerable groups', for example children, indigenous populations and people with intellectual disability, mental illness or cognitive impairment (Liamputtong 2007, 2010; see also Chapter 22). The present Australian guidelines carry a significant list in these respects (NHMRC 2007, Section 5). However, the danger is that identifying whole groups as 'higher risk' or 'unable to consent' may be a labelling issue that infringes the rights of at least some individuals in these groups to decide for themselves whether to take part (Ramcharan 2006, p. 184). It is then difficult to establish a balance between protection of the potentially vulnerable, and paternalism and stereotyping.

Such surveillance might be construed by some as a sinister attempt by powerful interests to control the free-minded. It also indicates a loss of trust: here **virtue ethics**, where judgments are made about a person (researcher) by their demonstrated moral character, and **deontological ethics**, in which a person acts in accord with (researcher) obligations and duties, have no place. Instead the dominant model is **utilitarian**, based on the assumption that it is possible to predict the likely consequences of an action (in this case, research) and the likely benefit it will have for the greatest number of people.

Having established many of the ethical principles and pointed to the ways in which they are made operational, it is important to recognise that decision-making by HRECs is a form of peer review. It is not a scientific process with an easily calculated answer. In this respect, the decisions made by committees are based on the information provided, and the case made will ultimately be subject to both the frailties and the benefits of human decision-making processes.

Virtue ethics: A situation where judgments are made about a person (researcher) by their demonstrated moral character.

Deontological ethics: An approach to ethics which holds that acts are inherently good or evil, regardless of their consequences.

Utilitarian: A model based on the assumption that it is possible to predict the likely consequences of research and the likely benefit it will have for the greatest number of people.

Summary

The framework for ethical regulation has come a long way since the Helsinki Declaration. There is now a system in place to which medical, health, behavioural and social care researchers are required to submit their research proposals for scrutiny. But there are a number of remaining issues, some fundamental and others of a more practical and evidential kind. First and foremost is the fundamental issue about the extent to which regulation is necessary at all. At one level, there are arguments here about the extent to which surveillance by regulatory bodies is itself infringing on freedoms: the freedom of some participants to make their own decision rather than having a formal body with the power to take away that right, and the freedom of thought necessary for researchers to break new ground and create knowledge.

But even if the utilitarian model is used, there are some really thorny problems. First, the decision of the HREC is made before the research begins: it is conceivable that the·researcher might comport him or herself in an unpalatable way during the research, particularly research among those who are most vulnerable, who have least voice and power. Second, no research evidence base drawing on previous research (again, particularly with vulnerable groups) has been used to demonstrate the ethical dilemmas that have actually been encountered. The problem here is that the regulatory system tends to operate from a worst-case scenario. The surveillance approach may therefore be highly inefficient, and unnecessary. Additionally, there is an issue of proportionality in the ethical regulation process. How dangerous is an interview or participant observation, compared to physically invasive research? Is the same level of regulation really necessary?

Since research and its associated methods change and adapt, so do the principles that guide the ethical regulation of research. For example, participatory and emancipatory research paradigms will involve the collection and use of data by the beneficiaries of the research. What new relationships are created when the researched become researchers, when they are privy to information and when they seek to publish their findings? As the world contracts through speedy transport and new media, how can we rethink regulation across national boundaries and fend off the cultural imperialism of frameworks imposed on other cultures and nations? If the majority of the population gain through technology and access to information on which they base everyday decisions, what responsibility do researchers have to record their reservations about such information, given their alternative perspectives and evidence? In a world of e-technology, artificial intelligence, robotics and cloning, what will be the implications for ethical regulation and who will be in a position to police these areas?

Paul Ramcharan

Practice exercises

1   In a group, a few students choose a recent empirical study from a doctoral thesis that is available in your library or from your tutor. Identify the ethical issues in this study. The other students should listen to the students relating the ethical issues that arise in this study, and question them about how they will resolve those issues.

2   As a group, write a wiki that outlines the key contemporary issues and debates on research ethics in health and related research.

3   Most health research is not invasive or ethically challenging. Ethics committees are therefore a waste of time and money. Debate.

4   Your tutor will provide one or more research proposals. Form HRECs (with different roles) and make a decision about the research, using the learning from this chapter. After you have made your decision in relation to the proposal(s), discuss how you feel about how the process operates and the difficulties HREC members may encounter in their role.

Further reading

Beauchamp, T.L. & Childress, J.F. (2001). *Principles of biomedical ethics*, 5th edn. Oxford: Oxford University Press.

Bulmer, M. (2001). The ethics of social research. In N. Gilbert (ed.) *Researching social life*. London: Sage.

Dickson-Swift, V., James, E. & Liamputtong, P. (2008). *Undertaking sensitive research in the health and social sciences: managing boundaries, emotions and risks*. Cambridge: Cambridge University Press.

Israel, M. (2015). *Research ethics and integrity for social scientists: beyond regulatory compliance*, 2nd edn. London: Sage.

Liamputtong, P. (2007). *Researching the vulnerable: a guide to sensitive research methods*. London: Sage.

Liamputtong, P. (2010). *Performing qualitative cross-cultural research*. Cambridge: Cambridge University Press.

Malone, S. (2003). Ethics at home: informed consent in your own backyard. *Qualitative Studies in Education*, 16(6), 797–815.

Mann, C. & Stewart, F. (2000). *Internet communication and qualitative research: a handbook for researching online*. London: Sage.

Mauthner, M., Birch, M., Jessop, J. & Miller, T. (2002). *Ethics in qualitative research*. London: Sage.

Punch, M. (1986). *The politics and ethics of fieldwork*. Beverley Hills, CA: Sage.

Shaw, I.F. (2003). Ethics in qualitative research and evaluation. *Journal of Social Work*, 3(1), 9–29.

Tollich, M. (2015). *Qualitative ethics in practice*. London: Sage.

Websites

www.nhmrc.gov.au/health_ethics/research/index.htm

The NHMRC hosts this useful website. It discusses research integrity, which suggests that the ethical conduct of research is a shared responsibility of researchers, organisations that employ the researchers, funding agencies and ethics committees. The NHMRC, which publishes guidelines about research, also has a crucial role in ensuring that research is conducted ethically.

http://en.wikipedia.org/wiki/Human_experimentation#History

This page contains some history on unethical human research.

www.who.int/ethics/research/en/

This webpage contains WHO's ethical standards and procedures for research with human beings.

http://ahcsa.org.au/research-overview/ethical-review-ahrec/

The Aboriginal Health Research Ethics Committee promotes and supports quality research that will benefit Aboriginal people.

QUALITATIVE APPROACHES AND PRACTICES

4

The In-depth Interviewing Method in Health

TANYA SERRY AND PRANEE LIAMPUTTONG

Chapter objectives

In this chapter you will learn:

- about the fundamentals of the in-depth interviewing method
- how to prepare the interview structure and sequence
- how to ask questions to elicit maximum information
- how to maintain empathic neutrality
- some practical considerations

Key terms

Empathic neutrality

In-depth interviewing

Interview transcript

Semi-structured interview

Introduction

> Interviewing is rather like marriage: Everybody knows what it is, an awful lot of people do it, and yet behind each closed front door there is a world of secrets (Oakley 2009, p. 93).

In-depth interviewing: A method of qualitative data collection. The interview does not use fixed questions, but aims to engage interviewees in conversation to elicit their understandings and interpretations.

Among qualitative research methods, **in-depth interviewing** is a well-established method of data collection and is widely employed in qualitative methodology (Kvale 2007; Minichiello *et al.* 2008; King & Horrocks 2010; Gubrium *et al.* 2012; Brinkmann & Kvale 2014; Morris 2015; Patton 2015; Bryman 2016). Conversation itself is a fundamental means of interaction among individuals in society. Through conversation, Kvale (2007) contends, individuals have an opportunity to know others, to learn about their feelings, their experiences, and the world in which they live. So if we wish to learn how people see their world and experience various phenomena, we need to talk with people (Brinkmann & Kvale 2014; Morris 2015; see also Chapter 9).

Interviews in social research are seen as 'special conversations'. In an interview conversation, the researcher asks questions or uses probing comments and then listens to what individuals say about their lived experiences, such as their dreams, fears and hopes. The researcher will hear about the interviewees' perspectives in their own words, and learn about their family, social life and work (Kvale 2007; Hesse-Biber 2014; Morris 2015; Patton 2015; Bryman 2016).

Most people, including researchers, will claim that they know about in-depth interviews, and that it is not difficult to ask questions and talk to people. But conducting a quality in-depth interview requires a lot more preparation and skill than just asking questions and talking to people. There are many salient matters and techniques that qualitative researchers must consider in order to elicit rich, detailed and accurate information from their participants (Brinkmann & Kvale 2014; Morris 2015).

What is an in-depth interview?

An in-depth interview is similar in many aspects to conversation, because it involves two participants who mutually observe and abide by widely accepted rules of verbal interchange and reciprocity (Brinkmann & Kvale 2014; Morris 2015; Patton 2015). Yet, as Cheek and colleagues (2004, p. 148) indicate, 'simply interviewing someone is not qualitative research'. There is a specific purpose to the in-depth interview (Ritchie & Lewis 2005). The interviewee typically contributes significantly more content to the conversation, while the interviewer is engaged in listening and facilitating the flow of conversation (Brinkmann & Kvale 2014; Morris 2015; Bryman 2016).

According to Taylor (2005, p. 39), 'the aim of the in-depth interview is to explore the "insider perspective," to capture, in the participants' own words, their thoughts, perceptions, feelings and experiences'. Through a partnership, researchers can delve into the 'hidden perceptions' of their research participants (Marvasti 2004, p. 21). For example, if researchers wish to examine people's attitudes towards euthanasia, in-depth interviews will allow people to adopt 'it depends' expressions. Instead of making people indicate whether they agree or disagree with assisted dying, they may say something like, 'It depends on the person, their illness and what their circumstances and personal beliefs were'.

STOP AND THINK

You need to find evidence about the safe sex practices of people living with an intellectual disability who reside in supported accommodation in Melbourne. You are interested in their understanding of sexual behaviours, their knowledge about safe sex practices, their sexual health, and their access to sexual health services in Melbourne.

- How would you go about finding out this evidence?
- Would the in-depth interviewing method allow you to find your evidence?
- How would the method help you to find the evidence?

Framework options for the in-depth interview

Patton (2015) describes three levels of structure in interviewing. The choice typically depends on the type of qualitative research undertaken. These options are the informal conversational interview, the interview guide or semi-structured interview, and the standardised open-ended interview. The informal conversational interview allows for vast flexibility but is best suited to ethnographically oriented qualitative research, by virtue of its informality and spontaneity (see Chapter 7). The standardised open-ended interview is carefully worded and ensures that all participants are asked similar questions, but it affords far less opportunity to explore themes and issues as they arise. The **semi-structured interview** provides a balance between the two more extreme approaches. Figure 4.1 depicts the options for structure in an in-depth interview, along a continuum.

> **Semi-structured interview:** An interview where the researchers elicit information from prepared questions, but allow the participants to elaborate on their responses.

FIGURE 4.1   Options for structure in an in-depth interview: a continuum

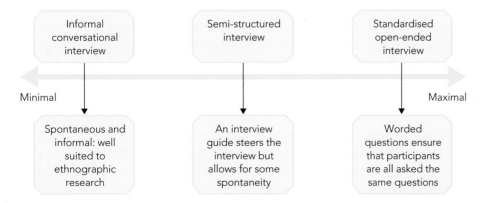

Tanya Serry and Pranee Liamputtong

We have chosen to focus primarily on the semi-structured interview in this chapter, for two reasons. First, in our experience, the semi-structured format is most commonly used in qualitative research in health and the social sciences. Second, since the semi-structured interview option takes the middle ground, it serves as a useful framework on which researchers can base an in-depth interview format adapted to their specific needs.

Questions and in-depth interviews

In order to create a comfortable and non-judgmental environment, the interviewer's language and specific jargon need to be used with care (Fontana & Prokos 2007; Hesse-Biber 2014; Morris 2015). For example, if exploring a specific phenomenon such as experience of facial scarring, we suggest starting the interview by asking the participant what they call or how they refer to this phenomenon. Similarly, we recommend summarising the purpose of your interview before you commence, even though this will have been covered as part of the consent process, and remind the participant about how you will be recording their interview. In our experience, attentive researchers intuitively use many of the attributes we outline below when formulating their questions. Our suggestions can facilitate your interaction style with participants for optimal information-gathering.

Open-ended questions

Questions should be dominated by an open-ended style rather than a closed format or one where forced options are given by the interviewer (Morris 2015). Open-ended questions can allow for 'unexpected turns or digressions that follow the informants' interest or knowledge' (Johnson & Rowlands 2012, p. 107). In making the question open-ended, you must use a succinct questioning format and speak as little as possible. This will allow the participants to talk about their lived experiences in their own terms (Low 2013; Hesse-Biber 2014; Morris 2015).

Active listening

This is crucial. It means listening not only to what is said, but to how it is said. Non-verbal features such as hesitations, pauses and volume changes will optimise your capacity to be actively engaged with the participant. Listening to what the participant is *not* saying will allow you to follow up with further prompts and explore unexpected territory.

Monitoring linguistic choices

Your linguistic style should vary with different participants. Liamputtong (2013) suggests that the interviewer should adapt their own vocabulary to meet the needs of the interviewee, while also ensuring that questions are grammatically clear and concise. To accommodate the diverse socio-cultural and linguistic needs of individual participants, she recommends avoiding the use of a fixed wording format.

Monitoring the use of jargon

The use of jargon should also be carefully monitored, as using too much or too little can rapidly derail an interview. You will need to make astute judgments based on participants' personal or professional backgrounds, and on how each individual presents at the interview.

The assumption of 'not knowing'

Questions presented with the implied assumption that the researcher 'doesn't know' or is 'being empathically inquisitive' are useful, as they provide an environment for the participant to talk freely and without assuming that the researcher is an expert in the field. When we explored the experiences of parents whose children have reading difficulty, we came to each interview with an intimate theoretical knowledge about the mechanisms underlying reading difficulty. Yet when asking parents how or why they think their child might have reading difficulty, we asked questions such as, 'Do you have any thoughts on how your child might have run into difficulty with reading?' This format allows parents to respond in any number of ways. For example, some parents may talk about a premature birth, while others may talk about their own history of learning difficulty and/or of experiencing low self-esteem. Others may lay blame on too much time spent on electronic games, or worry that they put too much pressure on their child. A poorly worded question that presents the interviewer as 'knowing' runs the risk of limiting such options.

Attention to participants' silences

Silence is important when conducting an in-depth interview, and it need not be feared. You need to be aware of the ramifications of silences in interviews. Charmaz (2002, p. 303) suggests that 'not all experiences are stories, nor are all experiences stored for ready recall. Silences have meaning too. Silences signify an absence—of words and/or perceivable emotions … [and] may … reflect active signals—of meaning, boundaries, and rules'.

Silences, as Low (2013) suggests, may also tell you that the participant is tired. Sometimes their illness or disability prevents them from speaking, or causes pain. Sometimes, silences reflect an intense emotional response to the content of the interview. Silence may also mean that you have said something that makes the participant fall silent or not wish to respond (Charmaz 2002). Silences should be recorded and used in the analysis of data.

Avoidance of appearing to 'test' the interviewee

A question such as 'Have you thought about XYZ as a possible cause?' may appear to put the participant 'on trial' by highlighting a fact that they may not have considered. Such questions may be perceived by a participant as disrespectful and lacking in sensitivity. Such questions also risk making the participant feel ignorant or naïve. Furthermore, you risk introducing bias to the interview data by presenting an idea that was not generated by the participant. Instead, you might ask, 'Have any other thoughts come to mind about possible causes?' or 'Has anyone else shared their views with you about this?'

Avoidance of leading questions

Similarly, asking leading questions that can influence responses should be avoided. Leading questions are those that force the participants to respond with specific answers; inevitably, they do not allow the participants to say what they really think. Instead of 'Do you think the school is just too under-resourced?' a more appropriate question would be 'What is your view on the resources available for parents in your situation?'

Avoidance of dichotomies

It is crucial to limit the number of questions that can easily be answered with a simple 'yes' or 'no' or a forced choice such as 'Do you think it was her idea or her partner's idea?' These are referred to as 'dichotomous questions', since there are only two possible answers to them. They do not encourage participants to continue their stories, and this will shorten the interview or not allow the researcher to elicit rich information.

The question 'Why?'

Researchers must be cautious about asking 'Why?' Often, participants may not know *why* they behave or think in a certain manner. As a result, they may feel confronted and respond defensively when asked to explain the reasons for their behaviour or viewpoint. This does not mean that the question should not be asked in an interview, but that it should be put in a different way. For example, instead of asking, 'Why did you choose to home-school your children?' you might ask, 'Can you tell me what things led to your decision to home-school your children?' Occasionally, simply saying 'How come?' or 'I wonder why' rather than 'Why?' can reduce any sense of confrontation felt by the participant.

Non-questioning responses

An in-depth interview, as in a regular conversation, is not solely a question-and-answer exercise. Researchers need to engage in a variety of methods, other than questions, to ensure that active listening and participant engagement are maintained. Strategies may include:

- verbal or non-verbal expressions encouraging the participant to continue
- retelling the interviewee's narrative as a tool to ensure that the researcher has understood the information correctly. For example:
  - 'So just so that I am clear on the sequence of events, first you approached the classroom teacher and when that was not so helpful, you felt you really had to take it further. Is that how it happened?'
- acknowledging difficult questions or topics. Recently, we were interested in asking our participants about sensitive terminology. We approached the topic by framing the question as follows:
  - 'It's a bit of an "elephant in the room" but I was just wondering what your views are on …'

- validating a participant's response delivered with **empathic neutrality**. Often, this may act as a springboard to further probing. For example:
  - 'You make a very interesting point about the program. Can you tell me …'
  - 'That's a very powerful experience that you've described'.

Empathic neutrality: This occurs in an interview where the researcher can validate the interviewee while remaining neutral to the content of what is being said.

STOP AND THINK

QUESTIONING EXAMPLES

Below are some questions that could be addressed to university students with dyslexia. Would you word anything a bit differently? If not, why not? If so, please attempt to do so.

- I'm wondering if you've got any thoughts about what it is that you've done, or what's got you to uni?
- I'm curious to find out how you think your dyslexia impacts on you as a university student, especially now that you are a postgrad student?
- I wonder if you could you tell me a little bit more about how you've sensed that stigma?
- Why did you avoid telling anyone about your dyslexia?
- Were there particular things that you thought were really helpful?
- Did you expect to struggle that much once you started uni?
- What else do you think could have made it easier for you?
- That sounds like a crushing experience. How did you manage to get over that hurdle?
- Do you think everyone should disclose their dyslexia when they start university?
- Why did you think it was important to speak to the subject coordinator?

Types of questions

Researchers can use different types of questions for different purposes. The following question types combine suggestions made by Kvale (2007, pp. 60–2) and Bryman (2016, pp. 476–8). Table 4.1 describes a variety of question types and provides examples.

TABLE 4.1 Question types available for the in-depth interview

QUESTION	USEFUL FOR	EXAMPLES
Introductory or opening question	Allows the participant to talk at great length, typically offering spontaneous and rich descriptions Participants can provide what *they* see as the main issues or phenomena under investigation	In your own words, please tell me about receiving that diagnosis. How would you describe your experience of becoming a single mother?

(continues)

TABLE 4.1   Question types available for the in-depth interview (*continued*)

QUESTION	USEFUL FOR	EXAMPLES
Follow-up question	Encourage participants to say more about the answer they have just given Participants' responses can be further elaborated Usually asked as a direct question	Do you mean you had a negative experience with your doctor? You said earlier that you'd prefer not to adopt a child. Could you tell me more about this?
Probing question	Researcher probes for further discussion so that they have a clear understanding of the matter being examined	Can you give me some more examples of this issue? Can you say more about what you have just told me? What happened? When did it happen? How did it happen?
Specifying question	Similar to follow-up questions; asking more specific questions so that a more explicit response can be obtained	How did you react when the physician told you how serious this was?
Direct question	Used to clarify the issues or some ambiguity during the interview Should be left until later in the interview, when participants have offered their own explanations Researcher is sure that the topic of the direct question is of key importance	Have you ever experienced discrimination from others in your workplace? What stops you from looking after your baby as you would like to do?
Indirect question	Several indirect questioning techniques, such as projective and contextualising questions, can be used. Although the participant will typically talk 'outside him/herself' in response, their own attitudes may be revealed to some extent Further careful questioning is essential in order to accurately interpret participants' responses to indirect questioning	How do you think other men would react to domestic violence? What do other teachers say about feeling physically intimidated by some of their students? What do you think may make your experience different from that of others?
Structuring question	This type of question assists the participant to move on to the next line of questioning Researchers should indicate to the participants when the topic of the previous question has been dealt with Also useful when the participant gives a long discussion of matters that may not be directly relevant to the research	The researcher may summarise their understanding of the answer given by the participants then say, 'I would now like to introduce another topic …' (Kvale 2007, p. 61). When the participant pauses momentarily, the researcher may introduce the next line of questions as a way of bringing the participant back to topic.

QUESTION	USEFUL FOR	EXAMPLES
Clarifying question/ statement	This type of question assists the researcher to ensure that the interviewee's comments have been understood Researchers should indicate to participants that this is the intention of such a question. It may involve the researcher reflecting back to the participant what s/he has just said Clarifying questions can also be a useful but indirect prompt to the interviewee to provide a clearer and more succinct response	It sounds like the feeling of shame was what prevented you from seeking support earlier? Can I just be clear on the order of the steps you undertook to help your baby's sleep patterns?
Interpreting question	Questions that assist researcher to interpret or clarify what the participants have suggested May simply be rephrasing the participant's response	Is it correct that you feel that he is being discriminated against at school?

FUNNELLING TECHNIQUES MINIMISE BIAS

We have often used a funnelling technique, as described by Smith (1995), for our in-depth semi-structured interviews. To do so, we start with an introductory question such as, 'Could you start by telling me about your panic attacks?' Such an open question aims to put the interviewee at ease but, importantly, also helps to ensure neutrality in the researcher (Liamputtong 2013). We maintain that a funnelling technique minimises the bias that might arise if we had set the structure and themes for the interview by probing specific points at the outset.

Typically, we find that interviewees tend to respond to our introductory question with rich, detailed and lengthy responses. We are then able to funnel questions to probe specific issues that were raised. The funnelled questions may be of any format (direct, prompting, indirect, etc.) and allow us to pick up on key issues raised by the participant in tandem with following up points pertinent to the research. Our sense of this technique, based on reading our transcripts, is that it is a rather gentle and respectful way to seek in-depth information.

RESEARCH IN PRACTICE

Examples of questions

Here are examples of some questions Pranee used in research with women living with HIV/AIDS in Thailand. You will see that most are open-ended, but occasionally there are some direct questions about their feelings. Pranee used introductory questions, followed by some probing, specifying, direct and indirect questions:

- Can you please tell me about your thoughts about HIV/AIDS?
  - In your view, how do people get HIV?
  - Is there any way people can prevent it?
  - In your view, what can people do to prevent it?
  - Some people may say that it is difficult for them to prevent HIV. What do you think about this?
- I would like to ask you about health care or treatment of HIV/AIDS that people might have.
  - Have you ever received any health care or treatment for HIV/AIDS?
  - If yes, what type of treatment have you received?
  - Can you please tell me more about this?
  - Where did you seek health care?
  - How did health care providers treat you?
- As a woman and a mother, can you please tell me about your experience of living with HIV/AIDS?
- Is there anything we have not discussed that you would like to tell me more about?
- Is there any advice you would like to give to other women who are in the same situation as you?

Doing an in-depth interview: the sequence

Below is a typical sequence for conducting your in-depth interview, from meeting your participant until the time you leave. In presenting this, we have considered some strategies such as how to facilitate a flowing interaction, managing and containing a verbose participant, and how to provide closure at the end of the interview.

On arrival and introduction

- Engage in 'small talk' and make the participant feel comfortable in your presence.
- Feel free to accept or acknowledge the hospitality of the participant as a way of developing rapport.
- Introduce the research and explain the purpose of the study and the participant's involvement.

- Reassure them of confidentiality, and ask for consent. Request permission to record, even if this has been mentioned in a written consent form.
- You are now ready to commence the interview.

Beginning the interview

- Using your interview guide, start with an opening question (see previous section). Encourage the participant to keep talking by using probes and strategies as suggested earlier.
- Be mindful of your body language and your verbal cues. These can act as subtly powerful markers for your participant to continue talking, showing that you are interested in hearing their stories.
- You may wish to take brief notes as a way of following up or clarifying issues. If you plan to do this, inform your participant beforehand to avoid uncertainty about what you are doing.
- Let the interview flow as naturally as possible. Although some responses may seem irrelevant to the questions, it is essential that you allow the participant to finish their story.
- Often, participants want to tell their stories, and researchers should acknowledge this need (Barbour 2008, 2014; Hesse-Biber 2014). In our experience, many participants have actually stated their appreciation about being given the opportunity to tell their story without the normal constraints of time pressure and/or judgment by others.

Ending the interview: some options

- You may choose to summarise some of the main points the participant has given.
- You may indicate that you have no further questions, then ask if the participant would like to add anything further. For example, 'I have no further questions. Is there anything else you would like to bring up, or ask about, before we finish the interview?' (Kvale 2007, p. 56). When interviewing university students with dyslexia, Tanya ended each interview with something like, 'Perhaps I end by asking you if someone with your profile was starting university next year, what advice would you give that person?'
- Barbour (2008, 2014) suggests ending on a positive note, such as asking participants to share advice for others in the same situation.
- These options may give closure to the interview, but further valuable data may arise when you initiate the end.

After the interview

- You may need to debrief with the participant. Make sure the participant is left feeling like their interview was valued.
- It is important not to underestimate how moving and powerful it may be for participants to disclose information about their world.

Tanya Serry and Pranee Liamputtong

- It is likely that some participants will experience distress during or at the end of an interview. It is important not to rush off. Occasionally, you may need to refer someone for appropriate support. This should be in your research plan and it is likely that, for a project that requires ethical approval, a support plan will have been documented should a participant experience distress.

- You may ask the participant about their experience of the interview. Often, we have found that the participant initiates such a reflection.

- Take time to thank the participants and reconfirm how their contribution will help your research (Daly 2007).

- It is valuable to keep a reflective journal of your interviews and to complete this as soon as possible after the completion of each interview. Your reflections may well contribute to your data and inform your final research findings.

Practical issues in doing an interview

Preparing an interview guide

An interview guide will help you cover the issues you wish to explore. It will contain these general issues to be covered in your questions. However, you are unlikely to follow the guide strictly. Depending on the responses of the participants, you will probably ask additional questions based on the progression of each interview (Taylor 2005; Kvale 2007; Brinkmann & Kvale 2014; Morris 2015). You may need to rephrase questions and change their order. We present some key suggestions that can help you plan an interview guide:

- Construct the guide to help you address what puzzles you or what you have identified as crucial to your research (Daly 2007).

- Prepare an individual interview guide for each participant. By doing so, you can also use the interview guide page to record a person's socio-demographic details and other relevant information.

STOP AND THINK

Recently, a doctoral student began to explore experiences of challenges associated with maintaining fluent speech following speech pathology intervention for stuttering. Here is a subsection of the interview guide that was used with participants:

- expectations of your speech fluency after treatment
- views or beliefs about what might trigger a relapse into stuttering
- advice for other people who stutter, about maintaining stutter-free speech after treatment.

Location of the interview

The interview location requires careful consideration. As a practical measure, Bryman (2016) recommends selecting a quiet setting so that recording quality is not marred. To protect the confidentiality of the participants, the setting should also be private so that others cannot overhear the conversation.

As far as possible, we ask participants where they would feel most comfortable being interviewed (Liamputtong 2010, 2013). Participants tend to nominate their own home as the most comfortable and practical location for the interview. Sometimes they prefer to be interviewed away from home for reasons such as privacy, shame or suspicion from others. Researchers have conducted interviews in cafés, libraries, health care centres, parks, playgrounds and supermarkets, wherever participants suggest. If you conduct interviews in participants' homes, steps must be taken to ensure your own safety. We advise sending a text message to a colleague or a research supervisor on arrival at and departure from a participant's home. In some circumstances, interviewing a participant in their home may not be appropriate.

RESEARCH IN PRACTICE

FINDING A SUITABLE VENUE FOR INTERVIEWING

As a novice researcher, one of Tanya's projects necessitated interviewing school staff. It was usually possible to find a quiet space but on one occasion, an interview had to be conducted in the staff room because there were few available rooms. This became a problem due to other staff walking in and out, which in turn appeared to restrict the natural flow of the conversation.

Tanya became aware of a number of limitations with the interview. First and foremost, there was the matter of privacy. Although it was teaching time, various staff members did go in and out of the staff room, typically focused on their own tasks. Nevertheless, the presence of a particular person appeared to constrain the participant's dialogue. As subtly as possible, Tanya asked the participant if she felt some discomfort with certain people in earshot of the conversation. She indicated that was all right, even though her body language did not seem to convey this. Tanya used that observation as data, although she believes she may have missed out on some valuable data. Second, it became somewhat distracting for both researcher and participant when people walked in and out. And finally, the photocopier in the background made listening to the recording rather a challenge. Although interviews in cafés and other public places can be noisy and distracting, the effect was greatly exacerbated in the staff room experience when the distractions were from peers and colleagues.

Recording interviews

It is strongly suggested that you record an in-depth interview, preferably using a digital recorder. Since you need to pay close attention and respond accordingly to what participants say, it is difficult to write down the conversation at the same time (O'Reilly & Kiyimba 2015). Kvale (2007, p. 94) says that 'taking extensive notes during an interview may be distracting, interrupting the free flow of the conversation'. He points out that a benefit of recording is that 'the words and their tone, pauses and the like are recorded in a permanent form that it is possible to return to again and again for re-listening' (p. 93).

Recording equipment

In the past, researchers had to rely on cassette tape-recorders. Nowadays digital audio recorders, which are small and not intrusive, give excellent sound quality and can record for many hours without interruption. Digital recorders also allow you to transfer audio files directly to a computer. Software is available to assist with transcribing interviews from digital recordings. We use an easily downloadable and free program called Express-Scribe (www.nch.com.au/scribe) to transcribe audio files. Features such as keypad controls for rewinding and slowing the speed of the recording make Express-Scribe a very useful tool. There are also a number of transcription programs that can be purchased.

Audibility

Poor audibility of recorded interviews has been a problem for many researchers. If indoors, ensure that the interview room does not have too much background noise. In an open space or a café, noise can obscure or distort the conversation. Be mindful of how you set up seating and positioning for such an interview. Fortunately, many digital recorders are able to cope well with background noise.

Consent to record

Sometimes researchers may feel it is unethical to record the interview as it is too intrusive for the participants. Consent must be sought before recording a participant. Most often, participants will agree to have the conversations recorded. However, some participants may refuse for various reasons and this must be respected. For example, women from some ethnic groups may suggest that their religion forbids their voices being recorded, or being heard by anyone other than their husbands (Liamputtong 2007, 2010).

Non-recorded data

Sometimes a participant wants to give information after the tape is turned off (Bryman 2016). It may be that they forgot to talk about something during the interview, or they feel more able to speak freely when the tape is not running. Daly (2007, p. 149) calls this the 'door handle disclosure' and it presents the researchers with an ethical dilemma. However, this dilemma can be solved by asking participants for consent to include the unrecorded content in their research,

Transcribing interviews

Interview data must be transcribed into written form to enable data analysis. This written form of data is called an **interview transcript**. Transcribing interviews is in fact your initial data analysis (Gibbs 2008; Rapley 2007; Bailey 2008; Liamputtong 2013). Transcribing interview material is time-consuming, tiring and even stressful (Kvale 2007). An hour-long interview may take an experienced transcriber up to six hours to transcribe (Daly 2007; Gibbs 2008; Liamputtong 2013).

Interview transcript: The written record of an interview that has been transcribed from the verbal conversation. It is used for in-depth data analysis in qualitative research.

Who should transcribe the interview?

We recommend that the researcher or interviewer should transcribe their own interviews, as they 'will learn much about their interviewing style; to some extent they will have the social and emotional aspects of the interview situation present or reawakened during transcription, and will already have started the analysis of the meaning of what was said' (Kvale 2007, p. 95).

Some researchers may wish to have a research assistant or pay for a transcription service. If you choose this option, you must ensure that interviews are transcribed verbatim (Rapley 2007) with regard to verbal and non-verbal features (see below).

How should interviews be transcribed?

We suggest that each interview is transcribed verbatim (word for word), keeping all the informal conversation style and emotional expressions, such as pauses, emphases, laughter and sighing, and non-lexical sounds like 'hmm', 'oh', 'ah'. Importantly, both questions and answers must be transcribed for contextual clarity. What the questions were, how the researchers ask the questions and how the participants answer are all important.

PARTICIPANT REVIEW OF TRANSCRIPTS

We routinely offered participants the opportunity to view the written transcript before conducting our analysis. We informed participants that they were welcome to delete, add or modify any of their content. Our primary motive was to ensure that participants knew they could delete content that they now felt was too sensitive—because of the topic of discussion, sensitive information was often discussed.

A substantial number of participants took up the offer to review an electronic version of their written transcript, and some requested changes or added further information. More often than not, people were shocked at how their spoken output appeared as a written transcript. These were the types of comments we received from people—usually in jest: 'My goodness, I can't believe I say um so much!' 'I sound so ungrammatical.' 'You poor thing, having to listen to me talk so much.'

RESEARCH IN PRACTICE

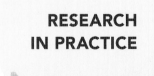

>>

Tanya Serry and Pranee Liamputtong

People use far more informal language in speech than they would in written form. It is only when people (including ourselves as interviewers) are confronted with their spoken words on paper that they realise that they may habitually use 'um', or filler phrases like 'you know' and so forth. It may be useful in some cases to gently alert people that their written transcript is unlikely to be perfectly grammatical and fluent.

Summary

In-depth interviewing is the method most commonly employed in qualitative research. A skilful performance from the researcher is required to obtain sufficient, detailed and rich information. We conclude by presenting a list of key attributes that we believe are essential foundations for conducting in-depth interviews. Researchers need to be well-informed and well-organised when approaching an interview. In order to optimise the interview process, we need to have strong investigative skills and a well-developed capacity to draw people out (Miles *et al.* 2013). We should be actively engaged in listening and responding to the interviewee in a supportive and non-judgmental manner. It is essential to facilitate the flow of conversation and be attentive to verbal and non-verbal cues from the interviewee. It is also crucial to ensure the interviewee has sufficient time and opportunity to respond to questions. Last, we should bring empathic neutrality (Patton 2016) to the interview, which means that we validate the interviewee while remaining neutral about what they're saying.

Practice exercises

You are planning to investigate how people who have had a traumatic brain injury learn to live with their physical and/or cognitive disability. You want to explore your participants' views on their altered self-identity and you have chosen to use in-depth interviews to gather data.

1   What interview framework will you choose? Think about the rationale for your choice.

2   What questions will you use to elicit information from the participants? Make a list of some potential questions. Identify what types of questions they are.

3   How will you ensure that you will obtain in-depth information? Think of some strategies that you might use.

4   Write down your plans and your question guide, which will help you to have more focus on your research.

Further reading

Bird, C.M. (2005). How I stopped dreading and learned to love transcription. *Qualitative Inquiry*, 11(2), 226–48.

Davies, P. (2000). Doing interviews with female offenders. In V. Jupp, P. Davies & P. Frances (eds), *Doing criminological research*. London: Sage, 82–96.

Fontana, A. & Prokos, A.H. (2007). *The interview: from formal to postmodern*. Walnut Creek, CA: Left Coast Press.

Gubrium, J.F., Holstein, J.A., Marvasti, A.B. & McKinney, K.D. (2012). *The Sage handbook of interview research: the complexity of the craft*, 2nd edn. London: Sage.

Hopkins, T., Clegg, J. & Stackhouse, J. (2015). Young offenders' perspectives on their literacy and communication skills. *International Journal of Language & Communication Disorders*. doi: 10.1111/1460-6984.12188

Kvale, S. & Brinkmann, S. (2008). *Interviews: learning the craft of qualitative research interviewing*. London: Sage.

Minichiello, V., Aroni, R. & Hays, T. (2008). *In-depth interviewing*, 3rd edn. Sydney: Pearson Prentice Hall.

Morris, A. (2015). *A practical introduction to in-depth interviewing*. London: Sage.

Ogden, J. & Cornwell, D. (2010). The role of topic, interviewee and question in predicting rich interview data in the field of health research. *Sociology of Health & Illness*, 32(7), 1058–71.

Patton, M. (2016). *Qualitative research and evaluation methods*, 4th edn. Thousand Oaks, CA: Sage.

Pooley, J., Breen, L., Pike, L.T., Cohen, L. & Drew, N.M. (2008). Critiquing the school community: a qualitative study of children's conceptualizations of their school. *International Journal of Qualitative Studies in Education*, 21(2), 87–98.

Websites and online clips

www2.pathfinder.org/site/DocServer/m_e_tool_series_indepth_interviews.pdf

> This website links to the Pathfinder International Tool Series. It includes a report on the use of an in-depth interviewing method.

www.nch.com.au/scribe

> A program called Express-Scribe used to transcribe audio files.

www.youtube.com/watch?v=hNNKCD2f4qw

> This clip provides a concise summary about how to conduct an in-depth interview for research.

www.youtube.com/watch?v=9t-_hYjAKww

> This clip briefly describes the key attributes of a competent qualitative researcher. Two interviews are shown, one with many flaws and one with many strengths.

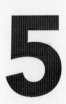

5

Focus Groups in Health Research

PATRICIA M. DAVIDSON, ELIZABETH J. HALCOMB AND LEILA GHOLIZADEH

Chapter objectives

In this chapter you will learn:

- the value of the focus group method in nursing and health research
- about the advantages of obtaining a group perspective in health research
- methodological principles of the focus group method
- the importance of preparation and promoting methodological rigour in the conduct and reporting of focus groups
- about professional development strategies to assist you in undertaking focus groups

Key terms

Data analysis

Focus groups

Moderator

Qualitative research

Thematic analysis

Theme

Introduction

As we strive to provide health care services that are specifically targeted to the needs of individuals, communities and key stakeholders, obtaining their views and perspectives is crucial. This is important not only for assessing needs and evaluating health issues, but also in developing and evaluating interventions. When the researcher's intention is to enquire, explore and probe, a qualitative research approach is often most appropriate. There is a range of qualitative approaches (see Part II) but when the research question requires shared and socially contextualised information, focus groups can be a highly lucrative source of rich and meaningful data.

Originating from market research, **focus groups** play an important role in health and nursing research for both exploration and evaluation (Morgan 1997; Halcomb *et al.* 2007; Liamputtong 2011). The focus group can be used as a single method in qualitative research, but it is also increasingly used within mixed methods research designs and evaluation research (Sandelowski 2000; Johnson & Turner 2003; Tashakkori & Creswell 2007; Larkin *et al.* 2014). Increasing numbers of published studies demonstrate evidence of the utility of focus groups to elicit a range of views and opinions in a moderated setting. Some innovative approaches to the focus group method have emerged, particularly with the use of online media and the growing power of social media (Schneider *et al.* 2002; Gaiser 2008; Liamputtong 2011; Walker 2013). Online focus groups can be both synchronous and asynchronous, and require the same attention and focus as face-to-face methods of group interviews (Fox *et al.* 2007; Liamputtong 2011). In contrast to other methods, such as interviews and surveys (see Chapters 4, 13), focus groups generate data through group interaction to provide a collective perspective and socially generated knowledge. It is often through the lens of others and through synthesised views and opinions that new insights can emerge and there can be a collective interpretation of a phenomenon. Not only can this method provide data from a collective experience, it can illustrate the polarity and diversity of opinions within a group and generate conversations about sensitive issues.

Focus groups: A data collection method based on group discussion. The participants express their views by interacting in a group discussion of the issues.

Although debate continues on the value and merit of focus groups, like most approaches to research, high-quality focus groups are dependent on planning and adherence to methodological rigour and effective reporting (Tong *et al.* 2007). Ensuring methodological rigour, confidentiality and promotion of truthful disclosure are key concerns of focus groups. Increasingly, online focus groups are addressing these issues in vulnerable populations who prefer the anonymity that this media provides (Liamputtong 2011; Stover 2012; Walker 2013).

Due to the complexity of the social process, planning for the event is just as important as the development of the proposal, data analysis plan, report writing and manuscript preparation. In focus groups, planning includes the logistics of recruitment, organising venues and managing group dynamics. Reporting each of these factors, particularly how the participants were recruited and engaged, is crucial, not just in determining the meaning of data but also to the generalisability of findings. In this chapter we will outline the rationale for choosing focus groups as a method of data collection, the advantages and disadvantages

Patricia M. Davidson, Elizabeth J. Halcomb and Leila Gholizadeh

of this approach, and the steps involved in planning and conducting a focus group in nursing and health research.

Why choose focus groups as a method of enquiry?

All research focuses on establishing new knowledge and is a prospective, systematic form of enquiry. Since qualitative research is an inductive process, the intent is exploration and the questions are open-ended (see Chapter 1). It assumes a partnership and reciprocity with participants. Exploring knowledge, attitudes, beliefs and experiences is important for developing health care interventions and services, as well as for evaluating interventions. The focus group method sits neatly within this framework. Significantly, group discussions provide information and insights that would be less accessible without the interaction between participants. As health care is provided in a social context and moderated through social, political and economic factors, obtaining a collective perspective is often very useful (Davidson *et al.* 2003). In focus groups, by witnessing other people's perspectives, individuals are prompted to decipher and filter their own views and opinions. Moreover, experiences which are confronting and disturbing, such as stigma, racism and bullying, may be validated by the views and opinions of others.

PURPOSES OF FOCUS GROUPS
- assessing needs
- providing a voice for participants
- using discussion to filter and decipher views and opinions
- describing contexts
- eliciting knowledge, attitudes and beliefs on a group basis
- evaluating health care interventions
- exploring knowledge, attitudes and beliefs
- generating hypotheses
- elucidating quantitative data
- developing survey items and item banks

Focus groups can be used in many ways. The box summarises the purposes of focus groups. Although practical matters are important in choosing a research method, the choice of a specific approach should be driven by study objectives, characteristics of the health condition or social situation, and participant characteristics. As this chapter emphasises, focus groups are particularly useful if the intent is to explore an individual's perspective within a social context.

When planning and conducting research, it is important to consider the feasibility of selecting an appropriate methodology. The collective perspective and the capacity to capture multiple participants' views in a single interview setting make focus groups a prudent use of limited research resources. However, this view has been contested by some researchers, who have found focus groups to be more time-consuming than individual interviews (Coenen *et al.* 2012). Ideally, focus groups consist of five to fifteen participants. This number is recommended as it allows all participants to meaningfully contribute, facilitates group management, and promotes cohesion within the group (Papastavrou & Andreou 2012). However, the size of a focus group can vary depending on the research topic and social context of the participants.

Focus groups should, where possible, consist of a homogeneous group with similar characteristics, such as social standing, professional group or education level (Liamputtong 2011; Acocella 2012). It is important to remove power differentials and ensure that participants are comfortable expressing their opinions in front of other members of the group. At the same time, it is important to ensure that the group is not so homogeneous that it does not allow some variation in perceptions (Acocella 2012; Liamputtong 2013). If there is a wide heterogeneity in power relationships and social class within the groups, it is advantageous to conduct separate groups with each subgroup individually. For example, front-line workers may feel intimidated expressing views in front of managers. Usually, more than one focus group should be conducted with each participant type to ensure that findings are common across groups. The number of focus groups conducted, therefore, should be determined by the number of participant types within the study. For example, in their study of women with endometriosis from different ethnic groups, Denny and colleagues (2011) conducted separate focus groups for women from each of the five ethnic groups that they included in their research. As is traditional in qualitative research, data should be collected from focus groups until saturation is achieved. That is, until no new data is emerging from subsequent groups (Liamputtong 2013; see also Chapter 1).

STOP AND THINK

Many health researchers seek to engage individuals in health care interventions by accessing people in religious settings such as churches and mosques. Recruiting participants in this setting assists in identifying people who share a common religion, as well as demonstrating the endorsement of community leaders, which may encourage participation. In this setting, exploration and evaluation occur in a social, collective context.

Can you describe why focus groups may be useful in this setting?

The interaction between participants and the socially derived knowledge is the novelty and strength of the focus group method. Responses of individuals and the direction of the moderator prompt reflection of views and perspectives. Hence, focus groups are useful in obtaining information on perceptions, insights, attitudes, experiences and beliefs. Focus groups are also advantageous in gathering unique subjective perspectives, particularly as they pertain to collectives or groups (Liamputtong 2011). As a consequence, this method is often used to derive views on shared experiences, such as being assessed for cognitive impairment (Disler *et al.* 2015) or communicating about end of life issues (Gillett *et al.* 2016).

This collective perspective is achieved by creating an opportunity for group members to stimulate each other to comment and question. For example, Halcomb and colleagues undertook a series of fourteen focus groups to inform the development of new professional practice standards for nurses in Australian general practice (Australian Nursing and Midwifery Federation 2014). The initial focus groups sought to explore the current and potential roles, as well as the scope of nursing practice in this setting. Barriers to and enablers of the nursing role were also explored. Subsequent focus groups worked to develop, test and achieve consensus on various aspects of the new standards. Given the significant variations in practice and the potential impact of the new standards across the profession, gaining a group perspective and buy-in from the nurse stakeholders was important. The focus groups provided an opportunity to explore variation in practice between general practice settings, while enabling the identification of common elements of nursing practice. Such comparison and contrast would not have been possible from individual perspectives alone.

The focus group method also allows access to research participants who may find individual interviews intimidating or threatening (see Chapter 4), or where it may not be culturally appropriate to interview individuals alone (Halcomb *et al.* 2007). This principle has been extended to the online environment, where matters of greater sensitivity can be explored in greater anonymity. In online focus groups, a predetermined set of questions is posed with a chat room or discussion group, with or without an online moderator (Walker 2013). In order to be considered a focus group, online studies need to adhere to the principles of distilling and synthesising views and opinions in a group context.

Focus groups are particularly useful as a research method when studying underrepresented and marginalised populations such as women and those who are not part of the mainstream culture (Liamputtong 2007, 2010, 2013). They are suited for research investigating cultural perspectives because they provide a collective experience from which both consensus and polarised opinions are derived (Halcomb *et al.* 2007). In these participant groups, the method can be tailored to meet situational factors and the needs of the target population. For example, focus groups can be conducted in community settings and at times convenient to participants. The use of community leaders and cultural brokering can also assist in recruiting participants and ensuring that structure and process are commensurate with participants' value systems and cultural views and beliefs (Norris *et al.* 2005). In culturally and linguistically diverse populations participants' a range of approaches can be used, and focus groups can be undertaken via interpreters or in participants' original language (Quintanilha *et al.* 2015).

Risks associated with the focus group method include susceptibility to moderator bias and the potential for the discussion to be dominated by a vocal minority. However, these risks can be minimised with effective planning and strategies for ensuring the integrity of qualitative data, such as the critical analysis of audiotapes to assess the moderator's role (Morgan 1998c). The focus group method does not allow for probing of in-depth information at the individual level; if this is the intention of the research, other methods should be employed.

It is the moderator's responsibility to protect the vulnerability of individual participants within the collective approach. The contextual and socially derived nature of focus groups means that the information derived from group interviews is not representative of other groups, so the ability to generalise findings is limited. Nevertheless, an expanding literature illustrates the potential of this method to evoke crucial perspectives to inform health care delivery.

The focus group method can be a primary form of enquiry where the data generated are the sole source, or a part of a mixed methods enquiry where focus groups are complementary to quantitative data collection in order to further elucidate findings (Liamputtong 2011). Considering potential risks to rigour in the planning stages of your research can maximise the data yield from focus groups and minimise potential distress to participants and the researcher.

In spite of these limitations, an important advantage of the focus group method is that it is suited to investigating cultural perspectives and diverse views (Halcomb *et al.* 2007; Liamputtong 2010, 2011). Facilitating social interaction and maximising group dynamics can encourage and stimulate the participants to share their beliefs and ideas with those of similar socio-economic or cultural backgrounds (see 'Research in practice' below). The assumption of commonality and acceptance often increases the utility of focus groups in investigating cultural perspectives. It has been suggested that when researchers use quantitative methods they often explore, and therefore interpret, the experiences of participants from other cultures from the viewpoint of their own cultural beliefs and values. This can lead to inaccurate assumptions regarding knowledge, practices and experiences. Therefore the use of qualitative methods, particularly when members of the target group are involved in the development, conduct and evaluation of focus groups, makes it much more likely that the data will allow the participants to have a voice (van Berckelaer *et al.* 2012; see Chapter 1).

IMPROVING PALLIATIVE CARE SERVICE DELIVERY

Although palliative care is widely endorsed across both malignant and non-malignant conditions, many individuals do not have access to this important service for a range of patient, provider and health care system factors. The taboo associated with death and dying and the cultural dimensions of this experience mandate exploratory methods to determine the most appropriate service. Led by a Māori organisation, Oetzel and colleagues (2015) explored optimal strategies for communication between Māori carers/patients and palliative care workers. Hosie and colleagues (2015) explored nurses' perceptions of the feasibility of integrating the Nursing Delirium Screening Scale into practice within an inpatient palliative care setting. Each of these studies have reached out to key stakeholders in delivering palliative care services to engage them in shaping and formulating health care services.

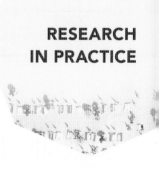

RESEARCH IN PRACTICE

>>

The advantages and challenges of the focus group method are summarised in Table 5.1. It is important to remember that careful planning and appraisal of risks is vital to minimising these challenges (Morgan 1997, 1998c).

TABLE 5.1 Advantages and challenges of the focus group method

ADVANTAGES	CHALLENGES
Provides a collective perspective on the topic of interest	It is challenging to control for confidentiality issues and to manage issues that are distressing to individual participants
Allows access to groups that may not always access traditional data collection methods such as surveys because of language difficulties	Conflicts may arise in the group that are challenging without skilled moderation
Facilitates cultural brokering, engagement and developing culturally appropriate strategies	Group dynamics may influence participants' level of involvement
Allows for the clarification and synthesis of views and opinions through a group perspective	The success of the focus group is dependent on the skill of the moderator
Facilitates access to a large number of participants for lower resource expenditure than individual interviews	The monitoring of verbal and non-verbal responses is challenging because of the number of participants

STOP AND THINK

You need to evaluate women's experience of accessing a women's refuge.

Evaluate the strengths and weaknesses of conducting focus groups in this setting.
List three advantages and three disadvantages.

Planning the focus groups

As in all research, the research questions should drive the choice of study method as well as the planning and organisation of the focus group. These questions will inform the question route for the group and determine the number and characteristics of participants and the interview setting. These matters are also important when choosing whether to use electronic media such as online focus groups (Liamputtong 2011). Moderating online focus groups requires skills and competencies that are different from those used in face-to-face methods. It also evokes a number of ethical issues. For example, when reading online responses it may not be as easy to sense whether a participant is distressed, and it is more challenging to control the access to and use of data (Gaiser 2008).

As discussed, these challenges should not deter you from using a particular method. In fact, the internet has provided unprecedented capacity for engagement with communities and data collection: for many vulnerable groups such as lesbian, gay and bisexual people, it has provided a source of support and community (Hillier *et al.* 2012). But it is important to consider the open nature of the internet, where the perceived lesser control of the moderator underlines the importance of risk assessment and risk mitigation strategies (Gaiser 2008). For example, the moderator needs to be prepared to remove inappropriate discussion from conversation threads. The use of the online medium can avoid transcription costs but this should not overshadow the importance of getting the right data collection method for the study being undertaken.

During the planning process, the recruitment of participants needs to be considered. In many instances, engaging key stakeholders, such as community leaders or clinical champions, can be crucial in recruiting participants. When using online media, considering recruitment methods using specific strategies may be necessary (Boydell *et al.* 2014). Getting together a group of participants who meet the inclusion criteria involves careful planning and can often take considerable time. In the online environment, similar considerations apply and many groups may initially be reluctant to engage in online research. It is also important to explore the ethical implications of the research and take the time to consider matters that may impact on the welfare of participants (Kitzinger 1995). As many of the issues affecting individuals can be confronting, considering the needs of participants should be paramount in your planning. Often, brainstorming potential risks within the research team and finding solutions will maximise the chances that all will go well in your focus group discussions. Refer to Chapter 3 to help you work through ethical issues that may arise in planning your research.

There are two aspects of data collection that must be considered. First, it is often useful to obtain basic demographics of participants, such as age and gender. The depth of socio-demographic data collection will depend on the study questions and may require the completion of a brief questionnaire (see Chapter 13). In some groups with low literacy, participants may need assistance in completing data collection. Demographic data are important as they can help to describe the community of interest and interpret individual responses. Massey (2011) discusses a range of latent themes emerging from focus group analysis: articulated, attributional and emergent themes. Therefore, having some contextual data on participants may help in interpreting and synthesising the data. Second, many focus groups take part in natural or social sessions, which means that determining the optimal number of participants is challenging. A number between four and twelve is considered to be optimal (Carlsen & Glenton 2011).

Developing the focus group guide is an important step that leads researchers through key steps of the data collection process and increases the likelihood that the data collected will be rich, meaningful, address research questions and are true to the views and descriptions of participants (Krueger & Casey 2009). Table 5.2 provides a guide for planning the question route. It includes the framework of introductory and transitional questions and, importantly, the potential for summation and conclusion. It is also important to consider the need for questions that probe points raised by participants and to search for explanation and meaning. In some instances, theoretical frameworks can drive the question route and focus discussion (Drayton-Brooks & White 2004). If the questions asked within a group discussion are superficial, the data emerging from the study will lack depth and may fail to adequately address the study questions.

Patricia M. Davidson, Elizabeth J. Halcomb and Leila Gholizadeh

TABLE 5.2 Examples of a focus group question route to evaluate a bereavement support group after death of a spouse

Introductory question	Can you please tell us about your experience of attending the bereavement support group?
Transition question	Can you tell us how attending the bereavement support group influenced your experience of grief?
Transition question	What made you decide to attend the bereavement support group?
Focus questions (these should be based on research questions)	What are the greatest needs faced by people following the death of a spouse? What can health professionals do to help people cope and adjust following the death of a spouse?
Summarising question	As you know, we are evaluating this bereavement support program to assist those who have recently experienced the loss of a spouse. Think back on your experiences and our discussions today and tell us what we can do to improve the care people receive.
Concluding question	Is there anything else that anyone feels we should have talked about today but didn't? Please feel free to share these thoughts.

Source: Adapted from Halcomb *et al.* (2007).

Developing the question route should focus on promoting cohesion and emphasis in the group, and promote engagement and participation by all focus group members. Strategies such as round-robin questions, where each participant answers a basic question about themselves or offers their opinion in turn around the circle, can be invaluable in promoting comfort and confidence within the group. However, subsequent questions need to facilitate group interaction rather than promote individual responses if the full benefits of the focus group approach are to be achieved (Acocella 2012). See also Chapter 4 for questions used in interviews. Further, the level of structure and direction depend on the purpose of the focus groups. In some cases the questions can be exploratory, for example, 'What is your view of asylum seekers?' When evaluating a program or experience, often the question route and interview may have a narrower focus. It is important to consider that, in focus groups, the data are the product of group interaction and dynamics that emerge from facilitated discussion, so the questions are important in focusing the moderator's actions (Acocella 2012).

Conducting the focus groups

The questions and the manner in which the focus group is facilitated depend on the participants and the study setting. It is often considered best practice to have a **moderator** and notetaker facilitating the group. The role of the moderator is to facilitate the discussion, raising the questions and probing for deeper responses, while the notetaker records field notes about the interaction to augment the audio recording. The role of the moderator is crucial in generating data from the focus group and skilfully navigating the discussion to derive rich

Moderator: A key person in focus groups, who may or may not be the researcher. A moderator leads and guides group discussions.

and meaningful information (Liamputtong 2011). In essence, the moderator becomes a tool not only to facilitate the group discussion, but also to generate the first level of analysis by providing their initial perceptions of participants' views. As the moderator can influence the outcome of focus groups, it is essential to ensure that this individual not only has knowledge, attitudes and competencies for the topic but also is acceptable to participants.

Ideally, the moderator should be someone with whom the participants feel comfortable, can potentially relate to and are likely to feel that they can openly disclose information to (Acocella 2012). For example, consideration of cultural expectations and customs is important when conducting focus groups with culturally and linguistically diverse groups. In some such groups it may be inappropriate to have a male moderator conduct focus groups with female participants (Halcomb *et al.* 2007).

The moderator should not only be skilled in facilitating group dynamics, but should have a genuine sense of reciprocity and respect for the target group. This is important for establishing rapport and trust. The moderator should be familiar with the issues being explored and any potential areas of sensitivity (Liamputtong 2011). In some instances, focus groups can have two moderators, although this will require careful planning and a cohesive and respectful relationship between them. The box 'Guidelines for moderators' gives some guiding principles for the moderator role.

Strategies should be implemented to ensure that offensive comments are minimised and that people's individual views and opinions are respected. It is also important that participants feel confident to express divergent views, as it is these differences of opinion that will yield rich data and deeper understandings. It is the moderator's role to address inappropriate comments and maintain mutual respect within the group. Doing role-plays as part of preparation for focus groups can be useful in preparing the research team to deal with the challenges of group dynamics. Similarly, anticipating the milieu of the online environment is important in ensuring that discussion is engaged, considerate, respectful and geared to focus on answering the research questions.

The notetaker also plays an important role in accurately representing discussion (Liamputtong 2011). This individual is responsible for recording field notes about their observations and perceptions during the course of the focus group, to augment the video or audio recordings. The notetaker can also assist in identifying any aspects of the conversation that the moderator has not probed sufficiently. Summarising the critical points at the end of each focus group and asking the participants to confirm their accuracy is an important way of maintaining the credibility of findings. This task is often undertaken by the notetaker, although it can be done by the moderator if desired. At the conclusion of each focus group, it is very helpful for the moderator and notetaker to reflect on the conversation and capture their thoughts. This is best done as soon as possible, while the ideas and discussion are still fresh in mind. The box 'Example of focus group data collection template' gives an example that may be useful for note-taking based on the question route given in Table 5.2.

It is useful for the moderator and notetaker to critically analyse the recordings of the focus groups to appraise their performance and to modify their technique and question route where appropriate. Questions to ask during preliminary analysis include: Is the moderator dominating the conversation and not allowing participants to discuss and debate? Is the

Patricia M. Davidson, Elizabeth J. Halcomb and Leila Gholizadeh

moderator successful in probing and clarifying positions espoused by participants? Is the conversation focused on addressing the study questions? As in all qualitative research, positioning of the researcher and reflectivity are of great importance.

'Research in practice' below describes how Aboriginal and non-Aboriginal researchers and health care workers partnered to explore barriers and facilitators to early childhood services for children with a disability. Aboriginal and Torres Strait Islander children in Australia experience a higher prevalence of disability and socio-economic disadvantage than other Australian children, and although early intervention is recommended, access is challenging (Green *et al.* 2014). As they were really interested in participants' views, the focus groups were conducted and moderated by experienced health professionals who were not actively involved in the delivery of health care services.

RESEARCH IN PRACTICE

FOCUS GROUPS USEFUL IN EVALUATING HEALTH SERVICES

Evaluating program delivery is a critical element of health services research. The use of a single method of evaluation, such as a survey (see Chapter 13), can be limited because of floor and ceiling effects of instruments—that is, when instruments capture extreme ranges of scores (Andrew *et al.* 2011). Focus groups are often useful for health service evaluation, as they provide both an individual and a collective picture. Using the focus group method, DiGiacomo and colleagues (2013) undertook focus groups for health and service providers and carers of Aboriginal children with a disability; these were held at an Aboriginal Community Controlled Health Service in Sydney, Australia. The focus groups were undertaken in collaboration with the local Aboriginal community which was an important factor in ensuring the engagement of participants. Despite dedicated disability services in an urban community, access was not optimal. Increasing awareness of services, facilitating linkages and referrals, eliminating complexities to accessing support, and working with families and Aboriginal community organisations within a framework of resilience and empowerment were identified as important for improving health services.

GUIDELINES FOR MODERATORS

Introduce yourself and your role and thank participants for agreeing to come. Explain the reason they were chosen and the main purpose of focus groups. Explain group guidelines, emphasising respect for others' opinions and the confidentiality of issues disclosed, and tell participants how long the focus group will last. The following is a sample of statements that could be used during the introduction of the focus group.

- We have the discussion scheduled for approximately one hour today. During the group we want to obtain your views on … [briefly describe the content area].

- My role is to facilitate the session today. You won't offend me, whatever opinions you give. We are interested in hearing *your* point of view even if it disagrees with others' opinions.

- It is my role to keep the discussion focused on the topic we are here to discuss, so I may need to move the conversation along so we can cover all the items and make sure that we get to hear from everyone here today.

- It is important that we maintain confidentiality and respect others' beliefs and opinions.

- We will be audio recording/videotaping the discussion, with your permission, because we don't want to miss any comments. It is important for you to realise that no names will be attached to the report or any publications. You can be assured of complete confidentiality in the report and publications.

- I would like to introduce you to my colleagues [notetakers and co-moderators].

- I would also like you to introduce yourselves [level of introduction and affiliations depends on the purpose and context of the focus group].

- If you find any of the matters discussed distressing, please come up to one of the research team and discuss your concerns.

STOP AND THINK

You are facilitating an online focus group.

- Consider how you will provide information about 'group rules' to promote confidentiality, respect and promotion of participants' well-being.
- Explain how you will ensure that these group rules are followed.

After briefing participants on the purpose of the focus group and allowing the group time to become acquainted, the moderator will pose the questions to the group and allow time for participants to respond to each other's comments. Some flexibility is required, to allow views to be expressed and to explore issues that may not have been anticipated by the researchers. It is also important to ensure that voices of all participants are heard and that vocal members do not dominate the conversation and prevent the group view from emerging. This is an important part of the moderator's role.

Practical considerations, such as ensuring that recording devices are working effectively and are optimally placed, are fundamental to ensuring that effective data are obtained (see also Chapter 4). In some instances, videotaping is conducted. Such recording requires additional planning and the explicit consent of participants. Before a decision is made to videotape a group, its potential impact on the participants must be considered.

Patricia M. Davidson, Elizabeth J. Halcomb and Leila Gholizadeh

Taking time at the end of each focus group to reflect and comment on the outcomes of the session is crucial, because transcription can be challenging when several participants are talking at once. Therefore, not only is the initial debriefing the first step in data analysis, it also contributes to the planning for subsequent focus groups where it may be necessary to probe emerging issues or add questions to draw out information more clearly. It is also a risk mitigation process in case of recording failure or difficulties in transcription. Assigning a research team member to take responsibility for both audiotaping and observing is important, since assembling the same participants and repeating the interview is not usually feasible.

Similar reflection and maintenance of rigour is necessary in the online environment. Critical analysis of discourse, close analysis of the text and trending of views and opinions are critical in ensuring the rigour of data collection, interpretation, synthesis and reporting. Documenting these steps is critical in the accurate reporting of methodological characteristics.

EXAMPLE OF FOCUS GROUP DATA COLLECTION TEMPLATE

Date: ....

Start time: ....

Stop time: ....

Moderator: ....

Notetaker: ....

Observer (s): ....

Venue: ....

Participants: ....

FOCUS QUESTION	RESPONSES	KEY ISSUES
What were the greatest needs or most important issues faced by people suffering bereavement following the death of a spouse?		
What are the barriers to and facilitators of recovery from the death of a spouse?		
What can health professionals do to help individuals adjust to life following the death of their spouse?		
Summary and reflections		

It is important that after each focus group the research team takes the time to reflect on the group and assess the efficacy of the question route as well as the dynamics of eliciting information. Scheduling adequate time between focus groups to allow preliminary data analysis is generally recommended, to ensure the focus of the interviews is adhered to and to optimise subsequent group interviews. The number of focus groups is determined by the depth of data required, the range of participants and whether the focus group is a primary, adjunctive or secondary data source. As in other forms of qualitative data, determining when data saturation has been reached is important; this underlines the importance of an iterative and reflective process. Generally, data saturation is said to occur when no or little new data emerges (Liamputtong 2011; see also Chapter 1). Although there is no rigid rule, it is generally useful to conduct another one or two focus groups, following the perception of data saturation, to ensure that saturation has indeed occurred. Optimally, you should conduct at least two focus groups with each type of participant or subgroup. It is also important to consider both within-group and across-group saturation. Theoretical and data saturation must occur both within each participant type and across groups of various participant types (Onwuegbuzie *et al.* 2009).

Data analysis

The method of data analysis should be driven by the study questions (see Chapter 23). Analysing focus group data should follow the epistemological and conceptual foundations of qualitative research, where the researcher becomes the instrument to provide a voice to participants. At first, **data analysis** is often mechanistic, looking for recurrent patterns and themes. In the next phase, the analysis is interpretive, searching for meaning and conclusions. At each step it is important that the research team remains aware of their positioning and maintains the credibility of the data. Maintaining a reflective journal can provide a useful audit trail and assist in verifying and validating emerging themes.

Data analysis: The way that researchers make sense of their data. In qualitative research, it means looking for patterns of ideas or themes, whereas in quantitative research data are analysed by counting various response alternatives.

As in all forms of qualitative data analysis, the process of the researcher immersing themselves in the data is crucial to truly understanding participants' perspectives. Massey (2011) argues for a more critical approach when eliciting data that are specifically articulated compared to those which are attributed. When using qualitative approaches, the researcher acts as a research instrument to give a voice to participants and is pivotal to data analysis and interpretation. As a consequence, declaring the values, perspectives and experiences that the researcher brings to the research process is important. Researchers should consider any of their assumptions, biases and experiences that might shape the research process and the degree of acceptance by participants, and that might influence analysis and interpretation (Malterud 2001). Although qualitative methods can yield subjective, biased and unreliable findings, the closeness of the relationship between a qualitative researcher and the participants' experience is more likely to achieve a better understanding of the subject under investigation, particularly if the premises of methodological rigour are observed.

In focus group studies, data collection and analysis should be concurrent (Liamputtong 2013; see Chapter 23). Delaying analysis of one group increases the likelihood that its social context, mood and meanings may be lost among the data collected from subsequent focus groups (Krueger 1997; Krueger & Casey 2009). It is important to include as many members of the research team as possible in this fundamental stage of analysis. Data sources available for interpretation include the verbatim transcriptions of the data, field notes, and the thoughts of the moderator and notetaker following each group. Transcriptions should be reviewed repeatedly to facilitate immersion in the data. The field notes should include the individual researcher's reflections and perceptions as well as commentary on interactions and emerging issues. Methods of data management vary from paper notes through to qualitative data analysis software such as NVivo (see Chapter 24). It is important to note that, regardless of the method of data management, the researcher remains the tool through which the views of participants are filtered and synthesised.

Generally, **thematic analysis** is used to analyse focus group data (Liamputtong 2011, 2013; Bazeley 2013). This process classifies words and observations into categories based on their conceptual significance. In the initial phases of analysis, ideas, observations and concepts are coded. Subsequently, similar incidents, reflections and comments are grouped together (Liamputtong 2011, 2013; Bazeley 2013). It is important to continually return to recordings, transcripts and field notes to verify reflections and observations. Using predetermined codes (e.g. aggression and anxiety) can force emerging themes in qualitative data (Gomm 2004). This is particularly the case where each individual focus group influences subsequent interactions. Being open to the messages of the qualitative data and providing a voice to participants is a hallmark of good qualitative research.

Once data is organised into categories based on groups of words with similar meanings, common issues and meanings described as **themes** can emerge. The search for commonality should not mean disregarding the range and diversity of experiences and perceptions. As focus groups and data collection progress, initial themes should be validated and explored in subsequent groups to seek confirmation and completeness of understandings. Emerging themes and the degree of relevance to the study questions should be considered within the context of field notes, personal notes and discussions within the research team. Similar approaches should be used in online focus groups, where a reflective and iterative approach should be taken with close adherence to the textual data source. See more detail in Chapter 23.

A reflective and iterative process should be used to maximise the validity of data interpretation and minimise external bias, although it is important to consider that the moderator inevitably becomes part of the social interaction. The need to ensure rigour as a measure of reliability and validity in qualitative research has been well recognised (Liamputtong 2013; see also Chapter 1). Some qualitative researchers argue that the reliability of qualitative research should not be judged by quantitative criteria, and suggest an alternative terminology to describe different concepts of qualitative studies, such as trustworthiness, whereby researchers attempt to show that their research process is auditable so that the reader will be able to track and verify the research process (Liamputtong 2013). This emphasises the importance of reporting. Accessing the consolidated criteria for reporting qualitative research (COREQ), a thirty-two item checklist for interviews and focus groups, early in the planning stage can not only assist in the planning but serve as a reminder for collecting important data to ensure the transparency and accountability of the research process (Tong *et al.* 2007). The research is trustworthy if the results reflect the experiences of the participants as much as possible. Trustworthiness includes credibility, which reflects the accuracy of presenting the data and, specifically, participants' views (see Chapter 1). Dependability relates to reliability

Thematic analysis: The identification of themes through a careful reading and rereading of the data.

Theme: A grouping of data that emerges from the research and to which the researcher gives a name.

and transferability of the data. A study is said to be trustworthy when the data have been presented accurately and truthfully (Miles & Huberman 1994). Member checking, where participants are asked to review and comment on study findings, is one way of assessing for credibility (Liamputtong 2013). The process of member checking may not, however, be feasible in the context of multiple focus groups. Instead, using subsequent focus groups to explore initial findings can be a substitute for individual groups checking their own transcriptions.

SUMMARY OF STEPS TO ACHIEVE RIGOUR IN FOCUS GROUPS

1. Develop a protocol involving a comprehensive and critical literature review.
2. Outline the roles and responsibilities of the research team.
3. Generate focus group questions that will collect data that address the study aims.
4. Engage key stakeholders' support and submit for ethical approval.
5. Develop a risk management plan that considers participants, study setting, protocol, researchers and an implementation plan.
6. Anticipate ethical issues and implement appropriate strategies, such as access to counselling if necessary.
7. Consider unique issues relating to culture, gender and socio-economic circumstances.
8. Declare researchers' stance in relation to the target population and the study project.
9. Plan for participant recruitment, participation and identification of appropriate and accessible venues.
10. Audio/videorecord focus groups and document observations of interactions, in particular non-verbal communication and group dynamics.
11. Ensure that notetaking by observers and that field notes and summary templates are included in the data analysis plan.
12. Summarise critical points at the end of each focus group and ask participants to confirm their accuracy.
13. Have a debriefing session between the moderator(s) and observer(s) immediately after each focus group to capture initial impressions and highlight similarities to and differences from preceding focus groups.
14. Plan for a systematic process of data analysis, to ensure credible representation of participants' views.
15. Make careful documentation of study processes such as planning, data collection, analysis and dissemination of findings.
16. Consider issues of translation of transcripts, in the validation of data content.
17. Ensure that the report of focus group findings addresses transparency and accountability to ensure interpretation of data and assessment of study quality.

Patricia M. Davidson, Elizabeth J. Halcomb and Leila Gholizadeh

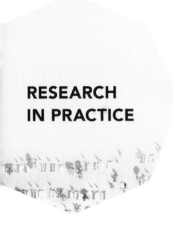

RESEARCH IN PRACTICE

A PRACTICAL CASE STUDY AND REFLECTIVE ACCOUNT OF THE USE OF FOCUS GROUPS

Leila Gholizadeh (2009) is a nurse born in Azerbaijan. She worked as a cardiovascular nurse and nurse educator in Madani Heart Hospital, Azerbaijan, for seven years. During this period she encountered patients and carers who had limited knowledge of risk factors for heart disease and inaccurate perceptions about their personal risk factors, and who made inaccurate causal attributions about their heart disease.

Health professionals were also struck by some patients' low adherence to prescribed medical regimens. For example, one patient was rehospitalised for another heart attack after being discharged from hospital just two weeks before. He had resumed high-intensity manual work on his farm, against health care recommendations. In another instance, Leila was explaining to a patient about his heart attack and the importance of reducing risk factors. During the encounter a relative of the patient pulled Leila aside and told her that she was not supposed to tell the patient about his diagnosis, as his doctor would not approve. This stance of non-disclosure challenged many of her assumptions of what the accepted best practice in cardiovascular care, involving emphasis on providing information and empowerment.

For her PhD program in Australia, Leila investigated factors impacting on Middle Eastern women's perception of cardiovascular disease. Focus groups were used to describe the views of immigrant Turkish, Persian and Arabic women regarding their perceptions of the risk of heart disease, their causal attributions and risk-reducing behaviours. Leila was able to reach out to women through community-based groups and interact with women who do not commonly interact with the health care system. Themes emerging from the focus group discussions were: (1) Middle Eastern women underestimate the risk of cardiovascular disease; (2) stress is a pervasive factor in the lives of Middle Eastern women; and (3) Middle Eastern women face many barriers to reducing their risk of cardiovascular disease. Overwhelmingly, participants underestimated their risk of cardiovascular disease. The women in this study attributed the risk of cardiovascular disease to psychological status rather than lifestyle factors.

Findings from this study have implications for health care services to develop culturally and linguistically competent programs for Middle Eastern women while taking into account cultural differences in beliefs and traditions. Leila has built upon her research training and her bilingual skills to mentor and develop other researchers to provide a voice to vulnerable populations of immigrants (Shishehgar et al. 2015).

STOP AND THINK

You want to engage a community of which you are not a member.

- Consider the strategies that you will have to undertake to gain access to the group. Are there any ethical issues to consider?
- What characteristics of the moderator are most likely to facilitate rapport and address study objectives?

Developing proficiency in conducting focus groups

As in most scenarios, practice makes perfect. If you intend to use focus groups as a method of data collection, it is important that you take time to dissect the anatomy of this method of data collection, identifying the elements that make focus groups successful (Liamputtong 2011). As well as reading about techniques, practise them. The practice exercises in this chapter are a good place to start. The important considerations in perfecting the focus group technique are preparing the research questions, taking time to understand the dynamics and nuances of the target group, preparing the setting and data collection methods, and undertaking a process of self-reflection to ensure that the moderator becomes the voice of the target group and ensures the well-being of participants. In some instances, a very directive questioning style can be appropriate, whereas in others a less directive approach is warranted. It is also important to validate with the group if an issue is sensitive or distressing in any way.

Preparation and planning for focus groups includes not only the physical setting and organisational aspects but also considering factors such as group dynamics and anticipating the needs and perspectives of participants (Liamputtong 2011). Implementation and dynamics of focus groups may be related to participants' views on authority, gender, class and culture. For example, do not be dismayed if some participants decline to have sessions audio- or videorecorded (Liamputtong 2011). In some cultural groups this can be perceived as authoritative, with potentially punitive consequences. Denying participants a voice and access to potentially valuable data by sticking rigidly to protocol can be a limited view. This underscores the need for the moderator to be proficient and competent, and to have a notetaker present.

Devising strategies to understand the target group means that many of the challenges of focus groups can be anticipated and included in the study protocol. Being receptive to participants' needs, as well as maintaining methodological rigour (see Chapter 1), is part of the art as well as the science of conducting effective focus group interviews. Participating in role-plays and critical analyses of individual performances is important if the data yield is to be maximised. This requires critical self-reflection in order to improve quality. Further understanding of the online milieu is critical in conducting online focus groups (Walker 2013). In this instance, the textual analysis is very important (Gaiser 2008).

Critical analysis of audio/videorecordings and transcriptions, for example calculating the ratio of participant to moderator dialogue, is one example of a strategy to elicit high-quality data. It is also important to consider non-verbal factors of communication and strategies for achieving group perceptions and how these will be included in the process of analysis and interpretation. Other strategies, such as preparing standard phrases—'It is important that everyone has the opportunity to express their ideas, regardless of your individual perspective', or 'Thank you for sharing that opinion, but it is important that we consider everyone's view'—which can be used by the moderator to address various

Patricia M. Davidson, Elizabeth J. Halcomb and Leila Gholizadeh

situations within the focus group, can ensure that respect and reciprocity are prevailing themes of the focus groups. If an issue is controversial, it is important to anticipate how to manage a hostile participant.

The moderator needs to be prepared to deal with divergent and conflicting views, be able to deal with disagreements and be astute in targeting participants who appear distressed and may need follow-up. It is part of the researchers' responsibility and an ethical requirement to provide participants with contact details for counselling services if they appear distressed, or seem to require support or counselling. These considerations also apply in the online setting, where counselling services and resources can be provided via the internet.

Therefore taking the time to understand the group you are targeting, particularly from a cultural perspective, allows you to anticipate potential challenges. Having a risk management plan is an important part of your research planning. For example, what to do if there is an equipment failure? How to react to distressed or hostile participants? Developing templates and effective forms of data management, as outlined in this chapter, are vital considerations in preparing for focus groups. They can make your experience of these groups less stressful and more likely to generate rich and valuable data. Moreover, they will enable you to minimise risks to participants, which is an important consideration in planning research and obtaining ethical clearance for your project.

Summary

This chapter has demonstrated that focus groups are a useful strategy for obtaining the collective perspective of a group of individuals with common characteristics, particularly to elicit data of an exploratory or explanatory nature. Focus groups can be undertaken in a range of settings, including online, using a range of software tools. Most commonly, they are undertaken in a natural setting, such as a church, hospital or community group. However, the internet is increasingly becoming a source of community for many individuals; it is particularly useful in addressing hard-to-reach populations or investigating sensitive issues.

This chapter has emphasised that undertaking a focus group is a team activity and therefore the roles and responsibilities of the research team need to be delineated. It is crucial to understand the amount of planning required. The box 'Summary of steps to achieve rigour in focus groups' encapsulates important factors when preparing to conduct focus groups. Focus groups are particularly valuable in obtaining the views and perspectives of underrepresented and marginalised individuals where issues such as low literacy prevent participation in many other forms of research, such as surveys. This also increases the complexity of research, in particular protecting vulnerable participants. In health research, the focus group method can be informative in exploring issues as well as useful as an evaluation technique. Focus groups are a powerful research tool. When conducted effectively and with rigour, they have the potential to elucidate rich data and provide a voice for participants.

Practice exercises

1 A successful focus group is contingent on planning and coordination. Another crucial factor is the proficiency of the moderator. As a group, identify the ideal characteristics of a moderator. Discuss how you might be able to identify the facilitation of the moderator, by listening to audiotapes and reviewing transcripts. What are attributes of a moderator for particular target groups?

2 Describe the strategies you would use to facilitate engagement of all participants in focus group discussions. What are some statements that you could use to maximise participation?

3 Identify issues in undertaking focus groups online. What are important strategies in moderating groups in an online environment?

4 Discuss the process of data management in focus groups. Identify strategies for data recording, transcription and analysis. What strategies would you employ to achieve methodological rigour?

5 Review the COREQ guidelines. How will the data management strategies discussed above facilitate the quality of reporting?

Further reading

Acocella, I. (2012). The focus groups in social research: advantages and disadvantages. *Quality and Quantity*, 46(4), 1125–36.

Gaiser, T.J. (2008). Online focus groups. In N. Fielding, R.M. Lee & G. Blank (eds), *The Sage handbook of online research methods*. London: Sage, 290–307.

Krueger, R.A. & Casey, M.A. (2009). *Focus groups: a practical guide for applied research*, 4th edn. Thousand Oaks, CA: Sage.

Liamputtong, P. (2007). *Researching the vulnerable: a guide to sensitive research methods*. London: Sage.

Liamputtong, P. (2011). *Focus group methodology: principles and practice*. London: Sage.

Marková, I. (2012). *Dialogue in focus groups*. London: Equinox Books.

Phillips, J.L. & Davidson, P.M. (2009). Focus group methodology: being guided along a pathway from novice to expert. In V. Minichiello & J. Kottler (eds), *Qualitative journeys: student and mentoring experiences with research*. Thousand Oaks, CA: Sage, 255–76.

Patricia M. Davidson, Elizabeth J. Halcomb and Leila Gholizadeh

Websites

Community Tool Box: http://ctb.ku.edu/en/table-of-contents/assessment/assessing-community-needs-and-resources/conduct-focus-groups/main

> This website provides important information to consider when undertaking focus groups, particularly in a community setting.

Usability: gov www.usability.gov/methods/analyze_current/learn/focus.html

> This website describes important features in ascertaining perspectives on usability.

Instructional Assessment Resources: www.utexas.edu/academic/ctl/assessment/iar/research/plan/method/focus.php

> This website gives step-by-step resources for undertaking a focus group.

www.sjsu.edu/people/fred.prochaska/courses/ScWk242Spring2013/s2/New-York-State-Teachers-Focus-Groups.pdf

> This site provides resources on program evaluation using the focus group method.

Center for Disease Control: www.cdc.gov/healthyyouth/evaluation/pdf/brief13.pdf

> This site provides guidelines for undertaking focus groups.

6

Narrative Enquiry and Health Research

PRISCILLA ENNALS AND LINSEY HOWIE

Chapter objectives

In this chapter you will learn:

- about the nature of narrative enquiry
- how to use narrative enquiry in qualitative research
- about the narrative enquiry method: sampling, participants, data collection and analysis
- what steps to take in narrative analysis and analysis of narratives

Key terms

Analysis of narratives

Data analysis

Discourse

Metaphor

Narrative analysis

Narrative enquiry

Plot

Purposive sampling

Snowball sampling

Introduction

As occupational therapists and academics, we have been drawn to qualitative research methods, the potential they offer to explore our interest in people's lives, and the links between what people do, their occupations, and their states of health and ill health. Exploring the range of qualitative methods available, **narrative enquiry** has potential to answer questions relevant to understanding people's occupational lives and their experiences in receiving occupational therapy and other health services. We have come to appreciate the value that narrative enquiry places on people's lives, their individual experiences and responses to specific events, circumstances, relationships and environments. We connect with the views of Robert Atkinson (2007, p. 224), a scholar of human development who specialises in narrative methodologies, who asserts that 'we are the storytelling species. Storytelling is in our blood. We think in story form, speak in story form, and bring meaning to our lives through story. Our life stories connect us to our roots, give us direction, validate our own experience, and restore value to our lives'. Narrative enquiry, as Pinnegar and Daynes (2007) observe, 'begins in experience as expressed in lived and told stories'(p. 5). With its focus on enabling storytelling to reveal people's experience, narrative enquiry is a method that foregrounds what people bring to matters of importance to them. Having origins in the humanities and literary scholarship, and an established background in social disciplines, including anthropology and sociology, narrative enquiry has more recently been embraced by the major allied health professions (Spector-Mersel 2010). It offers the opportunity for research participants to describe in detail the wider context shaping their experience of the phenomenon in question. The narrative researcher studies particular stories elicited through a wide range of methods to facilitate the in-depth telling of pertinent experience (Liamputtong 2013).

Our reading of the works of leading authors in this area (especially Bochner & Riggs 2014; Clandinin 2013, 2007; DeFina & Georgakopoulou 2015; Goodfellow 1997; Mishler 1999; Polkinghorne 2005; Riessman 2008) has informed this chapter. Our experiences of using a narrative framework while conducting research and supervising honours and higher degree students is included in the form of exemplars, tutorial exercises and reflections on past studies in occupational therapy (see Cussen *et al.* 2012; Ennals & Fossey 2009; Feldman & Howie 2009; Howie *et al.* 2004; Kelly & Howie 2007).

Narrative enquiry:
A research method that focuses on the structure and nature of the narratives, or stories, produced.

STOP AND THINK

The word 'experience' is used widely in debates about narrative enquiry.

- What does the word mean to you?
- Make a list of a few of your most recent experiences.
- Do your examples resonate with a view that experience is not something 'we *have* as a private possession, but something we *do* in relational participation' (Gergen & Gergen 2011, p. 380)?

What is narrative enquiry?

The field of narrative enquiry can be confusing to the beginning researcher, or the seasoned researcher coming to qualitative research methods for the first time. While narrative studies can be traced to origins in hermeneutics and phenomenology (Josselson 2006), it has been widely adopted in history, anthropology and sociology, and across a variety of professions such as law and education, medicine, psychology, nursing, social work and occupational therapy (Liamputtong 2013; Riessman 2008). The 1980s saw what is described as a 'narrative turn' in the human sciences—a push back against the reductionist positivist traditions dominant at that time and a way of reclaiming a view of human life as storied and complex (Bochner & Riggs 2014). Narrative methodological approaches have developed since the early 1980s in a range of fields, resulting in some confusion as to what constitutes narrative enquiry. Writing about a special issue in *Narrative Inquiry*, devoted to understanding contemporary uses of the method, Smith (2007, p. 392) notes how narrative enquiry can 'mean different things to different people'. He adds, 'Narrative enquiry might therefore be best considered an umbrella term for a mosaic of research efforts, with diverse theoretical musings, methods, empirical groundings, and/or significance all revolving around an interest in narrative.' Riessman (2008), for example, distinguishes between storytelling practices, narrative data and narrative analysis, and Bochner and Riggs (2014) highlight differences between narrative analysis and narratives-under-analysis.

This is useful to keep in mind. There are many ways to conduct a narrative enquiry and, while the literature is extensive, it is characterised by disparate views as well as corresponding ideas (see Liamputtong 2013). This section offers one way of understanding narrative enquiry; other authors will have different perspectives or different emphases. This does not give researchers free rein to do whatever they like. Rather, it invites you to read widely and think carefully about how to construct a narrative study.

Schwandt's definition (1997, p. 98) draws attention to the centrality of story to this method: 'Narrative inquiry is concerned with the means of generating data in the form of stories, means of interpreting that data, and means of representing it in narrative or storied form.' Josselson (2006, p. 4) reminds us that narrative research 'strives to preserve the complexity of what it means to be human and to locate these observations of people and phenomena in society, history and time'. Polkinghorne (2005, p. 5) describes it as a 'subset of qualitative research designs in which stories are used to describe human action'. However, to distinguish narrative enquiry as a research method from the word 'narrative' commonly used in qualitative research, he emphasises that 'narrative' in narrative enquiry 'refers to a discourse form in which events and happenings are configured into a temporal unity by means of a plot'. Goodfellow (1997, p. 61), on the other hand, describes narrative in this context in terms of 'a form of natural **discourse** in which the narrator conveys the nature of what has been experienced through the sequential telling of that experience'.

Three further elements of narrative enquiry are important to grasp at this point: the significance of meaning-making in people's use of stories, and the relevance of plot and

Discourse: In this chapter it means 'communication of thought by words, talk or conversation' rather than its specific meaning in the social sciences.

Plot: The narrative structure of a story, indicating how people extract understanding from past events to make sense of present circumstances.

Metaphor: Used in narrative enquiry to enhance the meaning of stories by suggesting an analogy with something familiar.

metaphor to this process. Josselson (2011, p. 225) reminds us that 'meaning is not inherent in an act or experience, but is constructed through social discourse'. Kielhofner and colleagues (2008, p. 110) say that humans 'conduct and draw meaning from life by locating themselves in unfolding narratives that integrate their past, present, and future selves'. **Plot**, they maintain with reference to Gergen and Gergen (1988), is a 'forestructure of narrative' indicating how people think in recounting stories and revealing the meaning and significance of various story elements. Plot also indicates how people extract understanding from past events to make sense of present circumstances. The use of **metaphor** in narratives also enhances the meaning of stories by suggesting an analogy with something familiar, or emphasising the meaning of experience that might be difficult to understand or convey in any other way. Savin-Baden and Niekerk (2007, p. 464), however, challenge the need for structure and a coherent plot, suggesting that narratives are 'interruptions of reflection in a storied life'. They argue that lives can present unpredictable disruptions that can change the direction of stories. This is frequently seen in narrative research conducted in health, where illness, disability or life events interrupt expected narrative directions. The stories told and created with researchers in these situations are about experiences of loss and feeling swamped in the wake of the disruption, making sense of the disruption, or re-creating self and life following disruption. Plotlines of lived lives are always works in progress, but in these situations they require dramatic reworking.

The literature proposes many uses for narrative enquiry. Riessman (2008, pp. 8–9) reflects on narratives and people's everyday use of stories to 'remember, argue, justify, persuade, engage, entertain and even mislead an audience'. She emphasises that recalling past experiences supports individuals to make sense of painful or fragmented memories. This, she argues, is achieved through therapeutic processes, or through writing, reading, or dramatic or other cultural or political events. Narratives, she maintains, are 'strategic, functional and purposeful' and they can 'mobilise others into action for progressive and social change'. Gergen and Gergen (2006) note the uses of narrative practices in therapy and in organisational transformation and conflict reduction. They maintain that understanding narratives as embedded in social interaction in various contexts reveals the potential for stories to enhance relationships and produce personal and social change. Smith (2007, pp. 391–2) too observes that narratives are 'effective in social and individual transformation' as well as 'constructing selves and identities'. These examples illuminate the uses of narrative enquiry beyond the individual memoir or reflection on a particular experience, and invite discussion about how narrative research can be used to bring about social change or action.

Narrative researchers have varying views on what a narrative enquiry entails, but the literature appears to concur that stories, freely told, reveal human activity in all its complexity and these stories have the potential to enhance understanding of people in their environments. There is no absolute 'right way' to implement a narrative enquiry, but researchers are encouraged to record, discuss and debate their practices to expand knowledge of the potential for this research method to answer contemporary questions of individual or social importance. Stories are foregrounded in every aspect of a narrative enquiry: in data collection, in analysis and in the findings. The unpredictable nature of storytelling and the different perspectives that humans put on a story, depending on the audience or the moment of telling or the environment in which stories are communicated, are instructive ideas for all researchers undertaking a narrative enquiry. While certainty is not guaranteed, establishing procedures to guide the conduct of a narrative study can be very beneficial.

Narrative enquiry method

So, how do qualitative researchers set about designing and conducting a narrative enquiry? A reading of contemporary narrative studies confirms there are many ways to proceed. Smith (2007) notes the tendency of studies reviewed in the special issue of *Narrative Inquiry* (2006) and published as a book (Bamberg 2007) to distinguish between those that are more formulaic in structure and those that tend to be playful or more creative in method. We find this distinction helpful, but consider it more useful in the present context to describe a systematic approach to doing narrative research, and to present information gleaned from our reading and research experience over recent years.

Sampling procedures and participants

In line with most qualitative studies, the sampling method used in narrative enquiry will necessarily include participants who are rich in information and able to express their experiences or recall events in depth (see also Chapter 1). There are a number of sampling strategies assembled under the umbrella term 'purposive sampling' to guide researchers engaging participants in narrative studies. **Purposive sampling** is widely used to select small numbers of people who share perceptions, behaviours, experience or contexts relevant to the study aims (Liamputtong 2013; see Chapter 1). It allows the establishment of inclusion and exclusion criteria to ensure participants have the desired qualities or abilities. In narrative enquiry, it is usual to select participants without cognitive limitations, people who are able to recollect significant events and relationships, and people who are able to range freely around the research question. People with a good command of the language in which the study is undertaken are also valuable in this type of research.

> **Purposive sampling:** Looks for cases that will be able to provide rich or in-depth information about the issue being examined, not a representative sample as in quantitative research.

Selecting the right sampling method for a study largely needs common sense and a willingness to review the various types of sampling in order to select people who meet the study objectives. Purposive sampling includes criterion sampling, extreme case sampling, homogeneous sampling and **snowball sampling** (Liamputtong 2013; see also Chapter 9). The last of these begins by selecting one or a few participants with pertinent knowledge or experience and asking them to identify others with similar experience. We used this form of sampling in a study of psychiatric nurses to determine the influence of training in gestalt psychotherapy on their nursing practice (Kelly & Howie 2007). In another study (Feldman & Howie 2009), we used criterion sampling to select a particular group of older people who assessed themselves as in good health, were actively engaged in leisure occupations, and were able to reflect on their histories of occupational participation.

> **Snowball sampling:** Sampling that relies on existing participants to identify acquaintances who fit the inclusion criteria of a study in order to increase the size of the sample.

Data collection

During data collection in narrative enquiry, the researcher engages in thoughtful conversations with participants, in an attempt to enter their world and understand the story or stories at the heart of the study. Data collection may use various methods. In-depth interviews (see Chapter 4), journal and diary entries are common, but researchers might like to use graphic techniques, visual methods or electronic methods such as email, or narratives recorded by the participants.

Interview schedules guide researchers to stay on topic while simultaneously eliciting individuals' unique and nuanced stories through in-depth interviews. Schedules can vary from highly structured to minimalist, depending on the needs of the study and the experience and confidence of the interviewer. The five examples described here illustrate a range of structure levels in interview schedules and some more creative approaches to data gathering. Ennals and Fossey (2009) use the Occupational Performance History Interview – II (Kielhofner *et al.* 2004)—a semi-structured, occupationally focused, life-history interview—to gather information about the lives of people with mental illness and their experiences of recovery. This interview guide provides a comprehensive set of prompts that the interviewer can select from to build an understanding of a participant's occupational identity and experience over time.

The work of Cussen and colleagues (2012) uses a combination of two semi-structured interviews and photographs taken by participants, to create stories about participation in leisure activities by adolescents with cerebral palsy. The stories revealed commonality in aspirations held by adolescents with and without cerebral palsy, and the type of supports likely to be required if the young people are to achieve their aspirations as they move into adulthood.

A study by Hewitt and colleagues (2010) explores people's planning for and experience of occupation in retirement. The authors identify four central prompts (Table 6.1), or topics of interest to be covered in the interviews. The first author uses basic interviewing skills—reflective listening, paraphrasing, and open questions such as 'Can you say some more about that?'—to explore the topics in great depth.

TABLE 6.1   Interview schedule: plans for and experience of retirement

What was happening in your life and what prompted you to plan activities for your retirement?
What were the influences on this decision?
How did you set about preparing yourself for retirement?
What are your experiences of retirement now?

Source: Hewitt *et al.* (2010, p. 11).

In a narrative study of psychiatric nurses who did further training in gestalt psychotherapy (Kelly & Howie 2007), the authors want participants to freely develop their own account of the research topic, so a minimalist guide is developed to focus on the narrative as the participant is telling it and to seek the rich, complex and varied elements of each story. The final prompt asks participants to identify a word or metaphor to describe the influence of gestalt therapy training on their psychiatric nursing practice. This is a useful technique to elicit a spontaneous idea or ideas, and often generates further details to enhance understanding of the research question.

In a narrative study, Feldman and Howie (2009) use the Self Discovery Tapestry (SDT) (Meltzer *et al.* 2002), a life-history review tool during individual face-to-face interviews, to assist eleven participants aged eighty-one to ninety-nine to evoke past events, reflect on their long lives and consider how they are adapting to changing capacities and environments. The SDT, unlike autobiographical methods, uses a matrix and coloured pens to denote significant events or periods in a lifetime. It provides an orderly framework and immediate graphic representation to facilitate recollection.

WHEN RESEARCHERS QUESTION HOW THEY COLLECT DATA

Having collected data for a study of older people using the SDT to guide the research interviews in which a number of researchers were involved (Feldman & Howie 2009), the authors questioned what in the instrument did not support the participants to share their experiences in the way they had anticipated.

Our concerns

Howie reflected on her data collection procedures and participants' experience of them (Feldman & Howie 2009). First, it was apparent that 'reflecting on a long life and recalling significant events and relationships was not necessarily an easy experience for the participants'. Second, 'despite modifying the SDT to accommodate older participants in this specific study, it remained difficult for them to complete without considerable assistance. For instance, choosing a coloured pen to resonate with an experience, and an inability to "stay within the lines" of the matrix caused frustration and concern to some participants and most participants asked the researcher to fill in the matrix for them'. Third, 'some participants were also concerned to "get the facts right." The longevity of the participants' lives meant that for some it was difficult to recall exact dates and sequences of events. Even recalling major events such as weddings, births, the death of a spouse required extra effort and many could not indicate times of turmoil or confusion or when they were happy or unhappy' as the SDT asked them to do.

RESEARCH IN PRACTICE

What can we learn from this?

We have learnt that greater participation of the older people themselves in trialling the matrix, in the early stages of this study, would have been valuable in confirming the use of the SDT with this age group. It was not enough to rely on the literature or our experience with a younger population. We considered that 'conducting focus group research with older people would establish the value and appropriateness of the tool in exploring changes across the life course'. We also learnt that 'a matrix-based instrument which allows for more spontaneous recall of events, memories and dispositions identified by participants rather than insisting on linear recall could be more encouraging and less threatening to this age group'.

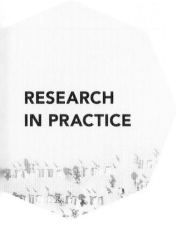

**RESEARCH
IN PRACTICE**

DESIGNING AN INTERVIEW SCHEDULE

Consider a research topic that is of interest to you. How would you know if it is suitable to be designed as a narrative enquiry? Does the topic lend itself to a story format with a beginning, a middle and an end? If so, imagine you are now ready to construct the interview schedule.

In an example encountered by an Honours student, Stapleton (2008), the challenge was how to construct an interview schedule for a study of older parents caring for an adult child with a long history of mental illness. She designed a schedule that had three sections: caring then, caring now, caring in the future. To begin with, she asked for some preliminary information about their role as carers and then about significant milestones in their lives (education, work, children, family, leisure interests, etc.). Next, she invited the participant to look back to the time of their son or daughter's diagnosis and the impact this had on their lives (caring then). Then she asked about their current experience, what caring involves now and how the demands of caring impact on their work, leisure and social relationships. Finally, she asked about their thoughts and plans for caring for their child in the future.

Data analysis

Following data collection, transcription of data and preparation of a master transcript (which includes de-identifying data, listening to the interview and editing the transcript to ensure accuracy, line numbering and page set-up according to standard qualitative research procedures), data analysis in narrative enquiry can begin (see also Chapters 4, 23). We prefer each line of the transcript left-adjusted, with 70 characters to a line (approximately), allowing room on the right-hand side to record your analytic response to the data.

Many beginning researchers become apprehensive in approaching **data analysis**, wondering how to assume responsibility for interpreting other people's stories (see Chapter 23). However, as Josselson (2006, pp. 4–5) reminds us, every aspect of narrative research is an interpretive act. She observes that from the initial choice of research question and participants, 'deciding what to ask them, with what phrasing, transcribing from spoken language to text, understanding the verbal locutions, making sense of meanings thus encoded, to deciding what to attend to and to highlight—the work is interpretive at every point'. This is helpful, as it reminds us that by the data analysis stage of a study we have already engaged in interpretive practices.

Data analysis, like data collection procedures, searches for the story inherent in the individual telling of experience. When you have the experience of transcribing an interview, you will observe that people do not usually recount experience in an orderly chronological fashion. It can be daunting to sit with pages and pages of narrative data and not have a clear

Data analysis: The way that researchers make sense of their data. In qualitative research it means looking for patterns of ideas or themes, whereas in quantitative research data are analysed by counting various response alternatives.

sense of how to begin or proceed with analysis (Liamputtong 2013). We propose a sequence of steps to guide data analysis. This may appear overly formulaic, but in our experience it is useful for researchers new to narrative enquiry. The steps we propose are drawn from the work of Goodfellow (1997) and Polkinghorne (2005) and include our experience of imposing order on narrative data, first by creating a storied account of the data (**narrative analysis**) (see Table 6.2) and second by deriving themes from the stories to demonstrate commonalities and dissimilar experiences (**analysis of narratives**) (see Table 6.3).

Narrative analysis: A method of creating a story by imposing order on narrative data.

Analysis of narratives: The type of data analysis where themes are derived from the stories to demonstrate commonalities and dissimilar experiences.

TABLE 6.2 Data analysis: Step 1, narrative analysis (story creation)

STEPS	RESEARCHER ACTIONS
1 Transcript review	• Read, and if necessary reread, the final or master transcript to get a sense of the whole interview. • Pay particular attention to what is being said that extends your understanding of the research question—what is familiar, or what offers a novel appreciation of the topic. • Notice how things are said, what the participant emphasises (the strength of words, use of metaphors or figures of speech). • Reflect on what is avoided or minimised. • Make file notes and record line numbers at particular points of interest. These notes support the deeply intellectual work associated with data analysis and will develop your central argument about the phenomenon in question.
2 Story preparation	• Create headings that permit a chronological or logical sequencing of the data into a story with a beginning, middle and end. • Ensure these headings will reflect data collected from all participants and will incorporate the central concepts, behaviours or events relevant to the research question. • Colour-code the transcripts to indicate the heading to which the data are best assigned. Note: some data may not be relevant to the research and will not be included. • Transpose the data to a separate document for each participant according to the matching headings.

(continued)

TABLE 6.2   Data analysis: Step 1, narrative analysis (story creation) (*continued*)

STEPS	RESEARCHER ACTIONS
3 Story creation	• Write a story for each participant using the headings identified in Step 2. • Write the story in the third person, past tense. For example, Stapleton's thesis (2008) on caring for an adult child with a mental illness begins Maggie's story under the heading 'Early Days' as follows: 'Maggie recalled that Emma (daughter) "loved primary school" but on entering high school she revealed, "it was shocking. She was bullied from the day she went" … Reflecting on that time, Maggie was saddened that she "couldn't protect her" from the other children and regretted having not done something about it at the time. "I should have put my foot down", she said. "It ruined everything" (p. 22). • Continue in a similar vein until you have written a short and lucid account of the participant's experience, inserting direct references to the transcript where appropriate. • Edit the story carefully and ensure that references to the transcript are accurate. • Send a copy of the story, neatly printed and soft-bound, to the participant. • Request feedback from the participant if ethics approval has been granted to do so.

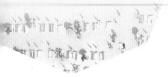

RESEARCH IN PRACTICE

WHEN RESEARCHERS HAVE CONCERNS ABOUT PARTICIPANTS' REACTION TO THEIR CREATED STORY

Sharing created stories with participants can present researchers with some concerns, particularly when participants have recounted traumatic or distressing experiences. Participants' potential reactions are part of a researcher's ethical obligations. It is appropriate to offer additional support or links to supports or debriefing if participants experience distress on reading their constructed stories. It should not be assumed, however, that reading accounts of distressing experiences in constructed stories will necessarily be distressing for participants. For some people, witnessing their lives as constructed into a story by a researcher can be affirming, enjoyable and empowering—this was our experience in sharing stories with participants in a recent unpublished study.

Similarly, in an Honours study conducted by Angell (2011) on five mothers caring for a young person with first-episode psychosis, we were concerned for the participants' reaction to reading their story as it involved their reflections on the circumstances surrounding their child's hospital admission and treatment. During the interviews the mothers had described traumatic experiences as their child became increasingly unwell, withdrawn and sometimes violent and destructive to others and themselves. While the focus of the study was on how the mothers' self-care, productive and leisure occupations were affected by their child's illness, we thought that their willingness to recount some extraordinary circumstances could not be overlooked in the final created story. In order to remain faithful to their narratives and provide participants with an accurate account of their experience, we discussed support mechanisms we had initiated at the research proposal stage for participants to seek counselling through their child's health service if they experienced upset or distress. In the end, our concerns did not materialise. The participants had not experienced distress in reading their story and had the opportunity at the second interview to correct any inaccuracies that did not fit with their experience. Further, it seems that in recounting their story of taking up a caring role they had not expected to give expression to thoughts and feelings that had been dormant in the face of demanding caring duties. Providing participants with their story written in the third person, past tense was seen as therapeutic, and a valued document that could potentially be shared with family and friends.

Note: the results of a narrative enquiry are presented in the form of individual stories created according to the steps outlined above.

Following this creative act of writing a story derived from the original transcript, the second step in analysis involves a shift in focus to analysing the individual story in conjunction with all the stories comprising the study. Josselson (2011, p. 239) refers to this two-stage process as deconstructing the story, followed by a reconstruction of the story. The reconstruction occurs 'in conversation with the theoretical and conceptual literature, either to critique existing concepts or to extend and deepen them', to arrive at a deeper understanding of the stated research question. A chapter by Josselson in Wertz *et al.* (2011) provides an example of the processes used in the narrative analysis of Teresa, a singer, and her experience of loss as a result of throat cancer. Josselson describes her method for identifying themes (p. 232) then shows the themes she identified from Teresa's story. Her description of the process of theme generation is helpful for less experienced researchers who may be seeking clearly defined themes that tend not to materialise. Josselson recounts her relief in noticing how the categories she has identified blur and intertwine; she takes this as reassurance that she has effectively captured the complex, layered and linked strands of the narrated life she is analysing.

The benefits of narrative enquiry

A concluding question relates to how narrative enquiry can be used. How might the findings of narrative studies benefit our understanding of people? In the context of this book, what does narrative enquiry add to our understanding of people's health and

TABLE 6.3   Data analysis: Step 2, analysis of narratives

STEPS	RESEARCHER ACTIONS
1 Transcript and narrative review	• In preparation for analysis of each story and the development of themes relevant to all the stories, revisit each transcript *and* story to fully appreciate the participants' experiences.
2 Story preparation for analysis	• Create a new document for each story, allowing 70 characters per line and two columns to the right of equal width to facilitate the next step in analysis.
3 Analysing the stories: first response to the story	• In the column closest to the story, enter your initial response to the details contained in each sentence. • Ask the question, 'What is this sentence about?' • Insert your interpretation in a few words or a phrase. • Repeat this process for the whole story. • Observe that the central column now has a distilled version of the story in your own words. • Repeat for all stories in the study.
4 Analysing the stories: developing provisional categories and creating a thematic schema	• Discuss this process with a supervisor or co-researcher to confirm the attribution of categories (and their definitions) to each story. Once you have verified these categories to your satisfaction, map out a categorising system to represent the relationship within and between each category. You will most likely develop a hierarchical categorising system to reflect these relationships. • You are now positioned to convert your categorising system into a thematic system or schema that provides you with the themes and subthemes relevant to the study findings. • For example, Stapleton's thesis on older caregivers of an adult child with a mental illness developed three themes: a) *Caring—A Productive Occupation*; b) *Caring and Growing Older*; c) *Influences on Occupations in Later Life*. Three of the five subthemes relating to the first theme were identified as: 1) Providing a home; 2) Managing and monitoring the illness; 3) Providing links to the community (Stapleton 2008, p. 43). • Write the discussion according to the themes derived from the stories and outlined above. The discussion follows a logical progression according to the themes and subthemes identified in this process.

experiences of health care? Frank (2000, 2010), Kleinman (1988) and others have argued that eliciting and sharing stories is valuable both for those who tell and those who listen. Indeed, narrative therapies (based on the work of White & Epston 1990) are founded on beliefs that storying and re-storying can liberate people from stuck or frozen narratives and facilitate healing and transformation. We argue that opportunities to share stories (and to read stories constructed sensitively by narrative researchers) can be rewarding, enjoyable, enlightening and even therapeutic for research participants. In our experience, most participants welcome the return of created stories in an attractively presented document and few request changes to researchers' interpretation of their story. This created story document provides a record of a participant's experience, skills or knowledge in a particular domain and evidences their commitment to the research project.

Charon (2012) argues that narrative understanding of people and their experiences of illness is required to stir empathic and human responses by health practitioners. Studies that generate narratives and translate understandings found within and across stories allow health practitioners access to the unknown worlds of health care recipients, and thus provide opportunities to respond in ways that better meet recipients' needs. The capacity of stories to hold an overall or holistic account of phenomena, as opposed to fragmented parts of the whole picture, is another benefit of narrative enquiry (Goodfellow 1997).

On the other hand, Josselson (2006, p. 3) has argued that small studies that produce 'highly individualised' accounts of phenomena in different locations, with different researchers, raise questions about how to 'build a knowledge base that can amalgamate the insight and understandings across researchers'. This is an important issue and one that warrants serious consideration in health sciences research. There are clear arguments for narrative studies in the health sciences to develop beyond individual accounts of experience if we are 'to understand the patterns that cohere among individuals and the aspects of lived experience that differentiate' them (p. 5). Josselson's article sets out a number of ideas that might contribute to this 'amalgamation of narrative knowledge' (p. 8) and invites researchers to enter conversations about how to enable this to happen. By extension, the challenge to expand the benefits and uses of narrative enquiry in the health sciences is worth taking up. In this historical moment, there are any number of health professionals engaging in narrative research supported by a proliferation of journals and texts on the subject. Bringing together a community of researchers to envisage integrating knowledge derived from multiple studies is both timely and essential. The effort of narrative health science researchers to deliver best practice and fully understand the range of human experiences and behaviours is worth pursuing.

STOP AND THINK

Have you ever questioned the value of small studies in qualitative research? What do you think about Josselson's comment about building knowledge from individual insights or from small studies?

- In your professional practice, are you aware of having developed insights into clients' experience of an illness or treatment from listening to an individual's story of rehabilitation or recovery?
- Briefly record what you have learnt from a specific client. Did this help you to understand other clients' experience?
- Do you have colleagues working in the same or similar professional area, with whom you could develop a 'community of researchers' to expand knowledge of your area of interest?
- Write brief notes on what you would be interested in researching and search the databases to see if there are any qualitative studies on that topic.

Priscilla Ennals and Linsey Howie

Summary

This chapter has introduced health science researchers to the main aspects of conducting a narrative enquiry. The method offers a creative means of studying a phenomenon while drawing on the strengths of individuals to recount their experience of events, and the researchers' skill in entering a dialogue in order to elicit the richness of individual experience. The chapter has provided a background to narrative enquiry, its origins and practical application. While it acknowledges the diversity of narrative methods, one specific procedure is outlined to support the conduct of research when research questions lend themselves to the exploration of experience through the story form.

The inventive and interpretive steps associated with this method can be disquieting to researchers steeped in positivist approaches to research. This chapter describes rigorous data collection and analysis procedures, and transparent reporting mechanisms to illuminate aspects of the method and guide the further development of narrative enquiry in the health sciences.

Practice exercises

1   You are preparing to conduct a narrative enquiry and want some experience of analysing data to create a story. In the first person, past tense write two to four pages on an everyday recent experience that you can readily recall, such as preparing a meal for friends or family, taking a trip to the zoo or going to the beach for a swim. Without too much thought, begin to write (word-process) your account of the experience beginning at a point that seems right to you. Continue to write in as much detail as you can remember about the experience: what you did, where it happened, who was present. Include your thoughts and feelings about the experience (to the extent that you are prepared to commit them to paper) until you reach a conclusion to your story. You now have a transcript with which to practise writing a story.

2   Follow Steps 1–3 outlined in Table 6.2 until you have written a short and lucid account of your experience in the third person, inserting direct references to your transcript where appropriate and adding interpretive details if they seem relevant, given a second or third reading of your story.

3   Let us assume your name is Mary and you chose to write about going to the beach. Your created story will be different from the transcript, but it will reflect the facts, situation, elements or mood in your original account and may provide insights not evident in your original telling of events. It might begin as follows:

Mary remembered that the night before she arranged to go to the beach with friends, the weather forecast had been for a hot summer day. She was not looking forward to the day. She had recently moved unexpectedly from interstate and she did not want to 'disappoint her new friends'.

4   This small excerpt raises questions about collecting and analysing data in narrative studies. You will be aware that there are many factors influencing an individual's experience and telling of events and that they are open to various interpretations, depending on a multitude of prior experiences, memories, cultural and societal values and other factors. In this passage, some researchers might be surprised that Mary did not eagerly anticipate going to the beach on a hot day. Others might question the relevance of her reference to a recent and unexpected move from interstate. Remember that the questions we choose to ask in research interviews (and how participants understand and respond to our questions), and what we bring to interpreting data, are central to the rigorous conduct of narrative enquiry and all qualitative research.

    (a) Are you familiar with the literature on reflexivity and ethical aspects of the research relationship in qualitative research?

    (b) Are you aware of the standpoint in narrative studies that researcher self-knowledge is of prime importance in all aspects of the enquiry?

    (c) If you would like to know more about this issue, see Cho and Trent (2014), Curtin and Fossey (2007) and Josselson (2007, pp. 537–66).

    (d) What areas of research are of most interest to you, what specific population, age group or gender, and why? How did you develop this interest? Why is this important to establish?

5   Reread your created story carefully and observe the impact on yourself of reading your story when written in the third person. In a few words, or a sentence or two, write about the impact on you, beginning with an 'I' statement and using the present tense: 'I am …' What have you learnt in completing this exercise:

    (a) as a researcher?

    (b) as a potential participant in a narrative study?

Further reading

Clandinin, J. (2013). *Engaging in narrative inquiry*. Walnut Creek, CA: Left Coast Press.

Cortazzi, M. (2014). *Narrative analysis* (Vol. 12). Milton Park: Routledge.

DeFina, A. & Georgakopoulou, A. (eds) (2015). *The handbook of narrative analysis*. Chichester: Wiley Blackwell.

Dollard, J. (1949). *Criteria for the life history*, 2nd edn. New York: Peter Smith.

Priscilla Ennals and Linsey Howie

Emden, C. (1998a). Conducting narrative analysis. *Collegian,* 5(3), 34–9.

Emden, C. (1998b). Theoretical perspectives on narrative inquiry. *Collegian*, 5(2), 30–5.

Feldman, S. & Howie, L. (2009). Looking back, looking forward: reflections on using a life history review tool with older people. *Journal of Applied Gerontology*, 28(5), 621–37.

Josselson, R. (2007). The ethical attitude in narrative research: principles and practicalities. In J.D. Clandinin (ed.), *Handbook of narrative inquiry: mapping the methodology*. Thousand Oaks, CA: Sage, 537–66.

Riessman, C.K. (2008). *Narrative methods for the human sciences*. Los Angeles: Sage.

Websites

www.clarku.edu/faculty/mbamberg/narrativeINQ

> *Narrative Inquiry* is the continuation of the *Journal of Narrative and Life History* (1990–97), and its focus on theoretical approaches and analysis of narratives is very useful for researchers in health sciences, nursing and social work.

http://qix.sagepub.com

> This website is a link to Sage Publications and the journals *Qualitative Inquiry* and *Qualitative Health Research*. It offers a free sample of an issue that can be printed but not saved to your computer.

7

Ethnography as Health Research

JON WILLIS AND KAREN ANDERSON

Chapter objectives

In this chapter you will learn:

- about the history and tradition of ethnography
- how ethnography applies to research in health care
- what are focused ethnography, institutional ethnography and ethno-nursing
- how to design an ethnographic study

Key terms

Case study in qualitative research

Culture

Emic

Ethnography

Ethno-nursing

Etic

Focused ethnography

Institutional ethnography

Key informant

Meta-ethnography

Netnography

Observation

Qualitative data analysis

Participant observation

Photovoice

Postmodern ethnography

Thick description

Introduction

Ethnography: A research method that focuses on the scientific study of the lived culture of groups of people, used to discover and describe individual social and cultural groups.

Ethnography is a research method that focuses on the scientific study of the lived culture of groups of people (O'Reilly 2012). The word is derived from two Greek words: εθνος (*ethnos*), meaning nation or people, and Γράφειν (*graphein*), meaning to write. It was first coined in 1834, and the method enjoyed considerable popularity and growth through its association with the profession of anthropology during the nineteenth century as a tool of colonial expansion through the auspices of the Royal Anthropological Society in Great Britain and the Smithsonian Institute in America (see Ellen 1984 for a brief survey of the very early history of the method). Although often conceived as a single method—the 'ethnographic method'—with a single object of study—culture—ethnography has historically developed as a suite of techniques of field data collection that include participant observation, key informant interviews, social network analysis (such as genealogical analysis), and social and other mapping. Equally, the focus of ethnographic study has shifted from the totalising gaze of early ethnographers on the culture of native groups in far-flung places. Ethnographers now seek to gain in-depth understanding of people and events within local cultures, whether these are the meaning-making practices of ethnic groups, or those of neighbourhoods, institutions or social groups defined without regard to ethnicity. In recent years, ethnography has begun to focus on the shared meaning-making of groups that transcend local and even geographical boundaries, for example the ethnography of multiple users in cyberspace. It has become increasingly useful as a tool for developing in-depth understandings of the workings of complex institutions, including those of the health care system (Savage 2000; Coates 2004; Liamputtong 2013).

A method with a long pedigree

Culture: The knowledge people use to generate and interpret social behaviour.

The notion of **culture** is central in ethnography and is based on the assumption that any human group that spends time together will develop a culture. Although there are many possible definitions, for the purposes of ethnography we suggest a broad definition of culture, such as that proposed by McCurdy and colleagues (2005, p. 8), who define culture as 'the knowledge people use to generate and interpret social behaviour'. In the mid- to late nineteenth century, early ethnographers such as Sir Edward Tylor, Lewis Henry Morgan and Sir James Frazer worked by analysing the published reports of missionaries, travellers and colonial officials to derive their understandings of the cultures about which those authors wrote. These researchers were mainly working in the academic tradition of Victorian natural science, and used a comparative method to show how all human societies passed through evolutionary stages. Their studies emphasised the ways in which the customs and beliefs of so-called primitive societies resembled each other and, by tracing a natural evolution to modernity, helped to justify colonial interference in those societies. These early ethnographers also began a tradition of exploring health beliefs and practices, particularly through the examination of 'magical' and religious beliefs and their relationship to modern science and medicine. At the same time, philosophers working in the French sociological tradition, such as Durkheim, Mauss and Levy-Bruhl, brought considerable scientific rigour to the comparative method and began to write ethnographic work that focused on the unique features of single societies.

In the early twentieth century, a new generation of professional anthropologists, as they were known then, grew out of the training opportunities afforded by the establishment of schools of anthropology at major universities such as Oxford (1884), Cambridge (1900) and University College London (1908) (Evans-Pritchard 1951). The Cambridge school is credited with some of the earliest ethnographic fieldwork, and advanced the discipline by sending multidisciplinary teams of researchers under the direction of marine biologist A.C. Haddon to remote locations (such as Melanesia and the Torres Strait in 1898) to conduct systematic fieldwork for the first time. Franz Boas began developing and teaching a form of ethnographic field research at Columbia University in the USA from 1899, based on his early experience of geographic studies on Baffin Island in the Arctic. These early university programs trained a generation of professional anthropologists who made significant advances in the development of ethnographic field methods; among them were Bronislaw Malinowski, A.R. Radcliffe-Brown, E.E. Evans-Pritchard, A.L. Kroeber, Edward Sapir, Ruth Benedict and Margaret Mead.

In these earliest renderings, ethnography continued to focus on a range of cultural practices and beliefs, and ethnographers regarded the local customs and social issues of small-scale societies as highly important. Malinowski was the first anthropologist to translate an abstract and inclusive concept of culture from a local language into a series of famous studies that coupled intensive field data with the conceptual and theoretical insights that are typical of modern ethnography (Hughes 1992; Baillie 1995). Malinowski developed the tradition that ethnography was conducted by living among other cultures for months, even years. He states that 'the final goal of which the ethnographer should never lose sight … is briefly to grasp the natives' point of view, his relation to life, and to realise his vision of his world' (Malinowski 1922/1961, p. 25). Malinowski's development of the ethnographic method was partly accidental—he became stranded in Melanesia when the First World War broke out and was forced to remain in the field for several years. Because of this involuntary sojourn, he was able to collect the ethnographic data that formed the backbone of his classic monographs *Argonauts of the Western Pacific* (1922/1961) and *The sexual life of savages in north-western Melanesia* (1932).

STOP AND THINK

- How would you go about grasping someone else's point of view?
- What is your vision of your world? How would you communicate it to someone else?

Other anthropologists were working in similar ways at the time. Radcliffe-Brown took the insights of Durkheim's sociological theory and applied them to field data he collected in the Andaman Islands and Central Australia to produce the classic monographs *The Andaman Islanders* (1922/1964) and *The social organization of Australian tribes* (1931). Evans-Pritchard, working in the Sudan among the Azande and Nuer tribespeople, combined the methodological insights of Malinowski and the theoretical complexity of Radcliffe-Brown to produce the first anthropological work that concentrated on medical practices and beliefs; he is often regarded as the father of medical anthropology. Evans-Pritchard's monograph on Azande religion, *Witchcraft, oracles and magic among the Azande* (1937), remains an important source of insight for any student applying the ethnographic method to scientific or medical beliefs.

The later work of Margaret Mead opened the door to a new generation of anthropologists who turned the ethnographic gaze back on their own societies. Although Mead began her ethnographic work by examining diverse foreign cultures, including those of Samoa (1961), highland New Guinea (1942, 1956, 1968, 1977) and Bali (Bateson & Mead 1942; Mead & Macgregor 1951), theoretical insights from these studies led her to examine similar areas of culture within her own society of the USA (1944). She became interested in education and socialisation (Mead 1951; Mead & Wolfenstein 1955; Mead & American Museum of Natural History 1970), in aspects of race (American Association for the Advancement of Science & Mead 1968; Mead & Baldwin 1971), and in women's place in the family in Western societies (Mead 1949, 1965; Mead & Heyman 1965). Mead's lead in applying ethnographic research methods to contemporary societies and problems was taken up by the sociology department at the University of Chicago (also known as the Chicago or Ecological School) from the 1920s onwards. After the Second World War, the Chicago School began a series of ethnographic studies known as the Chicago Area Project that contributed significant methodological developments to ethnography via the study of crime and delinquency, particularly through the use of ecological mapping techniques and of ecological theory as a frame of reference for their enquiries. Ethnographies such as Suttles' (1968) *The social order of the slum* and Hirschi's (1969) *Causes of delinquency* are examples of Chicago School contemporary ethnographies. In recent years, the tradition of urban ethnography in the classic style continues in the work of researchers like Philippe Bourgois, who has done complex ethnographic research in crack houses in East Harlem and among urban drug users in San Francisco (Bourgois 1995; Bourgois & Schonberg 2009).

Postmodern ethnography: Requires a traditional commitment to observation and the use of key informants as the basis for description and analysis of the social world.

Key informant: An individual who is able to provide in-depth information to an ethnographer, a notion used more often in ethnographic research than other qualitative methods.

The more recent innovations in **postmodern ethnography** continue to focus on conveying the cultural experience of another person (Marcus & Fischer 1999; Hammersley & Atkinson 2007). Postmodern ethnography still requires the traditional methodological commitment to observation and the use of **key informants** as the basis for detailed description and structural analysis of the social world. With realist ethnography, it shares a commitment to the use of cases, particularly cases of conflict where individual interests seem opposed to social forces, as in the work of Victor Turner (1968). What is distinctive in postmodern ethnography is an embedded sense of what it is like to live in the social world so described. The approaches used most commonly are life history (e.g. Shostak's *Nisa: the life and words of a !Kung woman* [1983] or Crapanzano's *Tuhami: portrait of a Moroccan* [1980]) and the lifecycle (e.g. Rosaldo's *Knowledge and passion: Ilongot notion of self and social life* [1980]). Ethnographers use these techniques in combination to provide greater ethnographic richness, as well as to improve the reliability of both data and interpretation. For example, the approach of Levy (1988, p. xix) in describing mind and experience in Tahiti involved a period of unstructured household observation and participation in village life, coupled with systematic, relatively formal interviewing of individual informants to establish life histories. Once his language was adequate to the task and he had achieved a strong degree of acceptance from his informants, he followed up with detailed but unstructured interviews with twenty informants, aimed at eliciting individuals' responses to their life history and to their present life. Shore (1982, p. xv), working in Samoa to unravel the symbols and meanings that give structure to social relations, based his work on observations over a seven-year period: household surveys, fifty-five two-hour interviews, a questionnaire delivered to 140 schoolchildren, and analysis of published materials and recordings made of meetings, speeches, songs, plays and other cultural performances. His use of a dramatic incident, a murder, like Geertz's cockfight (1973, pp. 412–53), provided a structure on which to centre his analysis.

As our notions of geography have expanded beyond the physical into cyberspace, so our notions of the social and cultural now take into account virtual experience, identity, interaction and community. Consequently, ethnographic innovation since 2010 has focused on collecting data on, and conveying, cultural institutions and experiences online, and the subdiscipline of virtual ethnography—*netnography*, a term coined by Kozinets (2002)—is emerging. Netnography has been particularly influenced by techniques developed in online marketing research, as well as traditional methods of participant and non-participant observation, reflective fieldnote-taking, and a variety of computer-assisted methods of data quantification and qualitative analysis. Because online activity is typically framed through text, the collection and analysis of naturally occurring text has formed a key part of these methods. The use of multiple techniques, however, distinguishes netnography from simple content analysis.

Ethnography in health settings

Despite the methodological, theoretical and disciplinary shifts over the past century, contemporary ethnography remains embedded in the traditions and practices of anthropology. 'Ethnography' nowadays refers to both the processes for accomplishing it—which generally involves conducting fieldwork and always requires the reorganisation and editing of materials for presentation—and the presentation itself, the product of that research, which usually takes form as prose (Wolcott 1990). Ethnographic approaches have been applied in a range of contemporary settings including hospitals, businesses, schools and communities—regardless of setting, the focus remains on culture (see Dykes & Flacking 2016). Ethnographic research is as useful to the study of problems defined and dealt with by human groups as it has traditionally been in the study of systems of belief, of religious frameworks or of world-views (O'Reilly 2012). Ethnographic approaches are also useful in the study of the structures that underpin how people organise their accounts of their social world (Wolcott 1990; O'Reilly 2012).

Because ethnography is used in a range of settings and disciplines, several approaches to ethnography have developed, including focused ethnography, institutional ethnography and ethno-nursing.

Focused ethnography

Ethnographers do not always have to be holistic, cross-cultural and comparative and do not need to spend extensive periods of time in the field when they wish to explore a problem or are asked a question. The tenets of traditional ethnography do not need to be followed faithfully, especially when researchers are working under the constraints of time and scope (Wolcott 1990; Higginbottom & Liamputtong 2015).

Focused 'micro-ethnography' concentrates on a single problem in a particular setting. Rather than attempting to portray an entire cultural system, **focused ethnography** draws on the cultural ethos of a microcosm to study selected aspects of everyday life. It gives emphasis to particular behaviours in specific settings and allows researchers to work within time and scope limitations by narrowing the focus and providing objectives that are more manageable. Focused ethnography is also known as specific, particularistic or mini-ethnography (Wolcott 1990; de Laine 1997; Morse & Richards 2002; Higginbottom & Liamputtong 2015).

Traditional and micro-ethnographic approaches can be applied to any social unit or isolated human group that is under enquiry, and is common in nursing (Leininger 1985, 1994; de Laine 1997; Liamputtong 2013). Ethnographic research in nursing can focus on a hospital, community health centre, nursing home, general practitioner's rooms or a hospital ward, and can assist researchers and practitioners in understanding 'cultural rules and norms as well as values as they are related to health and illness behaviour' (Morse 1994a, p. 172).

Focused ethnography can be used to explore special topics or shared experiences. It is different from traditional ethnography in that the topic is specific and can be identified before the researcher begins the study (Muecke 1994; Morse & Richards 2002). The use of focused ethnography in nursing research and health research is becoming more common. Along with time limitations, limitations in knowledge and experience may preclude the use of a more traditional ethnographic approach. A more focused approach allows the scope of the research to be clarified for the researcher and allows researchers to enter and experience the richness of the real world of people within a particular setting (Leininger 1985). **Netnography** has a particular value as a methodological approach in focused ethnography, and has been used most effectively to track emergent health-related trends, to examine peer and support networks for particular diseases and conditions, and to understand the penetration of health information and health word-of-mouth in specific consumer, patient or practitioner virtual communities.

Institutional ethnography

Institutional ethnography is a qualitative mode of social enquiry that was developed with the aim of discovering or exposing the chains of coordination and control in a social system or among settings of everyday life (Smith 1987; DeVault & McCoy 2002; Mykhalovskiy & McCoy 2002; Winkelman & Halifax 2007). According to Travers (1996, p. 544), the combination of 'institutional' and 'ethnography' implies the need to move away from the particular to an

Focused ethnography: Concentrates on a single problem in a particular setting.

Netnography: Collecting data on, and conveying, cultural institutions and experiences online.

Institutional ethnography: Its aim is to discover and expose the chains of coordination and control in a social system or among settings of everyday life.

explanation of the 'intersections of local practices [with] practices beyond immediate experience'. Although similar to other forms of ethnography, institutional ethnography is not empirically focused on 'experience' or 'culture', but rather on social organisation. It is concerned with exploring and describing the social and institutional forces that shape, limit and otherwise organise people's everyday worlds (Mykhalovskiy & McCoy 2002).

Institutional ethnography allows the researcher to access the possibility of explaining how institutional processes are embodied in people's everyday experiences (Kirkham 2003). It explores what is happening to people in local settings such as schools or hospitals, but is not limited to the designated organisational spaces. The aim is to explore how and what is happening to people in these settings, and how their experience is coordinated with and organised by organisational activities or work practices (Mykhalovskiy & McCoy 2002). The purpose of institutional ethnography is not to generalise about a group of people but to find and describe the social processes that might have generalising effects (DeVault & McCoy 2002).

Ethno-nursing

Ethnography has been used in a variety of ways to explore nursing and is continually being developed as a method for research (Laugharne 1995). Ethnography has also been used to study groups of students or nurses (MacKenzie 1992; Baillie 1995). For example, MacKenzie's study seeks to understand the learning experiences of district nursing students in the community setting and examines their learning using a series of interviews and observations.

Ethno-nursing is defined by Leininger (1979, p. 38) as the 'study and analysis of the local or indigenous people's viewpoints, beliefs and practices about nursing care phenomena and processes of designated cultures'. The use of ethnography as a method for research in nursing allows nursing to be studied within the natural setting and viewed within the context in which it occurs, as well as studying areas that have not been previously explored (Baillie 1995). It can be used to document, describe and explain nursing phenomena in relation to care, health, illness prevention and illness or injury recovery using information from nurses, clients and nursing or health institutions (Leininger 1985). It can provide in-depth data and detailed accounts of nursing phenomena or experiences, and it can give a holistic view not otherwise gained through other research methods (Aamodt 1982).

Ethno-nursing: A method where ethnography is used to document and explain nursing phenomena in relation to care, health, illness prevention and so on.

STOP AND THINK

- Think about the last time you were ill. What kind of things that happened were typical of responses to illness in your culture?
- If you consulted a doctor or a pharmacist as part of your illness, think about the consultation as a kind of cultural performance. What were the roles involved?
- Was the interaction culturally scripted in some way? Did all participants understand and play their roles according to the cultural script?
- What kind of language was used?

Jon Willis and Karen Anderson

The flexibility of ethnography allows its use in a variety of settings in the nursing discipline, so researchers can explore whole wards or units within the hospital setting. In addition, the use of a combination of data collection methods allows researchers to acquire enough information to present a comprehensive account of the phenomena being studied (Robertson & Boyle 1984; Baillie 1995). The nursing profession needs to develop a meaningful knowledge and theory base in order to allow nursing practice to evolve, and the use of ethnography as a research method has potential to contribute to this knowledge base (Robertson & Boyle 1984).

Meta-ethnography

Meta-ethnography: An approach that enables a rigorous procedure for deriving substantive interpretations about any set of ethnographic or interpretive studies.

Meta-ethnography was developed by Noblit and Hare (1988) as a way of conducting systematic reviews of ethnographic studies. Although their seven-step process is now more than twenty years old, it is increasingly popular in published studies in the health field (e.g. Campbell *et al.* 2003; Ring *et al.* 2007; Chapter 18). The object of meta-ethnography is to provide a new third-order interpretation of ethnographic data, incorporating not only the participants' published data and author interpretations from the original studies, but also reciprocal or refutational translation synthesis (e.g. comparing the experience of one condition against that of another, or one type of treatment against another, and identifying comparable as well as oppositional accounts) and then line-of-argument synthesis (weaving the examined similarities and differences between cases into an integrated line of argument that fits all the studies) (Mays *et al.* 2005). Meta-ethnography focuses on the translation of salient categories of meaning, so is focused not on pooling data from one study to another but on finding a new interpretation through thematic analysis and constant comparison techniques.

Designing an ethnographic study

Etic: An outsider's perspective. In ethnographic studies conducted from the etic perspective, the researcher has no knowledge of or experience in the culture they are studying.

Although the approach of ethnography does not have a primary focus on numeric measurements, it uses both qualitative and quantitative information to search for and find regularities in phenomena. The regularities it searches for are patterns of observed events that can subsequently be analysed in more detail using various tools, including quantitative methods (Hughes 1992). Ethnographic approaches employ various data collection and analysis techniques such as individual and group interviews, key informant and focus group interviews, structured and unstructured observation, and unobtrusive methods (including document analysis) (O'Reilly 2012; Liamputtong 2013; see also Chapters 4, 5).

Emic: An insider's perspective, that is, conducted in your own culture, such as an intensive care nurse conducting research within an intensive care ward.

The standpoint of the researcher in ethnographic studies can be either **etic** (outsider's perspective) or **emic** (insider's perspective). In ethnographic studies conducted from the etic perspective, the researcher has no knowledge of or experience in the culture they are studying. Studies conducted from an emic perspective are conducted in the researcher's own culture, such as an intensive care nurse conducting research within an intensive care ward (Byrne 2001). The ethnographer determines the epistemology on which ethnography is based, and this is usually determined by the techniques the researcher uses to acquire knowledge.

Knowledge that is acquired through an understanding of the meaning of behaviour according to the perceptions and interpretations of those who engage in that behaviour requires a methodology that explains how those engaging in the behaviour construct reality in their own terms (Pelto & Pelto 1978; Schwartz & Jacobs 1979). An etic epistemology assumes that the meaning of behaviour can be best interpreted and explained by the researcher within their own dimensions (Robertson & Boyle 1984; Barratt 1991).

STOP AND THINK

- What might be some of the differences between an emic and etic point of view of a cultural celebration like a birthday party?
- Make a list of the different ways a small gift like a bunch of flowers can be interpreted.

Neither approach should be employed alone, nor does one approach hold a higher or lower scientific status than the other (Robertson & Boyle 1984; de Laine 1997; Suwankhong & Liamputtong 2015). While the goal of good ethnographic research is to provide an analysis of society from an observer's point of view, human behaviour can usually be properly understood only in context, in the natural setting in which it occurs (Robertson & Boyle 1984; de Laine 1997).

THE TEACHING OF KNOWLEDGE AND SKILLS IN NURSING

In a recent study, Karen Anderson explored the health promotion knowledge and skills taught in a university nursing course and graduate nurses' health promotion practices. She writes:

The research was inspired by a need to increase insight into the teaching and practice of health promotion in nursing. Consistent with focused ethnography, my study focused on the subcultural groups of nursing students and graduate nurses and university and health care institutions. It also drew on an aspect of traditional ethnography in that the culture was unfamiliar to me. I was able to use principles of institutional ethnography to explore the designated organisational spaces such as university and hospitals, the social process in these organisations, and how they affect health promotion in nursing.

After conducting a literature review to explore how these areas have been dealt with by previous research, and to refine my research questions and approach, I designed a study in two phases. The first stage looked at how health promotion is taught in an undergraduate nursing degree, and the second focused on how graduate nurses use their health promotion skills in clinical practice.

In the first stage, I collected data through observations of health promotion units in the Bachelor of Nursing degree, document collection and analysis, and interviews with teaching staff and focus group discussion with nursing students. I selected these techniques for the different aspects they would capture of the teaching of

RESEARCH IN PRACTICE

health promotion in nursing. To be an unobtrusive observer, I worked on fitting in to my field setting in a number of ways. I made sure my behaviour was appropriate to the personal attitudes, values and beliefs of my informants. It was also about genuinely caring for their experiences, and also using my own personal experiences and history both as a university student and in health promotion to respond to informants. My knowledge of health promotion and experiences as a student assisted in establishing credibility and ensuring that a level of trust and rapport was established. As a researcher, I needed a level of intuitiveness to synthesise the experience of the informants through immediate contact and empathy, and to be receptive to the experiences of those providing the data, to be willing to be taught by the participants and always be open to their feedback. My participants were my co-researchers, so it was vital for there to be a sense of reciprocity. They needed to feel that I was on an equal footing with them and not exerting power over them. Sensitivity was also important, and my perceptions and experiences of the field setting needed to be seen, heard and reported accurately. As a participant observer, I was effectively the data collection instrument, so I had to be dynamic rather than static when measuring what was going on around me.

Gaining entry to the field

An important initial step in ethnographic research is gaining entry to the field. This involves more than just getting formal permission to conduct the research. One aspect of gaining entry into the field is identifying gatekeepers, especially within the formal structure of organisations (Hammersley & Atkinson 2007; Liamputtong 2013; Suwankhong & Liamputtong 2015). Gatekeeping is not a new or unusual phenomenon in health care or health care research. Gatekeepers can allow or deny researchers' access to the setting or to participants, and offer protection to vulnerable people, such as patients, their families and health care professionals. Gatekeepers can provide protection at an organisational and professional level (Holloway & Wheeler 2002; Lee 2005; Suwankhong & Liamputtong 2015).

STOP AND THINK

- Imagine you want to do a study of a local high school. Who are the gatekeepers?
- What kind of approaches might you use to get the gatekeepers on your side?

Working with gatekeepers can assist in increasing the trust and rapport with participants. Establishing rapport is an essential part of fieldwork, and develops an affinity between researcher and participants. Good rapport increases the validity and reliability of the fieldwork, as participants are likely to be more truthful and accurate in their responses (Liamputtong 2007, 2010, 2013). Gatekeepers play an important role in initial negotiations to conduct ethnographic research (Suwankhong & Liamputtong 2015). One of the problems here is that gatekeepers need to maintain the integrity of the organisation and the picture that the ethnographic researcher might create. As a result, they may block or limit certain paths of enquiry, which could limit the effectiveness of the research, or which may result in the researcher having to choose approaches that are alternatively secretive or deceptive (Hammersley & Atkinson 2007). Such approaches pose ethical difficulties that may discourage the researcher, damage their relationships or reputation, or damage the integrity and reliability of the research. Negotiating the research question and methods so that they satisfy the requirements of the gatekeeper, as well as complying with rigorous and ethical research requirements, is usually a better tactic (e.g. Willis & Saunders 2007, p. 102 ff).

Data collection and analysis techniques in ethnography

Regardless of ontological or epistemological framing (see Chapter 1), ethnographic research is well served by a range of qualitative techniques for data collection and analysis, particularly where researchers are interested in exploring multiple realities and experiences in the terms of those who are living them (Coates 2004; O'Reilly 2012; Creswell 2013; Liamputtong 2013). These include observation techniques such as participant and simple observation, a range of interview techniques such as key informant, life history and diary-interview techniques, focus and other group interview techniques, and case studies. In recent years, ethnographic techniques have also encompassed a range of visual, mapping and sorting techniques. See Chapters 4, 5, 6, 9, 10.

PARTICIPANT ASSENT AND OBSERVATION

In the first stage of Karen's research, she made initial contact with the Head of School, Nursing and Midwifery, and the Bachelor of Nursing Course Co-coordinator, to identify the relevant nursing units to observe and to identify the unit convenors. She talked to the convenor in order to gain approval to conduct observations in both of the identified units and to approach the other member of the teaching staff. She asked teaching staff in each unit to inform the students of the purpose of the research and observations and to gain their assent to observations being carried out in their presence, before the start of observations. She looked for students' verbal assent in the units being observed, as opposed to their informed consent. Participant verbal assent in observational studies is a common and accepted practice; activities or events are observed and recorded rather than data from or about participants.

Initial observations were carried out in each of the units when she first entered the field. Exploratory observations allowed her to observe and capture the big picture of the people and the events in the field. Further observations and a structured audit tool were used to narrow the focus of enquiry to the health promotion topics that were taught in each of the health promotion units. The audit tool was used to explore the health promotion theories and concepts that were taught as well as health promotion skills, student assessments and the links between the units and nursing competencies. Unobtrusive observations were carried out in each of the units. The nature of the lecture environments and class sizes meant that she was able to sit among other students and unobtrusively observe the teaching of health promotion in nursing. All observations in both lectures and tutorials were audio-recorded to increase the rigour of data collected and to aid in analysis.

RESEARCH IN PRACTICE

Jon Willis and Karen Anderson

Data collection methods

Observation has long been a technical mainstay of ethnographic data collection. Ethnographic fieldwork is typically framed around participant observation, in which 'the ethnographer enters the everyday world of the other in order to grasp socially constructed meaning' (de Laine 1997, p. 147). **Participant observation** requires the researcher to both participate and observe; the focus of this technique may include individual actions and interaction, social relationships and group life, as well as the motives that underlie action and the accommodation of action to the requirements of the social group (Liamputtong 2013). Simple observation may be structured or unstructured, and focus on the external signs of social life in the physical world, the locations and times in which action takes place, and the way that motives and beliefs are expressed through movement and language.

Observation: The process of collecting data by looking rather than listening.

Participant observation: A particular method of collecting data employed in ethnography. The researcher lives in a community, observes people's daily activities and witnesses first-hand how they behave.

STOP AND THINK

- What kind of privacy issues might be involved in participant observation?
- How would you deal with these issues as a researcher?
- How would you deal with these issues as a research participant?
- How would you check the accuracy of what you were observing?

Interview techniques range from structured, where questions follow a survey format and leave little room for individual variation, to completely unstructured, where the logic of the interview and the knowledge it generates derive from the social interaction between researcher and participant (see Chapter 4). Key informant interviews have a long history of use in ethnographic research. They require a research participant to take on the role of skilled and knowledgeable assistant to the researcher by explaining important aspects of what is observed or otherwise learnt from other participants. Life history interviews demand that participants structure their experience according to a chronological narrative logic by relating the history of their involvement in a social group (see Chapter 6). A related technique is the diary-interview, where informants are asked to keep a diary of their activities for a limited period such as a week, then are interviewed about the activities they have recorded (see Liamputtong 2007).

Focus and other group interview techniques are typically used to simulate a naturalistic setting for collecting information from a homogeneous group of participants (Liamputtong 2011). In focus groups, the group interview concentrates on specific questions, and the researcher provokes a discussion about a matter of interest in order to record how members of the community or organisation typically think about the matter. In focus group techniques, points of agreement and disagreement are of equal interest, and the researcher needs to be mindful of both what is said and what is left unsaid. Group interviews can be framed around collecting specific information without the requirement for a focused discussion; for example, a group may be asked to brainstorm an issue, or describe or map a typical aspect of their community or organisation (see Chapter 5).

Visual techniques, including photo-elicitation techniques such as **photovoice**, are increasingly used to elicit contextual information about health beliefs and practices (Keller *et al.* 2008; Liamputtong 2010). Typically, participants are asked to photograph important things in their lives, then explain their choices. Other creative techniques including poetry, song-writing or autobiography, and the production of visual art works, have been used by researchers to explore the unspoken content of cultural beliefs or practices (Liamputtong 2007). Visual techniques of ethnographic data collection encompass asking participants individually or in groups to produce maps or diagrams of their community and its resources. Such techniques have been used to explore, for example, caring relationships within communities, as well as concrete aspects of physical spaces such as the location of local plants or animals (see Sillitoe *et al.* 2005 for an extensive discussion of these alternative data collection methods).

Case studies in qualitative research are a typical way of recording and presenting ethnographic information. In this technique, in-depth information about a case of interest is collected using a range of techniques, then woven together to form an in-depth, contextualised and detailed whole. The case of interest may be a person or community, an agency, an organisation or one of its programs, or a particular event, period or incident. The data about the case may include interview data, observational data, documentary data, or impressions and statements made about the case (Liamputtong 2013).

Data analysis in ethnography

Data collected through ethnography is analysed similarly to other qualitative approaches (see Chapters 6, 8, 23). Three main approaches are typically used. In the first, the ethnographer presents data in the form of a dialogue with key theoretical points that are raised in a literature review, and so is able to confirm, contradict or extend the theoretical insights gained from the literature. The second approach uses categories and themes derived from the field data themselves as a framework for the analysis and presentation of the data, in a manner similar to that described in detail in grounded theory analysis. The third common approach treads a middle ground between these two, and is usually presented in the form of a critical incident from the field data which is then unpacked according to themes and categories derived from the literature review and from a thematic analysis of the field data, including the conditions under which the data were produced. This third approach is often referred to as cultural analysis or **thick description**, in deference to Clifford Geertz who originated the approach. His essay 'Deep play: notes on the Balinese cockfight' exemplifies this approach (Geertz 1973, pp. 412–53). Since both thematic and grounded theory analysis are covered in detail in Chapters 8, 23 and 24, we will provide only a reflective account of an example of the second approach here, in this case from Karen's research.

Photovoice: By using photography to record the concerns of their community, people who rarely have contact with those who make decisions over their lives can make their voices heard.

Case study in qualitative research: The study of a particular issue which is examined through one or more cases within a bounded system such as a setting or context.

Thick description: Descriptions that give ample detail and background information so that people's actions can be understood in the context of the experiences and patterns of meaning that influence them.

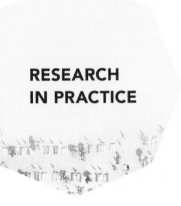

RESEARCH IN PRACTICE

Karen's early analysis of her data used open coding, which means searching for similarities and differences and making comparisons between events, actions and interactions, then labelling these in categories. Open coding at this stage helps to identify some of the main themes in the data. *In vivo* codes, which are taken directly from the data using lay terminology, were also coded during this stage of identifying and coding the data. She carried out open coding on interview and focus group transcripts and documents such as field notes, unit outlines and classroom handouts, with the assistance of a software program (NVivo) designed for qualitative data analysis (see Chapter 24). She moved between open coding of individual lines and sentences of text with the interview and focus group texts and paragraphs of text with document analysis.

Open coding of the text gave way to axial coding, which means putting the data back together in new ways and making connections between categories. Axial coding involves exploring the codes, and examining the relationships between the codes and developing categories and their subcategories. Karen then reviewed the data, which included revisiting the transcripts of interviews, the focus group and documents such as audit notes and unit outlines, and listening to audiotapes of interviews and classroom observations in order to verify the links between the codes and to search for any new codes. Finally, she began writing her account.

Themes and codes

Qualitative data
analysis: An ongoing,
cyclical process that occurs
from the very beginning of
the research.

Qualitative data analysis involves searching the data for themes that emerge and then become categories for further analysis (see Chapter 23). Ethnographic approaches involving descriptive or interpretive research encompass formally identifying themes as suggested by the data and demonstrating support for those themes. Thematic analysis techniques are similar to those of grounded theory, but do not include theoretical sampling. The process of thematic analysis involves coding, sorting and organising the data in themes that have not been decided before coding the data. Central to the data analysis process is coding, the process of identifying themes or concepts in the data in an attempt to build a systematic account of what has been observed and/or recorded.

Summary

Ethnography focuses on the description of practices and beliefs of groups of people, understood within the contexts of the shared cultures that they use to structure and derive meaning from their actions and interactions. Understood in this way, it provides unique insights into the ways that patients understand illness and the struggle for health, the ways that health practitioners organise and justify their actions, and the way societies privilege particular versions of health and illness while dismissing others. In this chapter we have explored the origins of ethnography in early twentieth-century anthropological practice, and charted its development as a methodological tool used in a range of social and health science disciplines. In particular, we looked at the specific uses of ethnography in the area of health through an examination of focused ethnography, institutional ethnography and ethno-nursing. Finally, we examined a range of data collection and presentation techniques including observation, individual and group interviewing, visual techniques and the use of the case study.

Practice exercises

1 Watch the teen movie *Mean Girls* (Waters 2004), which depicts the culture of US high school social cliques. Imagine that you are new girl and ethnographer Cady Heron. Your task is to describe the operation and culture of the clique known as the Plastics.

   (a) Critique the pitfalls of participant observation for the fictional Cady, depicted by Lindsay Lohan in the film. What strategies could you use to avoid these pitfalls?

   (b) You decide to use key informants to help you understand the social processes of the Plastics. What kind of differences in your understanding would you get if you chose the following as your informants: Janis Ian and Damien; Regina George; Gretchen Weiners and Karen Smith; Miss Norbury and Mr Duvall; Regina's mother?

   (c) One of the major documents produced by the Plastics is the Burn Book. How would you analyse the Burn Book to illuminate processes of meaning construction at North Shore High School?

   (d) The revelation of the Burn Book to the student body, Cady's party, the Mathletes' participation in the state competition, and the Spring Fling emerge as critical incidents in Cady's period of fieldwork. Choose one of these incidents and analyse the cultural meanings of the incident.

2 Identify an ethnographic study from the health literature and use it to answer the following questions.

   (a) What is the field site that the author has chosen for the study? How has this choice been justified?

   (b) What techniques does the author use to collect data? How are different perspectives accommodated by each method?

Jon Willis and Karen Anderson

(c) How does the author describe the process used to analyse the field data collected in the study? How are these data presented?

(d) How has the author dealt with conflicting or contradictory data in the study?

3   Think about an ethnographic study of your own.

(a) Describe your field site for this study. Whose culture(s) is/are represented in this field?

(b) What techniques would you choose to collect data for your study?

(c) Write a memo describing your study idea and data collection strategy.

Further reading

Atkinson, P., Coffey, A., Delamont, S., Lofland, J. & Lofland, L. (eds) (2007). *Handbook of ethnography*. London: Sage.

Bernard, H. (2011). *Research methods in anthropology: qualitative and quantitative approaches*. Lanham, MD: AltaMira Press.

Clifford, J., Maruse, G.E., Fortun, M. & Fortun, F. (2010). *Writing culture: the poetics and politics of ethnography*. Berkeley: University of California Press.

de Laine, M. (1997). *Ethnography: theory and applications in health research*. Sydney: McLennan & Petty.

Dykes, F. & Flacking, R. (eds) (2016). *Ethnographic research in maternal and child health*. Abingdon: Routledge.

Gobo, G. (2008). *Doing ethnography*. Los Angeles: Sage.

Jorgenson, D. (1989). *Participant observation: a methodology for human studies*. Newbury Park, CA: Sage.

Kozinets, R. (2015). *Netnography: redefined*, 2nd edn. London: Sage.

Liamputtong, P. (2013). *Qualitative research methods*, 4th edn. Melbourne: Oxford University Press.

Marcus, G. (1998). *Ethnography through thick and thin*. Princeton, NJ: Princeton University Press.

McCurdy, D., Spradley, J. & Shandy, D.J. (2005). *The cultural experience: ethnography in complex society*, 2nd edn. Long Grove, IL: Waveland Press.

O'Reilly, K. (2012). *Ethnographic methods*, 2nd edn. London: Routledge.

Suwankhong, D. & Liamputtong, P. (2015). Cultural insiders and research fieldwork: case examples from cross-cultural research with Thai people. *International Journal of Qualitative Methods*. doi: 10.1177/1609406915621404

Websites

http://eth.sagepub.com

This is the website for the journal *Ethnography*, one of the best peer-reviewed journals in publication. It features interdisciplinary and international articles focused on theoretically informed ethnographic research.

http://jce.sagepub.com

> The *Journal of Contemporary Ethnography* is another leading international and interdisciplinary peer-reviewed journal focused on contemporary research that makes innovative use of ethnographic methods.

www-rcf.usc.edu/~genzuk/Ethnographic_Research.html

> In this article, 'A synthesis of ethnographic research', Michael Genzuk from the University of Southern California gives a range of useful and practical tips for conducting ethnographic research, including summary guidelines for fieldwork and interviewing.

www.aiga.org/ethnography-primer/

> This presentation, from the American Institute of Graphic Arts, presents the steps in conducting ethnographic research in a straightforward and pragmatic way.

8

Grounded Theory in Health Research

PAULINE WONG, PRANEE LIAMPUTTONG AND HELEN RAWSON

Chapter objectives

In this chapter you will learn:

- why and when to use grounded theory
- the origins and historical background of grounded theory
- the common principles of using a grounded theory approach
- how to use analytical coding processes in a grounded theory study
- the divergent modes of grounded theory
- how grounded theory has been adopted in nursing research

Key terms

Coding

Constant comparative analysis

Data saturation

Grounded theory

In-depth interviewing method

Memos

Symbolic interactionism

Theoretical sampling

Theoretical sensitivity

Introduction

Decisions regarding the methodological approach and data collection methods used to perform a particular study are informed by the research aims and questions (Charmaz 2014; Corbin & Strauss 2015). A **grounded theory** method is appropriate to explore many health-related research questions. A major tenet of using a qualitative method is that there are concepts related to a particular phenomenon yet to be fully defined or adequately developed (see Chapter 1). Additionally, further exploration may be required to provide a more comprehensive understanding of the topic (Corbin & Strauss 2015). To gain the detail and complexity required to fully understand the research problem, the researcher needs to interact and speak directly with participants and listen to their rendering of the issue. This can be achieved through an **in-depth interviewing method**—a data collection method that is commonly used in grounded theory research (see Chapter 4). A qualitative approach is also relevant when there are inadequate theories for particular populations or 'existing theories do not adequately capture the complexity of the problem' (Creswell 2013, p. 48).

Grounded theory is a qualitative method most suited to research about which very little is known (Holloway & Wheeler 2013; Liamputtong 2013). The primary purpose of grounded theory is to generate explanatory models of human behaviour that are grounded in the data. The main focus of using this method is to explore social processes with the goal of theory development (Glaser & Strauss 1967). Grounded theory methods 'consist of systematic, yet flexible guidelines for collecting and analyzing qualitative data to construct theories from the data themselves. Thus, researchers construct theory "grounded" in their data' (Charmaz 2014, p. 1).

Grounded theory: A qualitative research method that uses a systematic set of procedures to collect and analyse data with the aim of developing an inductively derived theory that is grounded in the data.

In-depth interviewing method: A method of qualitative data collection. The interviewer does not use fixed questions, but aims to engage interviewees in conversation to elicit their understandings and interpretations.

A plethora of studies focus on families' needs and overall experiences in the intensive care unit (ICU), particularly in the USA, the UK, Canada and northern Europe. However, there is limited understanding of families' interactions within the context of an ICU in the Australian health care system, solely from the families' perspective. In addition, there is a paucity of literature that focuses on the interaction experiences of families more broadly in ICU. Further to the importance of knowledge about the manner in which ICU nursing staff interact with families, there is a dearth of research about families' perspectives on their interactions with: other staff in ICU, the ICU environment, their critically ill relative, families of other ICU patients and their own family members. Grounded theory is an appropriate method for this study due to the recognised gaps in the literature surrounding these aspects of families' experiences in ICU. As there are limited theoretical frameworks to guide clinical practice in these areas, the grounded theory method is most relevant (Charmaz 2014).

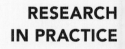

RESEARCH IN PRACTICE

Pauline Wong, Pranee Liamputtong and Helen Rawson

STOP AND THINK

In health disciplines, many questions related to care delivery, perception of illness and health utilisation can be answered using a grounded theory approach. This enables an understanding of the topic from the patients', family members' and clinicians' perspectives. What health-related research questions from your discipline could be answered using a grounded theory approach?

The historical development of grounded theory

The historical development of grounded theory is presented here, from its original conception in the mid-1960s to the divergent interpretations that have evolved since then. Two sociologists—Barney Glaser and Anselm Strauss—developed grounded theory as a way of 'discovering' theory that explained social processes inherent in human behaviour. Anselm Strauss trained at the University of Chicago, where he was influenced by interactionism (see below) and pragmatism and was inspired by writers such as John Dewey, George Herbert Mead and Herbert Blumer. Strauss contributed the following ideas to grounded theory:

- the need to get into the field to truly understand
- importance of theory, grounded in empirical reality
- nature of experience as continually evolving
- active role of the person in shaping the worlds they live in
- emphasis on change, process, variability and complexity of life
- interrelationships among conditions, meaning and action (Strauss & Corbin 1990, pp. 24–5).

His thinking also focused on the interrelationship between data collection and analysis and he developed **coding** paradigms to be used during the analysis (Strauss & Corbin 1990; see also Chapter 23).

Barney Glaser trained at Columbia University, influenced by Paul Larzarsfeld who was known for his use of quantitative statistics. Empirical research combined with theory generation was emphasised at Columbia. Based on his quantitative training, Glaser felt a need to develop a precise and systematic set of methods for coding and testing hypotheses generated during research (Schreiber & Stern 2001; Strauss & Corbin 1990).

As a result of their collaborative work and reflecting their respective Chicago and Columbia research traditions, Glaser and Strauss developed the grounded theory approach, which can be defined as:

> A qualitative research method that uses a systematic set of procedures to develop an inductively derived grounded theory about a phenomenon. The research findings constitute a theoretical formulation of the reality under investigation … Through this methodology, the concepts and relationships among them are not only generated but they are also provisionally tested (Strauss & Corbin 1990, p. 24).

Coding: Part of the data analysis process where codes are applied to chunks of data. It is the first step that allows researchers to move beyond tangible data to make analytical interpretations.

It was important that the theory was accessible to both professionals of the discipline and laypersons. To this end, the goal of grounded theory is to generate a theoretical framework that explains patterns of human behaviour that are 'relevant and problematic for those involved' (Glaser 1978, p. 93).

Symbolic interactionism

Symbolic interactionism is an interpretive approach that arose from the Chicago School of Sociology early in the twentieth century (Charmaz 2014). It is presented here as the theoretical framework from which the research method of grounded theory was developed (Holloway & Wheeler 2013). The US philosopher and social psychologist George Herbert Mead laid the foundations for an approach to the study of human society and human conduct known as 'symbolic interactionism' (Chenitz & Swanson 1986). A student of Mead, Herbert Blumer (1969), advanced the theoretical framework and based it on the following three assumptions.

First, 'human beings act toward things on the basis of the meanings these things have for them' (Blumer 1969, p. 2). Such things may include physical objects, other human beings or groups, institutions, guiding principles, the activities of others and situations encountered in everyday life. Thus, behaviour does not arise simply as a response to a stimulus, but individuals construct meanings for a situation or object, which then determines their action.

Furthermore, a person's world consists of objects, which may be viewed differently by different people. This is because the nature of an object is based on the meaning that object has for the person for whom it is an object, which will determine how that person acts toward it and talks about it. For example, a tree means different things to a botanist, a timbercutter, a poet and a home gardener. Therefore, in order to understand people's actions, it is important to identify their world of objects (Blumer 1969).

Second, the meanings of such things are products of social interaction. Meanings are not merely inherent within the object. Blumer (1969, p. 4) writes: 'The meaning of a thing for a person grows out of the ways in which other persons act toward the person with regard to the thing'. How we view the world is learnt from other people through shared meanings of objects with the people in our lives (Taylor & Bogdan 1998). The meaning of an object arises fundamentally out of the way it is defined to a person by others with whom they interact. The functioning of society, social organisations and other group life is based on a consensus of shared meanings between individual group members through a process of communication and common language (Chenitz & Swanson 1986).

Third, meanings 'are handled in, and modified through, an interpretive process used by the person in dealing with the things he encounters' (Blumer 1969, p. 2). Thus, people attach meanings to things, situations and themselves through a process of interpretation, which in turn guides action. The process of interaction is an intermediate step between meanings and the final action itself, or an indication to take a certain course of action. As people move

Symbolic interactionism: A theoretical perspective that explains human behaviour and human interaction through the use of symbolic communication and shared meanings. People interact with others and objects based on the meaning those things have for the individual.

through various situations in their day-to-day life, they are constantly interpreting, defining and redefining things and the situations (Taylor & Bogdan 1998).

Human beings interacting with one another do so in direct response to an interpretation they make of what the others are doing or about to do. A person is then forced to behave or handle their situation in terms of that interpretation. Thus, the actions of others have an influence on the formation of one's own behaviour. Depending on what others do, 'one may abandon an intention or purpose, revise, check or suspend it, intensify or replace it' (Blumer 1969, p. 8). Thus, individuals act predominantly in response to one another or in relation to one another. Social interaction guides human conduct.

Based on these three premises, it can be seen how symbolic interactionism can be used to explain why people may say different things and act differently in response to the same situation. People have had different experiences and learnt different social meanings. Hence, multiple views of reality are constructed, based on an individual's social interactions and the meanings that the individual has attributed to various things or situations. Taylor and Bogdan (1998) illustrate the way people who hold different positions within an organisation may view situations differently. The example presented is a situation whereby a student breaks the school cafeteria window. This is defined by the principal as a behaviour control problem, by the counsellor as a family problem, by the janitor as a clean-up problem and by the school nurse as a potential health problem; the student does not view it as a problem at all. The race, gender and class of any of the participants in a situation may influence their definition of the situation and how they define each other. People also act differently depending on different situations and the context within which they find themselves. When individuals generate and interpret meanings, the process of interpretation is constantly changing depending on the meanings available and how they are handled. Such meanings are situational and context dependent.

Therefore, symbolic interactionism is a theoretical perspective that explains human behaviour and human interaction through symbolic communication and shared meanings. Human behaviour is understood on an interactional level and on a symbolic level. Research conducted within this framework is directed towards understanding patterns of interactions and their consequences. The implicit and explicit meanings underpinning people's actions and interactions are explored, as well as the contextual situations with regard to settings and conditions that 'preclude the interaction ... to establish larger symbolic events that create definitions and shared meaning in the situation' (Chenitz & Swanson 1986, p. 6).

STOP AND THINK

Clinicians' interactions with patients, family members and other health care staff are an important part of care delivery and the therapeutic relationship. From a health-related perspective, how could clinical staff's experiences impact on their interactions with patients, family members and other health care staff?

Common principles of the grounded theory approach

An overview of the major tenets common to the grounded theory approach serves two main purposes. First, it explains the procedures and techniques commonly adopted in the conduct of a grounded theory study. Second, it lays the foundation for explaining the divergent interpretations of grounded theory that have emerged since it originated, in particular the versions further developed by one of the original founders, Anselm Strauss, when he collaborated with Juliet Corbin to develop a more prescriptive representation of how to conduct grounded theory research (Strauss & Corbin 1990; Corbin & Strauss 2008, 2015) and more recently the philosophical arguments underpinning a constructivist grounded theory approach, as put forward by Charmaz (2006, 2014).

Theoretical sensitivity

Theoretical sensitivity refers to the researcher's ability to have insight into the nuances inherent in the data, based on previous knowledge and experiences relevant to the area (Corbin & Strauss 2015). Sources of theoretical sensitivity may come from the literature and from personal and professional experience (Corbin & Strauss 2015). Professional background, knowledge and experience can help the researcher to understand significance in the data more quickly and to become more sensitive to relationships between concepts. They can provide a foundation against which the data can be compared, therefore allowing the researcher to focus on the participants' meaning in contrast to the researcher's understanding. Likewise, the literature can be used to enhance sensitivity during the analysis of a grounded theory study and as a source for making comparisons with the data (Corbin & Strauss 2015).

> Theoretical sensitivity: The researcher's ability to have insight into the nuances inherent in the data based on previous knowledge and experiences relevant to the area.

There is contention among grounded theorists about the most opportune time to review and incorporate the literature in a grounded theory study (Thornberg 2012). Glaser and Strauss (1967) argue that a grounded theory is to be generated through 'discovery' of the theory from the data. They warn against entering the research setting with 'preconceived' theoretical ideas or 'logically deducted, a priori hypotheses' (Glaser 1978, p. 3). They believe that preconceptions could limit or prevent the theory from emerging, due to the researcher's inability to look beyond the preempted concept, theory or idea. Instead, the researcher should remain open to what is happening in the data without the filtering lens of 'pre-existing hypotheses and biases' (Glaser 1978, p. 3). Consequently, Glaser (1978) contends that the literature surrounding the phenomenon under study should be reviewed only after the theory is sufficiently grounded and developed. The emergent theory is then related to the literature by integrating those ideas.

Thornberg (2012) presents several arguments against delaying the literature review, including the value of using relevant literature to enhance theoretical sensitivity.

He contests Glaser's position of pure induction and entering the field theoretically and value-free. Background knowledge of the relevant literature can prompt questions about the data during analysis, can direct theoretical sampling and allow the researcher to critically evaluate prior knowledge and current theories. Also, institutional review boards (IRBs) must approve research before it can commence. Therefore, it is not feasible to perform data collection or analysis for a grounded theory until a literature review has been conducted and submitted as part of an ethics proposal to the IRB. Doing the literature review at an earlier stage allows the researcher to avoid reinventing the wheel. By becoming aware of previous research on the phenomenon, methodological and conceptual errors can be avoided (Thornberg 2012).

Theoretical sampling

Theoretical sampling: The procedure for collecting data in order to generate theory. This involves the researcher adopting an iterative process of concurrently collecting, analysing and coding data to determine the type of data that should be collected next, so as to develop the emerging theory.

Theoretical sampling is defined as 'the process of data collection for generating theory whereby the analyst jointly collects, codes and analyzes his data and decides what data to collect next and where to find them, in order to develop his theory as it emerges' (Glaser & Strauss 1967, p. 45). Data is collected from places, people and incidents with the aim of developing the properties and dimensions of concepts and then identifying variations and relationships between them (Corbin & Strauss 2015). Thus, the processes of data collection using theoretical sampling and data analysis are intimately related and controlled by the emerging theory (Glaser 1978).

Apart from the initial selection of the study site, sampling decisions cannot occur in advance of data collection, as they must be theoretically informed by the emergence of a guiding theory (Dey 1999). Preliminary decisions are made about where and how to collect data based on the most likely sources of observational, interview or document data relevant to the study (Wuest 2007). Consequently, the first sample is determined according to the study phenomenon and where it is found to exist (Chenitz & Swanson 1986).

Theoretical sampling renders issues about sample size in grounded theory research superfluous. This is because the primary purpose of theoretical sampling is to collect data that will develop the analysis to make categories more conceptually dense, rather than reaching a predetermined number of participants.

Constant comparative analysis

Constant comparative analysis: An analytical technique used in grounded theory during which information obtained from data collection is constantly compared with the emerging categories and concepts.

Grounded theory is often referred to as the constant comparative method (Corbin & Strauss 2015). As a technique that is used in conjunction with theoretical sampling, **constant comparative analysis** directs what and where to sample next, by asking questions about the data in a way that seeks out comparisons with the data. The initial stages of data analysis involve generating categories and identifying the properties or characteristics of those categories. A 'category' is defined as a classification of concepts that is developed when concepts are compared and found to be similar to one another. The category is a 'higher level' and more abstract grouping of similar concepts (Corbin & Strauss 2015, p. 216). It is also considered a stand-alone conceptualised element of the developing theory, whereas a 'property' is a conceptualised attribute, characteristic or element of a category (Glaser & Strauss 1967; Corbin & Strauss 2015). The process of comparing information from data collection to the emerging categories is known as the constant comparative method (Creswell 2013).

Memo writing

The process of **memo** writing in a grounded theory study serves several purposes. First, it allows the researcher's ideas and thoughts about codes and the emerging theory to be documented. Consequently, there is an audit trail that delineates how the theory develops from data to grounded theory. Birks and Mills (2012) hold that memos are a valuable tool in maintaining an audit trail that documents the procedural steps of a grounded theory study. Reflexivity is also a necessary part of grounded theory; memos allow the researcher to demonstrate reflexivity by presenting written evidence of how their position, assumptions and perspectives may influence the enquiry (Corbin & Strauss 2008, 2015; Birks & Mills 2012; Charmaz 2014). Second, the researcher's ideas and conceptual analyses often progress during the memo-writing process, as analytical insights often emerge during the writing activity. Third, a researcher may note their reflections on aspects of the research journey that worked well and those that could have been done differently, thus enhancing their future research skills.

Memos: Memos are documented accounts of the researcher's thoughts, ideas and reflections about the research process. Memos provide an audit trail of the researcher's analytical decision-making and logistical details about research activities.

There are generally two broad types of memos—personal and theoretical memos.

Personal memos are regular journal entries about methodological processes, procedures, decision-making, challenges and emotional responses experienced throughout a study. A methodological log of memos provides a documented record of the entire research process. Entries are dated chronologically and labelled with a title to reflect the content of the journal entry. Personal memos may include critical reflections on certain research activities, such as in-depth interviewing. Dilemmas encountered during participant recruitment may be captured in the memos. Field notes and other contextual information about the interviews are also recorded in this way.

Theoretical memos are an essential part of the analysis in grounded theory and are used to help the researcher interrogate the data and ask questions about the codes, categories and developing theory (Birks & Mills 2012). In theoretical memos, 'the researcher discusses tentative ideas and provisional categories, compares findings, and jots down thoughts on the research' (Holloway & Wheeler 2013, p. 185). These memos help clarify, direct and focus further data collection. They become more detailed and analytical as the research progresses. Therefore, theoretical memos move the analysis forward by increasing the level of abstraction (Charmaz 2006; Corbin & Strauss 2008, 2015; Birks & Mills 2012).

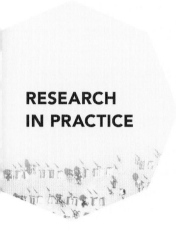

RESEARCH IN PRACTICE

Here, we provide two examples of the use of memos from our work.

In Australia, the reproductive and sexual health of young people are important issues, with childbirth and sexually transmitted infections being major contributors to overall morbidity among this age group. Many argue that greater effort is needed in service provision, health promotion and research to identify the interventions that are most likely to succeed in changing behaviours implicated in the production of 'unhealthy' practices and outcomes. However, while there is a wealth of literature on the sexual and reproductive health status and behaviours of 'young people', little work has specifically addressed young people from different cultural groups in Australia. Helen's PhD study sought to help fill this void by exploring the factors which influence the sexual behaviour of young people in Australia with a specific cultural heritage. In Helen's grounded theory study, she sought to understand how young Vietnamese Australian women navigated their sexual development and sexual health. In-depth interviews were used for data collection for this exploration, covering topics related to sexual behaviour, sexuality, sexual development and sexual health choices. The topic for this study was very sensitive, and it was necessary for Helen to have a link into the Vietnamese community so that she could recruit participants. Her two memos below relate to the process of establishing a link into the community.

Memo: Recruiting participants

Excellent contact with SS at the Vietnamese community group. She is very excited about my research. Keen to help with recruiting young girls for the study.

SS would love to have me participate in their youth projects.

A later memo addressed the same topic.

!!!!!! WHY??? After 5 months of being led up the garden path SS decides that she cannot see what benefit her organisation will get from this research. I feel desperate, angry and upset. How will I access potential participants now?

Contacted my supervisor at 8pm. She calms me down and says there are many pitfalls in research and this is just one of them. Meeting with her tomorrow to discuss participant recruitment.

In Pauline's PhD study about families' experiences of their interactions when a relative is admitted unexpectedly to ICU, the following concept, *Layman's terms*, emerged from interviews with several participants. The theoretical memo below is a compilation of two memo entries about this concept.

Memo: Layman's terms

Layman's terms are about making the complex simple, so that families can understand. Who uses layman's terms? Do only the nurses use them or do the doctors also use layman's terms? What constitutes layman's terms? Are they non-technical words? When are they used?

Family members describe the way health care professionals make it easier for them to understand aspects of the patient's treatment or care, particularly when they are in shock and may not be taking everything in, by using layman's terms.

Using layman's terms is about making complex medical terms and language simple. It's about simplifying information by saying it in another way, in 'non-technical' terms, so that a non-health professional, such as a family member, is able to comprehend the words used by health care professionals. Health care professionals use technical language and terms as part of their everyday communication. The technical language can sometimes be taken for granted by some health care professionals and they need to consciously be aware of the language used when speaking to families about their relative's condition.

Analytical coding procedures in grounded theory

Coding is the analytical process that develops concepts from the data (Corbin & Strauss 2015; see also Chapter 23). It comprises a set of operations during which data is 'broken down, conceptualized, and put back together in new ways … a central process by which theories are built from data' (Strauss & Corbin 1990, p. 57). Coding each incident found in the data generates a category, and each incident may be coded under many categories. Codes and categories emerge as each incident is compared with the previous incident then new incidents are compared with the emergent categories—constant comparative analysis (Glaser & Strauss 1967). As incidents are constantly compared, theoretical properties of the category are generated, whereby the dimensions, conditions, consequences, relationships to other categories and its other properties are identified (Corbin & Strauss 2015). As a result of making constant comparisons, including the integration of categories and properties, categories are developed at an abstract level but are 'indicated' by the data and provide meaningful images of the problematic area for the people whom the study is about (Glaser & Strauss 1967, p. 36).

Principles and techniques around coding processes have diverged since Glaser and Strauss (1967) established the original version of grounded theory. The following discussion outlines three main variants of grounded theory analysis as prescribed by the seminal grounded theorists, Glaser (1978), Corbin and Strauss (2008, 2015), Strauss and Corbin (1990) and Charmaz (2006, 2014). While each alternative offers a slightly nuanced version at each stage, the stages can be commonly classified as initial, intermediate and advanced coding (Birks & Mills 2012). Each stage represents a progressively higher level of conceptual analysis as the researcher progresses from initial to advanced analytical processes. Table 8.1 provides an outline of the coding stages of each approach.

The first stage of coding, 'open/initial coding' is a similar process in all three versions. Glaser (1978) describes open coding as 'coding the data in every way possible … for as many categories that might fit' (p. 56). He prescribes a set of rules to ensure it is performed successfully. These include asking a specific set of questions of the data, such as 'What is this data a study of?' and 'What category does this incident indicate?'; line-by-line data analysis; ensuring the analyst codes their own data; and interruption of coding to memo ideas. Both Glaser (1978) and Charmaz (2014) suggest coding with gerunds that focus on actions and processes in participants' accounts. Furthermore, remaining open to 'other analytical possibilities', sticking close to the data and treating initial codes as provisional all facilitate the development of codes that best fit the data (Charmaz 2014, p. 117).

TABLE 8.1   Variation of coding stages

ANALYTICAL STAGE	GLASER (1978)	STRAUSS & CORBIN (1990)/CORBIN & STRAUSS (2008, 2015)	CHARMAZ (2006, 2014)
Initial	Open coding	Open coding	Initial coding
Intermediate	Selective coding	Axial coding	Focused coding
Advanced	Theoretical coding	Selective coding	Theoretical coding/ integration

A core category is defined as the 'central phenomenon around which all the other categories are integrated' (Strauss & Corbin 1990, p. 116). At the intermediate coding stage, Glaser describes 'selective coding' as the process of identifying a core variable (or category) and restricting the coding to 'only those variables that relate to the core variable [which] ... becomes a guide to further data collection and theoretical sampling' (Glaser, 1978, p. 61). During the selective coding phase, data is collected for the sole purpose of delineating the core category and the categories around it (Skeat 2013). Focused coding is similar to selective coding. It requires the researcher to make decisions about which initial codes are most salient and 'make the most analytical sense to categorise [the] data incisively and completely. It also can involve coding your initial codes' (Charmaz 2014, p. 138).

Strauss and Corbin (1990) introduce axial coding as a coding paradigm that comprises a set of procedures to reconstruct the data in new ways after it has been fractured by open coding. The coding schema relates concepts to each other by reassembling the data and creating connections between categories and subcategories. They identify the types of categories that surround and are related to the core variable, as causal conditions, strategies, contextual/ intervening conditions and consequences. Strauss and Corbin (1990) argue that without the use of this coding paradigm the analysis would 'lack density and precision' (p. 99).

The final advanced coding stage diverges in focus among the three approaches but generally represents theoretical integration, during which the list of concepts is transformed into a grounded theory. Strauss and Corbin (1990) describe selective coding as a process during which propositions are developed that systematically interrelate the core category with other categories, relationships are validated with the data and a theory is established that explains a process, action or interaction about a phenomenon. It is not unlike axial coding but at a 'higher, more abstract level of analysis' (Strauss & Corbin 1990, p. 117). If a core category has not been explicated during intermediate coding, the analytical technique of producing a storyline is used to tell a conceptual story about the central phenomenon of the study and therefore select a core category (Strauss & Corbin 1990; Birks & Mills 2012; Creswell 2013; Corbin & Strauss 2015).

Theoretical coding uses advanced frameworks and theoretical codes as analytical tools to integrate focused/substantive codes, and conceptualise how they are related. Theoretical coding progresses the analytical story by enhancing 'the explanatory power of [a] storyline and its potential as theory' (Birks & Mills 2012, p. 123; Charmaz 2014). Glaser (1978) introduces 'theoretical coding families' that provide a framework to support what the grounded theory is about (p. 73). He describes eighteen sociological constructs, but suggests that theoretical frameworks taken from other disciplines can also be used to develop the theory.

The differences between these two methods of grounded theory, which have become known as Glaserian and Straussian, are highlighted by basic arguments articulated by Glaser in response to the methodological techniques that Strauss and Corbin developed in 1990 (Melia 1996; Charmaz 2000). One such argument centres on Glaser's emphasis on the emergence of the theory from the data, without imposing preconceived theories, questions or frameworks on it. According to Melia (1996), Glaser's critique of the axial coding paradigm is that it forces the data and analysis through the preconceived analytical questions and methodological processes of such a framework. He asserts that the method of constant comparative analysis is sufficient for the emergence of categories and properties. Furthermore, theoretical codes render axial coding unnecessary because they 'weave the fractured story back together' (Glaser 1978, p. 72).

Charmaz (2014) raises the tension concerned with the use of theoretical codes as prescribed by Glaser and Strauss (1967) and Glaser (1978), and whether they are applied to the developing grounded theory or are an 'emergent process' (p. 150). While Glaser (1978) directs that theoretical codes should be emergent, he also states that a researcher should use their prior knowledge of previous theoretical constructs to 'be sensitive to rendering explicitly the subtleties of the relationships in his data' (p. 72).

Thornberg (2012) reiterates the ambiguity addressed by Charmaz when he confirms that Glaser's position is not purely inductive because he advocates the use of coding families (extant conceptual frameworks) to facilitate the analysis. Many grounded theorists reject the idea that data can be collected and analysed from a starting point of no prior theoretical knowledge or preconceptions. Criticism of this *tabula rasa* approach (Thornberg 2012) is supported by the adage quoted by Dey (1999) that 'there is a difference between an open mind and an empty head' (p. 251). Researchers should make their underlying assumptions and preconceived ideas explicit, rather than hiding them or pretending they do not exist (Thornberg 2012).

Theoretical saturation

Theoretical saturation is the final consideration in theoretical integration (the last analytical phase). It is defined as the stage when no new categories/concepts are being generated and any further data collected fits within previously developed categories (Liamputtong 2013). According to Charmaz (2014), many grounded theorists assume their study has reached saturation because they misunderstand the term to mean the repetition of described events, actions and/or statements. She defines saturation to have occurred 'when gathering fresh data

Data saturation (theoretical saturation): Data saturation occurs during the final stage of analysis when no new categories or concepts can be derived from the data and any further data collected will fit within already developed categories.

no longer sparks new theoretical insights, nor reveals new properties of these core theoretical categories' (Charmaz 2014 p. 213). Once conceptual saturation has been reached, categories may be integrated to form a central theoretical framework around a core category, described by Glaser and Strauss (1967) as the main storyline of the study.

Data collection in grounded theory research

Grounded theory research can be performed using a range of data collection strategies, such as interviews, observations and documents, depending on the research question and where it leads the researcher. The significance of the analysis and the strength of the developing grounded theory are influenced by the ability to gather 'rich' data and 'thick description' that uncover the 'participants' views, feelings, intentions, and actions as well as the contexts and structures of their lives' (Charmaz 2014, p. 23).

The choice of data collection method depends on the nature of the research question asked and the phenomenon being explored, as well as the ontological and epistemological premises on which the research is based (see Chapters 1, 2, 20). Many qualitative researchers hold an ontological position that views social reality as constructed through meaningful interactions between the members of that society. The way we come to know about that reality is through understanding those meanings and interpretations (Minichiello *et al.* 2008). In-depth interviews are commonly used to collect data in grounded theory research, providing a method for the researcher to uncover those meanings and interpretations through the use of the participants' own words and language (Minichiello *et al.* 2008; Liamputtong 2013; see Chapter 4). This method of data collection is appropriate when the researcher cannot directly observe the situation under investigation. For example, if events occurred in the past or if practical constraints prevent the researcher from accessing activities or situations relevant to the research topic, accounts of interactions and experiences directly observed by the participants can be part of the interview process (Minichiello *et al.* 2008).

RESEARCH IN PRACTICE

In Pauline's grounded theory study, she sought to understand families' experiences of their interactions when a relative was unexpectedly admitted with a life-threatening condition to an Australian ICU. Ethical and practical considerations prohibited direct observation of the interaction experiences of the family members. Consequently, in-depth interviews were considered a more appropriate method of data collection.

Preparation to conduct in-depth interviews with family members included the selection of an appropriate site, building trust and developing rapport with participants over time, and preparing an interview guide. Establishing rapport with participants usually occurred over several meetings prior to the actual interview. During preliminary meetings, Pauline engaged in small talk to encourage a comfortable relationship and to discover more about their personal background. If it was appropriate, she offered information about her personal family situation as a way of building trust and strengthening the relationship through sharing common experiences (Liamputtong 2013). Johnson and Rowlands (2012) agree that it is not uncommon for an interviewer 'to bring some form of complementary reciprocity to the informant' to develop a sense of mutual trust (p. 104).

It is recommended that interviews be conducted in the participant's home or at a venue where the participant feels comfortable, in order to enhance the development of a positive relationship between the researcher and participant (Liamputtong 2007). In Pauline's study, while the potential power inequity between researcher and participants was recognised, practical concerns related to potential risks associated with the interview location and other factors also required consideration (Minichiello et al. 2004). There were two pragmatic reasons why interviews were not conducted in the participants' homes. First, at the time of conducting the interviews, patients were often still in ICU or inpatients on a general ward. This meant that families spent most of their time at the hospital visiting their relative. It is widely recognised that families need to be close to their critically ill relative (Engström & Söderberg 2004; Lam & Beaulieu 2004; Verhaeghe et al. 2005; McKiernan & McCarthy 2010; Vandall-Walker & Clark 2011; Plakas et al. 2014;). Therefore, in most cases it was more convenient for families to be interviewed on the hospital site. Second, as a novice researcher and unaccompanied woman presenting at the family's home, there would have been concern for Pauline's personal safety. The potential risk was related to the fact that some families of patients admitted to ICU following motor vehicle accidents or traumatic incidents have been known to become physically and/or verbally aggressive due to the stress of their situation or other

predisposing factors. It was a requirement of the institutional ethics committee that the interviews be conducted on the hospital site. Potential risks and threats to the safety of researchers during fieldwork and data collection, particularly when researching vulnerable and difficult-to-reach populations, have been documented in the literature (Dickson-Swift et al. 2007; Liamputtong 2007). The interviews took place in a building separate from the ICU but on the hospital site. It was a requirement of the ICU nurse unit managers that participants be interviewed in a place that was external to the ICU complex. This was to reinforce to families the position that Pauline's role was that of an independent researcher not affiliated with the ICU in any way.

A fundamental aspect of in-depth interviewing is to engage in spontaneous conversation with the participant, therefore, it could be considered counter-intuitive to use an interview guide. However, as Charmaz (2014) advises, without a guide a researcher who is inexperienced in this type of interviewing may become anxious. This could result in 'asking, poorly timed, intrusive questions that [they] may fill with unexamined preconceptions' (p. 63). In Pauline's study, relevant topics derived from the available knowledge and research objectives formed the basis of an initial guide. The topics were arranged in a logical sequence from broad to more specific (Kelly 2010). For example, the topic *Interactions with nursing staff* was a prompt for an introductory question, *'Can you tell me about your experiences interacting with nursing staff in ICU?'* Each subsequent guide opened with general questions but, in accordance with theoretical sampling, remaining questions were directed around themes that had arisen from previous interviews and required further exploration. Although the interview guide was used as a prompt, participants often addressed the themes spontaneously during the course of the conversation. They were encouraged to discuss in depth any aspect of their experiences interacting in ICU that they felt was important to them.

STOP AND THINK

As the choice of data collection method depends on the research question, it is important to have a clear understanding about what the research is seeking to address.

For example, in a study to understand how new migrants to Australia access health services, it is important to explore their health needs, their previous experience of health services and potential barriers to accessing health care. In-depth interviews with new migrants, migrant health workers and service providers would provide valuable insight that would address the topic.

Thinking of a health-related issue in your discipline, what question would you research and what data collection method/s would you use to explore the question?

Objectivist versus constructivist grounded theory

Whether a grounded theory study follows the methods developed by Glaser and Strauss in their original conception of the approach (Glaser 1978; Glaser & Strauss 1967) or the more formulaic techniques described by Strauss and Corbin (1990), it is apparent that canons of positivism and objectivism underpin both versions.

Charmaz (2000, 2006, 2009, 2014) argues for a constructivist grounded theory that offers an alternative to the objectivist approach. She positions the different versions at each end of a continuum. While they share some fundamental methodological strategies, such as theoretical sampling and constant comparisons, their underlying ontological and epistemological foundations differ. Constructivist grounded theory is derived from an interpretive tradition, while objectivist grounded theory is based on positivism (Charmaz 2011). Furthermore, the prescriptive nature of analytical techniques, such as axial coding and the conditional matrix that are characteristic of the Strauss and Corbin (1990) version, 'furthers the positive cast to objectivist grounded theory' (Charmaz 2000, p. 524). More recently, Corbin (2009) shifts the focus of the approach originally espoused by Strauss and Corbin (1990), with its objectivist underpinnings, to a contemporary version (Corbin & Strauss 2015). The philosophical foundations of the method have evolved and suggest more flexible and open guidelines based on social constructivist ideas (Corbin 2009; Charmaz 2014).

Aligned with tenets of qualitative enquiry, a constructivist grounded theory studies people in their natural settings while moving away from positivism. Charmaz (2014) contends that strict rules are not necessary, that flexible strategies can be used to conduct grounded theory. An interpretive understanding can be advanced by a focus on meanings and emergence within a symbolic interactionist framework while using constructivist grounded theory. Charmaz (2009) offers a constructivist grounded theory that assumes 'a relativist epistemology, sees knowledge as socially produced, acknowledges multiple standpoints of both the research participants and the grounded theorist, and takes a reflexive stance toward our actions, situations, and participants in the field setting—and our analytic constructions of them' (p. 129).

The objectivist approach assumes that data collection and analysis are performed uninfluenced by the researcher's biases or biographical context, and that the categories, concepts and theory have always been out there waiting to be discovered. In contrast, the constructivist approach recognises that the interaction between the researcher and the participant influences the emergent theory, because it is co-constructed based on the researcher's view as well as the participant's view of the situation. The interaction and the temporal, cultural and structural contexts of that interaction influence the reality that is discovered, as the researcher and the participant assign meaning to the interaction. The researcher becomes part of what is viewed and this in turn contributes to the analysis and theory generated (Charmaz 2014).

A constructivist grounded theorist does not assume there is one universal and eternal truth but a 'real' world does exist. Thus, a constructivist grounded theorist is a realist concerned with understanding human realities and holds the position that what is real, and therefore what is objective knowledge and truth, depends on one's own perspective. Consequently, the end product of a grounded theory study is the construction of '*a* reality, not *the* reality—that is objective, true and external' (Charmaz 2000, p. 523). It would seem obvious, therefore, that a constructivist grounded theory approach would align most appropriately with such a theoretical framework.

In direct contrast to constructivist grounded theory with its emergent and interactive principles, Charmaz (2011) highlights a 'positivist empiricism with researcher neutrality' (p. 365) that underpins the guidelines offered by the objectivist grounded theory approach of Glaser and Strauss (1967), Glaser (1978) and Strauss and Corbin (1990). An objectivist grounded theorist accepts the position of an external world that represents the truth and assumes that different people discover this world and view it in similar ways. They assume shared and similar meanings between researchers and respondents. Thus, only one reality exists, waiting to be discovered. They aim for context-free generalisations and abstractions that do not include the historical, social or situated circumstances that frame the study. Unlike the constructivist approach, an objectivist grounded theory does not account for the influence of the researcher or the interaction between researcher and participants (Charmaz 2014).

It is apparent from this that grounded theory has evolved from its original version to include the more prescriptive techniques of Strauss and Corbin (1990) and the more flexible approach of Charmaz (2006, 2014). The earlier versions are positioned in a more objectivist framework, assuming an external reality waiting to be discovered and a passive researcher who should remain objective and not allow their biases, reflections or interpretations to influence the emerging theory. The realist ontology and positivist epistemology are endorsed by the didactic and formulaic techniques prescribed by these approaches. In contrast, Charmaz (2014) views grounded theory methods as a set of principles and practices to be used as flexible guidelines, as opposed to strict methodological rules. She offers a social constructivist version of grounded theory, the assumptions of which align with the research paradigm underpinning most qualitative studies.

Pauline Wong, Pranee Liamputtong and Helen Rawson

Summary

In this chapter, we have presented a discussion of the use of grounded theory and how it may be applied to health research. The origins and historical background of grounded theory have been highlighted, before an overview of some common principles of using a grounded theory approach. This was followed by a description of the various analytical coding strategies used in a grounded theory study. We have also argued the divergent modes of objectivist versus constructivist grounded theory, based on fundamental epistemological beliefs underpinning qualitative research. Throughout the chapter, several applications of the tenets of grounded theory in nursing research have been presented to highlight how this approach can be used to explore health-related issues.

Grounded theory can offer health disciplines an understanding of care and service delivery, treatments and interactions from the multiple perspectives of patients, family members and health care staff. The outcomes can be used to inform evidence-based practice, health policy and education of staff, students and the community.

Practice exercises

1 Conduct a short (five- to ten-minute) interview with a friend or colleague about a health-related issue you are interested in exploring further.

    (a) Develop an interview guide with some broad topics/themes you could use to prompt questions that would provide some initial data on the topic.

    (b) If possible, audiorecord the interview. Otherwise, as soon as the interview is completed write down as many of the salient points you can recall.

2 Use theoretical sampling to determine what, where or how you will collect your next data, based on the responses you received from the short interview in Exercise 1.

3 After listening to your audiorecording or reviewing your notes about the interview, try to do some initial open coding by allocating some concepts to 'bits' of data obtained.

4 Alternatively, read the piece of transcript provided on page 155, then perform open coding by compiling a list of as many codes as you can create.

5   Ask a colleague to perform the task outlined in Exercise 4, then compare your lists of codes. Discuss the codes that were similar and those that differed from your own.

SAMPLE TRANSCRIPT

Mother: When we first arrived in the ICU I was all over the place. I couldn't really think and get my thoughts together. All I wanted to do was to see my son. I do remember a nurse coming out to speak to us not too long after we arrived in the waiting room … She kind of explained that [son] was still in the operating room and it would be quite a while before we could see him. She went through some of the things we would see when we came in. I think she was trying to prepare us for when we saw [son].

Interviewer: What was it like when you were able to see him?

Mother: Of course when we were finally allowed to go in to see him that first time, I don't think I really thought about what she had told us … It was such a shock when we saw him that first time. There were all these tubes and wires attached to him. He was surrounded by all this machinery and equipment. At first I was really scared because I didn't really understand what they were all for. I remember I started crying and all I wanted to do was hug [son] but I didn't know how to or whether I could touch him. It was really overwhelming that first time. As I said the nurse probably explained stuff to us but I think the whole situation just takes over and you can't really recall anything they told you.

Further reading

Birks, M. & Mills, J. (2012). *Grounded theory: a practical guide.* London: Sage.

Bryant, A. & Charmaz, K. (2010). *The Sage handbook of grounded theory.* Thousand Oaks, CA: Sage.

Charmaz, K. (2014). *Constructing grounded theory*, 2nd edn. London: Sage.

Corbin, J. & Strauss, A. (2015). *Basics of qualitative research: techniques and procedures for developing grounded theory*, 4th edn. Thousand Oaks, CA: Sage.

Glaser, B.G. & Strauss, A. (1967). *The discovery of grounded theory.* New York: Aldine Publishing.

Johnson, J.M. & Rowlands, T. (2012). The interpersonal dynamics of in-depth interviewing. In J.F. Gubrium, J.A. Holstein, A.B. Marvasti & K.D. McKinney (eds), *The Sage handbook of interview research: the complexity of the craft*, 2nd edn. Thousand Oaks, CA: Sage, 99–114.

Liamputtong, P. (2013). *Qualitative research methods*, 4th edn. Melbourne: Oxford University Press.

Plakas, S., Taket, A., Cant, B., Fouka, G. & Vardaki, Z. (2014). The meaning and importance of vigilant attendance for the relatives of intensive care unit patients. *Nursing in Critical Care*, 19(5), 243–54.

Vandall-Walker, V. & Clark, A.M. (2011). It starts with access: a grounded theory of family members working to get through critical illness. *Journal of Family Nursing*, 17(2), 148–81.

Pauline Wong, Pranee Liamputtong and Helen Rawson

Websites

www.groundedtheoryonline.com/what-is-grounded-theory

> A grounded theory website to support research students, higher degree supervisors and research committees and provide consultation to industry and professional researchers.

www.groundedtheory.com

> The website of the Grounded Theory Institute and the official site of Dr Barney Glaser and classic grounded theory.

http://groundedtheoryreview.com/

> *Grounded Theory Review* is an international, peer-reviewed, open-access publication that advances classic grounded theory research and scholarship,

http://qhr.sagepub.com/

> *Qualitative Health Research* is an international, peer-reviewed journal that provides a forum to advance the understanding of qualitative research in the health care context.

9

Phenomenology and Rehabilitation Research

CHRISTINE CARPENTER

Chapter objectives

In this chapter you will learn:

- to explore phenomenology as a methodological approach to conducting qualitative research in rehabilitation
- to consider the contribution qualitative methodological theory can make to developing a coherent and rigorous study design
- to discuss and critique the design and implementation of a phenomenological study
- to reflect on the central role of the researcher in phenomenological research
- to discuss the contribution of phenomenological research to evidence-based practice

Key terms

Bracketing

Descriptive phenomenology

Essence

Evidence-based practice

Hermeneutics

In-depth interviewing

Interpretive or hermeneutic phenomenology

Life-world

Method

Methodology

Multiple realities

Phenomenological reduction

Phenomenology

Positionality

Purposive sampling

Reflexivity

Semi-structured interview

Snowball sampling

Introduction

For the purposes of this chapter, I would like to take the opportunity to revisit and reflect on a phenomenological study I conducted a number of years ago (Carpenter 1994) from the perspective of what I learnt and what I would do differently given the research experience I have since acquired. That study derived directly from my practice as a physical therapist in spinal cord injury rehabilitation. I had been seconded from a physical therapy department to the position of research coordinator for a large study exploring issues of fertility after spinal cord injury. Clients who volunteered to be involved with the study shared with me their experiences of living with spinal cord injury in the community, some for many years post-injury. It was as a result of these privileged conversations that I came to recognise, for the first time in a long career as a physical therapist in rehabilitation, the significant discrepancies between the clients' and rehabilitation therapists' beliefs and understanding of life after spinal cord injury. I realised that, as a physical therapist, I interacted with clients in a relatively limited post-injury time-frame when they were in the process of assimilating the major changes caused to their lives, but that I had little opportunity to understand the impact on their long-term health or quality of life. It was these insights that led me to conduct the study discussed in this chapter.

Perhaps the most essential step in developing a research study is to generate a clear statement of purpose or question that can withstand scrutiny and critique. This takes the form of a declarative statement that 'reveals an area of interest or problem emerging from the researcher's professional and/or personal experience or the literature, where a gap of knowledge exists or where contradictory and unexplored facets are present' (Mantzoukas 2008, p. 373). The decision about which qualitative methodology to choose (if any) reflects the type of question being asked and, in turn, guides and contributes to a coherent and rigorous study design. For example, the purpose of this study was to explore the meaning of the experience of spinal cord injury from the perspective of individuals living in the community.

Methodology: A specific philosophical and ethical approach to developing knowledge; a theory of how research should, or ought, to proceed given the nature of the issue it seeks to address.

Method: The actual strategies and techniques that researchers use to acquire knowledge and collect data.

STOP AND THINK

Think of a situation in your work or student experience that could be explored using a phenomenological research approach.

• Develop a concise statement of purpose or question that could be addressed by an exploratory study.

Students and practitioners newly engaging in qualitative research are confronted with, as Creswell (2014) has described it, a baffling number of methodological traditions from which to choose. In addition, the terms **methodology** and **method** are not used consistently across disciplines. In this chapter I have adopted Hammell's definition of methodology as 'a specific philosophical and ethical approach to developing knowledge; a theory of how research should, or ought, to proceed given the nature of the issue it seeks to address' (2006, p. 167). In contrast, method is defined as 'the actual techniques and strategies employed to collect and manipulate data and acquire knowledge' (Hammell & Carpenter 2000, p. 2). In my opinion, 'an informed and explicitly described methodological approach lends coherence and consistency to the research design, and plays an important role in justifying the plan of inquiry' (Carpenter & Suto 2008, p. 46). It guides the research design and the analytic process, and enhances the credibility of the research. Some researchers do not articulate the theoretical approach that guides their study, nor do they justify the use of a qualitative approach. A critical appraisal of such studies often reveals a lack of understanding of the essential epistemological differences between qualitative and quantitative research, misuse of terminology, and a paucity of scientific rigour. Researchers, as Miller and Crabtree (2005, p. 626) assert, have the responsibility of creating 'methodologically convincing stories' by providing a cogent rationale for their research studies. The question of using methodological theory, however, continues to be vigorously debated by qualitative researchers. There is a concern that expecting researchers, particularly those with less experience, to ground their proposed research in methodological detail is excessive and that what is required instead is that researchers demonstrate a thorough understanding of the essential distinctions between interpretivist (qualitative) and positivist (quantitative) research (Avis 2003; see Chapter 1).

Phenomenology

Phenomenology is a methodological approach with a strong and dynamic philosophical and epistemological foundation that seeks to understand, describe and interpret human behaviour and the meaning individuals make of their experiences (Liamputtong 2013). There are a number of schools of phenomenological thought, the primary ones being descriptive phenomenology and interpretive or hermeneutic phenomenology, which have some commonalities and some distinct features (Dowling 2007). It is worth recognising the distinctions between the two approaches, however, a broad concept of phenomenology based on shared characteristics is most commonly applied in health-related studies.

Descriptive phenomenology

Edmond Husserl (1859–1938) regarded human experience as a fundamental source of knowledge and study in its own right (Dowling 2007) and developed phenomenology as an approach to studying 'things as they appear' (Dowling 2007, p. 132) in order to arrive at a rigorous and unbiased understanding of the essential human consciousness and experience. Descriptive phenomenologists such as Giorgi and Giorgi (2003) and Moustakas (1994) have perhaps the closest connections with Husserl's original conception of phenomenology, and focus on creating detailed descriptions of specific experiences of a phenomenon (Carpenter & Suto 2008). Central to **descriptive phenomenology** are the concepts of **phenomenological reduction** (or epoché) and **bracketing**. Phenomenological reduction is the central aim of this type of enquiry—to gain rich or 'thick' information that represents the essential nature of the individuals' experiences and that 'communicates the sense and logic of the phenomenon to others' (Todres 2005, p. 110) in new ways. Husserl was adamant that employing the technique

Phenomenology:
A methodological approach that seeks to understand, describe and interpret human behaviour and the meaning individuals make of their experiences.

Descriptive phenomenology: An approach to studying 'thingarrive at a rigorous and authentic understanding of the essential human consciousness and experience.s as they appear' in order to

Phenomenological reduction is the goal of phenomenological enquiry—to search for the multiple meanings attributed to a phenomenon and to provide a comprehensive and in-depth description of it rather than an explanation.

Bracketing: The suspension of all judgments and prior ideas in order to enter the unique world of the individual whose experience is the focus of the research.

of phenomenological reduction would allow for reflection in research while at the same time ensuring that the findings were not overly influenced or directed by the researcher's agenda (McConnell-Henry *et al.* 2009, p. 10). The process of bracketing can facilitate this type of reflection. Bracketing is the process by which the researcher identifies and attempts to hold in abeyance ideas, preconceptions and personal knowledge about the phenomenon of interest in order to authentically listen to and reflect on the lived experiences of participants (Lopez & Willis 2004). The feasibility and relevance of bracketing is the focus of much debate among qualitative researchers (McConnell-Henry *et al.* 2009). It is important, however, that researchers engaging in phenomenological enquiry have an in-depth understanding of the concept in order to justify its inclusion in or absence from their study design. Another assumption underlying the descriptive tradition is that there are features of any lived experience that are common to all persons who have had the experience; for example, most people would share commonalities of experience of the concepts of love and grief. The focus or subject of these emotions will differ in many respects, but an essential structure or **essence**, considered to represent the core nature of the phenomenon, can be discovered through the data collection and analysis processes. The 'essence' thus refers to the qualities that give an experiential phenomenon, for example spinal cord injury (Carpenter 1994), its distinctiveness and coherence (Todres 2005). Therefore an attempt is made to refine, as free as possible from cultural context, an understanding of the essential features of a phenomenon (Dowling 2007). In summary, the descriptive phenomenologist develops detailed concrete descriptions of experience.

Interpretive or hermeneutic phenomenology

In contrast, Martin Heidegger (1889–1976), a student of Husserl, developed an alternative philosophical approach called **interpretive or hermeneutic phenomenology**, which focused on 'deriving meaning from being' (McConnell-Henry *et al.* 2009, p. 8). Contemporary phenomenologists, such as van Manen (in education and pedagogy) and Benner (in nursing), use this methodology in applied or professional contexts to explore practical concerns of everyday living. Interpretive phenomenology focuses on a collaborative interpretation of the meanings attributed by individuals' 'being in the world and how these meanings influence the choices that they make' (Lopez & Willis 2004, p. 729). Researchers working in this tradition would encourage participants to describe interactions, relations with others, physical experiences and so on in order to place the lived experience in the context of daily life. This might involve an analysis of the historical, social and political forces that shape and organise individuals' experiences. In this tradition, the researcher's presuppositions or knowledge are valuable guides to enquiry, and in fact make the enquiry a meaningful undertaking (Lopez & Willis 2004). The word **hermeneutics** 'describes the process of establishing understanding of the text as a whole by constantly interpreting the individual parts in relation to the other parts and each in relation to the whole' (Carpenter & Suto 2008, p. 65). It is a core characteristic of phenomenological data analysis (Rapport 2005).

Essence: The essential structure of a phenomenon that would reflect the experience of people in general rather than that of individuals. The essence is derived through a rigorous analytic process during which the researcher brackets their habitual ways of perceiving the phenomenon.

Interpretive or hermeneutic phenomenology: Focuses on interpreting and describing the meanings attributed by individuals' being in the world and how these meanings influence the choices that they make.

Hermeneutics: A theory of the process of interpretation, used in qualitative research to examine the way people develop interpretations of their life in relation to their life experiences.

It is not possible, within the constraints of this chapter, to provide more than this simplified account of these important philosophical traditions. There are, however, a number of additional core concepts and principles characteristic of phenomenological research that differentiate it from other qualitative methodologies, such as grounded theory or ethnography, which readers may wish to explore further. These concepts—the **life-world**, **multiple realities** and essence— reflect the central interest of phenomenology in the individual experience, and the interlocking nature of these concepts is illustrated in Giorgi's (1997) descriptive method. The life-world can be described as the world of experience as it is lived by individuals, or a sense of lived life (Rapport 2005). The idea of multiple realities is that 'the same objects or situations can mean different things to different people, and that people and the worlds they occupy are inextricably intertwined' (Carpenter & Suto 2008, p. 66). The expression of these realities (the experience of a phenomenon) and the meanings attributed to them by research participants enables the researcher, through the analytic process, to distinguish the essence of the phenomenon. This essential structure enables us to gain an in-depth understanding of the depth and breadth of the phenomenon that is not available through individual accounts. This analytic process requires that the researcher engage in critical reflection in order to bracket habitual ways of perceiving the phenomenon. In this way, the researcher may assume 'a disciplined naivete' (Giorgi 1997), enabling the phenomenon to be viewed in as fresh a way as possible. The aim, as Giorgi (1997) suggests, is to offer a general detailed analysis, abstracted from the individual accounts, of a phenomenon such that it can be applied (or transferred) to other groups or individuals. While phenomenological findings cannot be generalised in any strict scientific sense to wider populations, they can prove relevant to other people and settings (Finlay 2009).

In summary, the aim of phenomenological research is to reveal the individual's lived meaning of the world. It does not assume understanding, but rather works to develop it, using the meanings constructed by the participant (Carpenter & Suto 2008).

Life-world: The world of experience as it is lived, our sense of lived life.

Multiple realities: The same objects or situations can mean different things to different people; people and the worlds they occupy are inextricably intertwined.

STOP AND THINK

Susan is a senior physiotherapist working in neurorehabilitation. She often says that, after all her years of experience, she has an excellent understanding of what it is like to live with a disability.

- How would you convince her that qualitative research, using a phenomenological approach, could contribute to her practice knowledge?

Designing and conducting phenomenological research in rehabilitation practice

The aim of my study (Carpenter 1994), as stated earlier, was to explore the experience of spinal cord injury from the perspective of individuals living in the community. At the time, I identified phenomenology as the appropriate methodological approach but did not attempt to further define the specific phenomenological tradition. In hindsight, I think the study aim is most congruent with descriptive phenomenology. However, the core concepts and principles were appropriately and consistently used to guide the study design and implementation. Ethical approval was obtained from the University of British Columbia Behavioural Sciences Research Ethics Committee.

Participant recruitment

Participants were recruited if they had sustained a traumatic spinal cord injury two to five years before the study and defined themselves as 'successfully rehabilitated' or 'back on track'. Initial access to a network of potential participants was gained through the sponsorship of a personal acquaintance. He had sustained a spinal cord injury, was educated as a social worker, and was involved in facilitating a peer-support group. His explanation of the study to that group resulted in three people volunteering to be involved. A further seven participants were recruited by a **purposive snowball sampling** technique, whereby the first participants interviewed were asked to recommend others who, in their opinion, met the inclusion criteria (see Chapters 1, 6).

Since conducting this study, I have frequently been asked to defend or justify its 'small' sample size. Questions like this reflect the assumptions of representativeness, normal distribution and generalisability that underpin quantitative and survey approaches. Phenomenological research focuses on determining the essence of an experience or phenomenon and is usually achieved by employing a rigorous purposive sampling strategy and conducting one to three in-depth interviews with a small number of participants. At the time, I justified the sample size of ten participants by referring to data or theoretical saturation (see Chapters 1, 6, 8). This concept originated in grounded theory but has been adopted more widely by qualitative researchers (Guest *et al.* 2006; see Chapter 8). Data saturation is presumed to have occurred when all the main variations of the phenomenon have been identified and incorporated into the emerging themes or theory (Guest *et al.* 2006; Liamputtong 2013; see also Chapters 1, 8). In reality, however, this concept is difficult to nail down, and there is little consensus in the literature to guide the decision about how many interviews to conduct. The broader the scope of the research question, the more participant interviews will be needed, the more data will be generated, and the longer it will take to reach data saturation. If the topic is fairly straightforward and uncontroversial, the data are more easily obtained and fewer participants will need to be involved. However, if the topic is more sensitive and difficult for the participants to talk about, or is 'difficult to grab', then the number of participant interviews may need to be increased (Morse 2000, p. 4). The dynamic nature of these decisions reflects the flexibility characteristic of qualitative research. In my study, data collection was curtailed more by the practical constraints of conducting research to fulfil the requirements and deadlines of a graduate program, and it is unlikely that data saturation was achieved. The key question in phenomenological research, when making sampling decisions, is whether the sample provides access to enough data and has the appropriate focus for the research purpose to be thoroughly addressed (Mason 2002). As a result, the initial sample size is an estimate rather than a fixed

Purposive sampling: This looks for cases that will be able to provide rich or in-depth information about the issue being examined, not a representative sample as in quantitative research.

Snowball sampling: This relies on existing participants to identify acquaintances who fit the inclusion criteria of a study, in order to increase the size of the sample.

number. All the participants I interviewed had considerable experience of living with a spinal cord injury, but some were more articulate and had clearly reflected on their experiences. In general, the better the quality of data acquired from each source, the smaller the sample size required (Carpenter & Suto 2008).

Data collection: conducting qualitative interviews

Single, fairly lengthy (sixty- to eighty-minute) **in-depth interviews** were the method I chose for my study (see Chapter 4). Bearing the aim of the study in mind, I developed a list of possible questions to guide the interview. I began with broad open-ended questions (see box) designed to encourage the participants to express their perceptions and understandings in their own words. As the interview progressed, I attempted to ask probing questions and reflect the participants' understanding back to them to ensure a full exploration of the experience. As a result, each interview was unique and did not follow 'a uniform, standardized, replicable process' (Taylor 2005, p. 40). The interviews gave the participants the opportunity to construct or reconstruct their experiences and, as such, were 'influenced by their ability to articulate, reflect on and recall experiences and the accompanying emotions' (p. 41). With the permission of each participant, the interviews were audiotaped; I transcribed the tapes as soon as possible after the interviews. These transcripts formed the main data for this study but were supplemented by field notes and analytic memos. I recorded field notes immediately after each interview and included them in each transcript. These notes enabled me to capture the meaning and context of the interview and to reflect on my participation in it. Throughout the process of planning the study, interviewing and reading the transcripts and related literature and data analysis, I continually experienced new insights and ideas that I wrote in the form of analytic memos. The compilation of such notes represents the sort of 'internal dialogue' or 'thinking aloud' (Hammersley & Atkinson 1995, cited in Carpenter & Suto 2008, p. 106) that is a core feature of phenomenology.

In-depth interviewing: A method of qualitative data collection that does not use fixed questions, but aims to engage the interviewee in a guided conversation to elicit their understandings and interpretations.

SAMPLE INTERVIEW QUESTIONS

- Imagine the years since your injury as a journey. Could you describe what was most significant for you (what influenced you the most) during that journey?
- Is there a particular feeling you have when you think of the experience of learning to live with a disability?
- Have your feelings about the experience of the past few years changed over time?
- Has there ever been a time when your way of thinking about the experience of spinal cord injury has seemed different from those around you?

Christine Carpenter

- Is there anyone you know who thinks about spinal cord injury and its consequences differently from you (e.g. other injured persons, health professionals, friends, strangers)?
- How do they think about it?
- How is that different from the way you think about it?
- What would you describe about your experience to someone newly injured or someone who knows nothing about spinal cord injury?

As a physical therapist, I considered myself experienced in conducting clinical interviews and taking histories as part of clinical practice. There is a danger, however, that the substantial differences between clinical or therapeutic and qualitative interviewing may not be recognised (Ryan *et al.* 2009). The aim of clinically oriented interviews is to acquire the information about a specific health problem needed to assess the problem accurately and develop treatment goals with the client. As a result, they are primarily oriented to the health care professional's agenda. In contrast, qualitative interviews are flexible and adaptable, and often characterised as a purposeful conversation. My thesis adviser did recognise the danger and insisted that I conduct two pilot interviews before embarking on the main data collection.

STOP AND THINK

Barry sustained a C6 complete spinal cord injury when he was nineteen. Since that time, he has lived independently and is working full-time as a learning resources counsellor at a major university. He uses a manual wheelchair, owns his own home and drives a van with hand controls. He has many interests and a well-established social life. He is now fifty and experiencing some of the consequences of ageing with a disability, such as repetitive strain shoulder injuries and collapsed thoracic vertebral bodies causing back muscle spasms. His health is generally excellent. He is seeking advice from the rehabilitation therapists.

- How might a qualitative interview exploring how Barry experienced spinal cord injury differ from a clinical interview?

The pilot interviews proved invaluable as they gave me the opportunity to assess the effectiveness of the interview questions and my interviewing technique, to manage the details of participant comfort, audiotaping and transcribing, to establish rapport with the participant, and to practise the authentic listening so essential to phenomenological research. The transcripts of these interviews were discussed with my thesis adviser and reviewed by the two participants to further refine the interview process. In the pilot interviews, it became apparent that the participants had redefined the direction of the interview, assuming that my primary interest as a physical therapist (which was known by all the participants) was their physical recovery from spinal cord injury in the formal rehabilitation setting. In fact, it was not my intention to explore their experiences in the rehabilitation system but to explore, from an adult learning perspective, individual conceptions of living with a spinal cord injury over time and the meaning these individuals attributed to the experience. As a result of insights gained from the pilot interviews, I refocused the questions on the meanings associated with a significant life event and was careful to omit the words 'rehabilitation', 'rehabilitation process' and 'treatment'. I also emphasised my connections, for the purpose of this study, with adult education rather than physical therapy.

The role of the researcher in phenomenological research

The interaction between participant and researcher is key to the data collection process in phenomenology and is influenced by how the participant perceives the researcher (Carpenter & Suto 2008). In this study, my background in spinal cord rehabilitation meant that I was perceived as knowledgeable, as someone who understood some of the realities of living with a spinal cord injury, or as someone who could be trusted to provide advice. Establishing a genuine rapport in phenomenological interviews is crucial and involves the concept of reciprocity. Reciprocity 'requires, on the part of the researcher, a genuine presence, self-disclosure, respect, and commitment to involving the participants in all phases of the research' (Carpenter & Suto 2008, p. 126; see also Liamputtong 2007, 2013).

Positionality

The concept of **positionality** is related to the 'position' from which one 'chooses' to speak. The research question or aim is developed from this position and to some extent lends credibility and authority to the study. Addressing my positionality meant giving a full explanation of the experience and knowledge I had accrued, as a physical therapist, about the research topic during a lengthy career in spinal cord injury rehabilitation. I also examined the theoretical lenses, in particular feminism, the social model of disability and the client-centred model of practice, that I had developed through clinical practice, professional conferences and an extensive reading of the literature.

Positionality: This is related to the 'position' from which one 'chooses' to speak. The research aim is developed from this position and lends credibility and authority to the study.

Reflexivity

Reflexivity is an essential strategy that makes explicit the deep-seated views and judgments that affect the research process, including a full assessment of the influence of the researcher's assumptions, perceptions, values, beliefs and interests in relation to the research topic of interest (Carpenter & Suto 2008). To address reflexivity, I systematically and critically reflected on and analysed all the decisions I made during the research process and constructed a reflective account in the form of analytic memos that my thesis adviser regularly discussed with me.

Reflexivity: A strategy that makes explicit the researcher's deep-seated views and judgments that influence and affect the research process.

In reflecting throughout the research process, my own assumptions became explicit; for example, about living with a spinal cord injury, the nature and impact of disability on a person's life, and the role of rehabilitation in assisting a person to get back on track after an injury.

Christine Carpenter

I was able to articulate how these had influenced the research design, particularly the data analysis process. I also experienced a major shift in my understanding of the psychosocial and political issues associated with living with disability. This has had a long-term effect on my rehabilitation practice and teaching.

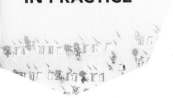

**RESEARCH
IN PRACTICE**

REFLEXIVITY AND PHENOMENOLOGICAL INTERVIEWING

With Peter Rowe (Rowe & Carpenter 2011), I conducted a qualitative study using a descriptive phenomenology framework to describe the experiences and challenges of Canadian military physiotherapists deployed to Afghanistan. Six military physiotherapists were recruited and interviewed by Peter. All interviews were conducted face to face, took place in different cities across Canada, and were between sixty and 142 minutes in length. Peter held a position of authority in the military and had twenty years experience as a military physiotherapy officer (PTO) in the Canadian Forces (CF). His interest in this topic derived from his involvement in the early planning phases of the deployment of PTOs to Afghanistan. He strongly believed that PTOs were essential on operational missions, despite the fact that there was considerable resistance from the CF operational mission planners, and planners in other militaries, to include PTOs in deployments for a variety of operational, clinical and doctrinal reasons. In order to ensure that Peter listened authentically to the participants during the interviews, it was essential that he engaged in rigorous critical reflection about his experiences as an advocate for the deployment of PTOs, and made explicit how the assumptions and values he held about the role of PTOs influenced the research process. Bracketing interviews were not conducted, but Peter aimed to be as transparent as possible about how he influenced the research, by keeping a reflective journal, conducting a pilot interview, and having discussions with me throughout the research process.

The concept of bracketing

The strategies of positionality and reflexivity are common to all qualitative research, whereas the related concept of bracketing is characteristic of descriptive phenomenology. In the original study I did not address the issue of bracketing; in writing this chapter I have taken the opportunity to revisit this concept. There is no consensus on the definition of bracketing—what it is, when it should occur, or the methods of bracketing. Bracketing has variously been defined as encompassing beliefs and values, preconceptions, biases, assumptions and presuppositions (Tufford & Newman 2010), and these definitions reflect the more general concept of reflexivity. The question is how the concept of bracketing, associated with descriptive phenomenology, can be differentiated from reflexivity. Tufford and Newman (2010, p. 84) suggest that bracketing is 'comprised of a multilayered process that is meant to access various levels of consciousness' that are 'difficult to access in the throes of conducting qualitative research'. Bracketing is not an attempt to be objective but rather an attempt to encourage researchers to set aside, as much as possible, their internal beliefs, experiences, understandings, biases, judgments and assumptions about the study topic so that they can authentically listen to the participants' perspectives and describe the essence of the phenomenon being studied. It is not a matter of simply articulating preconceptions, 'but a process of self discovery whereby buried emotions and experiences may surface' (p. 84) that begins before undertaking the research and continues through the research process.

More recently, I have been involved in bracketing interviews. This is a strategy in which researchers are assisted in the self-discovery process by a colleague or co-researcher in order to explore the impact of their personal and professional experiences during data collection and analysis. There is no consensus about when bracketing should occur, but Rolls and Relf (2006) favour making preconceptions explicit before starting the research project, and most agree that is an ongoing process. I have found it to be particularly useful when engaging in sensitive research where there are concerns about the personal, ethical and professional consequences for the participants, for example in exploring the impact of women's experiences of physical and sexual abuse on their relationships with health care professionals (Schachter *et al.* 2009).

Using the strategy of bracketing interviews

Bracketing interviews enable the development of a research-focused relationship between the researcher and an experienced bracketer (Rolls & Relf 2006). The bracketer is a person who has an understanding of the advisory nature of the relationship and the demands of qualitative research. Before conducting bracketing interviews it is important to negotiate the boundaries of the proposed interviews, for example differentiating the purpose of the interviews from other types of support that might be used by the researcher such as a mentor or peers, the timing of the meetings, and questions relating to maintaining confidentiality. In my experience, meetings between the researcher and bracketer took place as needed by the researcher and lasted for forty-five to sixty minutes. Each bracketing interview was treated as a form of data collection, being audiotaped and transcribed. In this way, the interviews were 'embedded in the research process' (Rolls & Relf 2006, p. 294). In being involved with bracketing interviews, both as researcher and bracketer, I have been guided by the four-session process described by Rolls and Relf (2006) (see box 'Research in practice').

THE SESSIONS OF BRACKETING INTERVIEWS

Before data collection

The purpose of this session is to establish an agreement about how to proceed and to explore the researcher's 'lack of neutrality' (Ahern 1999, p. 409). The interview focuses on accessing and making explicit the researcher's experiences, assumptions and value systems, and the emotions and feelings held about the research topic. The idea is for the researcher to reflect on experiences that might influence their ability to listen authentically to the participants and that might trigger judgmental or emotional responses to what they are hearing.

During the data collection

This session focuses on the experience of being the researcher and the interaction with the participants. Issues explored in this interview relate

RESEARCH IN PRACTICE

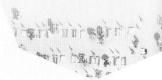

>>

Christine Carpenter

to actual or potential conflicts between the roles of physical therapist or academic and researcher, that is, managing 'boundary crossing' (Rolls & Relf 2006, p. 298). The researcher is encouraged to explore issues of reciprocity; that is, responding appropriately to questions posed by the participants, revealing personal information, and responding professionally and ethically during the study interviews.

During the data analysis

In this session, issues arising from the data analysis process related to representation are explored;

that is, accurately portraying the participants' experiences and perceptions (Carpenter & Suto 2008) in the emerging themes and in writing up the research.

At the end of the research

Rolls and Relf (2006, p. 301) suggest that this session is useful 'to consider any outstanding issues arising from the research and to review the bracketing process and reflect on its contribution to the study'.

The data analysis process

The analytical approach in phenomenology orients the researcher to an 'exhaustive, reflective and detailed analysis of each individual experience' (Carpenter & Suto 2008, p. 128; see also Chapters 6, 7, 8, 23). As Thorne explains, using the phenomenon of grieving as an example:

> Rather than explain the stages and transitions within grieving that are common to people in various circumstances … [phenomenological analysis] might attempt to uncover and describe the essential nature of grieving and represent it in such a manner that a person who had not grieved might begin to appreciate the phenomenon (2000, p. 69),

My analytical process began as I transcribed the interviews. I was guided by a series of interpretive stages that, I now recognise, reflect the framework developed by the phenomenologist Colaizzi (1978). These stages are described in Table 9.1.

TABLE 9.1   Application of Colaizzi's phenomenological framework in data analysis

STAGES OF FRAMEWORK	ANALYTICAL PROCESS
Stage 1: Acquiring a sense of each transcript	I read each interview transcript several times to get a sense of the data as a whole.
Stage 2: Extracting significant statements	Data chunks or fragments (units of meaning) were highlighted in the transcripts that identified or informed my understanding of each participant's experience of spinal cord injury. I labelled each statement with the participant's pseudonym, page and line number, then cut them from the transcript copy and assigned them initially to file folders and later on flipchart paper mounted on the walls.

STAGES OF FRAMEWORK	ANALYTICAL PROCESS
Stage 3: Formulation of meanings	I wrote my interpretation or restatement of the meaning of the significant statements distilled from the transcripts. During this stage I found it essential to consistently reflect on my own assumptions, reactions to the participants' narratives, and the connections I was making with the related literature, and to record these insights as analytic memos.
Stage 4: Organising formulated meanings into clusters of themes	Statements and associated formulated meanings that clearly represented a common focus were grouped together as a theme cluster (what I called a category). This stage of analysis resulted in approximately sixteen theme clusters. I presented the analysis at this stage to a colleague, who was knowledgeable in both qualitative research and spinal cord injury, to examine the emerging relationships between categories (a process called peer review) to ensure that the interpretive process was clear and accurately described. The sixteen categories were further consolidated to form three main themes—rediscovering self, redefining disability and establishing a new identity—that were common to all the participants' descriptions of their experience of spinal cord injury.
Stage 5: Exhaustively describing the investigated phenomenon	The three main themes were described in detail and illustrated by verbatim participant quotes (or data). This initial account was again discussed with my colleague (peer review). Differences in interpretive decisions occurred and these caused me to reflect on and re-examine my analytic process.
Stage 6: Describing the fundamental structure of the phenomenon	Colaizzi (1978) advocates that the theme descriptions should be further reduced to a statement of their fundamental or essential structure. It had become apparent to me that the three themes were informed by transformative learning theory and I developed an overall explanation of the themes framed by this theory.
Stage 7: Returning to the participants	Colaizzi (1978) suggests that the final validation of the data analysis should involve returning to the participants for another interview to ensure that they can recognise their own experience in the themes and for a final statement (a process called member checking). This was not feasible in this study.

Strategies of rigour

It is generally accepted that without rigour, research, whatever the methodological approach, fails to contribute to the professional knowledge base or to evidence-based practice. A number of strategies can be used to enhance the rigour of qualitative studies (see Chapter 1). These strategies do not themselves ensure the trustworthiness of the research. They need to be selectively employed, adapted and combined to achieve the purposes of specific studies, and their use is justified by linking strategy decisions with the research question, chosen methodology and study design (Carpenter & Suto 2008; Liamputtong 2013). Several strategies of rigour, congruent with the core concepts and principles of phenomenology, were incorporated into the study design.

Contribution to evidence-based practice

Evidence-based practice: A process that requires the practitioner to find empirical evidence about the effectiveness or efficacy of different treatment options then determine the relevance of that evidence to a particular client's situation.

Most rehabilitation professionals recognise that the complex issues inherent in rehabilitation practice have not been addressed in the most influential definitions of **evidence-based practice**, such as 'the conscientious, explicit, and judicious use of current best evidence in making decisions about the care of individual patients' (Sackett *et al.* 1996, p. 30). These definitions are impairment or disease-oriented, have a practitioner-centred focus, and promote the idea of a hierarchy of evidence that privileges randomised controlled trials as a sort of 'gold standard' (Hammell & Carpenter 2004; see Chapters 1, 15, 17, 19). Evidence-based practice can perhaps be better described as an approach to decision-making in which the practitioner uses the best available research evidence, in consultation with the client, to decide which option best suits that client. The need for greater methodological diversity in addressing the complex questions that arise from clinical practice, particularly where clients with chronic conditions and disability receive services from multiple health professions, is recognised. In turn, a combination of evidence generated by qualitative, survey and mixed methods research is now increasingly used to support clinical decision-making (Hammell & Carpenter 2004; Grypdonck 2006; Rauscher & Greenfield 2009), and more effective approaches to establishing the level of qualitative evidence continue to be debated (Kearney 2001a; Sandelowski & Barroso 2003; Sandelowski & Leeman 2012). In addition, 'research needs to be increasingly transdisciplinary—drawing from theory, knowledge and methods in the social sciences and humanities' (Gibson 2012, p. 357).

For qualitative research to make a significant contribution to professional knowledge and evidence-based practice, the findings of rigorously designed studies need to be disseminated in professional and public forums and by publication in peer-reviewed journals (Carpenter & Suto 2008). As Gibson (2012) argues, 'qualitative research at its best can help to address some of the most tenacious issues in health and rehabilitation' (p. 357). Phenomenology, the focus of this chapter, can contribute to evidence-based rehabilitation practice in a number of ways: by generating comprehensive descriptions of what it is like to live with a chronic condition or disability, the meaning that clients attribute to health and illness, their experiences of the professional services provided and the challenges and facilitators associated with quality of life and independence, what constitutes 'good' outcomes in rehabilitation and how these should be measured. The evidence derived from these studies raises important questions about the impairment focus of rehabilitation (which inevitably emphasises what clients cannot do rather than what they can do) (McPherson &

Kayes 2012, p. 382) and challenges the privileging of health care professionals' knowledge and expertise. Phenomenological research can also contribute to evidence-based practice and professional knowledge by investigating how health care professionals implement different models of practice and teamwork and by exploring their experiences of ethical and professional issues in practice and the challenges in providing services for specific client groups. Some of these contributions are illustrated in the following examples of phenomenological studies that address specific questions arising from practice about the client and professional experiences of rehabilitation.

Exploring rehabilitation clients' experiences

Redmond and Suddick (2012) explored the experience of freezing from the perspective of clients with Parkinson's. Freezing, described as a lack of voluntary movement or a sudden inability to initiate movement, is associated with Parkinson's and has a profound effect on functional ability and independence, particularly in the advanced stages of the condition. **Semi-structured interviews** were conducted with six participants who experienced freezing. The findings highlighted the heightened physical awareness and emotional cost of managing the uncontrollable and unpredictable nature of freezing, and identified a diversity of strategies the participants used to overcome or cope with it. This type of information helps rehabilitation practitioners to plan and evaluate individualised rehabilitation programs in collaboration with clients and this, in turn, contributes to the effectiveness of the interventions.

Semi-structured interview: An interview where the researchers have prepared some broad open-ended questions with the intention of eliciting in-depth information, while at the same time enabling participants to elaborate on their responses.

Paterson and Carpenter (2015) explored how adults with severe acquired communication difficulties experience and make decisions about the communication methods they use. Vulnerable client groups can all too easily be excluded from authentic partnerships with health professionals, in terms of establishing meaningful goals and making decisions. The lack of research involving adults with severe acquired communication difficulties may be attributed to the methodological challenges associated with data collection, consent, and participant and researcher fatigue. The flexible nature of qualitative research facilitated the implementation of some creative adaptations that enabled the researchers to effectively meet these challenges. Seven participants were recruited from a long-term care setting in a rehabilitation hospital. Data collection methods were face-to-face videorecorded interviews using each participant's choice of communication method, and email interviews. Four main themes were identified: communicating in the digital age (email and social media), encountering frustrations in using communication technologies, role and identity changes and influences associated with communication technology use, and seeking functional interactions using communication technologies. These findings provide the evidence needed to support assessment, training and the development of communication aids and highlight the importance of developing authentic partnerships between speech language therapists and clients.

Christine Carpenter

Janssen and Stube (2014) explore older adults' perceptions of participation in physical activity, in particular how it impacted productive ageing, with the aim of informing the development of an occupation-based physical activity program for older adults who live in the community, by occupational therapists. In this phenomenological study, fifteen community-dwelling older adults were recruited from a diversity of community locations, using purposive and snowball sampling. The data collection methods included two interviews with each participant. During the interview the researcher frequently engaged in the physical activity, for example raking the lawn while having a conversation with the participant, thus enabling the researcher to also observe the participant. The authors provide a detailed discussion of the findings, including a concept map. The primary finding is that older adults continue individual patterns of meaningful physical activity across their lifespan when they have support to adapt to age-associated limitations and there is a gradual decline in intensity during older years.

Exploring the professionals' experiences of rehabilitation practice

Phenomenological research that accesses the practice experiences of health professionals not only illuminates how practice is delivered in specific clinical contexts but can also explore the ethical and professional challenges faced by practitioners in increasingly complex and demanding health care systems. Jeffrey and Foster (2012) sought to understand how the personal experiences and values of physical therapists influence their decision-making when treating patients with non-specific low back pain (NSLBP). Using a hermeneutic phenomenological approach and practitioner-as-researcher model, they conducted eleven semi-structured interviews with physical therapists working in the National Health Service (NHS) in the UK. Three interwoven themes were identified: physical therapists believe that NSLBP has an underlying mechanical and recurring nature; physical therapists' attitude towards managing NSLBP is to empower patients to exercise and self-manage their pain and functional problems; and physical therapists experience feelings of tension between the advice and treatment they feel is best for their patient and the patient's own beliefs and attitudes. Conflict between patients' and professionals' different beliefs and attitudes about pain—the nature, impact and outcome of pain—needed to be negotiated in order to establish an effective decision-making partnership. The authors suggest that treatment decisions might be influenced when physical therapists modify their beliefs and attitudes to reduce this sense of conflict. Improving physical therapists' communication skills may help decrease feelings of conflict, enhance working relationships, and encourage a more consistent approach towards patients with NSLBP.

Over the last few years, there has been increasing concern regarding the apparent lack of compassion and caring in the NHS in the UK. The aim of Beckett's (2013) study was to explore nurses' and physiotherapists' understanding of the concept of care and how it is integrated into practice. She conducted in-depth interviews with twelve nurses and eleven physiotherapists in four demographically and geographically diverse NHS hospitals. Beckett (2013) reports that 'physiotherapists presented a distinct identity with caring both integral to the role and sustained by structural and organizational factors. In contrast, nurses had a diffuse identity with limited control within a biomedical and business model of care. They appeared "under siege" and were nostalgic for caring, which was frequently subordinate to other demands. Both nurses and physiotherapists faced challenges but nurses felt the context of their work was not conducive to caring' (p. 1118). This type of research promotes a deeper understanding of the frequently conflicting personal, professional, organisational and public expectations that practitioners must juggle in their efforts to provide care for patients within the NHS.

Rehabilitation services are provided in the private sector in many countries, and this practice environment presents a range of different ethical and moral issues for practitioners. Praestegaard and Gard (2013) used a hermeneutic phenomenological approach to explore the nature and scope of ethical issues as they are understood and experienced by physiotherapists in outpatient private practice. They conducted two in-depth interviews with twenty-two physiotherapists working in different private practices. The findings focused on issues associated with establishing equality in the professional–patient relationship, patient advocacy and transgressing boundaries (physical, cultural and privacy). In this instance, a phenomenological approach makes explicit the issues that need to be debated within a profession and that have implications for the therapeutic relationship and professional autonomy.

More broadly, phenomenological studies have the potential to illuminate the taken-for-granted and unexamined practices that characterise rehabilitation provision as well as 'the social, political and cultural forces that impact on health, function, and participation' (Gibson 2012, p. 357). In Sandelowski's opinion, 'qualitative research is the best thing to be happening to evidence-based practice' (2004, p. 1382). But conducting the research is only the first step. Qualitative researchers must also be accountable for moving research findings into practice and this means translating the knowledge represented by their findings into practice, encouraging understanding and critical appraisal of qualitative research (McBrien 2008; Ryan *et al.* 2007; see Chapter 27), and conducting metasyntheses (the term more commonly used in the qualitative research literature than 'systematic reviews') of qualitative research (Levack 2012; see Chapter 18).

Summary

Phenomenology is an established and influential research approach for examining therapy and rehabilitation practice from the client and professional perspective. In this chapter I reviewed two methodological traditions—descriptive and interpretive—both of which originated in the philosophical writings of Husserl. There are a number of schools of phenomenological thought, and the boundaries between phenomenology as a philosophy and research methodology can become blurred (Dowling 2007). As Finlay (2009) suggests, for some phenomenology is 'a rigorous, systematic, scientific method while for others, it is a fluid, creative approach with distinctly emotive, poetic sensibility' (p. 477). There is, however, consensus that phenomenological research seeks to explore the embodied experiential meaning, and to develop complex and rich descriptions of a phenomenon as it is lived by individuals. The key concepts associated with phenomenology—phenomenological reduction, bracketing, the life-world, multiple realities and essence—were discussed, and the argument was made that attention to the underlying philosophical theory strengthens the study design and coherence of the research. In this era of evidence-based practice it is imperative that new knowledge derived from rigorous qualitative research be effectively transferred into practice. It is my hope that the example studies illustrate the contribution that phenomenological research can make to rehabilitation practice.

Practice exercises

1   Ask some friends to individually describe, as fully as possible, what they mean when they talk of the phenomenon of 'love'. Identify the essence of the phenomenon reflected in these descriptions, that is, what elements are common to all their definitions. Compile these and share the result with your friends. Does this 'new' definition reflect their experience of the phenomenon?

2   If you were conducting a study exploring some aspect of your day-to-day practice, how would you describe your position in the research and how might you, in the role of researcher, influence the data collection and analysis?

3   If you wanted to include bracketing interviews in the design of a qualitative study, consider who you would ask (and why) to assist and what you would tell them about the role of the bracketer.

4   How would you involve the participants in a phenomenological study in enhancing the credibility (or rigour) of your research?

Further reading

Beckett, K. (2013). Professional wellbeing and caring: exploring a complex relationship. *British Journal of Nursing*, 22(19), 1118–24.

Braun, V. & Clarke, V. (2006). Using thematic analysis in psychology. *Qualitative Research in Psychology*, 3, 77–101.

Dowling, M. (2006). Approaches to reflexivity in qualitative research. *Nurse Researcher*, 13(3), 7–21.

Dowling, M. (2007). From Husserl to van Manen: a review of different phenomenological approaches. *International Journal of Nursing Studies*, 44(1), 131–42.

Gearing, R.E. (2004). Bracketing in research: a typology. *Qualitative Health Research*, 14(10), 1429–52.

Gibson, B. (2012). Editorial: beyond methods: the promise of qualitative inquiry for physical therapy. *Physical Therapy Reviews*, 17(6), 357–9.

Greenfield, B.H. & Jensen, G.M. (2012). Phenomenology: a powerful tool for patient-centered rehabilitation. *Physical Therapy Reviews*, 17(6), 417–24.

Janssen, S.L. & Stube, J.E. (2014). Older adults' perceptions of physical activity: a qualitative study. *Occupational Therapy International,* 21, 53–62.

Jones, F., Rodger, S., Ziviani, J. & Boyd, R. (2012). Application of a hermeneutic phenomenologically orientated approach to qualitative study. *International Journal of Theory and Practice*, 19(7), 370–8.

Levack, W.M.M. (2012). The role of qualitative metasynthesis in evidence-based physical therapy. *Physical Therapy Reviews*, 17(6), 390–7.

Lopez, K.A. & Willis, D.G. (2004). Descriptive versus interpretive phenomenology: the contributions to nursing knowledge. *Qualitative Health Research*, 14(5), 726–35.

Mantzoukas, S. (2008). Facilitating research students in formulating qualitative research questions. *Nursing Education Today*, 28, 371–7.

McBrien, B. (2008). Evidence-based care: enhancing the rigour of a qualitative study. *British Journal of Nursing*, 17(20), 1286–9.

McPherson, K.M. & Kayes, N.M. (2012). Qualitative research: its practical contribution to physiotherapy. *Physical Therapy Reviews*, 17(6), 382–9.

Moustakas, C. (1994). *Phenomenological research methods*. Thousand Oaks, CA: Sage.

Nicholls, D. (2012). Postmodernism and physiotherapy research. *Physical Therapy Reviews*, 17(6), 360–8.

Paterson, H. & Carpenter, C. (2015). Using different methods to communicate: how adults with severe acquired communication difficulties make decisions about the communication methods they use and how they experience them. *Disability & Rehabilitation*, 37(17), 1522–30.

Praestegaard, J. & Gard, G. (2013). Ethical issues in physiotherapy: reflected from the perspective of physiotherapists in private practice. *Physiotherapy Theory and Practice*, 29(2), 96–112.

Pringle, J., Drummond, J., McLafferty, E. & Hendry, C. (2011). Interpretative phenomenological analysis: a discussion and critique. *Nurse Researcher*, 18(3), 20–4.

Ryan, F., Coughlan, M. & Cronin, P. (2009). Interviewing in qualitative research: the one-to-one interview. *International Journal of Therapy and Rehabilitation*, 16(6), 309–14.

Ryan, F., Coughlan, M. & Cronin, P. (2007). Step-by-step guide to critiquing research. Part 2: Qualitative research. *British Journal of Nursing*, 16(12), 738–44.

Sandelowski, M. & Leeman, J. (2012). Writing useable qualitative health research findings. *Qualitative Health Research*, 22(10), 1404–13.

Shaw, J.A. & Connelly, D.M. (2012). Phenomenology and physiotherapy: meaning in research and practice. *Physical Therapy Reviews*, 17(6), 398–408.

Todres, I. (2005). Clarifying the life-world: descriptive phenomenology. In I. Holloway (ed.), *Qualitative research in health care*. Oxford: Blackwell, 104–24.

Christine Carpenter

Websites

www.phenomenology-carp.org/

> This is the home page of the Center for Advanced Research in Phenomenology (CARP), coordinated by the Department of Philosophy at the University of Memphis. This extensive site offers many valuable sources on phenomenological research.

www.phenomenologyonline.com

> This site, initiated by Max van Manen, offers public access to articles, monographs and other materials discussing and exemplifying phenomenological research.

www.bbk.ac.uk/psychology/ipa

> This is the home page of interpretative phenomenological analysis (IPA), developed by Jonathan Smith, Professor of Psychology at Birkbeck, University of London. It includes detailed explanations of IPA, references, and an opportunity to join an IPA discussion group.

http://hsl.mcmaster.libguides.com/c.php?g=306765&p=2044668

> The McMaster University Center for Evidence-Based Practice provides a number of very useful resources related to critical appraisal of research, guidelines and systematic reviews and metasyntheses, and links to other useful websites.

10

Clinical Data-mining as Practice-based Evidence

DAVID NILSSON

Chapter objectives

In this chapter you will learn:

- how data-mining is used as a research technique
- about its advantages and drawbacks in relation to other research methods
- how a health-based case study illustrates the application of data-mining

Key terms

Clinical data-mining

Data-mining

Practice-based research

Research-based practice

Secondary data analysis

Unobtrusive methods

Introduction

Academics are always searching for ways to encourage health and social care practitioners to engage in research in order to critically examine their own practice and ultimately to build practice knowledge and improve practice. Social work is no exception in this regard. Social workers are often immersed in their heavy client workloads and have little time to think about research, let alone carry it out. Therefore any research method that has the advantages of practitioners generating their own research questions for a research project, using existing data that has relevance to practice, and doing the bulk of the research themselves, has considerable benefits. The research method that is the subject of this chapter, **clinical data-mining** (CDM), has all of these advantages.

Data-mining: definition

Data-mining is the process of extracting and analysing data to uncover hidden patterns and useful information. It is commonly used in retail, marketing and fraud detection. Clinical data-mining has been defined by Auslander and colleagues (2001, p. 131) as 'involving practitioners in locating, conceptualising, retrieving, analysing and interpreting available clinical information to answer questions that emerge from and concern their own practice'. As clear and concise as this definition is, it does not mention a key element of CDM—that it is a form of research most often done by practitioners themselves, rather than external researchers. It also mentions possible foci for such research, but neglects to note the significant point that for this method practitioners can generate their own research questions or hypotheses that are designed to address practice issues and are aimed at informing their practice and that of other practitioners. So, more precisely, a definition of CDM should be the use of available client and agency information in social work to answer research questions about practice, particularly as related to intervention and its outcomes.

Data-mining is essentially a form of practice-based research using **secondary data analysis** (analysis of data collected for purposes other than for a specific piece of research) (Kellehear 1993; Smith 2008). In the qualitative approach, data-mining sits neatly within **unobtrusive methods** (Kellehear 1993; Liamputtong 2013). In contrast to evidence-based practice (see Chapters 16, 17), CDM is striving to provide practice-based evidence, that is, evidence or information derived from practice. Such evidence 'highlights the importance of experiential knowledge in clinical decision-making and its contribution to establishing broad-based best practice models' (Merighi *et al.* 2005, p. 710).

Context for its use

Social workers in all settings inevitably, and often perhaps to their annoyance, collect and record large amounts of information in various forms on client characteristics and their assessed presenting and ongoing problems, as well as their own interventions, and the

---

Clinical data-mining: Provides practice-based evidence that underscores the importance of experiential knowledge in clinical decision-making and its contribution to establishing broad-based best practice models.

Data-mining: The process of extracting and analysing data to uncover hidden patterns and useful information.

Secondary data analysis: An analysis of data collected for purposes other than for a specific piece of research.

Unobtrusive methods: These do not require direct contact with informants. They use data that have been published or are available in libraries, the press or other media.

responses and outcomes for clients as a result of those interventions. These data are primarily used for clinical, administrative and supervisory purposes and for accountability to funding bodies. Such information, while often voluminous, is easily accessible and non-intrusive yet its utility to social work research is often overlooked or even rejected.

It is often rejected for research purposes because utilising such data would not be seen as 'proper research'. But this information can be used to answer valuable questions for social workers. What are the characteristics of the clients we are seeing? What is happening when they are being seen? What are we actually doing for them? What seems to work in producing better outcomes for these clients? What produces more negative outcomes?

There are numerous examples of CDM studies involving a range of areas, for example, termination in an adolescent mental health service (Mirabito 2001), liver transplant mortality (Epstein *et al.* 1997), assessing a hospital support program for family caregivers (Dobrof *et al.* 2006), social work practice with renal dialysis patients (Auslander *et al.* 2001), single-session social work in hospitals (Plath & Gibbons 2010), and reviewing medical records of patient deaths in hospitals to assess utilisation of social work services (Pockett *et al.* 2010). More broadly, social work documentation can be a rich source of research material. It has been used as a means of research in social work practice in studies such as those by Floersch (2000, 2004) and Cumming and colleagues (2007).

STOP AND THINK

Jane is the chief medical social worker in a large suburban public hospital. She has fifteen social workers in her team. She would like to know more about the patients that these social workers see. She has access to patient medical records and the social workers' client files.

Generate five research questions that Jane could use with these sources of data.

VIDEOTAPES EXPLORE BEREAVEMENT EXPERIENCE

CDM is seen in practice in a study by Chow (2010). She used a rather unusual source of data: videotapes of social workers' clinical sessions with clients to explore the bereavement experience of Chinese people in Hong Kong. Such tapes are commonly made in Hong Kong for use in clinical supervision and for individuals or families to review. From analysis of the data, a pool of items was generated and used to develop a thirteen-item grief reaction inventory. The data were also used to generate hypotheses about effective clinical practice and contribute to theory-building in grief and bereavement.

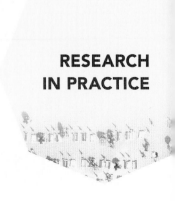

RESEARCH IN PRACTICE

Comparison with other research methods

The evidence-based practice (EBP) movement has been a major influence on the conduct of both research and practice in health for the last twenty years (Nathan *et al.* 1999; Sackett *et al.* 2000; Nathan & Gorman 2002). Social work has been slower to come on board in adopting EBP (Murphy & McDonald 2004; Ryan & Sheehan 2009), often because of a series of legitimate concerns about this approach to research (Gibbs & Gambrill 2002; Plath 2006). EBP emphasises the importance of practice being based on, and supported by, sound empirical research, with the preferred 'gold standard' being the conduct of randomised controlled trials (see Chapters 1, 15, 16, 17, 18).

Research-based practice: RBP is deductive (concepts derived from theory) and relies on standardised, quantitative research instruments.

Epstein (2001, p. 17) characterises **research-based practice** (RBP), like EBP, as having the following emphases:

- it is deductive (derived from theory)
- it seeks causal knowledge, therefore it gives priority to experimental, randomised control group designs
- it is prospective
- it relies on standardised, quantitative research instruments
- while it is collaborative, research requirements tend in the main to outweigh practice considerations.

Practice-based research: PBR is inductive (concepts derived from practice wisdom) and tends to rely on instruments tailored to the needs of social practice.

On the other hand, **practice-based research** (PBR), which includes clinical data-mining, according to Epstein (2001, p. 18), has the following essential attributes:

- it is inductive (concepts derived from practice wisdom)
- it makes use of non-experimental or quasi-experimental designs
- it seeks descriptive or correlational knowledge
- it may be either retrospective or prospective
- it may be quantitative or qualitative, but tends to rely on instruments tailored to the needs of professional practice rather than external standardised research instruments
- it is collaborative in nature and practice requirements tend to outweigh research considerations.

Epstein (2001, p. 18) goes on to emphasise that the fundamental distinction is between 'research *on* practice (RBP)' and, for PBR, 'research *in* practice'. For the former, the starting point is 'the research canon' and for PBR it is 'practice wisdom', that is, what practitioners know based on reflection on their experience of practice.

The crucial distinction is not between RBP being quantitative and PBR being qualitative. While RBP, which includes CDM, privileges a quantitative approach, CDM has a preference for seeking quantitative data, but is amenable to the combination of quantitative and qualitative data, and to qualitative data on its own (see Chapter 1). CDM incorporates the ideas of Argyris and Schon (1974) on the reflective practitioner (see also Schon 1983), and their ideas are not incompatible with those of some of their successors (see Fook *et al.* 2015; Fook & Gardner 2007) on reflective research and critical reflection.

USE OF CLINICAL INFORMATION TO STUDY SOCIAL RELATIONSHIPS AND GOALS

A study by McDonald and colleagues (2005) utilised clinical information routinely collected and used in joint planning with young people with early psychosis to study their social relationships and goals. Such goals included wanting more social opportunities, larger networks, more peer relationships and more social opportunities.

The findings of the study contributed to the existing knowledge base, particularly in relation to social networks and friendship, and had implications for service delivery, such as greater emphasis on social goal-setting in the intake assessment process.

RESEARCH IN PRACTICE

Clinical data-mining: its advantages and drawbacks

Clinical data-mining has a number of key advantages for social work practitioners wanting to research their own clinical practice. As Epstein and colleagues (1997, p. 225) point out:

> In comparison with studies based on original data generation, available information studies are likely to raise fewer ethical problems, are faster and less costly to complete, are less disruptive to existing staff and patient care routines, and make use of compliance on outcome indicators that are likely to be more agency and practice relevant.

To this list could be added the advantage that the analysis of available information is non-intrusive, which is ensured as long as the identity and identifying information of the client is carefully protected. This means that no ethical problems are presented and the research can be considered to be non-reactive (Kellehear 1993; Liamputtong 2013; see also Chapter 3).

On the other hand, CDM does have its problems. Finding information that will actually answer your research questions may be the first hurdle. Even if the information is there, it may not be pertinent to your chosen key variables because data on them simply has not been collected, which may well serve to highlight problems and issues with an agency's current collection of information. At the least, CDM can serve to highlight such omissions.

Of even more concern from a research purist's perspective is the reliability and validity of available information (see Chapter 1). Numerous questions can be raised about the data in relation to these two matters. Is what is written actually what practitioners have done?

David Nilsson

Have things been done that have not been recorded? Do practitioners consistently do things or assess things in the same way? If more than one practitioner has entered data, have their assessment and recording practices been consistent? These are legitimate concerns that need to at least be acknowledged as limitations in reporting the results of research using CDM.

Other drawbacks are that CDM can be labour-intensive. Locating old client information, retrieving it then going through it carefully seeking your particular foci of interest can take many hours of painstaking and laborious work. The work involved may mean that strategic decisions have to be taken on sampling, that is, which pieces offer the most complete and relevant source of data.

Despite the drawbacks, we believe that CDM is a legitimate way of conducting research that is relevant and useful to social workers. As Epstein (2001, p. 23) writes, 'problems of data quality … can be dealt with like any other applied research problem, i.e. with strategic compromise'.

STOP AND THINK

In examining the two sources of data available to her (patient medical records and social workers' case files), Jane finds that social work input and/or acknowledgment of their contribution is minimal in the medical records. In contrast, social workers' case file notes are detailed and rich.

- Can you suggest possible reasons for this discrepancy in the two sets of records?

Clinical data-mining: the process

The following steps are involved in the process of actually carrying out CDM (based on Epstein 2001, p. 28).

1   Locate a research site to inspect and take small samples of all available information sources to ascertain what kinds of information are generally available to you.

2   Assess the degree of accessibility, credibility, connectivity and (if handwritten) the legibility of this information.

3   Determine the unit of analysis you are going to examine, the time-frame, and the likely staging of this information-gathering.

4   Carry out a literature review to help conceptualise appropriate research questions and/or hypotheses, as well as identify concepts, theories/models and methods of data analysis in the current literature.

5   Conduct a detailed inventory of potential variables, distinguishing between predictors (e.g. demographics, health and psychosocial risk factors, resiliency factors), intervening variables (e.g. medical and psychosocial interventions) and dependent variables (e.g. mortality, morbidity, quality of life, client/patient satisfaction, etc.).

6   Develop initial data extraction forms that list all possible variables and categories.

7 Conduct studies of samples of key variables to ascertain their validity, reliability, accuracy and completeness until satisfactory levels are reached or some variables are excluded.

8 Construct finalised forms for data retrieval then extract the data from the records.

9 Create your own database (whether written or computerised, e.g. on Excel spreadsheet or SPSS [Statistical Package for the Social Sciences] data file) and enter the data. Run frequencies on variables to ascertain which are suitable for descriptive, bivariate or multivariate analysis (see Chapter 25).

10 Conceptualise, plan and conduct further studies based on the available data.

In relation to this research process, Epstein (2001, p. 29) identifies six important methodological lessons he learnt by doing CDM.

1 Have workers who are most familiar with the information/cases carry out data extraction in order to maximise validity and reliability.

2 Check for an agreement on key variables through multiple data sources (triangulation).

3 Identify strength, resilience and recovery factors as well as deficits and risk factors within the available information.

4 Describe in detail what is involved in the 'black box' of social work intervention.

5 Choose realistic intervention outcomes for your data.

6 Involve social workers at each stage and task (except tedious work like data entry) of the CDM research process. This enhances involvement and utilisation of collected information and findings and their later application.

STOP AND THINK

Jane obtains funding to carry out a small research project using CDM. She decides to engage a firm of external consultants to carry out the project. These consultants have a background in psychology and nursing and specialise in program evaluation.

What issues could arise by adopting this approach to the project?

ANALYSIS OF CASE RECORDS

In a study of positive family reunification outcomes in a New York City foster care agency, Condero (2004) used an examination of eighteen families' case records. Through this analysis she was able to identify the association between positive family reunification outcomes and three specific casework practices of the workers involved. From these findings, practice implications for refinement of foster care best practices were identified.

RESEARCH IN PRACTICE

David Nilsson

Clinical data-mining: a case study

This case study is based on a small piece of research that was carried out at the Royal Children's Hospital in Melbourne, within the Diabetes Unit where I previously worked as a social worker. The social work service to this unit focused mainly on two areas: assisting newly diagnosed children and their families to adjust to this significant event, and assisting children and their families who were experiencing difficulties post-diagnosis.

The Diabetes Unit included a strong multidisciplinary focus with twice-weekly biopsychosocial ward rounds, one of which focused on children in the adolescent ward. One morning the medical consultant let out a loud sigh upon reviewing the inpatient list. He had recognised the names of two teenagers whom he noted as being readmitted to hospital with disconcerting regularity despite the best efforts of medical staff and the diabetes clinical educator. Such patients had been dubbed 'frequent fliers'.

The consultant wondered whether there was something we were missing about these clients. He noted that there were a number of other adolescents like these who also seemed to be 'frequent fliers'. Was there some social or psychological aspect that was driving the frequent readmissions? He asked, 'As a social worker, what do you think? Is there something else we should be doing?' I was not sure, but said maybe I could look into it and get back to him. And so began an exploratory research process.

The first step was to review the medical records of the two teenagers. In doing so, however, I realised that I was unsure what I was looking for. I decided that it might be better to look at the published literature to get some clues. It was surprising to find how little literature there seemed to be in this area, especially in the local Australian context. The international literature did, however, identify some psychosocial factors that possibly contribute to poor diabetes control, which can be broadly divided into individual factors and family-related factors. Family-related factors included non-traditional family structures, family cohesion, family stress, family conflict (including teen–parent disputes and sibling rivalry), family resources, parenting skills and parental self-esteem. Individual (intra-psychic) factors that were identified as possible contributors included learning difficulties, psychiatric status, personality characteristics, body image, health locus of control, knowledge of juvenile diabetes, coping styles, stress, and the effects of recent personal life events.

The literature identified a condition termed 'brittle diabetes' (Tattersall 1985), which referred to patients with extremely unstable diabetes control that can lead to longer-term medical complications. This encompasses about 1 per cent of juvenile cases (Moran *et al.* 1991). While many studies aimed at understanding the relationship between psychosocial factors and diabetes control, the true nature of these relationships remained unclear.

To answer the medical consultant's broad question, I needed to come up with a plan to systematically review the available evidence at the hospital—a research project was conceived. The research questions emerged directly from the medical consultant's enquiry. Who are these 'frequent fliers' and how many of them are there in the clinic population? Do they share psychosocial factors that may affect their diabetes management, and if so what are they? Could we provide useful psychosocial interventions to overcome these factors? Could we use these factors to screen for earlier identification of potential problems and provide preventive interventions?

While a number of possible factors had been identified through the literature review process, I also wondered if there might be factors unique to this hospital clinic or to Australian children with diabetes. I felt it was important to be open to other possibilities so decided to incorporate a grounded theory approach in which the researcher uses inductive rather than deductive reasoning (Strauss & Corbin 1998; see Chapter 7). I aimed to be open to new and unique possibilities, attempting to approach the data without any preconceived ideas. This was quite difficult since I had already consulted the available literature.

In thinking about how I might answer the research questions, I had to consider how to gather relevant data. Existing hospital records provided an obvious source of readily available data. These included the patients' medical records, social work files, and the case records from a separate in-house mental health service. Clinical data-mining offered a logical way of exploring existing information without having to carry out time-consuming and intrusive interviewing or surveying. The next step was to identify how many and which patients were experiencing multiple readmissions to hospital. Fortunately, hospitals have excellent recording systems and I requested a report from the Hospital Records Department on average readmission rates for the Diabetes Clinic over the preceding three years. I discovered that the average readmission rate was 0.85 (i.e. less than one readmission per patient over the three years). In order to select an appropriate sample, I needed to identify a cut-off point that represented an unusually high number of readmissions. After consulting with other diabetes team members, we decided that four or more readmissions within the three-year period would represent a substantially higher than expected readmission rate.

A review of the Diabetes Clinic database using this criterion revealed that out of almost 750 Diabetes Clinic patients, only 18 (2.4 per cent) had four or more hospital readmissions over this period. These eighteen patients represented 8.7 per cent of the total number of patients requiring a readmission, but the total combined number of bed-days (610) used by these patients represented a disproportionate 21 per cent of total bed-days for all readmitted diabetes patients.

Reviewing the demographics of this small group of patients revealed that all but one was a teenager. Ages at the time of data collection ranged from ten years eight months to nineteen years eight months. There were twelve females (66.6 per cent) and six males (33.3 per cent). The females were on average older (median age eighteen years nine months) than males (median age thirteen years ten months).

With the sample group identified, the next step was to review all available related hospital documents. This was a slow and methodical process, as many of the patients had extensive medical records comprising several volumes. Each section was read to see what psychosocial issues or themes might be present that could impact on the patient's condition.

The file reviews revealed that psychosocial difficulties were indeed prevalent within the sample. Seventeen patients (94.4 per cent) were previously known to the hospital mental health program and sixteen (88.9 per cent) had social work files.

When reading the files, I took notes of all the psychosocial issues identified then constructed a list of common issues. Where issues were similar, they were collapsed into themes. This thematic analysis (see Chapter 23) resulted in thirteen key themes being identified for this group of patients:

1 patient identified as having learning difficulties

2 patient identified as having a psychiatric condition

3 patient identified as having body image issues

4 non-traditional family structure (e.g. single parent and/or divorce/blended family)

5 marital conflict

6 parental psychological problems (e.g. anxiety and/or depression)

7 financial difficulties

8 family communication difficulties

9 parent–child relationship problems of overinvolvement (e.g. enmeshment, overindulgent, overcontrolling practices)

10 parent–child relationship problems of underinvolvement (e.g. lack of interest, neglect, rejection)

11 sibling relationship difficulties

12 multiple other losses experienced by patient

13 general family stress reported.

With the key psychosocial factors identified, I then created a matrix table to map the relative frequency of each factor against the sample of eighteen patients. Analysis of these results revealed a range of interesting findings and confirmed the practice wisdom that the cases involving multiple readmissions were indeed complex and multifactorial in nature.

These patients had on average 5.2 different identifiable psychosocial factors associated with their readmissions. Some noticeable differences emerged when the results for females were analysed separately from those for males. Issues of greater relative prevalence for females included parent–child relationships of overinvolvement, general family stress, parental psychological problems and sibling relationship difficulties. For males, those identified were parent–child relationships of underinvolvement, learning difficulties, marital conflict, psychiatric disorder, non-traditional family structure, family financial difficulties and family communication difficulties.

While these results were not statistically significant because of the small sample size and it was not possible to infer causality within the data, they did identify some useful factors for targeted social work intervention and further investigation.

One such factor is learning disorders. While the number of patients with identified learning disorders (seven) did not reach statistical significance, the proportion in this sample (38.8 per cent) appeared greater than that expected in the general population and was indeed higher than results found in another, more general, psychological study (Northam *et al.* 1995) on the same clinic population. This would seem to suggest that patients with learning difficulties may have an increased risk of developing diabetes control problems, leading to more frequent readmissions to hospital. Schade and colleagues (1985) have noted that learning deficits and communication disorders are difficult to detect, and may go undiagnosed for long periods. It is possible that, undetected, these deficits may compound the effects of other psychosocial factors and negatively impact on diabetes control. Targeted screening for learning difficulties in patients who have more than one unexpected readmission to hospital may allow early remedial interventions.

Another psychosocial factor is parental psychological problems, which were identified in 61.1 per cent of the sample. Again, this was substantially higher than that found in Northam and colleagues' (1996) study, in which parental mental health problems ranged between 22 and 24 per cent. As this was the second most frequently occurring factor, it might be useful to carry out remedial interventions or provide appropriate referrals. Support programs and/or education sessions might appropriately address issues such as managing feelings of anxiety and depression.

Other frequently occurring factors also appeared to relate to family functioning. These were non-traditional family structure, general family stress, marital conflict, and parenting problems of overinvolvement. Parent-focused interventions might provide an important avenue for addressing the underlying problems associated with frequent patient readmission for poor diabetes control. Given the large proportion of families with a non-traditional family structure, it might be appropriate to establish specialist mutual support groups focusing on the particular challenges for sole parents and parents of blended families.

The findings of this study also suggested that educational initiatives for parents may need to focus on gender differences: girls in the study appeared to be more sensitive to general family stress and sibling relationship difficulties, whereas boys appeared to be more sensitive to marital conflict, financial difficulties, non-traditional family structure, family communication problems, learning difficulties and psychiatric disorders. The other key gender difference was that girls were more affected by parenting issues of overinvolvement and boys by parenting issues of underinvolvement.

The psychosocial factors that were identified in this study could be conceptually categorised with three different intervention foci: patient-focused, family relationships-focused, and parent-focused. There are several alternative therapeutic possibilities including individual therapy or casework with patients or parents, group work with adolescents or parents, and family-centred therapy. Since most patients had multiple factors that spanned more than one category, it seems unlikely that any single intervention approach would 'solve' these problems.

The findings of this study provided at least a partial answer to the questions of the medical consultant. The diabetes team discussed the findings and how they might incorporate them

David Nilsson

into practice. One of the changes the team made was to revise its adolescent group education program in light of some of the identified issues, so that they better addressed family-related issues as well as individual ones. The team also incorporated a new parents group that was run in tandem with the adolescent group.

This relatively simple CDM exercise provided valuable new insights into a difficult client group, not only for me as a social worker but also for my multidisciplinary colleagues. I subsequently published my findings in the journal *Social Work in Health Care* (Nilsson 2001).

The example of this study clearly suggests that CDM provides a logical, practical, inexpensive and non-intrusive method of investigating a difficult practice issue and can offer new and useful information to improve professional practice.

Summary

In this chapter I have outlined the nature and process of CDM for social work practitioners, as well as providing a case study of its use. Clinical data-mining has considerable potential for generating practice research based on currently available clinical information that has relevance and direct utility to social workers. With increasing computerisation of records in health and human service agencies, large and small, there will be greater opportunity for social workers to mine these rich sources in order to generate practice knowledge that can help to produce better client outcomes.

Practice exercises

You are a social worker who works as a case manager in a mental health service. You have noticed that some clients in your caseload do considerably better than others. You are keen to learn what factors predict positive outcomes for clients across the agency, including your own. Your agency collects basic demographic information and records case notes on all clients.

1 How might you go about exploring this information through data-mining to discover why some clients do better than others?

2 What are some of the possible ways of de-identifying client information in the use of CDM?

3 How could information from social work case records be triangulated when doing CDM research?

Further reading

Epstein, I. (2001). Using available clinical information in practice-based research: mining for silver while dreaming of gold. *Social Work in Health Care*, 33(3/4), 15–32.

Epstein, I. (2010). *Clinical data-mining: integrating practice and research.* New York: Oxford University Press.

Epstein, I. & Blumenfield, S. (eds) (2001). *Clinical data-mining in practice-based research: social work in hospital settings.* London: Haworth Social Work Press.

Fook, J. (ed.) (1996). *The reflective researcher: social workers' experiences with practice research.* Sydney: Allen & Unwin.

Kellehear, A. (1993). *The unobtrusive researcher: a guide to methods.* Sydney: Allen & Unwin.

Lalayants, M., Epstein, I., Auslander, G.K., Chi Ho Chan, W., Fouche, C., Giles, R., Joubert, L., Rosenne, H. & Vertigan, A. (2012). Clinical data-mining: learning from practice in international settings. *International Social Work*, 56(6), 775–97.

Nilsson, D. (2001). Psycho-social problems faced by 'frequent flyers' in a paediatric diabetes unit. *Social Work in Health Care*, 33(3/4), 53–69.

Smith, E. (2008). *Using secondary data in educational and social research.* Maidenhead, UK: McGraw-Hill Open University Press.

Websites

No websites could be located that are specifically related to CDM for social workers, but the websites below provide information on data-mining more generally, which may be useful for readers.

http://en.wikipedia.org/wiki/Data_mining

Data-mining (Wikipedia).

www.anderson.ucla.edu/faculty/jason.frand/teacher/technologies/palace/datamining.htm

Data-mining: *What is Data Mining?*

www.maths.anu.edu.au/~johnm/dm/dmpaper.html

Data-mining from a statistical perspective.

QUANTITATIVE APPROACHES AND PRACTICES

11

Measure Twice, Cut Once: Reliability and Validity of Clinical Measurement Tools

CHRISTINE IMMS AND SUSAN GREAVES

Chapter objectives

In this chapter you will learn:

- about two different methods of test development: classical test theory and item response theory
- what research studies are required to develop a valid and reliable measure
- how to apply criteria to evaluate methods used to validate an outcome measure or assessment tool
- how to critically appraise the methods used to establish reliability of a measure
- how to interpret reliability statistics
- how to identify the key criteria for selecting an assessment for use in clinical practice or research

Key terms

Assessment

Descriptive tests

Discriminative tests

Evaluative tests

Interval data

Measurement

Nominal data

Ordinal data

Population

Predictive tests

Ratio data

Reliability

Theoretical assumptions

Validity

Introduction

This chapter aims to provide readers with a basis for choosing and appropriately using measurement tools for either research or clinical practice. This knowledge will support the clinician's own practice and assist in interpreting the quality of research they read from the perspective of measurement selection.

Accurate, reliable and meaningful measurement is essential for providing an authoritative basis to explain and support research and to offer recommendations (American Educational Research Association *et al.* 2014). The choice and use of appropriate measurement tools should be fundamental to logical, empirically based research in health (Bond & Fox 2007). As clinical practice is an iterative process of assessing the need for intervention, applying an intervention, evaluating its effect and adjusting, continuing or ceasing the intervention, accurate assessment and measurement are equally important in the clinical context. Valid and reliable measurement is one of the foundational requirements of evidence-based practice (see also Chapters 1, 13, 15, 16, 17).

Throughout the literature, varying terms are used to describe the process of gathering data, such as 'evaluation', 'assessment' and 'measurement', and the instruments used to gather data, such as 'assessment', 'outcome measure' and 'measurement tool'. In this chapter, we will use **assessment** or 'evaluation' to describe the process of gathering data in general. **Measurement** will be used when the instrument or tool meets the requirements for being a measure; that is, it is capable of measuring the magnitude of the attribute under evaluation using a calibrated scale.

Assessment: The process of gathering quantitative data in general; also referred to as evaluation.

Measurement: This may describe the use of an instrument that is capable of measuring the magnitude of the attribute under evaluation, using a calibrated scale.

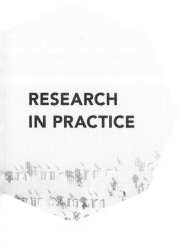

RESEARCH IN PRACTICE

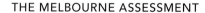

THE MELBOURNE ASSESSMENT

The *Melbourne assessment of unilateral upper limb function* (Melbourne Assessment; Randall *et al.* 1999) and the updated Melbourne Assessment 2 (Randall 2009; http://www.rch.org.au/ot/melbourne_assessment_2/) are used throughout this chapter as the primary examples demonstrating specific aspects of measurement theory and test development research. The Melbourne Assessment was developed out of a clinical and research need to quantitatively measure quality of movement of the upper extremity of children with cerebral palsy and other neurological impairments (Johnson *et al.* 1994). The tool was developed in the late 1980s when there were no valid reliable measures of the construct 'quality of upper limb function',

although there was a need to measure the construct before and after intervention that aimed to change upper limb movement (Johnson *et al.* 1994).

GATHERING EVIDENCE FOR VALIDITY OF A TOOL

Over time, evidence for validity of an assessment is gathered. Concurrent validity of the Melbourne Assessment was evaluated with the Quality of Upper Extremity Skills Test, which theoretically evaluates a similar construct. A high positive correlation between scores (Spearman's Rho = 0.90, *p* = 0.001) provided evidence that both tools evaluate similar constructs (Randall *et al.* 2012). This provided support for the validity of the Melbourne Assessment as a measure of upper limb quality of movement.

STOP AND THINK

The Melbourne Assessment 2 (Randall 2009) evaluates quality of upper limb movement in children with neurological conditions.

- What is quality of movement?
- What would you see?
- How would you describe it?

How do we measure?

Measurement involves the process of description and quantification. It means recording physical or behavioural characteristics by assigning a value to aspects such as the quality, quantity, frequency or degree of these attributes. Some attributes, such as joint range, can be measured directly. But many characteristics, such as quality of movement, are not directly observable; they are more abstract. Abstract characteristics are evaluated by conceptualising a relationship between the original characteristic and a construct that is assumed to represent it. Thus we measure the 'effect' of that characteristic (Portney & Watkins 2009). For example, range of movement around one joint is directly observable and can be measured, though not with perfect precision, using a goniometer. As quality of movement is not directly measurable, it was conceptualised within the Melbourne Assessment as comprising range of movement around multiple joints, fluency or smoothness of movement, accuracy of movement, and dexterity of grasp and release (Randall *et al.* 1999). So these attributes were observed and scored during the assessment on the assumption that quality of movement affects them.

Numerical values are typically used to describe the frequency or degree of the attributes assessed. These numbers help us score the level of the performance succinctly. However, not all numbers that are assigned during an assessment have mathematical properties. Specific criteria, called levels of measurement, have been defined to differentiate between types of numbers (Stevens 1946, as cited in Bond & Fox 2007).

Nominal data occur where objects or people are assigned to named categories according to some criterion, such as male/female. These categories may be given arbitrary numerical values; for example, boys = 1, girls = 2. In terms of the definition of measurement given above, these data are observations, not measurements.

Ordinal data also occur where objects or people are assigned to categories, but in this case the categories can be rank-ordered on the basis of predetermined level. Common examples are the Likert satisfaction scales ranging from very dissatisfied = 1, dissatisfied = 2, neutral = 3, satisfied = 4 and very satisfied = 5. While the rank order describes an increasing amount of the attribute (in this case satisfaction), the intervals between ranks may not be consistent or even known. Ordinal data also have limited statistical flexibility; the data remain as observations, not measurements as per the definition above, because we are unable to determine the magnitude of the difference between values. The scale is not calibrated (Bond & Fox 2007).

Nominal data: Where objects or people are assigned to named categories according to some criterion, such as male/female.

Ordinal data: These result when observations are rank-ordered and values are assigned sequentially to reflect the logical ordering of categories, e.g. Likert scales, which rank responses from low to high.

Christine Imms and Susan Greaves

Interval data: These have
the property of a rank
order, and distances or
intervals between the units
of measurement are equal.

Ratio data: These have
the same properties as
interval data, and have an
empirical rather than an
arbitrary zero.

Interval data also have the property of a rank order, and distances or intervals between the units of measurement are equal. For example, the thermometer measures temperature in equal interval units called degrees. A difference of 1°C is exactly the same at any point on the scale. This scale, however, does not have a true zero. Zero degrees does not mean an absence of temperature; rather, it is the point at which water freezes—the zero is criterion-referenced. Interval data meet the criteria for measurement because it is possible to define the distance between values and therefore identify how much one individual or group differs from another.

Ratio data have the same properties as interval data, and have an empirical (absolute) rather than an arbitrary zero. For example, range of movement as measured by a goniometer has equal intervals between units of measurement (in degrees) and an absolute zero: 0° flexion means there is no flexion around that joint and 20° is half the range of 40°. This is the highest level of measurement. Data from ratio scales have the greatest statistical utility, because of their mathematical properties.

There are many examples of tools using ordinal data where equal distances or intervals are assumed. For example, the original Melbourne Assessment comprises thirty-seven items on which performance is rated using ordinal scales (Randall *et al.* 1999). These ordinal data are then summed and converted to a percentage score as if they were interval data. Interval data are the minimum requirement for many statistical analyses, and Bond and Fox (2007) assert that it is not appropriate to pretend that ordinal data are the same as interval data. See also Chapters 13, 25, 26.

STOP AND THINK

Can you give other examples of scales that use nominal, ordinal, interval and ratio data?

How are assessment tools developed?

Developing valid and reliable tools demands considerable time, effort and fiscal resources. The study of methods for developing and evaluating assessment tools is referred to as 'psychometrics'. The goal of psychometric analysis is to establish the extent to which the conceptualisation of an attribute, which cannot be measured directly, is represented by the items in the tool (Hobart & Cano 2009).

Many aspects of this complex process will become apparent through this chapter. We will begin by describing some of the basic concepts in two models of test development, classical test theory (CTT) and item response theory (IRT). Both models initially involve processes designed to select items that measure a construct of interest. This will be described later in the chapter.

Classical test theory has for many years underpinned the way that measurement instruments have been developed. This theory rests on the premise that the observed test score (X) is made up of a true component (T) and a random error component (E), so that $X = T + E$. There are three assumptions within this theory:

- true scores and error scores are uncorrelated (not related to each other)
- because random errors are normally distributed, the expected mean value of the error is zero
- error scores on parallel tests are uncorrelated.

Generally speaking, the aim of CTT is to understand and improve the reliability of an assessment tool (Kline 2005).

Item response theory, also referred to as latent trait theory, is model-based measurement. This means that, to be valid, the test that is being developed must fit the mathematical model. In IRT, the amount of an underlying ability (trait) depends on both the person's responses to test items and the degree of difficulty of the administered items (Embretson & Hershberger 1999). IRT is based on two 'hard' assumptions. First, the scale is unidimensional; that is, all the items in a test evaluate a single latent trait or ability. If a rating scale is unidimensional, scores of each item can be summed to produce an overall score. Unidimensionality is a fundamental requirement for construct validity (Streiner *et al.* 2014). The second 'hard' assumption is local independence, which is a property of the items. Local independence means that the probability of success of people with the same amount of the trait on any one item is independent of their probability of success on any other item.

One IRT model used frequently in the rehabilitation sciences is the Rasch measurement model (e.g. Fisher & Fisher 1993; Greaves *et al.* 2013; Holmefur and Krumlinde-Sundholm 2015). The Rasch model conceptualises a measurement scale like a ruler. On the right-hand side, items are ranked along the measurement scale according to their difficulty. Less difficult items are located at the bottom of the scale, and the most difficult items are at the top. People (on the left-hand side) are located on the same measurement scale according to their ability or their level of the trait of interest. People with a low ability are located at the bottom of the scale, and those with higher ability are located at the top. The Rasch model has two additional assumptions:

- all people are more likely to achieve easier items than more difficult ones
- all items are more likely to be achieved by people with high ability, or more of the trait, than by those of low ability, or less of the trait.

The location or position of items and people along the measurement scale is estimated by the model from the proportion of responses of each person to each item. The Rasch model uses a logarithmic transformation of the raw scores into log-odds information units called logits. The scale resulting from the analysis has the properties of an interval scale with known and equal distances between the units, and is therefore a measure.

THE RASCH MEASUREMENT MODEL

The Rasch measurement model was used to revise the scale attributes of the original Melbourne Assessment in the mid 2000s. The result of this revision is a valid interval measure comprising four subscales. Figure 11.1 shows the person–item map from the range of movement scale of the Melbourne Assessment 2 (Randall 2009).

The premises underlying CTT and IRT are different and therefore the processes used to validate tools differ. A summary of the advantages and disadvantages of each method is presented in Table 11.1.

RESEARCH IN PRACTICE

FIGURE 11.1   Person–item map from the range of movement subscale of the revised Melbourne Assessment

LOCATION	PERSONS	ITEMS (uncentralised thresholds)	
6.0			
	0000		
5.0			
	0000000		
	0		
4.0	11.1(3)		11.1 Reach to brush from forehead to back of neck
	00000		
	0		
			8.1 Release of pellet
3.0	00 8.1(3)		6.1 Release of crayon
	00000 6.1(3)		
	0		
	00000		
			12.1 Palm to bottom
2.0	000 12.1(2)		
	00000000 15.1(3) 12.(1) 3.1(3) 16.1(3)		15.1 Reach to opposite shoulder
	000000000 13(4)		3.1 Reach sideways –
	00		16.1 Hand to mouth & down
	0000000000 2.1(3) 13(3) 1.1(3)		
1.0	00000		13 Pronation / Supination
	00000000000000		2.1 Reach forward - elevated
	00000000		1.1 Reach
	0000000000		
0.0	000000 11.1(2) 6.1(2)		
	000000		
	0 15.1(2) 8.1(2)		
	0000000000		
	00000000000 13(2)		
–1.0	000 13(1) 16.1(2)		
	00		
	000 3.1(2) 15.1(1)		
	00000		
	00000 2.1(2)		
–2.0	0 16.1(1) 8.1(1)		
	11.1(1)		
	0 1.1(2)		
	2.1(1)		
	3.1(1)		
–3.0	0000 6.1(1)		
	0		
	1.1(1)		
	000		
–4.0			
	0		
–5.0	0=1 Person		

Source: Unpublished data, personal communication M.J. Randall, 27 March 2009

Location = logit scores for the subscale; ° represents one person; Items indicated by test item on score sheet. Item 11 (reach to brush from forehead to back of neck) is the most difficult item; item 1.1 (reach forward) is the easiest item.

TABLE 11.1   A comparison of advantages and disadvantages of two methods for developing scales

THEORY	ADVANTAGES	DISADVANTAGES
CTT	Classical test analyses are based on a number of 'weak' assumptions (e.g. that random errors around a true score are normally distributed) that are easily met by traditional testing procedures. Analyses employ relatively simple mathematical procedures and are relatively easy to interpret. Analyses can be performed with smaller representative samples of individuals, which may be particularly important when field-testing an instrument. In analyses undertaken with very large samples, violating assumptions around the use of ordinal data is reported to have a minimal effect on the results.	Item and scale statistics are both sample-dependent, and should only be interpreted for that sample. It is difficult to separate the properties of the test from the attributes of the individuals taking it. That is, it is not possible to separate the ability of the person from the difficulty of the items. It is often assumed that scores from scales can be treated as interval data. However, items are commonly ordinal and the distance between response options may not be equal. Interpreting changes in scores using ordinal data is difficult, other than identifying the direction of change. Inferential analyses using ordinal data should be undertaken using non-parametric statistics. Different forms of a test are considered parallel only after considerable effort to demonstrate their equality.

(continued)

Christine Imms and Susan Greaves

TABLE 11.1   A comparison of advantages and disadvantages of two methods for developing scales (*continued*)

THEORY	ADVANTAGES	DISADVANTAGES
IRT	The scale derived from IRT analyses is an interval measurement, and parametric statistics can be used legitimately. Rasch analysis allows for test-free and sample-free measurement. That is, individuals can be compared even if they take different items from a test, and the scale can produce stable item estimates regardless of the sample of people used to calibrate the items. The hierarchical structure developed during Rasch analysis provides a clinically useful 'item map' by ranking items from difficult to easy. This can be used to monitor progress and develop programs that target clinically relevant areas of difficulty.	The 'hard' assumption of unidimensionality of the scale items may be difficult to achieve. Complex constructs such as quality of life or those affected by a number of potentially unrelated facets cannot be combined into an overall score. While the scale can be initially developed using relatively modest sample sizes, validation of the measure often requires large samples (e.g. 400–500 people) to provide a stable measure.

Psychometric (measurement) properties

The taxonomy described in this section is based on the COnsensus-based Standards for the selection of health Measurement INstruments (COSMIN), which are internationally agreed properties that should be reported for health measurement instruments (Mokkink *et al.* 2010a). The COSMIN taxonomy of measurement properties consists of three quality domains, with each domain containing one or more measurement properties.

Domain one: reliability (internal consistency, reliability, measurement error)

The need to evaluate reliability is based on the premise that measurement instruments possess some measurement error, and that humans are fallible when measuring and can produce inconsistent responses. In general, **reliability** refers to the extent to which a measurement instrument is dependable, stable, consistent and free from measurement error when repeated under identical conditions (McDowell & Newell 1996). Establishing the reliability of an assessment tool is an essential component of determining the instrument's adequacy (Streiner *et al.* 2014).

Variability (error) in measurement can come from many sources, such as the individual who is being measured or the rater who is completing the measurement process (Streiner *et al.* 2014). Reliability evaluates the extent to which scores for people who have not changed are the same for repeated measurements under several conditions. For example:

1 test–retest reliability describes the extent to which a stable evaluation of the attribute or behaviour can be obtained on two different occasions when no change is expected

2 intra-rater reliability describes the extent to which the same person can rate the same performance consistently

3 inter-rater reliability is the extent to which different people rate the same performance consistently.

Intra-rater reliability is higher than inter-rater reliability. For this reason, repeated measures in research and in clinical practice should be undertaken by the same rater whenever possible. In self-rated measures, intra- and inter-rater reliability estimates are not relevant; in these circumstances, test–retest reliability is estimated.

Another aspect of reliability is internal consistency. This evaluates the degree of interrelatedness among the items within the tool. It measures the extent to which individual items in a scale are correlated with each other and the total scale score (Streiner *et al.* 2014). Thus it provides evidence of homogeneity or unidimensionality of the scale. This is an important property of tools that aim to measure hidden constructs. In the Rasch measurement model, this is a required property of the tool. In CTT, some tools aim to measure constructs that are caused by a range of unrelated attributes (e.g. quality of life measures); these tools are not required to have high internal consistency (Streiner *et al.* 2014).

Estimating reliability. As previously described, in CTT the observed score comprises a true score and an error component. As it is not possible to know the true score, the true reliability of a test cannot be known. Rather, we estimate reliability based on the statistical concept of variance; that is, a measure of the variability among scores within a sample. Reliability is expressed as a ratio of the true score variance to the total score variance:

R = True score variance/True score variance + Error variance = T/T + E

Thus reliability is the proportion of the total variance in the measurements which is due to 'true' differences between subjects. Measurement error is the systematic and random error of a person's score that is not attributed to true changes in the construct to be measured.

Reliability estimates can be understood in terms of consistency and agreement. In general, a high level of consistency is required for instruments that are used to discriminate between individuals, and a high level of agreement is required for measures that aim to evaluate change.

Reliability: The extent to which a measurement instrument is dependable, stable and consistent when repeated under identical conditions.

Christine Imms and Susan Greaves

Consistency. Many reliability coefficients are based on correlation. Correlation reflects the degree of association between two sets of scores, or the consistency of position within the two distributions. The statistic is called a correlation coefficient.

Agreement. While correlation tells us about the relationship between two sets of scores, it does not tell us whether the actual values obtained by the two measurements are the same. To do this, we need to consider the agreement between scores (Terwee *et al.* 2007).

Intraclass correlation coefficients (ICCs) provide an estimate of reliability using indices of both consistency and agreement, thus taking into account the magnitude of the difference between scores as well as the relationship (Streiner *et al.* 2014). ICCs are the appropriate statistic when calculating reliability for continuous data. They range in value from 0.0 to 1.0, higher values associated with higher reliability. When data are nominal (simple agreement or disagreement between scores) the Kappa coefficient is appropriate. When data are ordinal, weighted Kappa is the appropriate coefficient.

Measures of agreement such as Bland and Altman's limit of agreement (LOA) plots (Bland & Altman 1986) and standard error of measurement (SEM) are expressed on the actual scale of measurement, which can aid clinical interpretation. An example using the LOA method is shown in Figure 11.2.

The standard error of measurement can be calculated using the standard deviation (σ) and the reliability coefficient (R) as follows: SEM = $\sigma \sqrt{1-R}$. The SEM can be used to draw a confidence interval around an individual's observed score (*Xo*). This would be shown as *Xo* ±

FIGURE 11.2   The Bland and Altman plot of intra-rater reliability data from the original Melbourne Assessment, showing difference between occasions on the y-axis and the average of the two scores on the x-axis

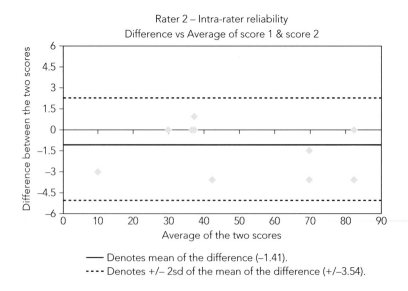

Rater 2 – Intra-rater reliability
Difference vs Average of score 1 & score 2

— Denotes mean of the difference (–1.41).
---- Denotes +/– 2sd of the mean of the difference (+/–3.54).

Although a slight bias towards higher scores on the second occasion is evident, clinically, the mean difference between occasions of –1.41 points in a scale of 100 points appeared negligible.

Z (SEM) where Z is the value from the normal curve associated with the desired confidence interval (e.g. 1.96 for 95 per cent confidence interval) (Streiner *et al.* 2014). Using the Melbourne Assessment as an example, an SEM of 2.56 points for total raw scores of trained raters (Cusick *et al.* 2005) means that an individual's observed raw score has a 95 per cent confidence interval of ± 5.02 raw score points. This gives an indication of how much error we might expect within the scoring of the individual's performance on the Melbourne Assessment on that occasion. Therefore, for individuals, score differences of more than 5.02 raw score points can be interpreted as representing a true change, beyond that due to error.

Domain two: validity (content validity, construct validity, criterion validity)

Establishing the **validity** of an instrument, or the extent to which an instrument measures what it is intended to measure, is vital (Streiner *et al.* 2014). Evaluating the validity of a tool is especially important when we are measuring constructs that are not directly observable, as is often the case in allied health.

Validity is not inherent to an instrument, but rather evaluated within the context of the test's intended use and specific **population** (Streiner *et al.* 2014). Validity is not an all-or-none concept; evidence that supports an instrument's validity is gathered over time. Methods used to evaluate various forms of validity are summarised in Table 11.2. Types of validity that are evaluated are generally found within the following categories.

1   *Content validity* is the extent to which an instrument covers all the important aspects or domains of interest that it intends to measure, and does not include items that are irrelevant to what is being measured. For example, the procedures used to develop the original Melbourne Assessment enhanced the content validity of the tool. The authors reviewed the literature on upper limb function, as well as clinical assessments of related upper limb constructs, and held workshops with expert clinicians. Item generation and selection were based on clearly defined criteria relating to the construct and the intended population (Randall *et al.* 1999). *Face validity* is a form of content validity that indicates that an instrument appears to evaluate what it is supposed to and seems plausible to the users of the tool (assessors and respondents). This judgment is made after the assessment tool has been constructed. It should not be considered sufficient evidence of a test's validity and is not always required, for example in instruments that are designed to obtain information about socially undesirable behaviours (Portney & Watkins 2009; Streiner *et al.* 2014).

2   *Construct validity* reflects the ability of an instrument to measure an abstract concept. It is the degree to which the scores of an assessment tool are consistent with predefined hypotheses based on the assumption that the tool validly measures the construct of interest (Mokkink *et al.* 2010b). Hypotheses can evaluate aspects such as internal relationships of the assessment tool, relationships of the scores to other instruments, or differences between relevant groups. Establishing construct validity has three steps: explicitly describing the theoretical concepts and how they relate to each other,

Validity: The degree to which a scale measures what it is intended to measure.

Population: In statistical research, the group or cases from which the sample in a research project is selected.

Christine Imms and Susan Greaves

developing an assessment tool that can measure the theoretical construct, and testing the relationship between the constructs and the observed behaviours that represent it (Streiner *et al.* 2014). In IRT, the third step is evaluated by how well the data gathered using the tool fit the measurement model and thus provide evidence that performances reflect a single underlying construct (Bond & Fox 2007).

TABLE 11.2   Examples of validation processes used in CTT and IRT

FORM OF VALIDITY	CTT	IRT MEASUREMENT MODELS
Content validity	Involves a range of methods for generating and selecting items for a scale. For example, a panel of experts may generate and view the items and decide if they satisfy the content domain. This often requires several revisions of the test following pilot testing with a specific sample. Qualitative studies may be used to generate items from key informants, or content analyses undertaken of observations of performance.	Similar to CTT.
Criterion validity (concurrent and predictive validity)	Correlation between the target test and a criterion test conducted either at the same time or at a future point in time. For diagnostic tests, accuracy, sensitivity and specificity are evaluated in comparison to a gold standard.	Differential item functioning (DIF) analysis: this determines whether items in the scale function the same way regardless of the characteristics of the person taking the test. Test linking: a process of determining whether two tests, or alternative forms of the same test, measure the same construct.

FORM OF VALIDITY	CTT	IRT MEASUREMENT MODELS
Construct validity	Factor analysis: an analytical method aimed at reducing the number of categories of measurement, e.g. combines multiple items into groups of factors that measure common variables. Known groups method: a method of determining whether a test can discriminate between a group known to have a disorder and a group that does not, or between groups with known levels of the attribute. Hypothesis-testing.	Internal scale validity assesses how well the items in the scale fit the measurement model (fit statistics). Principal components analysis: another term for one form of factor analysis. Rating scale structure: a method of determining the order of score thresholds for each item.
Internal consistency	Cronbach's alpha: an estimate of the correlation between items within the scale.	Person separation index: an estimate of reliability examining how well persons can be differentiated on the scale.

Source: Portney & Watkins (2009); Streiner et al. (2014); Bond & Fox (2007); Fawcett (2007); Holmefur (2009).

3   *Criterion validity* concerns the correlation of one tool (the target test) with another criterion measure, which is ideally a 'gold standard' test that has been widely used and accepted in the field of interest. Both tests are administered to the same group of people and, if the scores are found to be highly correlated, then the target test is said to be a valid predictor of the criterion score (Portney & Watkins 2009). One difficulty with this form of validity is the availability of tools that truly are gold standards. Criterion-related validity is often separated into two further subdomains dependent on the time-frame in which the predictions are made.

- *Concurrent validity* is evaluated by administering the target test and the gold standard at the same time, with an expectation that scores are highly related.

- *Predictive validity* is established by evaluating performance using the target test at a specified time-point (e.g. baseline, diagnosis, discharge) and following the target group over time until the outcome to be predicted occurs and the gold standard is administered. These studies determine the accuracy of the measurement tool to predict future outcomes (De Bie 2001).

When tests are diagnostic, that is, designed to determine if a condition is present or not, then a specific type of criterion validity study is conducted to establish the accuracy of the test in comparison with a gold standard. Data from these studies are not simply correlation statistics, but also describe the sensitivity, specificity, positive and negative predictive values and likelihood ratios. Greenhalgh (2014) gives a good overview of these studies and the data generated.

Domain three: responsiveness

Responsiveness concerns the ability of an instrument to measure change following an intervention or over time (Terwee *et al.* 2007; Streiner *et al.* 2014). Methods for evaluating responsiveness as well as the terminology reported in the literature are quite varied and include terms such as 'minimal clinically important change' and 'smallest detectable difference' (Beckerman *et al.* 2001; Hajiro & Nishimura 2002; Terwee *et al.* 2007). Within some of the definitions of these terms is an evaluation of how much change is required to be classified as 'important' and, correspondingly, who should be the judge of the importance (the clinician or the client) and under what circumstances (Hajiro & Nishimura 2002).

The underlying test property that contributes to the ability of a tool to be responsive is reliability (Beckerman *et al.* 2001; Streiner *et al.* 2014). Tools with high reliability, thus low measurement error, are likely to be more responsive (Streiner *et al.* 2014). One method of evaluating the ability of a tool to detect change is the estimate of the smallest detectable difference (SDD). The SDD is equivalent to calculating a confidence interval around the standard error measurement that takes into account both measurement occasions (SDD = SEM × 1.96 × √2) (Beckerman *et al.* 2001; Klingels *et al.* 2008). Tools with high levels of reliability, however, will not necessarily be responsive; the ability of a tool to detect change must also be evaluated within research. Typically, this involves using the tool, along with other instruments known to be responsive, within a clinical trial in which change in the attribute is expected.

Interpretability

An additional characteristic that is not considered to be a measurement property but which is an important attribute for an assessment tool is interpretability (Mokkink *et al.* 2010b). Interpretability is the degree to which one can assign qualitative meaning—that is, clinical or commonly understood connotations—to an instrument's quantitative scores or change in scores (Mokkink *et al.* 2010b).

Criteria for selecting tests and measures in research and practice

Theoretical assumptions underlying choice of tests and measures

Determining what is to be measured should be guided by the **theoretical assumptions** that underpin the research or practice appropriate to each health discipline. The International Classification of Functioning, Disability and Health is a universal model that describes the relationships between a health condition, body structures and function, activity performance, participation, environmental and personal factors (WHO 2001). If the intention is to improve participation, then participation must be carefully defined and measured. If the intention is to investigate relationships between constructs within the model, for example the relationship between impairments of body function and participation, then both elements must be evaluated. Careful consideration of the theoretical assumptions under investigation (in practice and research) is an essential component of all test selection.

Theoretical assumptions: Hypothetical statements that explain, or are used to predict, certain phenomena. Theoretical models are diagrammatic explanations of hypothetical relationships.

The reason for measuring (purpose of research or assessment)

Criteria to consider when selecting the measure or test to be used in research or clinical practice are related to the aim, the construct or attribute to be measured, and the population in whom it is to be measured. The tests listed below describe the different purposes for which assessments and outcome measures can be validated (Hanna *et al.* 2005). For each of these purposes, the level of measurement required for valid interpretation might differ. Tools may be validated for more than one purpose.

- **Descriptive tests** describe the difference between individuals within a group. An example of a descriptive measure is the Gross Motor Functional Classification System (Palisano *et al.* 2008), which classifies the gross motor function of children and youth with cerebral palsy into five different levels of ability based on their self-initiated movement.
- **Discriminative tests** distinguish between individuals with and without a characteristic or trait. For example, the Alberta Infant Motor Scale (Piper & Darrah 1994) discriminates between infants with normal and atypical motor development.
- **Predictive tests** aim to assess individuals in terms of their likely future outcomes. For example, hospital admission scores on the Functional Independence Measure were used to predict length of stay and discharge scores (Heinemann *et al.* 1994).
- **Evaluative tests** are designed to measure change over time and are often called outcome measures. To accurately measure the amount of change, evaluative tools need to collect data at interval or ratio levels, for example the Assisting Hand Assessment (Krumlinde-Sundholm & Eliasson 2003).

Descriptive tests: These describe the difference between individuals within a group.

Discriminative tests: These distinguish between individuals with and without a characteristic or trait.

Predictive tests: These aim to assess individuals in terms of their likely future outcomes.

Evaluative tests: These are designed to measure change over time and are often called outcome measures.

Christine Imms and Susan Greaves

STOP AND THINK

The last time you were assessed for a particular purpose (e.g. a medical appointment, a university examination), what was the purpose of the test? Was it a descriptive, discriminative, predictive or evaluative test?

- Can you think of examples in your own life of tests that you have undertaken which were descriptive, discriminative, predictive or evaluative?

The construct or attribute of interest

Carefully defining the construct of interest helps to determine how complex it is and whether a single item or measure can adequately capture the phenomenon or whether multiple behaviours must be measured. Complex constructs may need to be measured by more than one tool. However, it is important to have strong reasons for the inclusion of each measure and not to select too many measures, thus avoiding redundancy of measurement and burden for the client or research participants. At this point a systematic and comprehensive search for existing measures should be made.

Required properties of the tool

Validity for purpose

A tool is valid for your purposes when:

- it measures the attribute or construct of interest appropriately, that is, there is evidence of the tool's content, criterion or construct validity
- it meets the measurement property requirements for your research or practice needs, that is, it is descriptive, evaluative, discriminative or predictive as needed
- it was developed or subsequently validated for the population of people for whom you wish to use it. For example, the original Melbourne Assessment was not valid for children under five; the Revised Melbourne Assessment, which was developed in response to a growing research need for a measure that spanned a wider age range, is valid for children as young as (but not younger than) 2.5 years (Randall *et al.* 2008, 2012)
- the tool is used as it was designed to be used, that is, the tool is administered and scored as instructed. This means that items cannot be extracted and used in isolation, or in combination with items from another tool, without further research into whether valid inferences can be made from the results.

Reliability

If possible, researchers and clinicians should select tools with evidence of reliability in their population of interest because reliability estimates vary depending on the population in whom they are determined (Streiner *et al.* 2014). Although a tool may have demonstrated reliability, there is no guarantee that the same degree of reliability will be achieved in every situation. Researchers often perform pilot studies to establish the reliability of a measurement tool before the commencement of data collection. Additionally, the actual reliability is only as good as the person administering and scoring the test. To be reliable, the user must undertake appropriate training and administer and score the test or measure as prescribed.

Clinical utility

There are a number of characteristics that influence the clinical utility of a tool (Law 2004; Fawcett 2007), each of which need to be considered when selecting tests and measures. Criteria to consider include:

- clarity of instructions for administering the assessment, which also affects validity and reliability of administration of the tool

- format in terms of whether the tool is a self-report survey, interview, observation of performance or administered test. Some formats are more invasive than others and require higher levels of active participation from the individual and special equipment, all of which must be considered

- time to complete, including administration and scoring

- examiner training and/or qualifications required to administer or interpret results and cost in time and money

- cost of the tool including any equipment or software, score sheets and other expendable items

- amount of effort required by both the clinician and the client or research participant

- acceptability of the test to the clinician and the client or research participant.

Criteria for evaluating studies that examine the measurement properties of a tool

Like any other type of research, the utility and believability of the results of measurement studies depend on the methods used to obtain them. Thus the discerning reader will make a judgment about the internal validity of the study before examining the actual data reporting on the results. (Reminder: internal validity of a study is the extent to which bias is reduced by the design and methods used within the study.)

The COSMIN initiative aims to improve the selection of health measurement instruments by providing critical appraisal tools (checklists) for evaluating the methodological quality of studies on measurement properties (www.cosmin.nl). There are twelve possible checklists (labelled boxes in COSMIN) that can be used. Nine boxes evaluate whether a study meets the standards for methodological quality for the following measurement properties: Box A = internal consistency, Box B = reliability, Box C = measurement error, Box D = content validity, Box E = structural validity, Box F = hypothesis testing, Box G = cross-cultural validity, Box H = criterion validity and Box I = responsiveness. A further box contains standards for studies on interpretability. The final two boxes are checklists that contain general requirements for articles in which item response theory (IRT) methods are used, and general requirements for the generalisability of the results.

RESEARCH IN PRACTICE

APPLYING THE MELBOURNE ASSESSMENT TO SMALL CHILDREN

In the mid-2000s it was determined that the Melbourne Assessment could be modified and further developed to be applicable to children younger than five years (Randall *et al.* 2008, 2012). To achieve this, a number of studies were undertaken to establish the validity of the modified version of the Melbourne Assessment. Face and content validity were established in a four-phase process. Phase one involved reviewing item content and mapping against developmental literature the skills a child would require to achieve all items. Items that required modification to enable younger children to achieve them were adapted by changing the instructions or the scoring rubric or by making minor changes to the object used in the assessment. Following this, a three-round iterative survey was used to obtain

expert opinion about the changes and their suitability for measuring quality of upper limb function in children aged two to four years, with further modifications made during each round. Phase three involved administering the modified tool with thirty-two children aged two to four who did not have any known impairment, to validly test three hypotheses related to content. The first three phases were reported in a 2008 publication (Randall *et al.*). In phase four, the structural validity of the modified Melbourne Assessment was further assessed by administering the tool to thirty children with neurological impairment who were aged two to four and undertaking analyses to test three a priori hypotheses. In phases three and four children were also tested using the Quality of Upper Extremity Skills Test (QUEST; De Matteo *et al.* 1991) as a comparison measure.

To provide an example of using the COSMIN checklists to rate methodological quality of a measurement study, we have rated the paper by Randall *et al.* (2012) using Box Generalisability and Box F: Hypothesis Testing from COSMIN (see Tables 11.3 and 11.4).

The hypotheses tested in the Randall and colleagues 2012 study were that:

- there would be moderate to high and positive relation between children's scores on the modified Melbourne Assessment and the QUEST
- children would have comparable time requirements and compliance with both tests
- children rated as having a severe impairment would score significantly lower on the modified Melbourne Assessment in comparison with those rated as moderate, and that those rated as moderate would score significantly lower than those rated as mild.

TABLE 11.3   Generalisability of the findings from the Randall *et al.* (2012) study
of structural validity of the modified Melbourne Assessment

BOX GENERALISABILITY: DOES THE PAPER PROVIDE THE FOLLOWING INFORMATION	RANDALL *ET AL.* (2012)
Median or mean age (with standard deviation or range)	Range 2–4 years: Mean 42.7 months (SD 10.8); 10 children in each of three age groups (2-year-olds, 3-year-olds, 4-year-olds)
Distribution of sex	19 males, 11 females
Important disease characteristics (e.g. severity, status, duration) and description of treatment	Cerebral palsy = 22; acquired brain injury = 8 Distribution of motor type and topography reported Severity: mild = 16; moderate = 7; severe = 7
Setting(s) in which the study was conducted (e.g. general population, primary care or hospital/rehabilitation care)	Paediatric hospital
Countries in which the study was conducted	Australia
Language in which the HR-PRO instrument was evaluated	English
Method used to select patients (e.g. convenience, consecutive or random)	Convenience
Percentage of missing responses (response rate)	Unknown

Source: Generalisability table from Mokkink *et al.* (2010b).

The study found a Spearman's rho correlation of 0.90 ($p = 0.001$) between the modified Melbourne Assessment and the QUEST. Time and compliance demands of both assessments were equivalent, and there was strong evidence that the modified Melbourne Assessment could discriminate between children rated as having a severe (mean score = 38.1; SD = 12.1) or moderate (mean = 58.9; SD = 7.2) impairment ($p = 0.001$) and between those with moderate or mild impairment (mean = 83.4; SD = 8.0; $p = 0.01$).

TABLE 11.4   Quality rating of the study by Randall *et al.* (2012) to establish the construct validity of the modified Melbourne Assessment

BOX F: HYPOTHESIS TESTING	EXCELLENT	GOOD	FAIR	POOR
Design requirements				
1 Was the percentage of missing items given?	Percentage of missing items described	*Percentage of missing items not described*		
2 Was there a description of how missing items were handled?	Described how missing items were handled	*Not described but it can be deduced how missing items were handled*	Not clear how missing items were handled	
3 Was the sample size included in the analysis adequate?	Adequate sample size (≥100 per analysis)	Good sample size (50–99 per analysis)	*Moderate sample size (30–49 per analysis)*	Small sample size (<30 per analysis)
4 Were hypotheses regarding correlations or mean differences formulated a priori (i.e. before data collection)?	Multiple hypotheses formulated a priori	*Minimal number of hypotheses formulated a priori*	Hypotheses vague or not formulated but possible to deduce what was expected	Unclear what was expected
5 Was the expected direction of correlations or mean differences included in the hypotheses?	*Expected direction of the correlations or differences stated*	Expected direction of the correlations or differences not stated		

BOX F: HYPOTHESIS TESTING	EXCELLENT	GOOD	FAIR	POOR
6 Was the expected absolute or relative magnitude of correlations or mean differences included in the hypotheses?	*Expected magnitude of the correlations or differences stated*	Expected magnitude of the correlations or differences not stated		
7 For convergent validity: Was an adequate description provided of the comparator instrument(s)?	*Adequate description of the constructs measured by the comparator instrument(s)*	Adequate description of most of the constructs measured by the comparator instrument(s)	Poor description of the constructs measured by the comparator instrument(s)	No description of the constructs measured by the comparator instrument(s)
8 For convergent validity: Were the measurement properties of the comparator instrument(s) adequately described?	Adequate measurement properties of the comparator instrument(s) in a population similar to the study population	Adequate measurement properties of the comparator instrument(s) but not sure if these apply to the study population	*Some information on measurement properties (or a reference to a study on measurement properties) of the comparator instrument(s) in any study population*	No information on the measurement properties of the comparator instrument(s)

(continued)

Christine Imms and Susan Greaves

TABLE 11.4   Quality rating of the study by Randall *et al.* (2012) to establish the construct validity of the modified Melbourne Assessment (*continued*)

BOX F: HYPOTHESIS TESTING	EXCELLENT	GOOD	FAIR	POOR
9 Were there any important flaws in the design or methods of the study?	*No other important methodological flaws in the design or execution of the study*		Other minor methodological flaws in the design or execution of the study (e.g. only data presented on a comparison with an instrument that measures another construct)	Other important methodological flaws in the design or execution of the study
Statistical methods				
10 Were design and statistical methods adequate for the hypotheses to be tested?	*Statistical methods applied appropriate*	Assumable that statistical methods were appropriate, e.g. Pearson correlations applied, but distribution of scores or mean (SD) not presented	Statistical methods applied not optimal	Statistical methods applied not appropriate

Note: Quality rating of the study is indicated by bolded italics.

STOP AND THINK

- What is the risk of bias in the Randall and colleagues 2012 study?
- How might potential bias influence your interpretation of the results?

Summary

Health professionals use tests and measures frequently in practice. We use the data obtained to support practice, to understand the condition of the client, to determine intervention choices and to measure change. We must know how, and for what purpose, a test or measure was developed so we can choose the right measure for our intended use. Understanding the psychometric properties of the tool is crucial to knowing how much trust we can place in the findings. Reading validity and reliability research critically will enable you to determine the relative validity and reliability of a tool. Conducting rigorous research when investigating the psychometric properties of a tool is an important contribution to the knowledge base of health professionals. Selecting (or developing) psychometrically sound measures when conducting other forms of research is essential to our ability to develop knowledge in the field.

Practice exercises

1   Understanding validity. Locate three assessments that are relevant to your profession or field of study.

(a)   Decide the main purpose of the assessment tool. This may be defined in the manual or in papers describing the assessment tool.

(b)   Is there a secondary purpose for which the assessment tool has been validated and/or used?

(c)   What measurement properties are necessary to make this a good assessment tool for its intended purpose? To what extent does this tool have these measurement properties?

2   How reliable are you? This is a short exercise in evaluating intra-rater and/or inter-rater reliability.

(a)   Using a goniometer, measure the range of elbow flexion and hip extension in at least ten individuals.

(b)   Record your measurements but do not look at them again.

(c)   At least thirty minutes later, measure both joints again.

(d)   Using the limits of agreement method, plot the level of agreement between occasions of scoring for both joints. Use a hand-held or computer-based calculator for calculating means and standard deviations. Draw a plot similar to that shown in Figure 11.2 by hand.

Christine Imms and Susan Greaves

(e) What do the results tell you about your reliability?

(f) Can you identify sources of error? Could you have performed the measurement differently to reduce your error?

3   Evaluating measurement properties. Select a test or measure used within your field of practice. Locate the primary publication(s) describing the tool (maybe the test manual).

(a) Using the COSMIN guidelines, evaluate the quality of the research undertaken to develop the tool.

(b) What forms of validity were studied, and how? What types of reliability were tested, and how? Can you trust the findings?

(c) What were the results of the validity and reliability studies? How do these results influence the confidence with which you would use the tool?

Further reading

Bond, T.G. & Fox, C. (2007). *Applying the Rasch model: fundamental measurement in the human sciences*, 2nd edn. New Jersey: Lawrence Erlbaum Associates.

De Bie, R. (2001). Critical appraisal of prognostic studies: an introduction. *Physiotherapy Theory & Practice*, 17, 161–71.

Greenhalgh, T. (2014). *How to read a paper: the basics of evidence based medicine*, 5th edn. London: BMJ Books.

Streiner, D.L., Norman, G.R. & Cairney, J. (2014). *Health measurement scales: a practical guide to their development and use*, 5th edn. Oxford: Oxford University Press.

Terwee, C.B., Bot, A.D.M., de Boer, M.R., van der Windt, D.A.W.M., Knol, D.L., Dekker, J. *et al.* (2007). Quality criteria were proposed for measurement properties of health status questionnaires. *Journal of Clinical Epidemiology*, 60, 34–42.

Websites

www.casp-uk.net/

For those who wish to critique research that investigates the accuracy of an assessment tool, the Critical Appraisal Skills Program (CASP) of the UK NHS Public Health resources unit has a downloadable diagnostic studies appraisal guide, available from this site.

www.rasch.org

This is a very good web-based resource for understanding the Rasch measurement model, particularly the section on definitions of measurement. Research papers are available on the site.

www.socialresearchmethods.net/kb/index.php

For further reading online, this web-text provides definitions and examples of a number of research methods: W.M.K. Trochim (2006), *Research Methods Knowledge Base*. The Measurement section provides additional detail about validity, reliability, scaling and measurement issues. This section of the book is located at:

www.socialresearchmethods.net/kb/measure.php

12

Single-subject Experimental Designs in Health Research

MIRANDA ROSE

Chapter objectives

In this chapter you will learn:

- how to define single-subject experimental designs (SSEDs), describe their basic components, and outline their origins
- how to describe SSEDs within the context of other research designs used to investigate treatment efficacy
- how to highlight the phase and stage of research and the type of research questions SSEDs are best suited to
- how to summarise basic statistical and visual analysis techniques commonly employed in SSEDs

Key terms

Alternating treatment design

Meta-analysis

Multiple baseline design

Multiple probe design

Randomised controlled trial

Single-subject experimental design

Introduction

Every day, health and welfare practitioners make intervention and management strategy recommendations to their clients, patients and colleagues in health care and welfare teams. Increasingly, with the advances of evidence-based practice, practitioners want to base their recommendations on high-quality research evidence rather than rely solely on their own clinical experience or advice from more experienced colleagues (Reilly 2004; Hoffman *et al.* 2010; Foster *et al.* 2014). When contemporary health science students are asked to think about the type of research evidence on which practitioners base their treatment recommendations, they will often mention the so-called 'gold standard' of scientific treatment evidence, the **randomised control trial** (RCT) (see Chapters 1, 9, 15, 16, 17).

Many health and welfare students have had formal education and incidental community exposure to the concepts and methods involved in RCTs. For example, students usually know about the classic drug trial RCTs where participants are either treated with the drug under investigation (e.g. a blood pressure medication) or given a control placebo drug. Differences in the group (treated versus placebo) results (usually the group average score/mean) are analysed for their statistical significance (in terms of how likely any differences in group results were obtained by chance) and recommendations are made about the effectiveness of the drug under investigation. See Chapter 15 to learn more about RCTs.

Some of the important issues about RCTs are now listed.

- Researcher bias and contamination are minimised through the random allocation of experimental participants to either treatment or no-treatment groups, and the researchers are blinded as to which participants are receiving the experimental or the control treatments.

- Large samples of participants are recruited so that the sample is more likely to be a true representation of the overall population of interest than a special unrepresentative subgroup, and therefore the results of the study are generalisable to similar groups of people beyond those investigated in the study.

- The behaviours or physical measures (e.g. blood pressure, grip strength) being studied are carefully defined and the measurement devices used to take the pre- and post-treatment measures are valid and reliable.

Randomised controlled trial: A clinical trial where participants are randomly assigned to groups in order to receive different interventions. This randomisation removes many of the effects that may bias the true result.

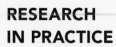

RESEARCH IN PRACTICE

CHRIS

Chris, a physiotherapist working in a rehabilitation centre, has been using two types of treatment for strengthening hand grip in patients with hemiparesis following stroke. A search of the scientific treatment literature fails to show strong evidence for either treatment. Chris knows that many of her physiotherapy colleagues use the two techniques and report good results. She has also seen positive results in patients with both of the techniques. However, she is concerned about having a stronger evidence base to support the use of the techniques in her clinical practice. She would also like to know if one of the techniques is more effective than the other. How could she get the evidence she needs?

David

David is an occupational therapist and academic staff member undertaking research at a university. He wants to investigate the efficacy of sensorimotor integration treatment for preschool children with general developmental delay. One option is for David to design a large-group comparison study where participants are randomly allocated to a treatment or a control group. However, David knows that it is very difficult to recruit large numbers of children with developmental delay, so he thinks a group comparison study will be very difficult to mount. What other research design options does David have?

- Other factors/variables that might influence how participants respond to treatment are carefully defined and controlled (e.g. other medications, diet, exercise, age, gender).

- Replication of the trial is possible because the study protocols are so well defined and clearly described.

Are RCTs and group designs always the designs of choice?

While the above characteristics of RCTs are usually true, I argue that there are some serious limitations in using RCTs for investigating the effectiveness of many physical and behavioural interventions that might be recommended by health and welfare practitioners (e.g. relaxation therapy for stress disorder, massage for chronic knee pain, word meaning therapy for aphasic word retrieval errors, diary use for memory loss after head injury). An RCT is generally not a suitable research design in some circumstances.

- The conditions we are treating are complex and multifaceted and the client/patient group has a high degree of variability. For example, people with aphasia (a language and communication disorder following brain damage) present in extremely variable ways with a huge range of severity and type of symptoms. Therefore, treatments for aphasia need to take account of the large range and type of aphasic symptoms: one size (therapy) does not fit all! Such high variability in the client group creates two major problems in employing an RCT to investigate treatment effectiveness.

  - RCTs generally require large numbers of participants in order to be effective. When client/patient conditions are complex and multifaceted and there are many variables that require control, it is even more important to have a large number of participants so that the power of the study is high. Unfortunately, when investigating complex conditions, it is very difficult or may be impossible to recruit a large enough group of participants with the same type of impairment.

  - In RCTs, the difference between the responses of the experimental and control groups to the treatment is examined with a powerful parametric statistical test (such

Miranda Rose

as Student's t-tests or an analysis of variance) (see Chapter 25). These statistical tests have a set of requirements (assumptions) about the nature of the data. One assumption is that the amount of variability in the groups being compared is similar (the assumption of homogeneity of variance or equality of variance; see any textbook on parametric statistics, e.g. Portney and Watkins [2009], or websites devoted to explaining statistics in plain language, e.g. <http://davidmlane.com/hyperstat/A45619.html>). When the samples being studied have unequal amounts of variability, we violate one of the assumptions of using the parametric statistical test. There are some mathematical ways to attempt to overcome this problem. However, when we start to compare the mean differences of two groups with very different amounts of variability, the overall results become difficult to interpret and apply to the 'average' client we might be seeing in the clinic or workplace (see also Chapters 25, 26).

- We are trying to carry out research in the clinical/working environment and not in an experimental environment, and we do not have the funding for a large-scale clinical trial or group study of treatments for complex conditions that require hundreds or even thousands of participants. In the clinical setting, we also may not have the flexibility to adapt our treatment protocols beyond the current accepted regimens.

- There are simply too few individuals with a particular rare condition who can be recruited to form a group study.

- The nature of the study is too onerous to expect large numbers of individuals to want to participate.

- The therapeutic procedures are too expensive to run across large numbers of participants.

- The investigation of a treatment is in the early phases of development. In the early stages of research (called Phase One research) into a particular treatment, we are often unsure about how potent the new treatment will be and what sort of treatment effects we will obtain. This lack of knowledge makes it very difficult to make a sensible calculation about the number of participants that need to be recruited in order to make the study powerful and meaningful. There is a danger of designing the study on too large a scale and spending unnecessary money and resources on it, or making the study too small and finding that the results are not meaningful. In Phase One research, we are often unaware of what variables require control and what factors determine candidacy for treatment. Therefore, in the early stages, pilot-level research work is undertaken to answer some of these questions. Sometimes small-group comparison studies (rather than large RCTs) are carried out.

- It is important to observe how participants respond to treatments over time (e.g. how quickly or slowly they respond, how variable the response is over time, that is, the nature of their learning/change). In RCTs, measures of participants are typically taken once before the treatment and a second time when the treatment finishes. This enables a simple two-snapshot window into the response to treatment. With the large numbers of participants required for RCTs, taking multiple measures of each participant over time becomes impossible or unrealistically expensive to mount (see Chapter 15).

Fortunately, there are alternatives to RCT and large-group experimental designs for investigating the efficacy and effectiveness of various treatments. One powerful alternative is the single-subject experimental design (SSED). SSEDs are being increasingly reported in the health science experimental literature, so it is important for students to gain an understanding of their strengths and limitations. Many clinicians who undertake research in the clinic or workplace use SSEDs routinely and students will be exposed to them during their clinical practice experiences.

STOP AND THINK

Imagine you are a GP with a patient presenting with severe osteoarthritic pain. This patient has a complex medical history and several rare additional medical conditions, likely to affect the effectiveness of medication. The results from the available RCTs concerning medication for osteoarthritic pain do not contain patients with these rare conditions.

- How applicable do you think the RCT results will be to your particular patient?
- Could you do a type of single subject design to measure the impact of a drug you wish to prescribe?

What are SSEDs?

A **single-subject experimental design** (SSED) is an experimental research method that focuses on a single individual and their response to treatment(s) over time. SSEDs always have at least a baseline phase (usually denoted as the A phase) where measurements of the behaviour (or system) to be treated (the dependent variable) are taken on several occasions during a no-treatment phase. This tells us what the participants' abilities are like before treatment commences and if there is any variability in the pre-treatment ability over time. SSEDs always have a treatment phase (usually denoted as the B phase) where measurements continue to be taken while the behaviour is treated (see the first two panels in Figure 12.1 for an example using mock data). There is an enormous range of SSED designs beyond this basic and rather weak A-B design, some of which are quite sophisticated and will be explained in the next section. In many studies, the researchers carry out a series of SSEDs so they can replicate the findings from a single SSED (it worked for this person, does it work for a second, a third etc?) and create better evidence for generalising the findings beyond a particular individual. In studies where several replicated SSEDs are reported, the data are first analysed individually. Sometimes the strength of the treatment effect demonstrated in each individual study is combined in a **meta-analysis** to create an overall effect size for the particular series of SSEDs.

Single-subject experimental design: An experimental research method that focuses on a single individual and their response to treatment/s over time.

Meta-analysis: A statistical technique that combines the results of similar studies into a single result that provides an estimate of the overall effect.

Miranda Rose

Figure 12.1   Example of A-B-A-B withdrawal design

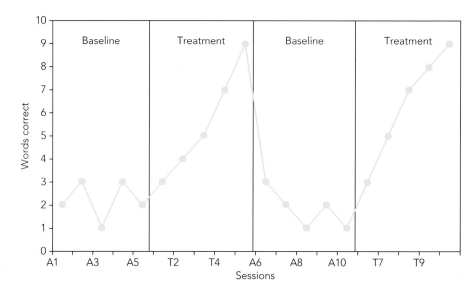

Terms used for SSEDs

Several terms have been used interchangeably for SSEDs. These include:

- single-case designs or single-case experimental designs
- single-subject designs
- interrupted time series designs
- N-of-1 trial
- small N designs.

SSEDs versus case studies: they are not the same!

There is an important distinction between two terms (and two types of research) which students and practitioners often use interchangeably but which in fact produce very different levels of research quality. These terms are 'SSEDs' and 'case studies'. In well-designed SSEDs, there is careful and rigorous control of the behaviour or attribute that is being treated (the dependent variable) (e.g. muscle strength, finger dexterity, picture-naming skills) and of the actual treatment being investigated (the independent variable) (e.g. strength training, dexterity training, word retrieval training). There is also a significant attempt to minimise the influence of any other variables that might influence the outcomes in treatment, such as improvements resulting from clients who simply get better over time, differences in skills between the treating therapists, and the varying motivation of the participants at different stages of the experiment. This careful control of experimental and extraneous variables means that the word 'experimental' in the term 'single-subject experimental design' is warranted. In other words, the investigator starts with a testable hypothesis, operationally defines the dependent and independent variables, carefully measures them, and attempts to minimise bias in the study.

In case studies, however, clinicians report detailed observations and measurements from a particular patient/client/case, usually in natural situations without directly manipulating or controlling variables. Therefore SSEDs are true empirical research designs because, when carried out well, we can be reasonably certain that any treatment effects demonstrated are a direct result of the treatment and not a result of some confounding variable. In case studies, on the other hand, it is very difficult to know what caused any observed and documented changes in behaviour. In the clinical and research fields, case studies are useful in highlighting possible therapeutic effects that require more rigorous investigation. Unfortunately, many people use the terms 'case study' and 'single-case design' or 'single-subject experimental design' interchangeably. It is important to consider whether a study you are reading is actually a case study or a true SSED because the strength, utility and generalisability of the evidence they produce are very different.

STOP AND THINK

A psychologist encounters a client with a previously undocumented reaction to a traumatic childhood event. The psychologist trials a novel treatment with the client, who reports feeling relieved of symptoms following a ten-week period of treatment. The psychologist writes up the experience, including a detailed case history and client description of symptoms, a measure of client anxiety before the treatment, a description of the treatment, and a measure of client anxiety after the treatment.

  • Is this an SSED or a case study?

When is an SSED the research design of choice?

SSEDs are the research design of choice when any of the following are true:

- The investigation of the effectiveness of a treatment is in the early stages (Phase One studies).

- The nature of the condition or the treatment is complex and the participants that can be recruited to research investigations are highly variable.

- The treatment is being investigated in the context of a rare condition.

- We want to understand the nature of the participant's response to the treatment (how fast, how variable) over time, not just at two discrete points (before and after treatment). In other words, we are very interested in the process of change over time, its patterns and variability, not just whether the change does or does not happen.

- The research is occurring in real-life clinical or community settings (Morgan & Morgan 2009; Portney & Watkins 2009).

Miranda Rose

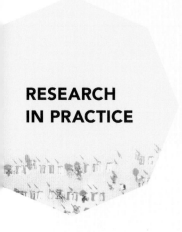

CHRIS

Chris wants to determine if one of the treatments she is using is better than another for the post-stroke patients she treats in the rehabilitation centre. When she did a literature search of the scientific treatment literature, she couldn't find evidence about either of the treatments. Chris is working in a clinical environment without access to large-scale research grant funds or research staff. Is an SSED appropriate to help her investigate her clinical question?

David

David wants to investigate the efficacy of a treatment for general developmental delay in preschool children, who present with delays of various types and severity and as a group are quite heterogeneous. As there is such a large degree of variability in the children, David knows he would need to design a group study with a very large N (number of participants) in order to take care of the number of variables he would need to control for. He knows it is very difficult to recruit such large numbers of children with developmental delay and also that he can't easily recruit large numbers of very similar participants. Would a series of SSEDs be an appropriate research design option for him?

When did SSEDs develop? Are they a popular design? Are they considered powerful?

Many students and practitioners think that SSEDs are a new or extremely novel research design. In fact, today's range of SSEDs originated in the early experimental work carried out by the famous behavioural scientist B.F. Skinner in the 1940s. Skinner and colleagues were interested in the ways in which animals learnt over time, and therefore the researchers needed an observational and investigative strategy that would allow multiple samples of behaviour to be analysed (Ittenbach & Lawhead 1996). Skinner was frustrated at the popular methods of the era, which involved group analysis of behavioural data. Skinner felt the group aggregating of the data created smooth learning curves that actually obscured the complexity and individual variability associated with true learning. At the time, there was a strong movement in the field of psychology towards group analysis techniques and parametric statistics (such as t-tests and ANOVAs; see Chapter 25), and the individual analysis methods of the behaviour analysts were seen by some as less powerful and inferior. This meant that often the research work of the behaviour analysts was not accepted for publication in the major psychology journals of the time, leading Skinner to start the now prestigious *Journal of the Experimental Analysis of Behaviour* (*JEAB*) in 1958. *JEAB* continues to publish work where the data are analysed individually rather than aggregated (Morgan & Morgan 2009). The power struggle between researchers using large-group studies with parametric statistics and small observational studies with no or non-parametric statistics continues to this day.

Between 1939 and 1963, Dukes (as cited in Ittenbach & Lawhead 1996) reported that 246 single-subject research papers were published, paving the way for the fields of education and psychology to emphasise the SSED in present-day treatment/intervention research. More recently, the disciplines within allied health, nursing and medicine have taken to SSEDs enthusiastically (Gabler *et al.* 2011). For example, when searching the speechBITE database (www.speechbite.com), a large database of speech pathology treatment studies, in February 2016, 39 per cent of the 4811 studies indexed were SSEDs. Many previous evidence hierarchies have ranked SSEDs low at Level 3 or 4 of a four-tier system (e.g. the NHMRC evidence hierarchy). More recently, the highly regarded Oxford Centre for Evidence Based Medicine ranked a systematic review of N-of-1 trials equal to a systematic review of RCTs (Level 1 evidence) in its 2011 Levels of Evidence Table (www.cebm.net/index.aspx?o=5653) for questions on treatment efficacy, common harms and rare harms. Clearly, there are differences of opinion in scientific circles concerning the strength of evidence obtained from well-conducted SSEDs and series of SSEDs, some of which still reflect the power struggles within scientific circles dating from Skinner's time. The rise in popularity of N-of-1 trials in medicine is having a significant impact on evidence hierarchies throughout the world. Clearly, the power of SSEDs to answer complex intervention questions is being recognised. Further, a rigorous approach is now being taken to the method quality ratings of SSEDs, with the recent publication of the Risk of Bias in N-of-1 Trial (RoBiN-T) Scale (Tate *et al.* 2013). The RoBiN-T Scale is a fifteen-item scale that helps to identify experimental from non-experimental single-case designs and reveals an overall method quality score. Reporting guidelines for SSEDs have also been recently developed and published (single-case reporting guidelines in behavioural interventions (SCRIBE); Tate *et al.* 2016).

STOP AND THINK

- How could systematic reviews of N-of-1 trials and systematic reviews of RCTs be considered equally strong evidence (Level 1) by the Oxford Centre for Evidence Based Medicine?
- In what ways are these two designs (RCTs and SSEDs) attempting to discover the same types of information? In what ways are they different?

Types of SSEDs

As mentioned earlier, there are various SSEDs structured to meet the particular type of research question, the nature of the treatment type(s) and the participant characteristics being investigated. I suggested that the basic A-B design is a descriptive/non-experimental rather than a truly experimental design (McReynolds & Kearns 1984). The A-B is a weak design because it is difficult to be sure that any change in behaviour noted in the B phase actually relates to the treatment and not to some other confounding variable such as general stimulation or natural recovery. A stronger, more commonly employed SSED is the A-B-A or A-B-A-B or withdrawal/reversal design. The logic of the A-B-A-B design is that after treatment stops, the behaviour under observation (e.g. number of angry outbursts in the classroom) will return to baseline or near baseline levels. Once treatment recommences in the second B phase, changes in the behaviour will occur that replicate those seen in the first B phase, thus supporting the view that it was the treatment that resulted in the behaviour change. Figure 12.1 shows an example of an A-B-A-B design. The participant's response to the baseline, treatment and withdrawal phases is shown by graphing the dependent variable (in this example, the number of words spoken correctly) along the *y*-axis and time (in this case the treatment session) on the *x*-axis.

However, in the social and health sciences it is rare for treatments to result in transient change. As many of our treatments result in more permanent or longer-lasting change, the A-B-A-B design is inappropriate as it is unlikely that the behaviours measured will return to baseline levels after the treatment stops. Further, it is often unethical to withdraw treatments. Fortunately, there are several more sophisticated SSEDs that take account of the more permanent changes in behaviour and states that are frequently achieved in our interventions. The next sections describe two of the more commonly employed SSEDs: multiple baseline experimental designs and alternating treatment designs.

Multiple baseline experimental designs

Multiple baseline design: In this design, the effects of treatment are replicated in several participants or in different target behaviours, and participants act as their own controls.

When it is unlikely that treated behaviours will return to baseline levels after withdrawal of the treatment, multiple baseline designs are frequently the design of choice. In **multiple baseline designs**, the effects of treatment are replicated in several participants or in different target behaviours. The design also allows for replication in different treatment conditions in a single participant so that the relative effectiveness of one treatment over another can be investigated. In multiple baseline designs, baseline data is collected and graphed in each condition (see Figure 12.2). Treatment is then applied to one condition while the other conditions are kept untreated. Once a set criterion is reached or a set number of treatments have occurred, treatment is applied to the second condition while the third (and perhaps fourth) is kept in baseline. Again, treatment continues until a set criterion is reached or a set number of treatments have been given. Finally, treatment is applied to the third condition. In this way, we can see the effects of the three treatment types in a stepwise manner while the other behaviours are kept in untreated baseline states. The multiple baseline design allows the researcher to see change in a treated behaviour while there is no or limited change in another related behaviour, making it more likely that any change seen in the first condition is a result of the treatment rather than an extraneous variable. In this way, participants act as their own controls. Further, because measurements are taken and graphed over time the researcher gains a clear view of the nature of any learning taking place in one condition as compared to another, allowing for assessments of the efficiency of the treatments and stability of any treatment effects.

Multiple probe design: A cost-effective alternative to the multiple baseline design. Some probes are taken on a predetermined and less frequent schedule or once a requisite skill is obtained.

A variation of the multiple baseline design is the **multiple probe design** (Horner & Baer 1978). Sometimes it is clear that a component of behaviour of interest (e.g. finger

FIGURE 12.2   Example of a multiple baseline design

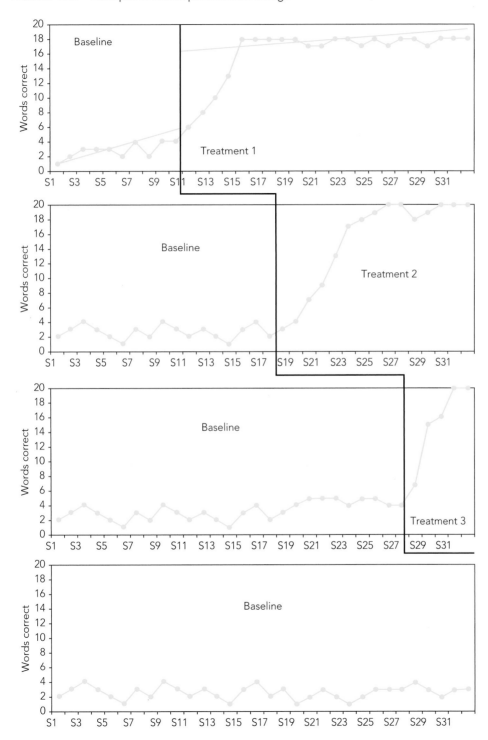

Dotted lines in panel 1 = celeration lines (indicating slope/rate of change)

Miranda Rose

grip strength of a patient with right hemiparesis following stroke) is a vital component of a larger behaviour (e.g. holding and writing with a pen). When this is the case, it seems rather pointless to repeatedly measure the participant's capacity to write a sentence if they are still unable to grip a pen. Similarly, it sometimes seems pointless to repeatedly measure a behaviour that is proving to remain incredibly stable during a study. The researcher has to weigh up the risks of taking unnecessary measures of behaviour and therefore adding an unnecessary burden to the participant, plus the costs associated with extra analysis and reliability measures, versus losing experimental control if an inadequate number of baseline measures are taken. The multiple probe design offers a cost-effective alternative to the multiple baseline design in these situations. Not all probes are taken in every session; rather, some are taken on a predetermined and less frequent schedule or once a requisite skill is obtained.

Alternating treatment designs

Alternating treatment design: Two or three treatments are provided in rapid succession and in an alternating format. The results are graphed together to show the difference in rate and stability of learning.

Another useful design when wanting to compare multiple treatments or placebo treatments is the **alternating treatment design**. In this, two or three treatments of interest are provided in rapid succession and in an alternating format either within a session, in a session-by-session format or in a day-by-day format. The results are graphed together to clearly show the difference in rate and stability of learning in each treatment condition (see Figure 12.3). Strictly speaking, in alternating treatment designs there is no need for the baseline phase. But including a baseline phase makes interpretation of the results easier because we can clearly see any treatment effects (in comparison with pre-treatment results), particularly if the effects of the treatments being compared are similar. One advantage of the alternating treatment design is that comparative results can be obtained more quickly than in multiple baseline or sequential designs (e.g. A-B-C-D-A designs). However, in order to take account of any potential order effects (where the order of the treatments is important), systematic counterbalancing or randomisation of the treatment sequence is required. The design is not suitable when we are expecting generalisation (or leakage) from one treatment to another.

An example of an alternating treatment design is given here, from a study investigating the comparative effects of three types of treatments for word production impairment (in this case an acquired apraxia of speech) in a man following a left hemisphere stroke. The treatments were a verbal (talking only) treatment, a gesture (hand movements only) treatment and a combined verbal + gesture treatment. Figure 12.3 shows the participant's response to the three treatments, and a comparison with the baseline phases and an untreated control group. Each of the three treatments was given in every treatment session, each treatment was applied to one of three carefully matched sets of twenty words. A fourth set of words was never treated; it formed the control set. The order of the three treatments was rotated each session to control for any possible order effects.

FIGURE 12.3 Example of an alternating treatment design

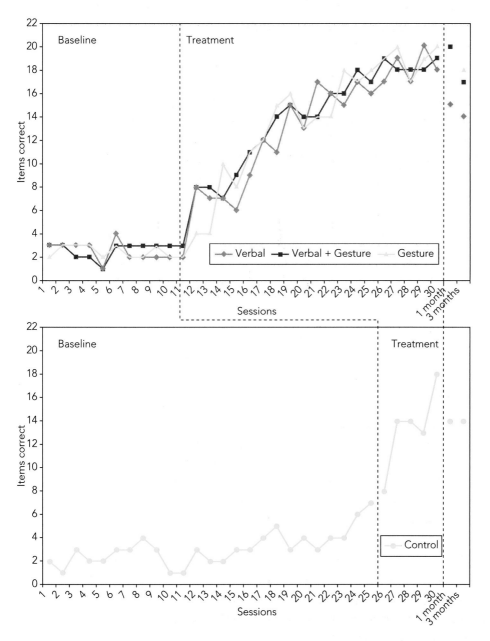

Source: Adapted from Rose & Douglas (2006).

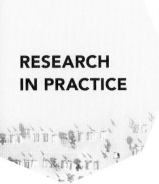

RESEARCH IN PRACTICE

CHRIS

An A-B-C-A design, where B is the first treatment phase and C is the second treatment phase, would be an appropriate design for Chris to investigate the relative effectiveness of the two different exercise treatments (treatment M and P) for hand grip strength. Following an initial stable baseline period where measures of hand grip (e.g. maximum squeeze pressure on pressure meter; maximum time for holding a 1 kg weight) are taken on three or four occasions, hand grip treatment M is implemented for, say, ten sessions. The hand grip strength measures are continuously probed throughout the design and graphically displayed. Following ten sessions of treatment M, ten sessions of treatment P would commence. Then the final A phase occurs, where the hand grip measures are taken to demonstrate whether improvements in grip strength are maintained or decline during the withdrawal phase. Comparisons are then made of the progress achieved during each of the treatment phases. The design could be strengthened by including a second probe measure of an impaired skill/behaviour not expected to be directly affected by the grip strength training but possibly affected by general therapeutic stimulation or spontaneous recovery of the nervous system after stroke, such as sitting balance. If positive changes are demonstrated in grip strength probes during the therapy but not the sitting balance probes, it is clearer that the specific treatment caused the changes in grip strength rather than other extraneous variables such as general stimulation. The design

would need to be replicated in several participants, alternating the order of treatments M and P to take account of possible order effects.

David

David could definitely use a series of SSEDs to investigate the effectiveness of the treatment for general developmental delay. Depending on how potent he thought the treatment was, and assuming there would be some return to pre-treatment behaviours during a withdrawal phase following a short burst of treatment, he could use an A-B-A-B design. In the first burst of treatment some improvement in target behaviours may be obtained, but not enough to reach desired criteria. Then, with a second burst of treatment where target levels of behaviour might be reached, he could demonstrate the effect of treatment over and above the baseline and withdrawal levels. However, if the treatment was potent and it was not expected that behaviours would return to baseline levels during withdrawal of treatment, a multiple baseline design across behaviours would be suitable. After a baseline phase measuring ball-catching skills, pencil grip and focused attention span during a storybook reading task, treatment would focus on, say, ball-catching skills first, while pencil grip and focused attention during a storybook task were kept in baseline. Then treatment would move to one of the remaining behaviours while the other two remained in baseline, and so on. The order of the treatments (for pencil grip, ball-catching, storybook attention) would need to be randomised across the series of participants to minimise potential order effects.

Analysis of SSED data

Visual analysis methods

The participant response to treatment (and during baseline and no treatment phases) is usually graphed on a standard case chart (Figures 12.1, 12.2, 12.3). The dependent variable (behaviour or physical attribute being measured) is graphed on the y-axis and the time-frame of the treatment (sessions, number or days, weeks etc.) is graphed on the x-axis. Visual inspection of the graphed results is by far the most popular analysis method (Portney & Watkins 2009). A visual analysis is made of the changes in the performance curves from baseline to intervention phases and between intervention phases. Three important aspects to review in the visual analysis are:

- the level of the graphed data (e.g. low, middle, high)
- the slope (or trend) of the graphed data (e.g. rising/accelerating, falling/decelerating, flat) and thus the rate of change
- the stability of the graphed data (degree of variability and pattern in the data).

These three aspects are reviewed within and across each phase of the study (e.g. baseline, treatment, withdrawal, maintenance etc.).

When relying on visual analysis techniques, during the initial baseline phase it is important that the participant response is either stable or moving in the opposite direction to what is expected during the treatment phases. For example, if we expect an increase in scores during treatment, it is preferable to have a flat or falling baseline. Then if the scores rise during the treatment phase, it is clear that the positive changes occurring during the treatment phases are not simply extensions of what was beginning to occur during the baseline. For example, when a slowly rising (accelerating) baseline leads into a slowly accelerating treatment phase the researcher is left wondering if the trend established in baseline (accelerating) is simply continuing during treatment, and therefore the treatment is not having a significant effect. Often researchers decide on achieving a pre-set criterion of baseline stability (e.g. no more then 5 per cent variability) before commencing a treatment phase. If the stability criterion is not met, a different behaviour (dependent variable) may need to be observed, measured and recorded or the study results will be difficult to interpret.

Fortunately, visual analysis can be improved by several design features and graphing techniques:

- baseline and treatment phase lengths should be roughly equivalent
- measures of the behaviour being studied (dependent variable) such as counts, percentages or times correct are plotted on the y-axis while the time measures such as day, week, or month are plotted on the x-axis
- celeration lines can be drawn for each phase. The celeration lines estimate the slope of each data phase and provide a visual aid to compare the slopes across the phases (Portney & Watkins 2009). These lines are drawn by calculating the median scores in

each half of each phase, drawing a horizontal line through the median scores in each half phase, drawing a vertical line through the middle score of each half phase, then connecting the two points of intersection between the horizontal and the vertical lines (see Figure 12.2, first graph).

Statistical analysis methods

It is important to realise that visual analysis has its critics. Threats to the reliability of visual inspection have been clearly documented (Matyas & Greenwood 1990). When there is high variability in the data or there are accelerating baselines, statistical methods are likely to be more reliable than visual inspection methods. A full description of possible statistical analyses is beyond the scope of this chapter, but Portney and Watkins (2009) provide a clear basic summary, and Franklin and colleagues (1996) provide a more extensive discussion. Recently, a promising new statistic, called Tau-U, has been reported for analysing treatment effects in SSEDs (Parker *et al.* 2011), and a robust but simple-to-calculate effect size including the ability to calculate confidence intervals, called the 'improvement rate difference', has been published (Parker *et al.* 2009). The effect size is a standardised expression of the amount of change seen between the baseline and intervention phase(s), so that we can compare effect sizes across studies. One thing to remember is that a combination of visual and basic statistical analyses may be powerful. For example, when visual inspection leaves some uncertainty, we can supplement the visual analysis with simple non-parametric tests. In a study to investigate the effectiveness of three treatments for aphasic verb retrieval impairments, we compared the last baseline score and last treatment score in each condition with the non-parametric McNemar's test (Rose & Sussmilch 2008). In a more elaborate statistical analysis of the response to treatments for noun retrieval impairment, we used curve-fitting techniques (Rose *et al.* 2002).

Some authors have attempted to integrate the results from several different SSED studies, all investigating treatment for a particular condition (e.g. aphasic word retrieval difficulty). Meta-analysis of single-subject experimental data is possible, particularly when using the overall effect sizes of interventions from each study, but there is considerable controversy about how to validly calculate effect sizes from SSED data. With the emergence of innovative methods, such as the improvement rate difference, we expect to see greater strength of evidence from combining data from series of SSEDs in the very near future (see Beretvas & Chung 2008 and Portney & Watkins 2009 for more details).

Reliability of the data

As SSEDs are true experimental designs, researchers must meet data reliability and validity standards expected in empirical research (see also Chapters 1, 11, 13). The reliability of the data is checked by having a second rater re-rate the behaviours measured in the dependent variable (e.g. number of positive statements per twenty-minute conversation) as well as the fidelity of any treatment provided. In treatment fidelity checks, a second rater views a videotape of the treatment sessions or live treatment sessions, and analyses how accurately the researcher employed the treatment protocol as specified in the study.

Summary

SSEDs are a type of experimental research design well suited to and commonly employed for the investigation of treatment efficacy, particularly the investigation of complex multistep treatments or for populations with a low overall incidence or high complexity and variability. SSEDs are very well suited to clinic-based research. A well-designed SSED with replication across participants or within one participant across behaviours or conditions provides evidence with strong internal validity. A series of well-designed SSEDs investigating a particular treatment for a particular condition, subjected to a meta-analysis, provides very strong evidence (Level 1 on the Oxford EBM rankings). There are various truly experimental SSEDs to suit a range of treatment efficacy questions including alternating treatment designs, multiple baseline designs and multiple probe designs. While visual analysis of the graphic display of participant response to treatments is common, the use of statistical analysis techniques is becoming more widespread. Further, statisticians are developing valid ways to carry out meta-analyses of series of SSEDs, which will assist in providing highly powerful treatment research evidence in the near future.

Practice exercises

1   You are a health practitioner who recently attended a seminar where a new treatment for memory loss following acquired brain injury was presented. The treatment is derived from sound theoretical principles but there is no current scientific evidence supporting it. The treatment involves learning and implementing several different strategies. It is suggested that clients require at least ten hours of treatment before they begin to acquire any of the strategies taught. Every year, you and your colleagues treat several clients with acquired brain injuries involving memory loss. The clients are diverse in their presentation and in other post-brain injury physical and cognitive difficulties. You want to know if the new memory treatment is more effective than the treatment that has been used in the clinic for some years, similarly with little published research evidence. Discuss ways of designing a research study to answer your question concerning comparative treatment efficacy.

Miranda Rose

2   Discuss the strengths and weaknesses of using an RCT versus a series of SSEDs to investigate the effectiveness of a behavioural treatment to improve eye contact during adult–child interactions for preschool children with autism. You might want to split your group into two teams: one team prepares the arguments for using an RCT while the other team prepares the arguments for using SSEDs. You could then hold a formal debate to compare and contrast the arguments.

Further reading

Kazdin, A.E. (2011). *Single-case research designs: methods for clinical and applied settings*, 2nd edn. New York: Oxford University Press.

Morgan, D. & Morgan, R. (2009). *Single-case research methods for the behavioural and health sciences.* Los Angeles: Sage.

Portney, L. & Watkins, M. (2009). *Foundations of clinical research: applications to practice*, 3rd edn. New Jersey: Prentice Hall Health.

Websites

davidmlane.com/hyperstat/A45619.html

A website providing interactive tutorials on basic statistics by Associate Professor Lane, Psychology, Statistics and Management at Rice University, USA.

www.cebm.net

The Oxford Centre for Evidence Based Medicine provides resources to help develop, teach and promote evidence-based health care.

13

Surveys and Questionnaires in Health Research

MARGOT J. SCHOFIELD AND CHRISTINE FORRESTER-KNAUSS

Chapter objectives

In this chapter you will learn:

- why we use surveys and questionnaires
- the main survey designs
- how measurement theory is applied to survey research
- how surveys are designed and structured
- how survey questions are constructed
- the main methods for administering surveys

Key terms

Cross-sectional survey

Funnel format survey

Interval data

Inverted funnel format survey

Likert scale

Longitudinal cohort survey

Measurement errors

Mixed format survey

Nominal data

Ordinal data

Questionnaire

Ratio data

Reliability

Standardised scale

Survey

Surveys to test intervention effects

Validity

Verbal rating scale

Visual analogue scale

Introduction

Survey: A descriptive research method where respondents are asked a series of questions in a standard manner so that responses can be easily quantified and analysed statistically.

Surveys are a common descriptive research method in the health and social sciences (Sarantakos 2005; Neuman 2006; de Vaus 2007; Ruel *et al.* 2015). Survey respondents are asked a series of questions in a standard manner so that responses can be easily quantified and analysed statistically. This enables the researcher to describe the characteristics of the sample being studied and to make generalisations to the larger population of interest. Surveys are particularly useful for collecting information about research phenomena that are not directly observable or measurable (Bowling 2005). They are also useful for collecting data from people who are widely distributed geographically, since direct contact between researcher and research participant is not necessary (Sarantakos 2005). Survey responses are derived primarily from self-completed surveys or through interview.

Questionnaire: A specific type of written survey made up of a structured series of questions. Questionnaires usually have highly standardised response options so that data can be easily analysed and compared.

A **questionnaire** is a specific type of written survey made up of a structured series of questions. Questionnaires usually have highly standardised response options so that data can be easily analysed and compared across individuals or groups (Bowling 2005). Surveys and questionnaires can also include more open-ended questions that invite respondents to write free responses. Many surveys include a mix of open and closed response options (de Vaus 2007).

The accuracy of information obtained through survey methods depends on many factors, such as the way the sample is selected and recruited, and how the questions are designed, asked and recorded. The validity of the data obtained also depends on the sensitivity of the questions asked, the motivation of the respondents to answer truthfully, and their ability to answer the questions accurately. Surveys can be a very efficient method of obtaining information about individuals but, like all research methods, have a number of limitations that researchers should attempt to minimise.

Why do we use surveys and questionnaires?

Surveys are a popular research method because they tend to be the most economical and efficient way of collecting data about a range of personal characteristics, health symptoms, history and behaviours. Large amounts of data can be collected in a fairly short time and responses can be recorded in ways that are easily entered into data files for analysis. The capacity to ask many questions around a particular research topic allows more sophisticated research questions to be asked and multivariate analysis to be undertaken on the data.

One important assumption underlying the use of survey research methods is that the survey respondents themselves are the best source of accurate information about these questions. This method is thus particularly useful for collecting information about social and psychological concepts such as beliefs, attitudes, opinions, expectations, knowledge, and satisfaction with health care (Bowling 2005). For such research questions, the individual is usually the best source of conceptual information.

In determining whether a survey is the best method of collecting information about a particular research question, the researcher must decide whether a subjective response will yield more accurate information than a more objective form of measurement. For instance, if you want to determine the extent of high blood pressure in a sample, you are likely to get a more accurate response by objectively measuring the blood pressure with a validated blood pressure monitor than by simply asking the sample (see Chapter 11). Similarly, for some problems, accuracy of response may depend on who is asked. For instance, asking a young child about the severity of their behaviour problems may not be the most accurate method. It may be better to ask teachers and/or parents to rate the child's behaviour over time.

There are, however, a range of practical and methodological reasons why a survey may be the method of choice, even for research topics where more objective methods are likely to yield more accurate data. For instance, if we take the blood pressure example, the choice of method depends on what we actually want to know about the blood pressure. If the question is, 'What is the incidence of high blood pressure in a particular sample?', then an objective measure will be the best method, since there are likely to be many people with high blood pressure who are unaware of this until tested, and the research question calls for a precise estimate of the incidence (see 'Research in practice' box).

If the question seeks to understand the knowledge, attitudes or behaviour of people who have been diagnosed by their doctor with high blood pressure, then a survey may well be the method of choice. In making this decision, we would need to assume that people know that they have been diagnosed with high blood pressure. There will be some error attributable to this assumption. However, this error will be outweighed by the benefits of economically identifying those who have been diagnosed with the condition, then administering a range of self-report measures. This is because the research question seeks to understand self-reported information associated with those who know they have high blood pressure.

SURVEY DESIGN IS LINKED TO THE RESEARCH QUESTION

Research on high blood pressure

The decision to choose a survey design depends on the aim of the study. Some examples are shown below.

Study question: What is the incidence of high blood pressure in a population?

Study design: The best method of answering this question is not through a self-complete survey, but by taking objective measures of blood pressure from a random sample of the population. This is because many people may have high blood pressure but be unaware of it. Therefore the most accurate method of answering the research question is to measure actual blood pressure using the most reliable measuring instrument for this purpose. If a survey was undertaken, it is likely that the incidence of high blood pressure would be seriously underestimated.

Study question: Among people diagnosed with high blood pressure, what are their attitudes towards medication?

Study design: A self-complete survey would be an appropriate method of answering this research question, since the sampling frame is limited to those who know they have high blood pressure and the main information sought (attitudes towards medication) requires a self-report response.

RESEARCH IN PRACTICE

Margot J. Schofield and Christine Forrester-Knauss

What are the main survey designs?

There are three main study designs in which surveys and questionnaires are used. The first is in cross-sectional research, where the primary purpose is descriptive. The second is in longitudinal cohort research, in which the primary purpose is to track changes over time. The third study design is experimental or intervention research, in which the primary question is whether a particular intervention or experiment produces change in outcomes. Each of these is described in more detail and the role of surveys explained.

Cross-sectional surveys

Cross-sectional survey: This gives a profile of the sample at one point in time. It yields a profile of the sample at that time and allows associations between variables to be explored.

A **cross-sectional survey** gives a profile of the sample at one point in time. It cannot make inferences about past or future, and relies largely on descriptive and correlational analyses (see Chapter 14). An example of such a survey is the National Health Survey conducted by the Australian Bureau of Statistics (ABS), shown in 'Research in practice' below (ABS 2009b). On a smaller scale, typical cross-sectional surveys commonly employed in health services include surveys of variables such as symptoms, pain, patient satisfaction and patient quality of life. In the broader community, surveys of health risk behaviours, health screening behaviours and use of health services or medications are common.

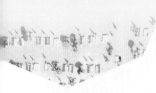

RESEARCH IN PRACTICE

EXAMPLE OF CROSS-SECTIONAL SURVEY

National Health Survey 2007–08

The ABS has conducted cross-sectional National Health Surveys every three years to track the state of health of the nation and trends in health service use (ABS 2009b). The survey is designed to obtain national benchmarks on a wide range of health issues and to enable changes in health to be monitored over time. These National Health Surveys are cross-sectional surveys, in that a new sample is selected for each administration. A comparison of trends can be made across time, however, because large representative samples are chosen on each occasion.

RESEARCH TOPICS

The National Health Survey collected information about:

- the health status of the population
- health-related aspects of lifestyle and other health risk factors
- the use of health services and other actions people had recently taken for their health.

Examples of particular health issues included:

- long-term illnesses experienced
- mental well-being
- injuries
- consultations with doctors and other health professionals
- health risk factors such as alcohol consumption, smoking, exercise, body mass and dietary practices.

Source: ABS (2009b)

SAMPLE

Approximately 20,000 people from all states and territories and across all age groups were included. The strategy included interviewing one adult (aged eighteen years or more) and one child (where applicable) from each sampled dwelling.

A cross-sectional survey can tell us what proportion of a sample or population reports certain symptoms, diseases or characteristics, and whether these are more prevalent among certain sections of the population. For instance, the 2007–08 ABS National Health Survey found that 63 per cent of males and 48 per cent of females were classified as overweight or obese based on their self-reported height and weight. Surveys repeated over time allow us to determine trends. For instance, the 1995 National Nutrition Survey found that 65 per cent of males and 48 per cent of females were overweight or obese (ABS 2006a). These results suggest that there was a concerning increase over the twelve-year period in the proportion of overweight or obese Australians.

STOP AND THINK

From the research described above:

- Why do you think that significantly more males than females are overweight or obese?
- What explanations can you come up with to explain the increasing proportion of adults who are overweight or obese over time?
- What type of research might best illuminate the causes of the increasing rate of being overweight?

Longitudinal surveys

Longitudinal cohort surveys administer the same set of questions to individuals on repeated occasions and seek to understand how individuals or groups change over time. They could be undertaken simply to monitor changes in health or some other variable over time, or to measure outcomes of certain interventions or treatments. A study demonstrating the first purpose (to monitor change over time) is the Australian Longitudinal Study on Women's Health. This large-scale prospective study has surveyed the same three cohorts of women (young, mid-aged and older women) every three years since 1996 (see Figure 13.1) and has monitored changes in health status and health care use over time (see <www.alswh.org.au>). See also Chapter 14.

Longitudinal cohort surveys: These administer the same set of questions to individuals on repeated occasions and seek to understand how individuals or groups change over time, allowing the researcher to predict outcomes.

FIGURE 13.1   Example of longitudinal postal survey: Australian Longitudinal Study on Women's Health

Cohort	Year of surveys					
	1996	98, 99, 00,	01, 02, 03,	04, 05, 06,	07, 08, 09,	...... 2015 +
Younger	☒	☒	☒	☒	☒	
Mid-aged	☒	☒	☒	☒	☒	
Older	☒	☒	☒	☒	☒	
	S_1	S_2	S_3	S_4	S_5......	

Source: Women's Health Australia (2005)

One advantage of longitudinal survey studies is that a greater range of research questions can be asked, predictive questions can be tested, and more complex statistical analyses can be made. Researchers can ask, for instance, about which factors at an earlier point in time can predict certain health outcomes at a later point. Such studies are able to shed light on both protective factors and risk factors for later illness or death. For instance, cohort-based studies have shown that certain diets are associated with development of cancer later in life (Bingham *et al.* 2003), and that smoking is linked to lung cancer (Doll *et al.* 2005).

Surveys to test intervention effects

Surveys to test intervention effects: These take measures before and after a treatment or intervention to determine whether the intervention produces change in outcomes.

Surveys to test intervention effects are administered before and after an intervention to test for changes in self-reported outcomes such as symptoms, subjective well-being, knowledge and attitudes, or health behaviours. This is similar to the longitudinal survey, in that measures are administered on repeated occasions with the intention of analysing scores for difference over time. However, in intervention studies, the measures are aligned to the purpose of the intervention or treatment and are designed specifically to test whether the intervention has produced hypothesised changes. For instance, if a particular treatment aims to improve certain symptoms, then a survey can be used to test whether these self-reported symptoms decrease in the projected time-frame after treatment. Surveys can be used alone or in conjunction with other diagnostic or objective measures.

How is measurement theory applied to survey research?

Before describing the process of constructing survey questions, it is important to have some understanding of measurement theory, that is, the set of rules that govern the way questions are constructed and responses recorded. See also Chapter 11.

Measurement can be defined as the process of assigning a number or symbol to an attribute or variable, according to a rule. It is a central aspect of research since it enables us to obtain data. Common measurement methods used for the collection of data are surveys, direct observation and interviews. Before we are able to measure a variable or construct, we have to operationalise it. In the process of operationalisation, the researcher must define how the variable or theoretical construct will be measured.

The researcher must also distinguish between different types of measures or data collection techniques. We can use measures that produce quantitative or qualitative data. Quantitative data are numerical values and qualitative data are pictures or words. The choice of measure depends on the research question and topic (see Chapters 1, 2). Since this chapter focuses on quantitative measurement as applied to survey research, we first describe the difference between discrete and continuous measures and then the four levels of measurement.

Discrete and continuous measurement

Variables can be differentiated as discrete or continuous. A discrete variable uses only whole numbers or units. Number of children is an example of a discrete variable. Height, weight and age are examples of continuous variables because there are values between units. Somebody can be 17.4 years old or 1.63 m tall, but a family cannot have 1.4 children. There are variables with two values, such as gender (female and male), and variables with multiple values, such as age or marital status. Age is a continuous measure, whereas marital status is a discrete measure—there is a fixed number of categories and there cannot be a score between those categories.

In terms of the broadest definition of measurement, there are four different levels of measurement or four different types of measurement scales—nominal, ordinal, interval and ratio (see Chapters 11, 25). Each of these is described in the following section.

Nominal data/categorical measurement

For **nominal data** or categorical measurement, we have different categories and allocate a value to each category representing a variable. Examples of nominal measuring are the allocation of a value to gender categories, country of birth, first language or religion (see Table 13.1). If the variable is gender, you could allocate the value 1 to female and 2 to male. The categories that individuals are allocated to are distinct and not continuous. It would not make sense to have the value 1.4 in relation to the variable gender.

Nominal data: These occur where objects or people are assigned to named categories according to some criterion, for example male/female.

A further characteristic of nominal/categorical measurement is that the category values are not in a particular order. We can freely decide if we allocate the value '1' or the value '2' to female. The value simply describes the category and the difference of the variable; it does not stand for a specific quantity. The numbers have no quantitative meaning. The fact that a nominal/categorical scale cannot be ordered and has no quantitative meaning has consequences for the analysis. It would not make sense to calculate an average. For nominal/categorical data, we can report frequencies or percentages of individuals. In our example with

Margot J. Schofield and Christine Forrester-Knauss

TABLE 13.1   Levels of measurement

LEVEL OF MEASUREMENT	EXAMPLE	POSSIBLE VALUES
Nominal/categorical	Gender	1 = female 2 = male
Ordinal	Satisfaction with treatment	1 = not at all satisfied 2 = slightly satisfied 3 = moderately satisfied 4 = very satisfied
Interval	Body temperature	36.9° 37.3°
Ratio	Weight	60.5 kg 75.7 kg 85.3 kg

gender, this would mean that we might report that the sample consisted of ten females and ten males or of 50 per cent women and 50 per cent men.

Ordinal measurement

Ordinal data: These result when observations are rank-ordered and values are assigned sequentially to reflect the logical ordering of categories, e.g. Likert scales, which rank responses from low to high.

Ordinal data result when observations are rank-ordered and values are assigned sequentially to reflect the logical ordering of categories. For variables like satisfaction with a treatment or degree of racism, the different attributes represent relatively more or less of the variable. We could assign a value to an individual that would stand for their degree of satisfaction with a certain treatment. The more satisfied the person is with the treatment, the higher the value. According to the values, the individual could be rank-ordered. We would know that some individuals reported more satisfaction with treatment than others. The categories of the variable can be clearly ordered, but are also distinct and not continuous. It does not make sense to calculate a mean score for ordinal measures, because the differences between the scores on the scale do not have meaning. If the value '1' stands for 'Satisfied with the treatment' and the value '2' for 'Very satisfied with the treatment', we would not be able to interpret the difference between the two values in terms of people who answered with '2' being two times more satisfied than people who answered with '1'. The differences between the values are meaningless. The value just describes the rank order for ordinal measurement, therefore the value '2' stands for a higher rating than '1'.

Interval/ratio measurement

Interval data: These have the property of a rank order. In addition, distances or intervals between the units of measurement are equal.

Ratio data: These have the same properties as interval data. In addition, they have an empirical rather than an arbitrary zero.

The **interval/ratio** scale is used in measuring variables for which the interval between the values on the scale has meaning. The distance between the attributes expresses meaningful standard intervals. Familiar variables for interval/ratio measurement are height or temperature. The distance between 10 cm and 15 cm is the same as that between 15 cm and 20 cm.

Ratio scales have the same characteristics as interval scales, but they have a true zero point representing the absence of the variable measured. For example, for the variable height, zero stands for the absence of height. A further example of a ratio measurement is IQ. The differences between the values have meaning—the difference between an IQ of 90 and 100 would be the same as that between 100 and 110 as there is a true zero point. In the measurement of temperature, however, zero does not stand for the absence of temperature and it is therefore an interval measurement, not a ratio one.

The choice of an appropriate method of data analysis depends on the level of measurement. If you are planning to calculate a mean, an interval or ratio measurement level is required (see Chapter 25). It is important to keep in mind that the necessary level of measurement needs to be chosen before you start your research because it is not possible to convert a lower-level measurement to a higher-level measurement. If you have decided to choose an ordinal measure, it will not be possible to convert it to an interval measure.

How are surveys designed?

Surveys are usually designed with three components: a cover (invitation) letter, some instructions on how the survey should be completed, and the set of questions to be answered.

Participant information letter

The participant information letter aims to inform the respondent about the purpose of the survey and about the researchers conducting the study, as well as to engage their interest and motivate them to respond. Ethical guidelines governing institutional research specify a number of aspects that must be covered in an information letter to ensure informed consent (see Chapter 3). Typical content of a participant information letter includes:

- a clear statement of the aims and significance of the research
- the names and contact details of the research team
- the funding source of the research
- reasons why respondents should complete the survey
- what is involved in completing the survey, such as maximum time
- assurances of confidentiality, and anonymity, if relevant
- a statement that participation is voluntary and that participants can withdraw after agreeing to participate
- information about how the survey results will be used
- information about how to gain further information or make a complaint.

Instructions

The instructions are important to ensure that participants know what they need to do so that the survey is completed correctly. It is usual to encourage participants to attempt to answer

Margot J. Schofield and Christine Forrester-Knauss

all questions. If the survey is largely about attitudes, the instructions might emphasise that there are no right or wrong answers and that an opinion is what is required. Participants can be informed about how to answer particular types of questions, and examples of correct and incorrect responses may be given. The instructions section should indicate how respondents should return the completed survey, for example 'Please return the completed questionnaire to the Researcher in the enclosed reply-paid envelope within two weeks'. Each question should also have instructions to clarify the type of response option: for example 'Tick one box only' or 'Tick all that apply' or 'Select the response that most closely reflects your views'.

What steps are involved in constructing the survey?

Constructing a survey takes much more effort than designing individual questions. It involves consideration of the overall structure, flow and coherence of the survey, and testing the adequacy of the developed questions. Typical steps (modified from Sarantakos 2005), include those discussed below.

1 Preparation

The researcher defines the survey objectives and key constructs to be measured, searches for relevant measures, and assesses their reliability and validity and whether they meet the needs of the study. If an appropriate measure is found, the researcher decides whether it requires adaptation. Note that if questions are adapted, this may diminish validity or reliability.

2 Constructing and critiquing the first draft

The researcher selects the available measures and/or constructs questions to address the key variables to be measured. It is usual to include a number of questions that describe the socio-demographic characteristics of your sample. The researcher then reviews the draft questions to determine whether they adequately capture the constructs, and whether they meet the general rules for questionnaire construction such as being relevant, unambiguous and in plain language, and whether they are logically ordered.

3 External review and revision

After revision, the draft survey is reviewed by other experts in survey construction or the research topic, and feedback obtained. On the basis of that feedback, the researcher revises the questions and perhaps reorders items. If substantial changes are required, the survey should go back to external review before moving on to the next step.

4 Pre-test or pilot test of the revised survey

Once a satisfactory revised draft is available, the researcher should pilot-test the whole instrument with a small sample similar to the intended study sample. Respondents may be asked to provide specific feedback on how they experienced the survey and whether they thought any questions were ambiguous or difficult to answer.

5 Further revision based on pre-test

Pre-tests or pilot studies will usually lead to further revision of the survey. If a major revision is required, further external review and pilot-testing of the revised version may be required.

6 Second pre-test or pilot test

The revised survey instrument will then undergo further pilot-testing of the survey or pre-testing of the revised component to determine if further revisions are required before the final draft of the survey.

7 Formulation of the final draft

At this point, the researcher stands back and considers the feedback from the various sources outlined above, together with a review of the overall study objectives and methodology, and makes the final changes. Often at this stage, questions of length, flow, coherence, structural components, layout and presentation will be reviewed. Any acknowledgments and instructions must be incorporated. A final proofread is required before finalising for printing.

How are surveys structured?

Researchers must decide how to present and order the questions in the questionnaire in a way that will enhance its acceptability and ease of completion. Questions should be presented in a logical order with a sense of a smooth transition from one section to the next. The overall design and logic of the survey is related to the likelihood of achieving a higher response rate. Furthermore, the order and logic will affect the meaning given to certain questions.

There are various approaches to the ordering of items within a survey. One common approach is the **funnel format**. Other formats include the **inverted funnel format** and the **mixed format**.

Funnel format

In this model, the questions move from a broad focus to more specific content, from non-sensitive questions to more sensitive questions, and from more impersonal to more personal. The rationale is that it is best to warm respondents up with general non-threatening questions, and as they become more engaged with the survey they will be more inclined to answer more personal questions. This also allows people time to reflect on topics at a more general level then at the more personal level, and suits respondents who are likely to think at a more abstract level.

Inverted funnel format

In this format, questions move from more specific to more general, from more sensitive to less sensitive, and from personal to impersonal. This format may be useful for respondents

Funnel format survey: Where the questions move from a broad focus to more specific content, from non-sensitive questions to more sensitive questions, and from more impersonal to more personal.

Inverted funnel format survey: Where the questions move from more specific to more general, from more sensitive to less sensitive, and from personal to impersonal.

Mixed format survey: Where the questions are organised in sections or domains and particular formats are applied within domains.

Margot J. Schofield and Christine Forrester-Knauss

who are primed to answer personal questions and where limited time demands that the more specific questions need to be focused on first.

Mixed format

This is particularly relevant for longer surveys covering a number of domains. Here, the questions are organised in sections or domains and particular formats are applied within domains. For instance, a funnel format may be used within each section, so that overall the survey moves from general to specific, and this pattern is repeated through various sections of the survey.

Structured and semi-structured formats

A structured format means that there is a set ordering of questions for respondents to work their way through. Every respondent is thus responding to the same set of questions in the same order and usually with set response options. This helps to avoid differences in responses that may be due to ordering effects. Semi-structured questionnaires are usually used in interview format; they allow for a more flexible ordering of items and often involve more open-ended response formats.

STOP AND THINK

Survey topic in area of interest

Think of a research question or topic in your area of interest that would be suitable to study using a survey format. Define the research question.

Structured questions

How would you phrase the main questions for a structured questionnaire and what response options would you provide?

Semi-structured questions

How would you phrase the questions in a semi-structured, more open-ended way?

Length of the survey

The length of the survey is an important consideration, as response rate is likely to decline with increasing length. It is therefore important to be disciplined in determining how essential each question is for the study. One strategy is to rate all the proposed questions as essential, desirable or optional, then decide how many questions or the maximum period for completion of the questionnaire. If items must be removed, the rating system will suggest which ones to remove. If items are removed, the overall flow and transition must be reconsidered. In general, fifteen to twenty minutes is considered the maximum length for general surveys unless participants are likely to be highly motivated.

Strategies for helping respondents navigate the survey

For longer surveys, a strategy that will enhance respondents' navigation through the survey is to put clear and engaging headings at the start of each section so that there is an overall sense of structure.

It can also help to provide feedback at certain points, which tells respondents how far they are through the survey. For instance, in a long survey, respondents might be told when they reach the halfway point and might be encouraged to have a break or a cup of tea before going on to the next section. Some researchers may even include a teabag! Small gestures acknowledging the burden on respondents can increase completions and goodwill.

Internet-based surveys usually include a little graph on each page showing the percentage of the survey completed. This provides more regular reinforcement, goodwill and encouragement to respondents (Toepoel 2015).

How are survey questions constructed?

Types of question content

Questions can be classified in a number of ways depending on the type of content and the type of response options. Dillman and colleagues (2014) suggest that there are five main types of question content: behaviour, beliefs, attitudes, knowledge and attributes.

- Behaviour questions ask what people do. For example, 'Do you currently smoke cigarettes?'
- Belief questions ask what people believe to be true or false about topics. For example, whether they think smoking is harmful to health, or whether they think peer pressure or parental example is more influential in determining smoking uptake among adolescents.
- Attitude questions seek to establish what respondents think is desirable. For example, whether they agree with a statement such as 'Airports should provide a smoking room for smoking travellers' or 'Hospitals should refuse to perform cardiac surgery on smoking patients'.
- Knowledge questions seek to determine what people know about particular topics. In relation to assessing knowledge about smoking, we could ask what they know about the harmful health effects of smoking on women, or the effects on unborn babies of mothers' smoking during pregnancy.
- Attribute questions seek information about more objective characteristics of respondents, such as their age, gender, occupation and place of residence. Many of these attribute questions can be sourced from major published surveys such as those run by the ABS in Australia.

Margot J. Schofield and Christine Forrester-Knauss

The types of question that ask about more subjective information, such as beliefs, attitudes, values and perceived quality of life, pose particular design challenges. Because these questions are less objective, researchers often use a standardised scale since these have been shown to increase reliability and validity (McDowell 2006) and there may be some normative data that you can compare with the results you obtain. Standardised scales are discussed in more detail in the next section.

STOP AND THINK

- Think about a particular health topic you are interested in.
- Construct a clear, simple question related to your topic for each of the following categories: behaviour, belief, attitude, knowledge and attribute.

Standardised scales

Standardised scale: This provides a scientific form of health assessment that is useful for measuring subjective constructs such as pain, mood and level of symptoms.

Reliability: The extent to which a measurement instrument is dependable, stable and consistent when repeated under identical conditions.

Validity: The extent to which the scale measures what it is supposed to measure (content and construct validity).

Standardised scales provide a scientific form of health assessment that is particularly useful for measuring subjective constructs such as pain, mood and level of symptoms. Standardised scales are made up of a series of self-report questions, ratings or items that measure a specific concept. The response categories are in the same format and can be summed or aggregated in some weighted form. The scale can then produce a number on a standard interval or ratio scale such as 0–100, to reflect a level of functioning, symptoms, pain, affect or beliefs. The process of standardisation means that the number assigned can be compared statistically either within or across individuals or groups. Standardised scales can be used to test for change over time, for instance as a result of treatment, or to look for differences between groups.

The concepts of **reliability** and **validity** are important for standardised scales (see also Chapters 1, 11, 12). 'Reliability' refers to the ability of the scale to provide consistent stable information over time and across respondents. For instance, if someone completes the scale today and again in two days' time, do you get essentially the same responses? 'Validity' refers to the degree to which the scale measures what it is supposed to measure (content and construct validity). For instance, does it have a good correlation with another gold standard measure?

Standardised rating scales cover a wide range of purposes. Some of the commonly used ones are diagnostic scales, symptom-based scales, quality of life scales, functional-level scales and client satisfaction scales. There is also a wide range of scales that assess psychosocial factors such as attitudes and beliefs, social support, optimism or loneliness. Many scales have a number of subscales as well as an overall scale score. An example is the widely used quality of life scale, the Medical Outcomes Study Health Survey Short-Form 36 items (SF-36). This is a well-validated scale comprising eight subscales as shown in Table 13.2. Each of the eight subscales contribute differing weights to the calculation of the physical and mental health component scores.

There are good sources that provide an overview of established scales for health research (e.g. Bowling 2005; McDowell 2006; Sajatovic & Ramirez 2012). These can help researchers to

TABLE 13.2 Standardised scale: Medical Outcomes Study Health Survey Short Form (SF-36)

8 SUBSCALES	2 COMPONENT SUMMARY SCORES
Physical functioning	
Role—physical	
Bodily pain	Physical component summary
General health	
Vitality	Mental component summary
Social functioning	
Role—social	
Mental health	

Source: Ware *et al.* (1994)

select appropriate measures for different studies since they include information on the content, scoring, validity and reliability of many different health measures. A thorough overview of constructing standardised scales can be found in Osterlind (2006).

Constructing your own survey questions

If you decide that there are no established questions for your purpose, you will need to construct your own questions. This is a complex task (de Vaus 2007) but it can be guided by a number of important principles as outlined in the box.

PRINCIPLES FOR CONSTRUCTING SURVEY QUESTIONS

- Use simple everyday language typical of the respondent group.
- Avoid jargon, technical terms and abstract concepts.
- Avoid ambiguity and double-barrelled questions.
- Avoid double negatives.
- Avoid making suggestive statements or assumptions about respondents.
- Provide sufficient instructions and probes.
- Pre-coded questions should offer sufficient response categories.
- When asking people to record past events, provide a temporal frame, e.g. 'Over the last four weeks' or 'In the past year'.

Response formats

Questions can be classified as open or closed depending on how respondents are asked to respond. Open questions simply ask the question and invite respondents to give an answer in

Margot J. Schofield and Christine Forrester-Knauss

whatever way seems most appropriate to them. This can yield rich data that may be missed if only closed response options are provided, but responses need to be coded before analysis can be made—a time-consuming process. Closed questions provide a set of predetermined response options and respondents choose which option applies to them—an economical method.

Some of the main types of response formats are summarised in the next 'Research in practice'. At the simplest level, there are Yes/No or Yes/No/Don't know response formats. These are closed questions with little room for participants to give finely discriminated responses. They are particularly suitable for questions where there is a relatively straightforward factual response, such as 'Have you smoked in the last week?'

Verbal rating scales are commonly used where a question is asked and a range of verbal response categories is provided; the participant has to circle the response that most closely represents their view. This is an example of categorical or ordinal data. To make such responses suitable for statistical analysis, the verbal categories are assigned to numbers that can be entered into data files as shown in the Verbal + Numeric Rating Scale in 'Research in practice'. Note that these numbers represent a rank-ordered scale, not an interval scale.

Likert scales are used to measure subjective variables such as attitudes. The researcher generates a number of statements (e.g. attitudes) and wishes to measure the extent to which participants agree or disagree with the statements. The scales typically ask each respondent to rate each item on a response scale that has discrete options, such as a 1–5 (or 1–7) response scale. A typical Likert scale is a 5-point scale. This can be unidirectional or have positive and negative (opposing) directions.

Visual analogue scales allow respondents to rate items on a continuous line between two end points. Typically, respondents are asked to mark a position on the line that goes from 0–10 or from 0–100. This has the advantage of providing an interval measure that can be analysed using a wider range of statistical tests. The continuous nature of this measurement scale differentiates it from discrete scales like the Likert scale, verbal or numerical scales, and it may produce a more sensitive and differentiated response under certain circumstances (Grant *et al.* 1999).

Verbal rating scale: Used where a question is asked and a range of verbal response categories is provided. The participant has to circle the response that most closely represents their view.

Likert scale: Used to measure subjective variables such as attitudes. The researcher generates a number of statements and wishes to measure the extent to which participants agree or disagree.

Visual analogue scale: This allows respondents to rate items on a continuous line between two end points.

RESEARCH IN PRACTICE

RESPONSE FORMATS

Yes/No/Don't know

In general, would you say your health is good?

YES	NO	DON'T KNOW

Verbal + numerical rating scale (categorical)

In general, would you say your health is:

EXCELLENT	VERY GOOD	GOOD	FAIR	POOR
1	2	3	4	5

Likert scale (ordinal)

In general, would you say your health is good?

STRONGLY AGREE	AGREE	NEITHER AGREE NOR DISAGREE	DISAGREE	STRONGLY DISAGREE
1	2	3	4	5

Visual analogue scale (interval)

In general, how would you rate your health?

MARK A POSITION ON THE LINE FROM 0 (VERY POOR) TO 100 (EXTREMELY GOOD)
0..100

Open-ended question

In general, how would you rate your health?

....

....

....

Designing response options to closed questions

While closed questions are helpful in producing numeric data for analysis in the most efficient way, it can be problematic to define the appropriate response categories. In designing response categories, it is necessary to ensure that categories are mutually exclusive, and that all or most options are catered for. An example of designing response options for marital status is given in the next 'Research in practice' box.

RESPONSE FORMATS

Suppose you want to know about marital/relationship status. You could look up the ABS question format and find that it is more complex than you first thought.

The ABS distinguishes between 'Registered marital status' and 'Social marital status'. The standard question for registered marital status is:

Q. What is your present marital status?

- Never married
- Separated
- Widowed
- Married
- Divorced

However, it is clear that this question alone will not tell you anything about the large number of people who live in de facto relationships or in same-sex relationships. The ABS has developed a series of additional questions to explore 'social marital

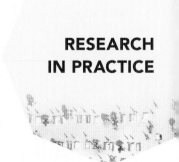

RESEARCH IN PRACTICE

Margot J. Schofield and Christine Forrester-Knauss

status', which are then matched to marital status responses to derive more defined categories. To simplify this for a survey, you could include |additional response options to the basic ABS response options.

Question response options for social marital status (modified from ABS format) could be as follows.

Q. What is your present marital status? (*Mark one only*)

- Never married
- Married (registered)
- Widowed
- De facto relationship (opposite sex)
- Divorced
- De facto relationship (same sex)
- Separated

This example shows that even what we might think of as a relatively straightforward and objective piece of information, such as marital status, can be quite complex to think through and it can be difficult to ensure that all possible response options are included. Failure to do this will mean that a proportion of people answering your survey will feel that none of the response options provided apply to them. You will be missing out on valuable information.

Measurement error

Measurement errors: These happen when researchers do not measure accurately or when they measure a different variable from the one intended. They can be systematic or random, depending on whether or not they have a constant pattern.

Despite our best efforts to enhance validity and reliability, errors can occur at different stages of the research process and for different levels of measurement. Mistakes can happen, for example, by choosing the wrong sample, by having errors in the measurement process or by interpreting the results in an invalid way. **Measurement errors** happen when we do not measure accurately or when we measure a different variable from the one intended. Measurement errors can be either systematic or random, depending on whether or not they have a constant pattern. To minimise or avoid measurement errors, it is important to ensure that the measures used have acceptable reliability and validity, which means that they measure accurately and that they assess the variable they intend to assess. See also Chapters 1, 11, 12, 26.

Sources of measurement error in surveys

Because survey measures rely on self-report, there are certain types of measurement error that need to be considered. Survey measures may contain errors due to poor memory, failure to understand the question or response options, a desire to give a socially acceptable response, or having response options that do not match the respondent's response (Engel 2015).

Some measurement errors can be identified by including more than one way of measuring variables that are susceptible to error. For instance, self-report measures can be supplemented by having more objective measures and assessing whether there is evidence of systematic error. One example of this is shown in the next 'Research in practice', where self-reported weight category is compared with measured BMI.

Asking retrospective questions is another common source of error. People often have difficulty remembering when health events in the past occurred, and memory tends to degrade over time. Measurement error due to memory problems can be improved by including certain prompts to improve memory.

SELF-REPORT MEASUREMENT ERROR

Perceptions of weight

In the 2007–08 National Health Survey, self-reported (subjective) classifications of one's weight as normal, overweight or obese were compared with the more objectively measured Body Mass Index (BMI), calculated by a formula based on the ratio of weight to height (ABS 2009b). It was found that:

When BMI was calculated from measured weight and height, 68% of males and 55% of females were classified as overweight or obese. However, only 63% of males and 48% of females considered themselves to be overweight or obese. Under-estimation of BMI category were highest in the overweight and obese group, with 21% of those under-estimating their weight category (ABS 2009b).

Thus we can conclude that self-reported weight perception has a high degree of error. Under-estimation was evident mainly in the overweight and obese groups, while adults in the other weight categories were found to be relatively accurate. Clearly, actual measurement of height and weight is more reliable, particularly for higher risk groups.

RESEARCH IN PRACTICE

STRATEGIES TO ENHANCE ACCURACY OF SURVEY RESPONSES

1   Ask respondent to take accurate measurements.
2   Ask questions in various ways.
3   Use scales for subjective constructs.
4   Keep the survey as short as possible.

How are surveys administered?

There are several key methods for administering surveys: self-completion questionnaire, group self-completion, mail self-completion, internet-based self-completion, face-to-face interview, telephone interview and internet interview.

- Self-completion questionnaire. Participants are asked to complete the survey instrument and instructions are provided.

- Group self-completion. A researcher may administer a survey to a group, such as a class of school students. Participants will each complete their own survey, but the process is facilitated and the researcher is present throughout.

Margot J. Schofield and Christine Forrester-Knauss

- Mail self-completion. Surveys are mailed out to participants, who are asked to complete the survey and mail it back, usually in a reply-paid envelope provided by the researcher.

- Internet-based self-completion. Participants are invited to complete an internet-based survey and are given the web-link for accessing it.

- Face-to-face interview. The researcher may conduct a face-to-face interview using an interview schedule (list of questions or topics). The responses may be recorded manually or tape-recorded and later coded.

- Telephone interview. Telephone interviews are like face-to-face interviews but are conducted over the phone. Computer-assisted telephone interviews (CATI) are a popular method, in which the survey is programmed into the computer and an interviewer reads through the questions and types in the respondent's answers. This enters numeric or verbal answers directly into data files.

- Internet interview. Internet interviews are similar to telephone interviews but are conducted using internet-based voice software such as Skype or MSN Messenger. The interviewer either types in responses or voice-records the interview, using the computer software program.

STOP AND THINK

What are the advantages and disadvantages of using an internet-based survey?

Under what conditions would you prefer a mailed self-completion survey to a face-to-face interview?

What about the response rate? How do you think the method of administering your survey influences the response rate, and why?

Summary

Surveys are useful for obtaining information about topics that are not directly observable, and for collecting data without direct contact with participants or people who might otherwise be difficult to reach. They make it possible to quantify responses so we can use them for statistical analysis. When interpreting the results, it is important to consider the accuracy of the responses. We differentiate between cross-sectional surveys, longitudinal surveys, and surveys to test intervention effects. The type of survey used depends on the research question and the intended statistical analysis. Standardised scales help us to measure subjective constructs and to make results comparable. Several principles should be considered in the development and construction of a survey. A number of steps are necessary, such as decisions about the survey format, the specificity of the question and response options, and the length of the survey.

Practice exercises

Evaluate the effectiveness of an intervention offered to adults to lower their level of experienced stress by practising relaxation techniques.

1 What is your research question?

2 At what time-points would you ask participants about their level of stress?

3 What survey administration method would you choose?

4 What kind of measures would you choose and how would you go about choosing them?

5 How would you get information about the validity and reliability of your chosen measures?

6 What principles do you need to keep in mind if you decide to write your own questions?

7 What type of sample would you choose and how would you recruit your participants?

Further reading

Blair, J., Czaja, R.F. & Blair, E.A. (2012). *Designing surveys: a guide to decisions and procedures*, 3rd edn. Thousand Oaks, CA: Sage.

Bowling, A. (2005). *Measuring health: a review of quality of life measurement scales*, 3rd edn. Maidenhead, UK: Open University Press.

De Leeuw, E., Hox, J. & Dillman, D.A. (2008). *International handbook of survey methodology*. New York: Lawrence Erlbaum.

de Vaus, D. (2004). Structured questions and interviews. In V. Minichiello, G. Sullivan, K. Greenwood & R. Axford (eds), *Handbook of research methods for nursing and health science*, 2nd edn. Sydney: Pearson Education Australia, 347–93.

de Vaus, D. (ed.) (2007). *Social surveys 2*, 4 vols. London: Sage

Dillman, D.A., Smyth, J.D. & Christian, L.M. (2014). *Internet, phone, mail, and mixed-mode surveys: the tailored design method*, 4th edn. Hoboken, NJ: John Wiley.

Fowler, F.J. (2009). *Survey research methods*, 4th edn. Thousand Oaks, CA: Sage.

Lavrakis, P.J. (2008). *Encyclopedia of survey research methods*. Thousand Oaks, CA: Sage.

Ruel, E.E., Wagner, W.E. & Gillespie, B.J. (2015). *The practice of survey research: theory and applications*. London: Sage.

Sue, V.M. & Ritter, L.A. (2012). *Conducting online surveys*, 2nd edn. Thousand Oaks, CA: Sage.

Toepoel, V. (2015). *Doing surveys online*. London: Sage.

Tourangeau, R., Conrad, F.G. & Couper, M. (2013). *The science of web surveys*. Oxford: Oxford University Press.

Margot J. Schofield and Christine Forrester-Knauss

Websites

www.socialresearchmethods.net/kb/survey.php

> This site of the Web Center for Social Research Methods provides a comprehensive overview of survey research methods.

http://writing.colostate.edu/guides/research/survey/pop2f.cfm

> This site contains an annotated bibliography of survey research.

www.alswh.org.au

> The website of the Australian Longitudinal Study on Women's Health provides access to a wide range of survey questions on women's health as well as basic descriptive data, publications and reports on findings.

www.advancedsurvey.com/surveys

www.limesurvey.org/en/

www.surveymonkey.com

> The above three survey-hosting websites provide information on designing online surveys.

How Do We Know What We Know? Epidemiology in Health Research

MELISSA GRAHAM

Chapter objectives

In this chapter you will learn:

- how the principal questions in epidemiology can be used to answer population health questions
- to distinguish between observational descriptive and analytical epidemiological study designs
- how you can use sources of population health data to answer questions about population health

Key terms

Analytical cross-sectional studies

Analytical epidemiological studies

Case-control study

Cohort study

Cross-sectional study

Descriptive epidemiology

Ecological study

Epidemiology

Exposure

Longitudinal studies

Measures of association

Morbidity

Mortality

Observational epidemiological studies

Outcome

Population

Population health data

Prevalence rate ratio

Introduction

We often hear health research and statistics quoted in the media. For example: 12,000 Australian women are diagnosed with breast cancer each year; babies die in public hospitals, during labour or shortly after birth, at three times the rate they do in private hospitals; one Australian woman dies every eleven hours from ovarian cancer; and cervical cancer is linked to deprivation. Where do these numbers and statements come from and what do they mean? These numbers are derived from population data that we employ in **epidemiology**. Epidemiological approaches can help us to understand these patterns of health states and make sense out of their meaning.

Epidemiology is concerned with the study of the distribution and determinants of health states in **populations** (Last *et al.* 1995). It can help us to determine the extent of ill health or disease in the community, identify the cause of ill health and the risk factors for disease, understand the natural history and prognosis of ill health, investigate disease outbreaks or epidemics, evaluate existing and new preventive and therapeutic programs and services, and provide the foundation for developing public policy and regulation (Gordis 2009). Essentially, this means epidemiology can provide the answers to questions asked in the health sector such as, How much disease is there? Who gets it? Where are most people affected? When did they have it? What happens over time? More importantly, it is how we as health professionals apply this to prevent and control health problems. The main aim of this chapter is to introduce you to population data to help us answer the questions of 'who', 'where' and 'when'. Before we examine sources and types of **population-based health data**, let us look at the underpinning principles of observational descriptive and analytical epidemiology and how this data is generated—study designs.

Epidemiology: This is concerned with the study of the distribution and determinants of health states in populations.

Population: In epidemiology, 'population' is used to describe all the people who live in a defined area or country.

Population-based health data: 'Ongoing systems that collect and register all cases of a particular disease or class of diseases as they develop in a defined population' (Oleckno 2002, p. 349).

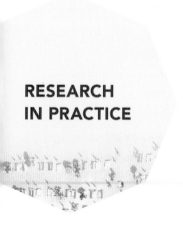

RESEARCH IN PRACTICE

SELECTING AN OBSERVATIONAL EPIDEMIOLOGICAL STUDY DESIGN FOR YOUR RESEARCH

The type of observational epidemiological study design you select for your research will depend on the research question you wish to answer. There are two broad types of observational epidemiology: descriptive and analytical. For example, consider the following research question: Is the prevalence of married female childlessness increasing in Australia? This question is concerned with describing what is happening over time in regard to the prevalence of childless women in Australia. We would use an observational descriptive epidemiological study design to answer this research question. However, what if we were interested in answering the question: Does being childless increase the risk of depression among Australian women? This question is asking us if there is an association (that is, does being childless increase or decrease the risk of depression) between being a childless woman in Australia and depression. To answer this we would use an observational analytical epidemiological study design.

The who, the where and the when

Population health statistics can give us useful information. When we hear health statistics or when we think about health and illness within our society, we often ask who are sick, where are they and when were they sick? These questions form the underlying principles of epidemiology and help us to answer many more questions about the population's health and well-being. Returning to our definition of epidemiology, we see epidemiology is the study of the distribution and determinants of health states or events in specified populations (Last *et al.* 1995). Health states or events are the diseases or conditions of interest. So, in epidemiology, when we investigate the distribution or pattern of a particular health state in a particular population, we are actually trying to answer the questions of 'who', 'where' and 'when'. In epidemiology, these questions are known as person (who), place (where) and time (when). We will now consider each of these questions and how they help us to understand the patterns of health within populations.

Person

Let's say we are interested in how many women have cervical cancer. The first question we ask ourselves in epidemiology is who has the condition or health state of interest—in this case, 'who' has cervical cancer? This question can be simply answered by counting the number of persons, in this case women who have cervical cancer. But often a simple count is not enough to answer our question adequately. This is because saying that X number of women have cervical cancer does not really tell us if this is a small group of women in the population or a very large group. We need to relate the number of women who have cervical cancer to the size of the population through the calculation of risks or rates (we will explore risks and rates later). Since populations are not usually a homogeneous group, we may want to express our counts in terms of the characteristics of the population. Commonly used characteristics of the population to describe subgroups include age and sex. In our example, we are interested only in women. In this case, it would also be useful to group our population of women by age—for example, women aged forty years or over in five-year age groups (i.e. forty to forty-four, forty-five to forty-nine and so forth). Other characteristics commonly used include socio-economic characteristics such as education, occupation or income; demographic characteristics such as geographic location, marital status or parity; or characteristics of health-related behaviours such as smoking, alcohol consumption and physical inactivity. Now that we know 'who', let's turn to the next question: 'where'.

Place

Following on from our example above, we may also wish to compare the number of people (women) with the health state (women who have cervical cancer) by place. By describing the geographic distribution of a health state, we can delineate those who may benefit from health-related interventions and provide information about possible determinants, risk or protective factors. Useful descriptors of place include place of residence, schools and workplaces, or birthplaces. Administrative descriptors of place such as local government area, city, state or country may also be useful. In our example, we may wish to look at the number of women who have cervical cancer in Australia or Victoria.

Time

So far, we have identified that we are interested in how many women aged forty years or over in Australia or Victoria have cervical cancer. Now, we turn to time—the 'when' question. What time-period are we interested in? Ever? A specific year? A time-range such as 2010 to 2012? The time variable can help us examine trends in health states over time and enable us to identify any changes in the patterns of the health state of interest. For example, has there been an increase or decrease in the health state at different points in time? Time can also help us predict what may occur in the future and provide clues to what is causing a change in the health state's occurrence. Finally, by examining patterns of health states over time we can examine the effectiveness of policies or programs that have been implemented to address the health state.

FIGURE 14.1   Percentage of women aged forty to forty-four years participating in the National Cervical Screening Program by remoteness area, 2012 and 2013

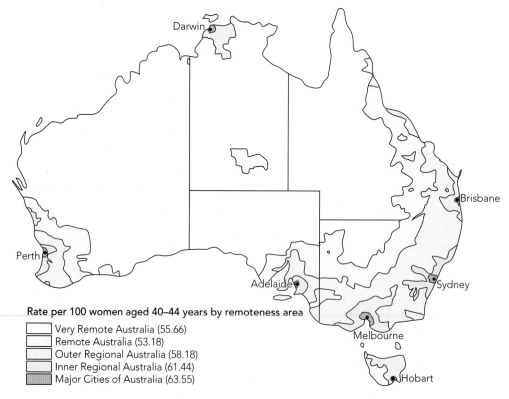

Rate per 100 women aged 40–44 years by remoteness area

- Very Remote Australia (55.66)
- Remote Australia (53.18)
- Outer Regional Australia (58.18)
- Inner Regional Australia (61.44)
- Major Cities of Australia (63.55)

Data source: AIHW (2015c)

Now that we have identified the building blocks of epidemiology enquiry, let's look at the types of epidemiological study designs we can use to answer our person, place and time questions.

STOP AND THINK

Figure 14.1 represents the percentage of women aged forty to forty-four years participating in the National Cervical Screening Program by remoteness area for 2012 and 2013 (AIHW 2015c).

- What can you conclude from this map in relation to person, place and time?

Observational studies: descriptive versus analytical epidemiology

Unlike experimental epidemiology, **observational epidemiological studies** do not seek to intervene or change people's exposure status. Rather, the aim is to collect information about people's exposure and health outcomes as they naturally occur within the population. Observational studies can be considered as either descriptive or analytical.

Descriptive epidemiology

Descriptive epidemiology focuses on describing health states and events and their distribution. They describe **morbidity** and **mortality** within the population using person, place and time variables. Descriptive studies do not have an *a priori* hypothesis that investigators set out to answer; rather, they focus on observing and describing what exists in the population. Given this, descriptive studies are helpful in determining the extent of ill health or disease in the community and studying the natural history and prognosis of disease. Descriptive studies are often carried out using pre-existing population health data.

There are two common types of descriptive epidemiological studies: cross-sectional studies and longitudinal studies (see Chapter 13).

Cross-sectional studies

A **cross-sectional study** involves the measurement of exposure and outcome simultaneously within the population of interest. Cross-sectional studies are often described as providing a snapshot of the frequency and characteristics of a health state in a population at a particular point in time. They are also referred to as prevalence studies. While cross-sectional studies are particularly useful for describing characteristics of the population, their main limitation is that **exposure** and **outcome** are measured at the same point in time. Therefore, it may not be possible to distinguish whether the exposure preceded or followed the outcome, and thus cause-and-effect relationships are not certain.

Melissa Graham

Observational epidemiological studies: These aim to collect information about people's exposure and health outcomes as they naturally occur within the population.

Descriptive epidemiology: This describes morbidity and mortality within the population using person, place and time variables.

Morbidity: The state of one's health, i.e. illness, disability, chronic disease and so on.

Mortality: Death.

Cross-sectional study: This gives a snapshot of the frequency and characteristics of a health state in a population at a particular point in time.

Exposure: A potential risk or protective factor for a health state—an actual exposure (environmental pollution), a behaviour (cigarette smoking) or an individual attribute (age).

Outcome: The health state that is under investigation and of interest.

PREVALENCE

Prevalence is the frequency of existing cases of a health state in a particular population at a specific point in time or time-period. Prevalence is calculated as:

$$P = \frac{\text{Number of people with the health state at a specified time}}{\text{Number of people in the population at the specified time}} \times 10^n$$

There are two types of prevalence: point prevalence and period prevalence. Point prevalence is the frequency of existing cases of a health state in a specific population at a point in time. Period prevalence is the frequency of existing cases of a health state in a specific population during a defined time-period (Szklo & Nieto 2007).

A large-scale population-based cross-sectional study (the second Australian Study of Health and Relationships), conducted in 2012–13, aimed to describe a range of sexual health factors such as contraceptive practices along with socio-demographic characteristics. This descriptive cross-sectional study found, in relation to heterosexual intercourse, that women (88.4 per cent) were significantly less likely than men (91.5 per cent) to report having ever used condoms (de Visser *et al.* 2014). The study also found that, among men and women, condom use for heterosexual activity in the previous year was associated with younger age, speaking a language other than English at home, bisexual identity, higher educational attainment, living in a major city (and, for men, a remote area), and having a lower income. As you can see, this example describes the distribution of condom use among a defined population at a specific point in time.

As cross-sectional studies are undertaken at a single point in time, they do not provide information on time trends. One way of obtaining information that includes the passage of time is to undertake a repeat cross-sectional study. This is similar to a cross-sectional study except that, instead of taking a single sample from a population at one time-point, a new sample is drawn from the population of interest at each time-point. Unlike longitudinal studies, repeat cross-sectional studies collect data from different individuals at each time-point. The most common form of cross-sectional study is the survey (see Chapter 13). For example, the Australian Bureau of Statistics conducts regular repeat cross-sectional population health surveys known as the National Health Survey, which collect 'information about the health status of Australians, their use of health services and facilities, and health-related aspects of their lifestyle' (ABS 2006a, p. 8). The purpose of the survey is to 'obtain national benchmark information on a range of health issues, enable trends in health to be monitored over time, and provide information on health indicators for national health priority areas and for important subgroups of the population' (ABS 2006a, p. 7). Findings from the National Health Survey can be accessed via the ABS website (www.abs.gov.au) in report format, aggregated (summary) data, or through the confidentialised unit record file (CURF). Access to CURF data requires approval as it is de-identified individual-level data. The Australian Study of Health and Relationships is another example of a repeat cross-sectional study, first conducted in 2000–01 then again in 2012–13 (Smith *et al.* 2003; Richters *et al.* 2014).

Longitudinal studies

Longitudinal studies are similar to repeat cross-sectional studies. But instead of drawing a new sample from the population at each time-point, the same group of people is followed over time. Longitudinal studies are useful to identify new cases (incidence) of a health state in a defined population and time-period. For example, an Australian longitudinal study that examined predictors of early motherhood found that women who become mothers early tend to live in rural areas, have low levels of education, are married or in a de facto relationship and not in paid employment (Lee & Gramotnev 2006). As you can see from this example, longitudinal studies allow us to follow a defined group of the population (women) over time to see if the socio-demographic characteristics of these women predicts the health state (early motherhood) of interest. We have described the distribution of the health state for women ('who') over 'time' (when) in Australia ('where'). As another example, analysis of longitudinal data from the Household, Income and Labour Dynamics in Australia study found that women without children experience poorer physical health during the peak reproductive years (thirty-four to forty-four) compared with mothers, but this was not the case for women of post-reproductive age. Never-married women without children experienced better physical and mental health than never-married mothers, while women without children experienced poorer health and well-being than mothers if they were divorced, separated, widowed or in a relationship (Graham 2015; see also Chapter 13).

Longitudinal studies: These follow the same group of people over time. They identify new cases of a health state in a defined population and period.

INCIDENCE

Incidence refers to the number of new cases of a health state in a particular population at a specific point in time. There are two types of incidence: cumulative incidence and incidence rate.

Cumulative incidence measures the risk of a person developing the health state in a defined time-period. Cumulative incidence can be calculated as:

$$CI = \frac{\text{Number of people with new health events during a specified time period}}{\text{Population at risk}} \times 10^n$$

Incidence rate is a measure of the rate at which new cases of the health state occur in the population during a specified time (Oleckno 2002). Incidence rate can be calculated as:

$$IR = \frac{\text{Number of people with the new health events during a specified time period}}{\text{Total person-time at risk}} \times 10^n$$

STOP AND THINK

Understanding the difference between incidence and prevalence can be confusing, particularly when it comes to identifying and applying the measures. Write down the characteristics of incidence (cumulative and incidence rate) and prevalence (point and period). In each of the following examples, identify the appropriate measure of incidence (cumulative or incidence rate) or prevalence (point or period).

- At the time of sentencing, tests conducted in Victorian prisons on 300 prisoners with sentences of at least two years revealed that seventy-one had a major psychological disorder. Follow-up testing eighteen months later showed that 165 were categorised as having a major psychological disorder. The person-time of follow-up between tests was 464 person-years.
- In a community with a population of 83,168 people, 657 developed high blood pressure during a one-year period.
- In 2009, a survey of 11,734 thirteen- to seventeen-year-old female secondary school students found that 37 per cent had smoked marijuana.
- In a survey of the reproductive histories of Australian women conducted in 2001, 24 per cent were found to have had at least one abortion.
- 1658 healthy women were followed for fifteen years; sixty-seven developed type II diabetes.

Analytical epidemiology

Analytical epidemiological studies: These are designed to test hypotheses about associations between an exposure of interest and a particular health outcome.

Analytical epidemiological studies are designed to test hypotheses about associations between an exposure of interest and a particular health outcome. Thus, analytical studies aim to identify or describe cause-and-effect relationships, or associations between exposure and outcome factors. In addition to the person, place and time variables, analytical studies can help us answer 'why' questions. Analytical studies can help identify if there is an association between two factors (e.g. cause and effect) and the strength of the association. In order to analyse associations between factors of interest, analytical studies involve planned comparisons between groups and generate measures of association.

Measures of association: Determine strengths of associations or relationships between exposures and outcomes.

MEASURES OF ASSOCIATION

Measures of association determine strengths of associations or relationships between exposures and outcomes. The measure of association used depends on the study design. Relative risks are a common measure of association and are primarily used for the analysis of associations in cohort studies. Relative risk is also known as risk ratio and can be calculated as:

$$RR = \frac{\text{Incidence in the exposed}}{\text{Incidence in the non-exposed}}$$

Another commonly used measure of association is the odds ratio. The odds ratio is mainly used in case-control studies; it is the 'odds' of exposure among the cases compared to the 'odds' among the controls. It can be calculated as:

$$OR = \frac{\text{Odds of exposure among cases}}{\text{Odds of exposure among controls}}$$

Chapter 14: How Do We Know What We Know? Epidemiology in Health Research

265

There are four main types of analytical studies: cross-sectional studies, ecological studies, case-control studies and cohort studies. The primary objective of analytical epidemiology is to identify reasons or causes for observed patterns of health states by studying associations between factors (exposures and outcomes) (Szklo & Nieto 2007). This means that, to begin with, we must identify the factors of interest in our analytical study—the outcome factor and the factor that may be related to (or be causing) the outcome of interest (exposure). The 'outcome of interest' is also often referred to as the 'dependent variable'. Other authors use the term 'disease'. In epidemiology, however, not all outcomes are diseases and in fact some outcomes may be desirable or favourable health states. It would be unfortunate and inappropriate to label these outcomes as disease. Therefore the terms *health state* or *outcome* are used throughout this chapter.

Analytical cross-sectional studies

Previously, I discussed cross-sectional studies as being descriptive, but they can have analytical purposes as well as, or instead of, descriptive aims. Like descriptive cross-sectional studies, **analytical cross-sectional studies** involve taking a snapshot or cross-section of the population at a particular point in time. Unlike descriptive cross-sectional studies, however, which do not involve looking at associations between exposures and outcomes, analytical cross-sectional studies aim to address questions about associations between exposures and outcomes. In analytical cross-sectional studies, the exposure and outcome are both measured at the same time-point and thus share the limitations of descriptive cross-sectional studies. Analytical cross-sectional studies allow us to describe the determinants (the 'why' question) of a health state and measure associations using prevalence rate ratios. For example, an analytical cross-sectional study that examined associations and potential modifiable risk factors for the management of sexual and reproductive health needs among women attending community mental health services found that an increase in smoking was associated with a decrease in the proportion of planned pregnancies, and that an increase in alcohol and other drug use was associated with an increase in sexual activity (Hauck *et al.* 2015).

> **Analytical cross-sectional studies:** These aim to address questions about associations between exposures and outcomes.

PREVALENCE RATE RATIO (PRR)

The ratio of the prevalence in the exposed to the prevalence in the unexposed. The PRR is calculated as:

$$P = \frac{\text{Prevalence in the exposed}}{\text{Prevalence in the unexposed}}$$

> **Prevalence rate ratio:** The ratio of the prevalence in the exposed to the prevalence in the unexposed.

Ecological studies

Ecological studies are different from the types of study designs we have looked at so far. In most epidemiological studies, individuals are counted and analysed in terms of their exposure and outcome status. In ecological studies, however, aggregates (groups) of individuals,

> **Ecological study:** An epidemiological study in which the unit of analysis is groups or aggregates rather than individuals.

areas or other larger units are analysed. The use of these aggregate measures means that associations can only be described at an aggregate level. For example, an ecological study has demonstrated a decrease in the incidence of high-grade cervical lesions in females younger than eighteen years of age, three years after the introduction of the human papillomavirus (HPV) vaccination program in Victoria, Australia (Brotherton *et al.* 2011). While this study suggests that there is an association between HPV vaccination and a reduction in the incidence of high-grade cervical lesions in young females in Victoria, we cannot conclude that this association exists among individuals. Inferring that group-level associations exist at the individual level is known as the ecological fallacy. Ecological studies commonly use pre-existing population health and other data.

Case-control studies

Case-control studies compare a group of people who have the outcome factor of interest (cases) with a group of people who do not (controls). Investigators look back through time to identify exposures in the two groups. The two groups are then compared using measures of association, most commonly the odds ratio. For example, a case-control study conducted in the UK to examine the factors associated with maternal death found that, compared with controls (survived child birth), cases (maternal death) had inadequate use of antenatal care, greater substance misuse, increased likelihood of any medical comorbidity, hypertensive disorders and previous pregnancy problems, and were of Indian ethnicity (Nair *et al.* 2015). By comparing a group of people with the outcome of interest with a group of people without the outcome of interest, and examining potential prior exposures, we can describe the distribution and determinants of health states. In doing so, we are able to establish cause-and-effect relationships because we know that the outcome followed the exposure. In case-control studies, it is essential that the cases and controls are comparable on all measures with the exception of the outcome.

Case-control study: A study that compares a group of people who have the outcome factor of interest (cases) with a group of people who do not (controls).

Cohort studies

Unlike longitudinal studies, where people are not categorised as exposed or not exposed, a **cohort study** follows over time a group (cohort) of people who have been exposed to a possible risk factor for a health outcome, and a group of people who have not been exposed. The incidence of the outcome in the exposed group is then compared to the incidence of the outcome in the group who are not exposed. This enables the relationship between the exposure and the outcome to be assessed. Cohort studies can be prospective or retrospective.

Cohort study: This follows over time a group (cohort) of people who have been exposed to a possible risk factor for a health outcome, and another group who have not been exposed.

A prospective cohort study starts with a cohort of people who do not have the outcome of interest. Participants are classified as 'exposed' or 'not exposed'. All participants are then followed forward in time until an outcome is established. Then, using the appropriate measure of association, the incidence of the outcome in the exposed group is compared to the incidence in the non-exposed group. For example, a prospective cohort study to examine whether social support during pregnancy affects postpartum depression (by comparing social support between women with and without depression) found that the women with both pre- and postpartum depression reported having less social support in terms of available supportive persons, along with lower levels of satisfaction with the social support they did receive, compared with non-depressed women (Morikawa *et al.* 2015). As you can see, prospective cohort studies allow us to examine the distribution and determinants of health states over time.

Retrospective cohort studies are conducted in the same way as prospective cohort studies except that they measure exposures from the past and outcomes in the present. Since exposures have occurred in the past, retrospective cohort studies often use sources of data collection such as hospital records. For example, a retrospective cohort study was undertaken to examine history of three or more miscarriages (exposure) and whether this was associated with adverse perinatal outcomes in a subsequent pregnancy. The study found, after controlling for known socio-demographic risk factors, an increased risk of preterm birth, very preterm birth and perinatal death in a subsequent pregnancy among women who had three or more miscarriages (Field & Murphy 2015).

We have looked at the types of observational epidemiological study designs that generate health statistics we often see in the media. Now let's turn to other sources of health statistics—population health data.

STOP AND THINK

So far in this chapter we have looked at a number of study designs used in observational epidemiology.

- What are the main differences between descriptive and analytical epidemiological study designs?

Population health data

A number of sources of **population health data** are freely available both nationally and internationally. Common sources of data that are routinely collected include census data and disease registries (e.g. births, deaths, cancer and infectious diseases). The collection of registry data is a national responsibility and often the data is provided to organisations such as the United Nations, the World Health Organization (WHO) and the World Bank. Other sources of data include regular surveys such as the National Health Survey and hospital records. There are a number of advantages to using existing population health data. For example, the data have already been collected and as a result are inexpensive to access. However, a disadvantage is that the data may be incomplete or of poor quality. This section will introduce a selection of population health data sources and some of their potential uses.

The WHO provides access to a range of indicators through the Global Health Observatory, including mortality, equity, health-related millennium goals, health systems, communicable diseases, non-communicable disease risk factors and much more over time, between countries

Population health data: Common sources of population health data include census data and disease registries (e.g. births, deaths, cancer and infectious diseases).

Melissa Graham

and within countries. We will consider the Millennium Development Goals (MDGs), which include maternal and reproductive health.

Figure 14.2 shows the maternal mortality ratio (annual number of maternal deaths per 100,000 live births) over time for selected countries. We can see that per 100,000 live births the maternal mortality ratio has increased between 1990 and 2013 in the USA and Canada, but it has decreased in Australia, Japan, New Zealand and France.

FIGURE 14.2   Maternal mortality trends, 1990–2013

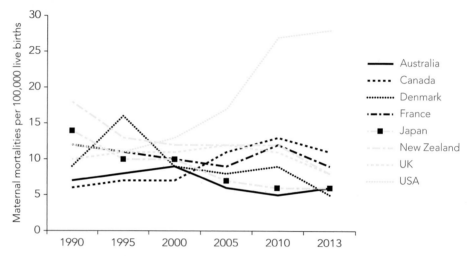

Source: WHO Global Health Observatory,
<http://apps.who.int/gho/data/node.main.MATMORT?lang=en>.
Note that the data are based on interagency estimates.

The World Bank also provides access to data by country, topic or specific indicator, for example health, education, social development, gender and so on. Data can be presented as graphs, maps or tables. Figure 14.3 shows that adolescent fertility rates are much higher in some parts of the world than in others.

As well as the National Health Survey previously discussed, every five years the ABS conducts the Australian Census of Population and Housing, which provides a detailed description of the population including age, sex, marital status, education, occupation, living arrangements and other characteristics (ABS 2006b). A range of census data products can be accessed at <www.abs.gov.au/Census>. The ABS allows you to search census data by area, topic or product type. Useful products include the QuickStats, Community Profile, TableBuilder, Longitudinal Dataset and DataPacks. The ABS also provides births data supplied by individual state and territory Registrars of Births, Deaths and Marriages (ABS 2009a). Births data are available via data cubes (data cubes are aggregate-level data available in spreadsheet table format). The ABS also provides customised data tables (at a cost to researchers). The next 'Research in practice' box demonstrates the use of ABS customised data tables.

The Australian Institute for Health and Welfare (AIHW) provides access to a range of data including alcohol and other drug treatment, cancer, chronic disease indicators, mental health,

FIGURE 14.3 Adolescent fertility rates (births per 1000 women aged fifteen to nineteen years) 2011–15

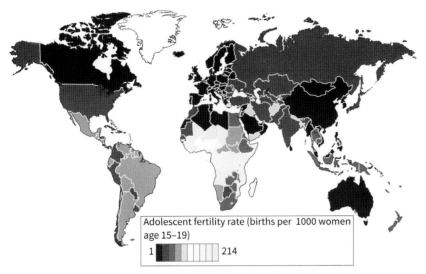

Adolescent fertility rate (births per 1000 women age 15–19)

1 ▮▮▮▮▮▮▮▯▯▯▯▯▯ 214

Source: World Bank social development indicators,
<http://data.worldbank.org/indicator/SP.ADO.TFRT/countries?page=1&display=map>.

disability, risk factors and National Hospital Morbidity data (AIHW n.d.). These data are drawn from a variety of sources. For example, the National Hospital Morbidity Database (NHMD) is collated from data supplied by the state and territory health authorities. It is a collection of confidentialised summary records for episodes of care in public and private hospitals in Australia. Procedures and diagnoses are recorded using the International Statistical Classification of Diseases and Related Health Problems, 10th revision, Australian Modification (ICD-10-AM) (AIHW 2009). The NHMD allows you to select a time-period, a health condition based on the ICD-10AM (diagnosis) and a procedure. 'Research in practice' gives an example of how you can use the National Hospital Morbidity data to understand patterns of health states.

CHILDLESSNESS IN AUSTRALIA

Customised data tables available from the ABS enable researchers to examine aggregate-level data on a range of indicators collected via the Census. Let us say we are interested in the prevalence of childlessness in Australia. Perhaps we are curious to see whether the prevalence is increasing or decreasing over time. Customised data tables for births by age were provided by the ABS. This enabled us to analyse the prevalence of childless women as a proportion of all women by age group in Australia in 1986, 1996 and 2006. Figure 14.4 shows that overall childlessness increased by 5 per cent from 1986 to 2006 (PRR = 1.05). The largest increase in the prevalence of childlessness

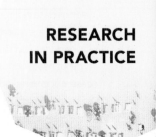

RESEARCH IN PRACTICE

Melissa Graham

was observed for women aged thirty to thirty-four years (PRR = 1.82). For women aged fifty years or

over there was a decrease in the prevalence of childlessness between 1986 and 2006 (PRR = 0.86).

FIGURE 14.4   The prevalence of childlessness in Australia, 1986–2006

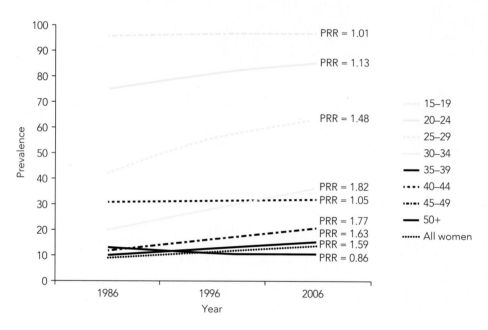

Data source: ABS (2007)

HYSTERECTOMY IN AUSTRALIA

Let us say we were interested in the incidence of all hysterectomies over time in Australia. Using the National Hospital Morbidity database, information on all females admitted to hospital for a hysterectomy can be extracted using the *Procedures* data cube. This data cube gives the number of hysterectomies by type of hysterectomy and age from 2000–01 to 2006–07. Each year of data needs to be selected separately. For each year of data we can select the ICD Procedure Chapter in which we are interested—in this case *XIII Gynaecological Procedures* and then *Uterus*. Now we can select the type of hysterectomy in which we are interested—in this case abdominal and vaginal hysterectomy (these need to be selected separately). These interactive data cubes

also allow you to export the data into Microsoft Excel. Using ABS population data, we are able to find out how many women there were in Australia during the time-period in which we are interested (2000–01 to 2004–05). We can now use the data from the NHMD (number of people with the health state) and the ABS population data (population at risk) to calculate the incidence of hysterectomy for each time-point. The hysterectomy incidence rate was 34.8 per 10,000 females in 2000–01 and 31.2 per 10,000 in 2004–05. This suggests an overall decrease in hysterectomy in that period. The data also allow us to examine the patterns of hysterectomy over time by age. As shown in Figure 14.5, women aged forty-five to fifty-four years had the highest rates of hysterectomy.

Chapter 14: How Do We Know What We Know? Epidemiology in Health Research

271

FIGURE 14.5   Incidence rate for all hysterectomies by age over time in Australia

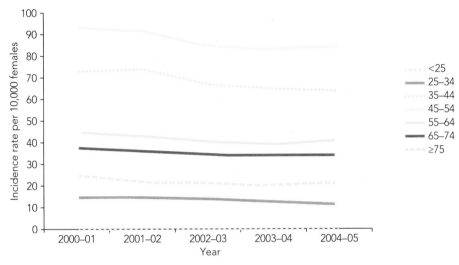

Source: Hill *et al.* (2010)

Mortality data for selected causes by age and sex are available via the AIHW General Record of Incidence of Mortality (GRIM). GRIM allows you to select cause of death, which can be examined by age, sex, time and so forth (AIHW 2015d). As shown in Figure 14.6, maternal mortality declined from 30.6 per 10,000 women in 1907 to 0.05 per 100,000 women in 2013.

FIGURE 14.6   Maternal mortality trends, 1907–2013

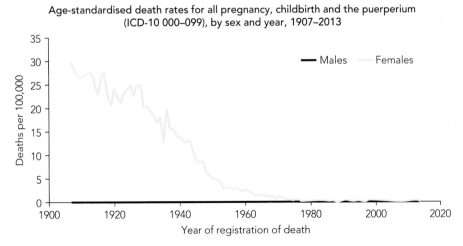

Age-standardised death rates for all pregnancy, childbirth and the puerperium (ICD-10 O00–O99), by sex and year, 1907–2013

Source: AIHW (2015d)

The Victorian Department of Health and Human Services provides morbidity and mortality data through the Victorian Health Information Surveillance System, which offers an interactive website that provides access to Burden of Disease data (life expectancy and disability-adjusted life years), avoidable mortality, ambulatory care sensitive conditions and much more (VDHHS 2015). Another source of population health data is the Victorian Population Health Surveys. These repeat cross-sectional studies are conducted annually by the Victorian Department of Health and Human Services.

Another source of data is the Australian Data Archive, which makes data from research undertaken in Australia available for secondary analysis. You will need to register with the Archive to access data that is freely available to download. Some data requires permission from the original contributor. There are a number of equivalent data clearinghouses internationally, for example the UK Data Archive (www.data-archive.ac.uk).

Summary

Epidemiology is the study of the distribution and determinants of health states in populations, and the application of this to the prevention and control of health problems. Person (who), place (where) and time (when) are key principles of observational epidemiology. Analytical epidemiology can also answer 'why' questions. Key measures used in epidemiology include prevalence, incidence and measures of association such as relative risks, odds ratios and prevalence rate ratios. The measure used is dependent on the research question and the selected epidemiological study design. Population health data is often readily and freely available and is a valuable source of information.

Practice exercises

1   A cross-sectional study conducted in 2008 of women aged thirty to thirty-four years in Australia found that of the 667 women in the study, 242 did not have any children. Calculate the prevalence of childlessness in Australia in 2008.

2   The Births Registry in Victoria, Australia, recorded 1652 births to females aged fifteen to nineteen in 2006. The population of females aged fifteen to nineteen for the same year was 169,593. Calculate the incidence of teenage births for females in this age group in 2006 in Victoria.

3   Explore the Health Status of Victorians webpage (www.health.vic.gov.au/ healthstatus/index.htm and click on 'Burden of Disease'). Generate a Burden

of Disease Life Expectancy report for your local government area. Repeat this for Victoria. Is the life expectancy in your local government area higher or lower than that for Victoria?

4   Explore the ABS website. What data sources do you think are most helpful? Why? How do you think you could use these population health data as a health practitioner?

Further reading

Bailey, L., Vardulaki, K., Langham, J. & Chandramohan, D. (2005). *Introduction to epidemiology*. Buckingham, UK: Open University Press.

Bonia, R., Beaglehole, R. & Kjellström, T. (2006). *Basic epidemiology*, 2nd edn. Geneva: World Health Organization.

Lee, P. (2016). Assessing the health of population: epidemiology in public health. In P. Liamputtong (ed.), *Public health: local and global perspective*. Cambridge: Cambridge University Press, 191–216.

Oleckno, W.A. (2002). *Essential epidemiology: principles and applications*. Long Grove, IL: Waveland Press.

Websites

Population health data discussed in this chapter are available from the following websites.

http://apps.who.int/ghodata/

WHO Global Health Observatory

http://data.worldbank.org/

World Bank

www.abs.gov.au

Australian Bureau of Statistics

www.aihw.gov.au

Australian Institute of Health and Welfare

http://dhhs.vic.gov.au/

Victorian Department of Health and Human Services

www2.health.vic.gov.au/public-health/population-health-systems/health-status-of-victorians#

Victorian Department of Health and Human Services, Health Status of Victorians

www.ada.edu.au

Australian Data Archive

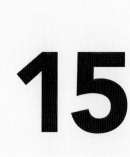

15

Clinical Trials: The Good, the Bad and the Ugly

KARL B. LANDORF

Chapter objectives

In this chapter you will learn:

- what makes a good trial and what makes a bad trial
- the effect of bias in clinical trials
- how to minimise bias and other threats to the internal validity of clinical trials
- whether the findings of a trial can be generalised to clinical practice (external validity)
- how to report clinical trials

Key terms

Allocation bias

Allocation concealment

Ascertainment bias

Assessment bias

Blinding

Citation bias

Clinical trial

Confounder

Confounding effect

CONSORT Statement

Explanatory trial

External validity

Generalisability

Intention-to-treat analysis

Internal validity

Outcome measures

Patient-reported outcome

Pragmatic trial

Publication bias

Quality assessment

Randomisation

Randomised
    controlled trial

Sample size

Selection bias

Stopping rule bias

Surrogate outcome
    measure

Types I and II
    statistical errors

Introduction

Clinical trials are conducted to determine if an intervention is effective; that is, whether it is beneficial to patients (Peat 2001). Clinical trials can be used to evaluate the effectiveness of interventions such as a pharmacological or physical treatment (what most health professionals would associate them with), although they are equally appropriate to evaluate other interventions. For example, a clinical trial could be used to evaluate the effectiveness of a behavioural intervention (Carding & Hillman 2001), a health education strategy, or a prevention program (Torgerson & Torgerson 2008). See also Chapters 16, 17.

Clinical trials can take many forms, from a simple case-series, where a series of participants receive the same treatment, to a more complex **randomised controlled trial** (RCT), where participants are evaluated after randomly being allocated a treatment. In the pharmaceutical industry, where clinical trials are frequently used, they are often classified into four phases: Phase I Trials—clinical pharmacology and toxicity; Phase II Trials—initial clinical investigation for treatment effect; Phase III Trials—full-scale evaluation of treatment; Phase IV Trials—post-marketing surveillance (Pocock 1983).

For the novice, it is hard to know which trials to believe and which ones not to believe. Like Clint Eastwood in the classic spaghetti-western film *The good, the bad and the ugly*, consumers of clinical trial research should be able to differentiate 'good' from 'bad', and they should also be able to decide when to dismiss a trial completely because it is truly 'ugly'! Accordingly, students, practitioners and researchers need to arm themselves with relevant knowledge to ensure that they are able to distinguish low-quality clinical trial research (the bad and the ugly) from high-quality clinical trial research (the good). The aim of this chapter, therefore, is to encourage you to be a wise consumer of clinical trials, not necessarily to teach you how to conduct clinical trials. To achieve this aim, the following discussion will focus on RCT methodology—the best available method to evaluate the effectiveness of an intervention.

Good trials versus bad trials

How does a consumer of research determine if a trial is good or bad? Let us return to the example of the simple case-series, where a series of participants receive an intervention (treatment) and the effect of that intervention is measured both before and after it is given. While on the surface it appears that this research design makes sense and would be relatively easy to conduct, it unfortunately has many problems that may make the measurement of the effect of the intervention inaccurate. For example, the placebo effect, where a patient responds positively to an inert intervention (i.e. an intervention designed to have no effect) is well known (Hróbjartsson & Gøtzsche 2010; Kaptchuk & Miller 2015). Many other **confounding effects** and biases can also cloud the true effectiveness of an intervention; these are likely if the trial is not well planned and controlled. Apart from the placebo effect, there are many other factors that may make the results of a poorly controlled clinical trial inaccurate, such as the Hawthorne effect, regression to the mean, and resentful demoralisation (Torgerson &

Clinical trial: A trial conducted to determine if an intervention is beneficial to patients.

Randomised controlled trial: A clinical trial where participants are randomly assigned to groups in order to receive different interventions. This randomisation removes many of the effects that may confound the true result.

Confounding effect: Distortion of the true effect of an intervention by extraneous, unwanted factors.

Karl B. Landorf

Torgerson 2008). Such effects need to be controlled for by: comparing interventions directly in parallel-group trials, employing appropriate randomisation into groups with allocation concealment to ensure groups have similar characteristics at baseline, and use of placebo/sham interventions (with blinding of investigators and participants).

In contrast, and at the other end of the spectrum from the case-series, is the RCT, where two (or more) groups receive interventions randomly. RCT methodology is currently considered the gold standard for evaluating the effectiveness of an intervention because it removes many of the effects that may confound or bias the true result (Straus *et al.* 2005; OCEBM Levels of Evidence Working Group 2011; see also Chapters 1, 12, 16, 17). Although RCTs are considered the gold standard for evaluating the effectiveness of interventions, an even better study design is the systematic review (OCEBM Levels of Evidence Working Group 2011; see Chapter 19). A systematic review combines many RCTs that have evaluated an intervention, thereby increasing sample size and improving the precision of the estimate of the effect of the intervention. But to conduct a relevant systematic review, we must have RCTs to include in the first place. It is important to note, however, that even RCTs, if conducted poorly, can result in inaccurate or biased findings, so thorough planning and execution is essential to ensure valid results.

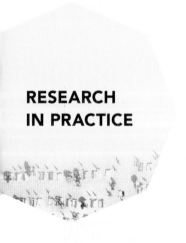

RESEARCH
IN PRACTICE

AN EXAMPLE OF CLINICAL TRIALS IN HEALTH CARE

Let us consider the results of two clinical trials, both of which I was involved in, that evaluated an adhesive tape to reduce pain in the heel of the foot (Landorf *et al.* 2005; Radford *et al.* 2006). Taping helps support the foot, which in turn takes force and stress away from the heel. In the first trial, a non-randomised trial (Landorf *et al.* 2005), a group of sixty-five participants received foot-taping (the intervention group) and forty participants received no taping (control group). However, data for the two groups were not collected simultaneously—data for the control group were collected approximately a year after the intervention group data were collected. Consequently, participants did not receive taping randomly and the two groups knew what intervention they received: the intervention group knew that they were receiving the taping treatment

to help their feet, while the control group knew that they were not receiving any intervention (i.e. the participants were not 'blinded'). Importantly, and to avoid not treating participants in pain, data were only collected on the control group for approximately two weeks (they then received appropriate advice and free shoe inserts/foot orthoses). In addition to the participants knowing what treatment they were receiving, the investigators knew as well; that is, there was no blinding of the investigators conducting the assessments in the study.

What did the study find? Well, interestingly, on a 100 mm visual analogue pain scale (a 100 mm line on a piece of paper by which a participant can indicate their level of pain, 0 mm = no pain and 100 mm = worst pain imaginable) the intervention group was on average 32 mm better off than the control group at the end of the comparison period. That is, the intervention group's mean pain level was 32 mm lower (= less pain) than the control group's mean pain level. What would the result have been if data had been collected on all participants (both the intervention and control groups) simultaneously and the intervention was truly randomised? Would the result have differed if the participants and the investigators were blinded to the intervention in question by adding a credible placebo or sham treatment (Sedgwick & Hooper 2015)? These are important questions, because non-randomised and poorly controlled trials, like the one outlined above, can overestimate the effect of a treatment (Schulz *et al.* 1995; Odgaard-Jensen *et al.* 2011).

In a follow-up taping study of ninety-two participants with heel pain (Radford *et al.* 2006), the investigators incorporated the features mentioned above into a higher-quality, and therefore more valid, RCT. To ensure blinding, both the intervention and control groups received sham ultrasound treatment to the painful heel (the ultrasound unit did not actually deliver any ultrasound but it appeared to do so). Because both groups were unaware that the ultrasound treatment was a sham, even the control group thought that they were allocated real treatment. Importantly, the only difference between the two groups was that the intervention group received taping, while the control group did not. At the completion of the study, the investigators found that the difference in pain on a 100 mm visual analogue pain scale was only 12 mm, much smaller than the original study that found a 32 mm difference. What could account for this difference, and why is it important for the accuracy of clinical trials that evaluate how effective an intervention is? This question leads us to the very essence of why RCTs are considered the gold standard method for evaluating whether an intervention is truly effective.

Randomised controlled trials

RCT methodology has been reported in medical science since the 1940s, although its initial use may have occurred fifty years earlier (Doll 1998; Hróbjartsson *et al.* 1998; D'Arcy Hart 1999). As mentioned previously, RCT methodology is considered the gold standard when evaluating the effectiveness of a treatment (Straus *et al.* 2005; OCEBM Levels of Evidence Working Group 2011). There are two key features to an RCT. In its simplest form these are that there is a comparison of a group receiving an intervention with one that does not, and there is random allocation to those groups (Pocock 1983). An RCT where two groups are being compared is sometimes referred to as a 'parallel-group RCT', as data are collected on both groups at the same time and participants receive only one of two (or more) interventions (Wang & Bakhai 2006). More complex trials are those where multiple interventions are compared (there are more than two groups).

A fundamental aim of using RCT methodology is to ensure as much as possible that the characteristics of the participants (the people who receive the interventions) at the beginning of the trial are similar across groups (Friedman *et al.* 1998). To illustrate why this is important, let us consider an RCT that sets out to evaluate the effectiveness of a dietary supplement on weight loss. It makes sense to ensure that both the intervention and control groups have similar weight at the beginning of the trial. Otherwise, any effect noticed over the course of the trial might be associated with the difference in weight at the beginning, rather than the dietary supplement being tested. Such a variable (in this example, weight) is known as a prognostic variable; that is, one that can affect the prognosis of the condition. If, however, appropriate randomisation is carried out and the two groups are similar at the beginning of the trial, confounding (unwanted effects that are not a result of the intervention being evaluated) will be minimised (Sedgwick 2015). Such confounding affects the **internal validity** of a trial, which can make the findings inaccurate (Odgaard-Jensen *et al.* 2011). It is important to explore these matters further in order to appreciate the power of RCTs. Knowledge of such issues gives practitioners the ability to assess trials on their quality, and consequently, whether their results are believable.

Internal validity: The truthfulness of the findings of a study based on the methods used in that study (are the methods used valid and reliable, and is there little chance of confounding or bias?).

Issues that affect the internal validity of a randomised trial

Random allocation

The key feature of RCTs is random allocation of participants to groups. This feature, as stated previously, promotes comparability among the study groups (Rosenberger & Lachin 2002), such that known and unknown prognostic variables will be similar (Friedman *et al.* 1998). Put more simply, **randomisation** is a powerful tool that ensures the groups at the beginning of the trial are as similar as possible except for the intervention being studied (Matthews 2006). Importantly, randomisation minimises confounding, which can lead to an inaccurate estimate of how effective an intervention is. When presenting the findings of a trial in a journal article, researchers should include a table comparing the groups in the trial on important participant characteristics that may influence the findings of the trial (see Table 15.1). This allows you to determine if similarity of the groups was achieved. If it was, then any differences in the outcomes of the groups at the end of the trial can be attributed to the interventions, rather than to differences in the participant characteristics.

Randomisation: A mechanism where participants are randomly allocated an intervention, e.g. the active test intervention versus a placebo or a sham intervention.

PARTICIPANT CHARACTERISTICS

Table 15.1 is an example of a table of participant characteristics showing that the two groups in the trial are similar at baseline (due to the chance of randomisation) on important variables that may influence the findings of the trial (Munteanu *et al.* 2011). This trial compared an intervention (a viscosupplement called hylan G-F 20) for osteoarthritis with a placebo.

RESEARCH IN PRACTICE

When looking at Table 15.1, compare each variable (e.g. age) for both groups to see how similar the two groups were at baseline.

TABLE 15.1   Participant characteristics comparing intervention (Hylan G-F 20) and placebo groups

VARIABLE	HYLAN G-F 20 (N = 75)	PLACEBO (N = 76)
Age, mean (SD), years	53.7 (11.3)	55.3 (11.2)
Gender, n (%), male	47 (62.7)	48 (63.2)
Height, mean (SD), cm	172.0 (9.7)	171.4 (9.7)
Weight, mean (SD), kg	80.4 (14.5)	80.3 (14.2)
BMI, mean (SD), kg/m²	27.0 (3.7)	27.2 (3.9)
Duration of symptoms, mean (SD), months	40.4 (35.8)	45.3 (59.0)
Side affected, n (left/right/bilateral)	25/30/20	20/35/21
Side treated, n (left/right)	32/43	29/47
Severity of OA, median, (IQR), (range)*		
Dorsal osteophytes	2 (1) (0–2)	2 (1) (0–2)
Dorsal joint space narrowing	1 (0) (0–2)	1 (0) (0–2)
Lateral osteophytes	2 (1) (0–2)	2 (1) (0–2)
Lateral joint space narrowing	1 (1) (0–2)	1 (0) (0–2)
Total score**	5 (4) (1–8)	5 (3) (1–8)

BMI = body mass index

IQR = interquartile range, which includes the middle 50% of values recorded when the values are rank ordered

OA = osteoarthritis

*Severity of OA graded using the radiographic atlas of Menz *et al.* (2007) where the presence of osteophytes was graded as absent (score = 0), small (score = 1), moderate (score = 2), and the presence of joint space narrowing was graded as none (score = 0), definite (score = 1), severe (score = 2) in the dorsoplantar and lateral views.

**Total score obtained by summing observations from all features in both views..

Bias

In any clinical evaluation, it is essential that the research method used ensures that the effect of a treatment is directly attributable to that treatment, and not to extraneous causes (Pocock 1983). For example, one common problem in clinical trials—even controlled trials—is that researchers may unknowingly influence or bias the outcome of a study (Chalmers *et al.* 1983; Schulz *et al.* 1995). Such bias can distort the results or conclusions away from the truth, the result being a poor-quality trial that underestimates, or more likely overestimates, the benefits of an intervention (Odgaard-Jensen *et al.* 2011). It is important to note that bias is different from confounding (discussed earlier), although both can lead to inaccurate estimates of an intervention's effectiveness. Some of the more common biases are discussed below.

Selection bias can arise if the investigators systematically manipulate enrolment into the trial (Greenhalgh 2006). For example, selection bias will occur if patients are selected using non-random methods or if they self-select themselves into groups (Peat 2001). This may make the recruits unrepresentative of the population with the condition being studied (it affects the external validity or generalisability of the trial) (Piantadosi 2005; see also Chapter 11). Selection bias can be minimised by careful sampling procedures and strict adherence to inclusion and exclusion criteria (Peat 2001).

Allocation bias is a type of selection bias. It occurs when the process of allocating participants to groups leads to differences in the baseline characteristics of those groups (Peat 2001). For example, if the allocation of participants to groups is not concealed from the investigators recruiting them, then the investigators may exclude certain potential recruits. This may occur, for example, if the investigators think that a potential recruit may respond poorly to the treatment they would be allocated (e.g. a placebo), so they exclude them or postpone their enrolment until they are certain the participant will receive the treatment they believe to be most beneficial (e.g. the new treatment under evaluation). This may result in differences in the baseline characteristics of participants in the groups to be compared (Chalmers *et al.* 1983), which is undesirable as the main purpose of randomisation is to ensure as much as possible that the characteristics of the participants at the beginning of the trial are similar across groups (Friedman *et al.* 1998). Allocation bias can be prevented by appropriate randomisation and concealment of the allocation schedule (allocation concealment) from trial staff involved in recruitment (Schulz & Grimes 2002a). Adequate concealment of the randomised assignment sequence is essential to prevent staff from deciphering the sequence, thus causing bias. Unfortunately, deciphering the randomised allocation sequence is more common than might be expected—staff involved in clinical trials often find it hard to resist 'cracking the code' (Schulz 1995). Trials that have inadequate allocation concealment often yield larger estimates of the effectiveness of interventions and are more likely to report significant findings (Hewitt *et al.* 2005; Odgaard-Jensen *et al.* 2011). Concealment of a participant's allocation to the intervention or control group can be simple—place the allocation in a sealed envelope that is opened only once the participant is recruited into the trial. A better method is remote allocation, where the person recruiting the participant must call a distant and separate randomisation service once the participant is recruited (Torgerson & Roberts 1999). When presenting the findings of a trial in a journal article, investigators should adequately report how they concealed allocation (Schulz 1996).

Assessment bias may occur if an investigator's assessment of a participant lacks objectivity (Pocock 1983). Subjective outcome measures are prone to exaggerate the effect of the intervention, particularly when there is a lack of blinding (Poolman *et al.* 2007; Wood *et al.* 2008). For example, if an investigator who assesses the participants in a trial is not blinded (they are aware of the group a participant has been allocated to), they may distort or misclassify

Selection bias: This arises if the investigators systematically manipulate enrolment into the trial.

Allocation bias: A type of selection bias that occurs when the process of allocating participants to groups leads to differences in the baseline characteristics of those groups.

Assessment bias: This occurs if an investigator's assessment of a participant lacks objectivity. Subjective outcome measures are prone to exaggerate the effect of the intervention.

the outcome measured. Bias may also occur from a participant's perspective; for example, participants may under- or overreport exposures, or not accurately report the outcomes being measured. Assessments, therefore, must be accurate and objective, and collected using standardised procedures. Objectivity is enhanced by blinding assessors and participants if possible, although this can be difficult with interventions that involve non-pharmacological interventions, such as physical treatments (Boutron *et al.* 2007).

Ascertainment bias occurs when the results or conclusions of the trial are distorted by the knowledge of which intervention each participant is receiving (Jadad 1998). For example, if the intervention for each participant is known, investigators may alter the types of co-intervention offered to participants or distort the outcomes being measured. Furthermore, if the investigators are not blinded they may alter the way in which they handle a participant who withdraws, drops out or violates the study protocol. For example, the investigator may ignore a participant's breach of protocol or allow participants to withdraw less easily if they know what intervention they have been allocated. Assessment bias, ascertainment bias and inappropriate handling of participants can all be minimised by blinding the investigators and the participants (Schulz & Grimes 2002b). When presenting the findings of a trial in a journal article, investigators should specifically report who was blinded (assessors, caregivers, participants, those involved in data analysis) and how they were blinded, not just the type of blinding, such as single-blind or double-blind, which are terms that are inconsistently interpreted (Schulz & Grimes 2002b; Haahr & Hróbjartsson 2006; Hróbjartsson & Boutron 2011).

Allocation concealment is not the same as **blinding**. Allocation concealment is where the randomised allocation sequence is concealed from the investigators who are involved in recruiting participants, whereas blinding is a technique to prevent assessors, participants or data analysis staff knowing which group the participant is in after they have been allocated.

Stopping rule bias can occur if a trial is stopped inappropriately. For example, it would be inappropriate if investigators are aware of the outcomes (the results) for each intervention and continue recruiting only until they obtain a positive or statistically significant result (see Chapters 25, 26). Accordingly, a prespecified (*a priori*) sample size (discussed later) should be determined and data collection should generally continue until that target has been reached.

Ascertainment bias: This occurs when the results or conclusions of the trial are distorted by the knowledge of which intervention each participant is receiving.

Allocation concealment: This refers to the randomised allocation sequence being concealed from investigators who are involved in recruiting participants.

Blinding: A technique used in RCTs to prevent assessors, participants or data analysis staff knowing which group a participant is in after they have been allocated.

Stopping rule bias: This can occur if a trial is stopped inappropriately.

STOP AND THINK

- How can a lack of allocation concealment lead to allocation bias?
- What methods are there to ensure concealment of the allocation sequence, and are some methods better than others?
- Can you think of a measurement (e.g. a physical test) that could be manipulated by an assessor in a clinical trial? Can you think of a way to avoid this potential for manipulation?
- What is the difference between allocation concealment and blinding?

Sample size

The size of the sample in a clinical trial is important because it can affect the meaningfulness of the statistical analysis that is conducted to compare groups. Researchers should conduct a prospective sample size calculation before the trial begins, to decrease the chance of **Type II statistical errors** (Moher *et al.* 1994). A Type II error (see Chapter 26) occurs when the investigators conclude that there is no significant difference between the groups (that the intervention being studied is not effective) although there may have been a clinically important effect, but the trial did not have a large enough sample size to detect it statistically (Portney & Watkins 2009). Appropriate sample size is fundamental to any clinical trial (Cohen 1977). With this in mind, all trials should recruit an appropriate number of participants to be able to detect clinically important effects (Altman 1980). **Sample size** is generally calculated using an appropriate formula (Friedman *et al.* 1998); there are many statistical programs that can perform this calculation. When presenting the findings of a trial in a journal article, researchers should include a paragraph on how the sample size was determined, including accurate reporting of parameters such as the clinically important effect that the study was statistically powered to detect (Charles *et al.* 2009; see also Chapters 1, 26). Below are two examples of sample size information (calculations) from randomised trials, both of which include relevant information on how the sample size was calculated.

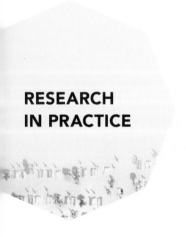

**RESEARCH
IN PRACTICE**

SAMPLE SIZE CALCULATIONS THAT WERE REPORTED IN TWO RANDOMISED TRIALS

1   A randomised trial evaluating an intervention to reduce falls in older people (Spink *et al.* 2011): 'An *a priori* sample size calculation, based on a falling rate of 60% in the control group, a 30% reduction in the proportion of fallers in the intervention group, a 15% dropout rate, 80% power, and a significance level of 5%, indicated that we needed 286 participants (143 per group).'

2   A randomised trial evaluating the effectiveness of an intervention for plantar heel pain (McMillan *et al.* 2012): 'Prospective sample size calculation indicated that 40 participants per group would provide 80% power to detect a minimal important difference of 13 points on the pain domain of the foot health status questionnaire (SD 20, $\alpha = 0.05$, 5% loss to follow-up). When doing this calculation we conservatively ignored the extra precision provided by covariate analysis.'

Outcome measures

Appropriate **outcome measures** should be used to measure the effect of an intervention (Roland & Torgerson 1998a). These should include **patient-reported outcomes**, where the patient, rather than the clinician, reports on the impact of a disease or intervention on the status of their health (Willke *et al.* 2004). Patient-reported health status measurement (or questionnaires), also referred to as 'health-related quality of life measurement', offers a broader investigation from the patient's perspective of the effect of an intervention, compared to **surrogate outcome measures** that are usually generated by the clinician (Jenkinson & McGee 1998; Bowling 2005; Landorf & Burns 2009). Clearly, when evaluating the effect of an intervention on a patient, the patient's perspective on whether or not that intervention is effective is most important (see also Chapters 11, 13).

Outcome measures should be both valid and reliable (Portney & Watkins 2009). When presenting the findings of a trial in a journal article, researchers should report in detail the outcome measures that were used (Poolman *et al.* 2007), and give details about the validity and reliability of the measures, particularly if they are not well known (see Chapter 11). Primary outcomes and the endpoints that they will be measured at should be nominated before the trial begins, to avoid selective reporting of outcome measures, which can lead to bias and overestimation of the effectiveness of an intervention (Chan *et al.* 2004).

STOP AND THINK

Think of a health problem or condition that you (or a family member) have had recently. What were the most important impacts of this condition on you? If it caused pain, did it cause mild pain or a lot of pain? Did it affect the way in which you could function? Did it affect your physical or mental state (or both)? Did it stop you doing things that you could normally do, like activities or socialising? How could you measure all these impacts?

Intention-to-treat analysis

An **intention-to-treat analysis** should be conducted as the primary analysis in a clinical trial. With this type of analysis, outcome measures are obtained regardless of compliance with the trial protocol, and data from all participants are analysed according to allocation, even if the participants had adverse events or unexpected outcomes (Fergusson *et al.* 2002; Schulz & Grimes 2002c). Intention-to-treat analysis maintains the balance of **confounders**, which reduces variability between groups (Newell 1992), thus maintaining the comparability of groups originally established by randomisation (Keech *et al.* 2007). Doing so provides a more pragmatic or real-life estimate of the benefit of a treatment (Hollis & Campbell 1999). When presenting the findings of a trial in a journal article, researchers should state whether they have analysed their results using the intention-to-treat principle.

Dropout rate

The dropout rate from a clinical trial should be kept to a minimum because excessive dropout may lead to distortion of results, particularly if more dropouts occur in one group. Trials with substantial loss to follow-up (e.g. greater than 15 per cent) should be viewed with caution (Lang & Secic 1997). Accordingly, investigators must ensure that only a minimum number of participants drop out of a clinical trial, although this is more difficult with intrusive interventions

Patient-reported outcome: An outcome where the patient, rather than the clinician, reports on the impact of a disease or intervention on the status of their health.

Surrogate outcome measure: An outcome that is measured from a source that is not directly from the patient; for example, a blood test or an x-ray measurement, which is used because it may have a relationship with change in the patient's health.

Intention-to-treat analysis: This is used in RCTs where outcome measures are obtained regardless of compliance with the trial protocol and where data from all participants are analysed according to allocation.

Confounder: An extraneous factor that distorts (or confounds) the true effect of an intervention.

Karl B. Landorf

and the longer the trial runs for. When presenting the findings of a trial, researchers should transparently indicate the dropout rate of the trial.

TABLE 15.2   Issues that affect the internal validity of an RCT

ISSUE	METHOD TO CONTROL ISSUE
Groups that differ in their baseline characteristics	Randomisation
Selection bias	Careful sampling procedures; strict adherence to inclusion and exclusion criteria
Allocation bias	Allocation concealment
Assessment bias	Blinding assessors; objective outcome measures
Ascertainment bias	Blinding investigators and participants
Inappropriate handling of participants who do not comply	Blinding investigators; intention-to-treat analysis
Stopping rule bias	Blinding investigators; prespecified sample size calculation
Small sample size	Prespecified sample size calculation that is large enough to detect a clinically important difference between groups
Inappropriate outcome measures	Use of valid and reliable outcomes that include patient-reported outcome measures

Explanatory trial: A trial that is highly controlled and hence reduces the number of variables that can affect the final outcome.

Pragmatic trial: One in which the investigators attempt to mimic common practice, thereby endeavouring as much as possible to make the results generalisable to everyday practice.

External validity: The extent to which the findings from a study relate to patients or clients in the real world (how much the results can be applied to the wider population). This relates to the generalisability of the findings of a study.

Generalisability: To ensure the findings of a clinical trial are generalisable, practitioners need to assess whether the participants, interventions and protocols employed in the trial are similar to their practice.

Issues that affect the external validity of a randomised trial

RCTs can either be explanatory or pragmatic (Schwartz & Lellouch 2009). An **explanatory trial** is one that is highly controlled, thus reducing the number of variables that can affect the final outcome. It therefore has more ability to explain what variable caused the result detected. However, because of the tight controls placed on the trial, the results of an explanatory trial may not necessarily be able to be generalised to everyday practice. In contrast, a **pragmatic trial** is one in which the investigators attempt to mimic common practice, thereby endeavouring as much as possible to make the results generalisable to everyday practice.

Pragmatic trials have become more common, in an effort to make clinical trials more meaningful to clinicians and the public (Zwarenstein & Treweek 2009). If a pragmatic trial is conducted, the participants, interventions, clinicians and study protocols should represent common practice as much as possible to ensure **external validity** and **generalisability**

(Roland & Torgerson 1998b). Some investigators conduct a survey of practitioners before beginning a trial to ascertain what common practice is or to obtain consensus on an intervention (Landorf *et al.* 2006; Cotchett *et al.* 2011). To assess a trial for external validity, practitioners should ask themselves the following questions. Were the participants in the trial of similar age and sex to those that would normally be treated with the condition in practice (Jüni *et al.* 2001)? Did they have a comparable severity of disease or number of co-morbidities? Was the intervention equivalent to what would be used in everyday clinical practice? Was the setting alike, that is, was the type of treatment centre or experience of the care providers comparable? Were the type of outcomes used and duration of follow-up similar?

Practitioners using the results of RCTs to inform their clinical decision-making must assess the extent to which each trial can be generalised to their workplace. A demonstrated beneficial effect of an intervention in an RCT in one group of the population (e.g. younger adults) may not exist with another group (e.g. older adults). Therefore, a practitioner who predominantly treats older adults may not experience the same beneficial effect from a treatment that was reported in an RCT because the participants from the trial are not comparable with the patients in their workplace. Practitioners need to keep this in mind when reading articles that present the findings of RCTs. They should appraise whether the characteristics of the participants, interventions and settings are similar enough to their situation (Jüni *et al.* 2001).

STOP AND THINK

There are many examples in the health research literature of young, healthy university students being enrolled in large quantities into research studies.

- What effect would this have on the generalisability of the findings from such studies?
- How could you improve the recruitment into these studies? What factors would you need to consider?
- What would the characteristics of participants need to be like if, for example, you wanted to study an educational program for children with a learning disorder, or an orthopaedic surgical intervention for people with severe osteoarthritis of the knee?

There is a final matter that practitioners need to be aware of when considering external validity—that the RCTs they encounter may be biased from a publication perspective. **Publication bias** occurs when a trial is published or not published because of the direction of its findings (Duley & Farrell 2002). Studies that find a positive result are more likely to be published; trials that find no difference between groups are, on average, less likely or will take longer to be published (Ioannidis 1998). **Citation bias** also occurs; in this, articles that have statistically significant findings are cited more often than others (Nieminen *et al.* 2007). Practitioners need to take into account the facts that they may be more likely to read about positive, statistically significant trials and that less positive trials are less likely to be published and cited.

Karl B. Landorf

Publication bias: This occurs when a trial is published or not published because of the direction of its findings. Studies that have a positive result are more likely to be published.

Citation bias: This occurs where articles that have statistically significant findings are cited more often than others.

TABLE 15.3   Components of an RCT that need to be considered by practitioners when assessing how generalisable the findings are to their practice

COMPONENT	ISSUE
Participants	If the patients in a practitioner's workplace have different characteristics from the participants in the trial, they might respond differently to the intervention
Interventions	If the intervention used in a practitioner's workplace is sufficiently different from that evaluated in the trial, the benefits of the intervention may not be the same
Settings	If the environment and experience of staff in a workplace are different from those of the trial, the benefits of the intervention for patients may not be the same
Outcomes	If the type and definition of the outcomes used to measure the effect of the intervention in the practitioner's workplace are different from those used in the trial, a different effect of the intervention might be perceived
Follow-up period	If the standard follow-up period for participants in a practitioner's workplace is inconsistent with that in the trial, the benefits of the intervention may be under- or overestimated
Publication	Positive, statistically significant trials are more likely to be published and cited, whereas less positive trials are less likely to be published and cited

Reporting RCTs

Bias may also occur during the dissemination process, both on the part of the authors and the readers of journal articles reporting the findings of RCTs. For example, insufficient information may be supplied in the article for readers to judge whether the study is of adequate quality for the results to be believable. To rectify this, researchers and editors involved in publishing scientific medical research developed the **Consolidated Standards of Reporting Trials (CONSORT) Statement** (Begg *et al.* 1996).

The CONSORT Statement aims to ensure accurate and complete reporting of the design, conduct, analysis and generalisability of trials, thus ensuring that the highest possible standards are met when clinical trials are published. To facilitate this process, a checklist was developed with items ranging from the title and abstract to methodological issues and reporting of results. A flow diagram is suggested to illustrate the progress of participants through the trial.

The CONSORT Statement has been revised (Moher *et al.* 2010; Schulz *et al.* 2010) and is widely recognised as the benchmark for appropriately reporting RCTs. It has been endorsed or recommended by many journals including the *New England Journal of Medicine*, *The Lancet* and the *Journal of the American Medical Association* (Laine *et al.* 2007). Following the CONSORT Guidelines (Moher *et al.* 2012) will ensure that researchers provide adequate details about a trial, thus giving clinicians and other researchers enough information to judge whether the findings are believable. This is important when making decisions about incorporating findings into clinical practice. A comprehensive guide to interpreting and reporting RCTs using the CONSORT Guidelines is available (Keech *et al.* 2007; see also Chapter 27).

Prespecification of important components of a clinical trial (e.g. inclusion and exclusion criteria, primary and secondary outcomes, data analysis) is now expected (Moher *et al.* 2010). To ensure that this is observed, most health and medical journals now demand clinical trial registration, where these important components of the trial are detailed, before the trial begins (International Committee of Medical Journal Editors 2012). In addition, the WHO (2012a) states that 'the registration of all interventional trials is a scientific, ethical and moral responsibility', and the World Medical Association's revised Declaration of Helsinki (2013, para. 35) states that, 'every research study involving human subjects must be registered in a publicly accessible database before recruitment of the first subject'. Clearly, if a trial is not registered, the investigators will have difficulty publishing their findings, particularly in high-impact journals.

Trial registration ensures that investigators commit to certain parameters for the conduct and analysis of their trial. Such scrutiny places tight controls over investigators and minimises the potential that they will cause bias. For example, a prespecified plan for data analysis prevents selective reporting of findings or data-dredging, where the investigators continue to analyse the data until they obtain significant findings, even from less important secondary outcomes (Chan *et al.* 2004). Testing multiple hypotheses that were not prespecified inflates the **Type I statistical error** rate, resulting in spurious and often implausible findings (Proschan & Waclawiw 2000; Austin *et al.* 2006; see Chapter 26). This causes bias and may lead the investigators to conclude that an intervention is effective, when it may not be. Similarly, multiple hypothesis tests on subgroups among the participants in a trial can lead to false positive results (Wang *et al.* 2007). When presenting the findings of a trial in a journal article, researchers should provide the registration details of the trial (the name of the registry and the registration number), so the way in which the trial has been conducted and analysed can be verified against what was prespecified. To help you understand the nature of clinical trial registration, the website address of a clinical trial registry is included in the Websites section at the end of the chapter.

Type I statistical errors: These occur when researchers mistakenly conclude that a finding was statistically significant when it may be a result of chance (due to overanalysis) rather than a real difference.

Assessing the quality of clinical trials

All of the above factors show that the quality of a clinical trial is clearly affected by a number of issues. Good trials are ones where most of these issues have been well thought through and addressed before the trial begins. Importantly, they minimise bias and are likely to report more accurate estimates of the effectiveness of interventions. In addition, as systematic reviews (see Chapter 19) become more common, thorough quality assessments of the included trials are recommended, to minimise bias from poor-quality trials (Egger *et al.* 2003).

Karl B. Landorf

Quality assessment: An evaluation of the methodological quality of a particular study or studies. A high-quality assessment rating is an indication that a study is not likely to be prone to confounding or bias, and is more likely to accurately reflect the effect of the intervention.

Once a clinical trial is published, though, how does a practitioner determine whether it is good or bad from a quality perspective? Fortunately, there are many quality rating scales. Two **quality assessment** scales that are commonly used are the PEDro Scale (PEDro 2009), used for clinical trials involving physical therapies (see also Chapters 17, 19), and the Jadad Scale (Jadad *et al.* 1996). Both these scales are more concerned with the internal validity of trials than with their external validity or generalisability to clinical practice. Nevertheless, they are useful for determining the trial's level of believability from a methodological standpoint.

STOP AND THINK

Think of some important methodological issues that can adversely affect the quality of a clinical trial. For each issue, can you think of a method to rectify it?

Summary

In the modern health care environment, practitioners must use the results of clinical trials to guide their practice when they want to know if an intervention is effective. While not always easy to detect, the quality of a clinical trial can be generally classified as good or bad, and some may even be considered downright ugly! RCTs are considered the gold standard to determine the effectiveness of an intervention. However, even an RCT, if conducted poorly, will be prone to bias, which will affect its internal validity. As such, the findings will not be accurate, precise or meaningful.

To avoid such bias, many issues need to be considered when conducting a trial, such as random allocation, allocation concealment, blinding of investigators and participants, use of valid and reliable outcome measures, appropriate handling of participants dropping out of the trial, and appropriate statistical analysis. When using the results of a clinical trial, practitioners must evaluate all these issues to assess whether a trial is of good quality, and therefore whether its results are believable. It is clearly not sensible to use findings from low-quality trials, as they do not reflect the truth about the effectiveness of the interventions they evaluate.

Investigators also need to report the results of an RCT in line with the recommendations outlined in the CONSORT Statement. Doing so makes it easier for practitioners to find key pieces of information easily, so they can quickly ascertain the effectiveness of the intervention being tested and the believability of its results (is it a high-quality trial?). Finally, practitioners need to assess whether the participants, interventions and protocols employed in a clinical trial are similar enough to their practice (are the findings generalisable?). By following the guidelines outlined in this chapter, practitioners will be able to avoid incorporating the findings from bad trials into their practice, concentrating instead on findings from good trials.

Practice exercises

1   What are the key reasons for conducting an RCT?

2   Discuss issues of bias in clinical trials and how they may affect the findings.

3   Discuss the effect a small sample size may have on an RCT.

4   What components of an RCT would you need to consider before generalising the results of the trial to your practice?

5   Go to the Australian and New Zealand Clinical Trials Registry (see website link on next page) and find a trial that interests you. Read through the trial's registration details to understand what information is required for a clinical trial to be registered before it begins.

6   Evaluate a published RCT to determine if the authors have satisfied the recommendations in the CONSORT Guidelines for reporting RCTs (see CONSORT website link on next page).

7   Assess the quality of a published RCT using the PEDro Scale (see the PEDro website link on next page). Once you have done this, assess a few more RCTs. How do their scores differ, and what issues were not addressed in the low-quality trials? What biases would these issues cause?

8   Think of an intervention that is used for a common condition you might encounter in practice. Try to design a high-quality RCT that would evaluate the intervention's effectiveness.

Further reading

Greenhalgh, T. (2014). *How to read a paper: the basics of evidence-based medicine*, 5th edn. Chichester, UK: John Wiley & Sons/BMJ Books.

Herbert, R., Jamtvedt, G., Birger Hagen, K. & Mead, J. (2011). *Practical evidence-based physiotherapy*, 2nd edn. Edinburgh: Elsevier.

Hoffman, T., Bennett, S. & Del Mar, C. (2013). *Evidence-based practice across the health professions*, 2nd edn. Sydney: Churchill Livingstone.

Peat, J.K. (2001). *Health science research: a handbook of quantitative methods*. Sydney: Allen & Unwin.

Torgerson, D.J. & Torgerson, C.J. (2008). *Designing randomised trials in health education and the social sciences: an introduction*. Basingstoke, UK: Palgrave Macmillan.

Karl B. Landorf

Websites

www.anzctr.org.au/default.aspx

A website for a clinical trials registry (the Australian and New Zealand Clinical Trials Registry).

www.cebm.net/index.aspx?o=5653

A website explaining where RCTs sit in the hierarchy of levels of evidence.

www.consort-statement.org

This website contains all relevant information about the CONSORT Guidelines for reporting randomised trials.

www.pedro.org.au

You can download a copy of the PEDro clinical trial rating scale from this website.

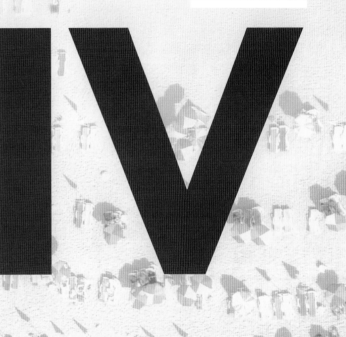

EVIDENCE-BASED PRACTICE AND SYSTEMATIC REVIEWS

16

Evidence-based Health Care

DEIRDRE FETHERSTONHAUGH, RHONDA NAY AND MARGARET WINBOLT

Chapter objectives

In this chapter you will learn to:

- appraise clinical guidelines
- describe how evidence can be implemented in practice
- develop strategies for success
- use audit to implement evidence-based health care

Key terms

Clinical audit

Evidence

Evidence-based practice in health care

Systematic review

Introduction

Evidence-based practice in health care: A process that requires the practitioner to find empirical evidence about the effectiveness or efficacy of different treatment options and then determine the relevance of the evidence to a particular client's situation.

'Everyone' is talking the talk of **evidence-based practice in health care**. According to Winbolt and colleagues (2009, p. 442) '[t]he move to evidence-based practice (EBP) has been driven by changing professional, government and consumer expectations as well as a need to justify the care given in terms of effectiveness and cost.' Health services say they 'do' EBP, but do we really know what it is? Are we using the same language and is there a shared understanding of what it means? We would argue for a resounding 'no' to all three questions. In this chapter we will unpick some of the myths, rhetoric and misunderstandings and try to clear the confusion. Having established what EBP is, we will explore some of the skills you need to determine confidently how good the evidence is and, just as importantly, how to translate it into everyday practice. The importance of leadership at every level will be emphasised.

Defining 'evidence'

Evidence: Evidence in the context of EBP is what results from a systematic review and appraisal of all available literature relevant to a carefully designed question and protocol.

When reviewing the literature for this chapter, one thing that became obvious is the confusion over what is meant by evidence-based practice. Indeed, most research papers appeared to confuse 'research-based' practice with EBP (Byham-Gray *et al.* 2005; Rubin & Parrish 2007; Ferguson *et al.* 2008; Scott & McSherry 2008; see also Chapter 10). Reading one, two or a dozen research papers and applying that to practice is *not* EBP. **Evidence** in the definition of EBP has a very specific meaning and is arrived at through a very specific and rigorous process. Evidence is what results from a systematic review (see Chapter 19) and appraisal of all available literature relevant to a carefully designed question and protocol; it is rated according to a hierarchy that determines 'how good' that evidence is or how confident the reader or practitioner can be in applying it (see also Chapters 1, 15, 17, 18, 19).

Taking this as the definition of evidence, to what extent do health professionals engage in EBP? It would seem to us that experience, tradition and (less frequently) research, rather than evidence, informs practice. Surveys often ask questions about the use of research, which is quite different from whether or not practice is evidence-based. Those papers that report health professionals being supportive of EBP often overestimate the extent to which what they do is actually based on the evidence.

STOP AND THINK

Think about your own practice:

- What informs your approach?
- Do you base your practice on what you learnt at university or on what is tradition in the workplace?
- How often do you actually read research papers?
- Do you know how to appraise a research paper and determine if it is high-quality research or do you just scan the paper and read the results or the abstract?
- Do you know how to differentiate a systematic review from a literature review?
- Could you appraise a systematic review?

Evidence-based practice

There are many definitions of evidence-based practice, but of note is the number that leave out what we see as perhaps most important, and that is the client. EBP evolved from evidence-based medicine (EBM) established by Archie Cochrane (1979), after whom the Cochrane Collaboration is named (see Chapter 17 for more detail). One of the acknowledged leaders in EBM is David Sackett, and if you go back to his definition (Sackett *et al.* 1997), which most writers do, you will find they always included clinician expertise and client (patient) choice. These aspects of the definition are often ignored, and then EBP is criticised as ignoring clinical expertise and client choice! Sackett and colleagues (1996, p. 71) define EBM as:

> the conscientious, explicit and judicious use of current best evidence in making decisions about the care of individual patients. The practice of evidence-based medicine means integrating individual clinical expertise with the best available external evidence from systematic research … and the more thoughtful identification and compassionate use of individual patients' predicaments, rights and preferences.

Further to this, they advocate that:

The practice of EBM is a process of life-long, self-directed learning in which caring for our own patients creates the need for clinically important information about diagnosis, prognosis, therapy and other clinical and health care issues in which we:

- convert these information needs into answerable questions
- track down, with maximum efficiency, the best evidence with which to answer them
- critically appraise that evidence for its validity (closeness to truth) and usefulness (clinical applicability)
- apply the results of this appraisal in our clinical practice
- evaluate our performance. (Sackett *et al.* 1997, pp. 2–3)

EBP reduces inconsistency in practice and increases efficiency and effectiveness, and has thus been accepted by government and funding bodies as essential to better health care (see Chapter 17). It is integral to clinical governance, which is now widely accepted as the responsibility of health organisations both nationally and internationally. Many definitions of 'clinical governance' exist, but one that is commonly quoted refers to it as the framework through which health 'organisations are accountable for continuously improving the quality of their services and safeguarding high standards of care by creating an environment in which excellence in clinical care will flourish' (Scally & Donaldson 1998, p. 62). Clinical governance is defined by the Australian Council on Healthcare Standards (2004, p. 4) as 'the system by which the governing body, managers and clinicians share responsibility and are held accountable for patient care, minimising risks to consumers, and for continuously monitoring and improving the quality of clinical care'.

Deirdre Fetherstonhaugh, Rhonda Nay and Margaret Winbolt

STOP AND THINK

Think about a practice from your workplace.

- Why it is practised in that way? If others practise differently in relation to this situation, on what do they base their decisions to practise their way?
- If you were required to justify your practice in court tomorrow, what would you use to mount your case?
- If your boss asked you to demonstrate that your practice was cost-effective, could you do so?
- If your client asked you to indicate other options and provide evidence as to why one option was better than others, how would you go about it?
- How do you determine if the practice is 'best practice' and acceptable to your client?

In the unhappy event that you end up in court, it would be far more convincing to be able to say, 'I based my decision on the best available international evidence, clinical experience and informed client choice' than 'Well, Your Honour, we have always done it that way and we know what is best for our clients'. You are also more likely to improve your budget situation if you can present reasoned evidence to your boss rather than simply argue from a position of emotion. Your clients have the right to make decisions about their health care and they are usually the best judge of what is best for them in their situation—but they can do this fully informed if you present to them the best available evidence and all options, rather than just your opinion.

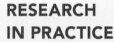

RESEARCH IN PRACTICE

QUESTIONS IN EBP

EBP usually begins with a question or problem from clinical practice. Examples may include:

1. Is this treatment better than usual care?
2. Can this education program improve health outcomes?
3. What are the barriers to reducing falls by 10 per cent?
4. How do older people and their families make decisions regarding end-of-life care?
5. What is the essence of pain?

Each question will be best answered using different research methods. Randomised controlled trials (RCTs) are the ideal way to answer questions 1 and 2—although ethical considerations may prevent the use of RCTs even for questions of effectiveness (see Chapters 3, 15). Grounded theory, ethnography or phenomenology will provide more appropriate answers to questions 3, 4 and 5 (see Chapters 7, 8, 9; Nay & Fetherstonhaugh 2012). Regardless of the question, however, EBP moves from the question to the development of a rigorous protocol that will determine what research will be included in a systematic review.

As you can see from Chapter 19, a **systematic review** is a major undertaking of finding all relevant evidence, appraising it and determining what recommendations for practice can be made. From this review, it is possible to know what, if any, evidence exists in relation to the question, how credible the evidence is and what recommendations can be made for practice. Good practice guidelines are then based on these recommendations rather than on the idiosyncrasies of the organisation or the most powerful ego on the health care team.

Systematic
review: A comprehensive
identification and synthesis
of the available literature
on a specified topic.
In a systematic review,
literature is treated
like data.

Misconceptions of EBP

Some detractors argue that EBP encourages practitioners to follow a kind of recipe book approach. This is clearly not the case. EBP provides the best available research evidence to inform your practice, but you must also individualise that evidence using person-centred care and your clinical expertise.

Another common criticism of EBP is that it is restricted to RCTs and meta-analyses and thus ignores important qualitative research (see Chapters 1, 9, 18). It is the case that EBM privileges RCTs. It is also true that most of the questions that medical practitioners ask are about the effectiveness of treatments, and these questions are best answered by RCTs (see Chapters 15, 17). However, other health practitioners, such as nurses and allied health professionals, are often interested in questions of meaning and/or how to change practice. The best available evidence must be related to the question asked (see also Chapter 1). So, for example, if you want to know how it feels to be told you are being 'placed' in a nursing home, you have a terminal illness or your baby has died, the best evidence will not come from RCTs but from qualitative research (see Chapter 1 and chapters in Part II). Arguing against EBP on the basis of how medicine has developed is baseless. The philosophy underpinning EBP cannot be debunked by critiquing how it is operationalised. Rather, non-medical practitioners (and medical practitioners interested in more than effectiveness) need to develop EBP to include the evidence that answers other relevant questions. This is happening. Indeed, the Cochrane Collaboration is now defining evidence more broadly and exploring ways of evaluating qualitative research.

SYSTEMATIC REVIEWS IN EBP

Systematic reviews may be of varying kinds, but all are based on rigorous protocols. An example of a qualitative review that undertook synthesis of findings rather than meta-analysis of data is that of Haesler and colleagues (2007, 2010) on constructive staff family relationships in care situations. This review (and its update in 2010) followed the system published by the Joanna Briggs Institute. It involved development of a strict protocol, searching and appraising according to that protocol then synthesising and ranking the evidence judged to be credible. A more recent and restricted example is that

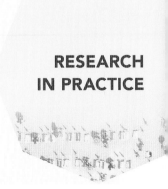

**RESEARCH
IN PRACTICE**

Deirdre Fetherstonhaugh, Rhonda Nay and Margaret Winbolt

of Dyer and das Nair (2012), that appraises only recent qualitative research from the UK. Both are useful, provided they are understood only in the context for which they are written and are not assumed to be unproblematically transferable.

It is worth considering whether the thalidomide tragedies or the deaths at the Bristol Royal Infirmary between 1988 and 1995 following paediatric cardiac surgery would have occurred if the related practice in each case had been evidence-based.

Further criticisms of EBP have been that clinical expertise and client preference are ignored. This is particularly so when EBP is interpreted and implemented as disease-oriented, and the guidelines and clinical recommendations have not been developed to answer the question about the most appropriate treatment or intervention for a particular patient or client at a particular time (Nay & Fetherstonhaugh 2007, p. 458). Evidence about the effectiveness of an intervention, that is, that it 'works' in a controlled population, does not answer the question about applicability or feasibility in a specific client–clinician context.

As already noted, EBP does not mean you have reviewed some recent papers from the library and/or that a group of experts drew up some guidelines. It also does not mean that you evaluate the care given at your place of work and base your practice on the 'evidence' gathered from that evaluation.

EBP includes client preference and clinician expertise; as 'Research in practice' tells us, the best available evidence must relate to the question asked.

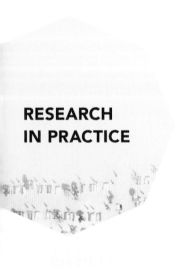

RESEARCH IN PRACTICE

BENEVOLENT OPPRESSION

Mrs Angus is living in the community on her own but with some community services. She has mild dementia and arthritis and has had a stroke. She frequently has constipation, for which she has always taken daily laxatives. She has lost 6 kg in the past three months. Mrs Angus' daughter Rhonda is concerned that her mother keeps coughing and spluttering and is worried that she will choke on her food; Rhonda wants the dietician to see her. Rhonda is also concerned about her mother coping at home alone. She cannot look after her mother as she works full-time and has young children. Rhonda asks Mrs Angus' GP to organise for her mother to be admitted to a residential aged care facility.

An Aged Care Assessment Service assessment finds Mrs Angus eligible for high care. Despite Mrs Angus' initial refusal to move, Rhonda convinces her mother that she needs 'looking after'. The social worker finds a 'nice place' which is 20 km from where she has always lived, so she has to change her GP. Mrs Angus is admitted to 'care'. The dietician orders vitamised food despite Mrs Angus' insistence that she would rather die than eat 'that mushy junk'. The 'new' GP prescribes the same daily laxatives for her constipation that she has always had and the practitioners give these to her religiously without review or assessment. Mrs Angus dies within a month of admission. Rhonda is distraught with guilt and feels that her mother just 'gave up'. The practitioners try to reassure her that what they all did was best for her mother and at least she died in care and not at home alone.

STOP AND THINK

How would you appraise the story above? Could it be seen as benevolent oppression, which Nay (1993) defines as taking away the rights of the person within a framework of believing it is 'best' for them? In short, could it be seen as 'killing with kindness'?

This vignette describes a fairly typical situation with which many people are familiar. How might EBP have resulted in a better outcome? There is available evidence about the effectiveness of various interventions that could have been implemented to address some of the clinical health issues that Mrs Angus experienced. The implementation of EBP, however, is not just about instigating interventions because they have been proved effective in controlled populations. Client choice and, where appropriate, the clinician's judgment and expertise are also important components of EBP. For Mrs Angus, her involvement and preferences would have been crucial factors in the effectiveness of any intervention. Appropriate assessment of swallowing status and the implementation of risk minimisation strategies, including modifying the way in which assistance with food was provided, ensuring that Mrs Angus sat upright when eating and drinking, and swallowed slowly, may have prevented the automatic vitamising of food that Mrs Angus so opposed (Joanna Briggs Institute 2008a).

Constipation is a common and often underrated clinical condition in older people (Department of Veterans' Affairs 2007) which requires assessment, evaluation and reassessment (Registered Nurses Association of Ontario 2005, 2011). The aim of any intervention to address constipation should be to restore regular bowel movements, and the choice of interventions should be tailored to the person's needs and situation (Joanna Briggs Institute 2008a; Chen 2013). Mrs Angus' routine daily laxatives were not effective. Neither the GP nor the staff administering the laxatives did an assessment or evaluation that took into account Mrs Angus' individual history and needs, which would have helped to determine an appropriate treatment. While the information provided here is not comprehensive enough to be in any way conclusive, it is likely that Mrs Angus may have been depressed since depression is common in older people (Neville & Byrne 2014). She was losing her independence and control and others were making decisions for her. The current situation with admission into residential aged care services in Australia requires the Cornell Scale for Depression to be used. It is only a screening tool, but a high score should flag the need for further investigation (Alexopoulos *et al.* 1988), so that if a diagnosis of depression is made the appropriate evidence-based interventions can be implemented. Mrs Angus may have benefited from such assessment. It is clear that an interdisciplinary approach (with Mrs Angus' consent) perhaps involving Mrs Angus, her daughter, the GP, nurses, dietician and physiotherapist would have resulted in a better outcome.

Appraising clinical guidelines

As the example of Mrs Angus demonstrates, the application of the best available international evidence, combined with client preferences and choices, can result in better outcomes for clients and their families. The example can also be used to show how good-quality clinical practice guidelines (CPG), developed from systematic reviews of the available evidence, can give health professionals access to the evidence in a ready-to-use format. Essentially, '[c]linical guidelines are systematically developed statements which assist the health professional and the patient to make decisions about what is the appropriate health care in specific circumstances' (Field & Lohr 1990, p. 38). CPGs are beneficial in that they clearly identify what should be happening in a given area of practice; they can bridge the gap between research and practice by providing easy access to the evidence, and they have the ability to increase consistency of both care and its outcomes. CPGs also have the ability to empower clients as they are readily available and make the evidence understandable to the consumer.

There are, however, some limitations surrounding CPGs. Most of these relate to poor development techniques and flawed or outdated practice recommendations. Factors that may contribute to poor-quality recommendations include a lack of evidence, poor-quality evidence, conflicting evidence, or the evidence not being applicable to the client population for whom the guideline is intended. There are numerous organisations and groups that develop CPGs relating to almost any area of health practice. The use of internet search engines means that these can be located with ease. But there is little information about the quality of these guidelines or the safety of implementing their recommendations. It is therefore important that health professionals are in a position to assess or appraise the quality of CPGs, and to determine the strength of the recommendations and create confidence in them prior to implementation.

A number of tools have been developed to assist health professionals appraise CPGs. Examples are the Appraisal of Guidelines Research and Evaluation (AGREE), the National Institute of Clinical Studies (NICS) and the National Institute for Clinical Excellence (NICE).

Regardless of the tool chosen, appraising a CPG essentially means identifying whether the key components of a good-quality guideline are present. A good-quality CPG should provide details of:

- the name of the developing organisation
- the names and credentials of the guideline developers
- the development method and any limitations identified by the developers
- the client group or population for whom the guideline has been developed
- the systematic review protocol and search strategy
- funding sources and any potential or actual conflict of interest
- the date it was published
- how the development team plan to review or maintain the currency of the recommendations.

CPGs should also contain clearly worded recommendations for practice, each supported by a discussion of the evidence on which it is based and an indication of the level or grade of the evidence. A brief summary of the recommendations should be included, and many guidelines now contain information written specifically for clients (see the Websites section at the end of the chapter). Taking this further, Vlayen and colleagues (2005) prefer a framework for guideline appraisal that suggests it involves not only ascertaining the presence of the above components, but also establishing the validity, reliability, clinical applicability, clinical flexibility, feasibility and clarity of the guidelines.

This framework can be applied by asking a series of questions of the CPG, as shown in Table 16.1.

TABLE 16.1   Questions to ask of a clinical practice guideline

Development team	Does the CPG: • tell you the name of the organisation that produced the guideline? • tell you who was on the development team? • tell you if consumers were involved in the development? • list who funded the development? • outline any conflicts of interest?	• You are looking to establish the credentials of the developing organisation and whether it has the appropriate credentials in guideline development, and whether the development team is appropriate to the topic and client population being targeted by the guideline. • You are also seeking to ascertain any potential or actual conflicts of interest between the development team, the funding sources and the recommendations.
Clarity	Is the CPG: • clearly worded and user-friendly? Does it: • include a summary of recommendations? • provide information for clients?	• The CPG needs to be clearly worded, understandable to the intended audience and user-friendly. • CPGs can be lengthy documents and are made clearer if a simple summary of recommendations is included. • Information written specifically for clients can promote their understanding of the evidence and can assist decision-making.
Validity	Does the CPG tell you: • how the evidence was collected? • the level of evidence supporting each recommendation? • about the potential risks and costs?	• You are asking whether there is enough information in the document for you to establish the source/sources of the evidence and exactly how it was collected and appraised, e.g. is the systematic review protocol given? Is the systematic review accessible?

(continued)

TABLE 16.1   Questions to ask of a clinical practice guideline (*continued*)

		• You are seeking some indication of potential risks in implementing the recommendations, either to the client or to your organisation. It is also valuable to know the potential financial costs associated with implementation.
Reliability	Could the CPG development be repeated by someone else and arrive at the same/similar outcome?	You are seeking to ascertain if the CPG gives enough detail about the development strategy to enable someone else to repeat it.
Clinical applicability	Does the CPG tell you: • what its purpose and aim is? • the topic it covers? • which client group it refers to? • which professional group it is aimed at? • the ethical considerations?	You need to be sure the CPG applies to the client group for whom you wish to implement it. You need to ascertain the exact topic and purpose before considering implementation, e.g. a CPG related to medical management of constipation in children may not be appropriate for nursing management of constipation in an older person living in a residential aged care setting.
Clinical flexibility	Does the CPG tell you: • who was included and who was excluded? • the role of client preferences?	This is linked to clinical applicability in that you can use this information to decide whether a CPG not written specifically for your client group is flexible enough to be adapted for your purposes. It is also important to know whether the guideline development team considered the role of client preference and choice, as this will enable you to make decisions about whether the CPG is flexible enough to support these.
Review	Does the CPG provide the issue date and have a plan stating how and when it will be reviewed?	CPGs rely on the latest available evidence and this can become dated very quickly. Outdated recommendations may put both the health professional and the client at risk, so it is important that you know when the CPG was issued. It is recommended that CPGs be reviewed and updated if necessary every three years (NHMRC 1999a).
Feasibility of implementation	Does the CPG give suggested implementation strategies and identify any policy and administration implications?	You are seeking guidance on any implications that implementing the recommendations might have on your organisation. You are also seeking the developers' thoughts on how their recommendations might be implemented.

| Dissemination strategy | Does the CPG explain how the development team planned to disseminate it? | This gives background information on how the development team intend to promote the CPG. |
| Evaluation strategy | Does the CPG explain how the development team plans to evaluate it? | This gives information on how uptake and effectiveness of the recommendations are to be evaluated. It may also assist you in developing an evaluation strategy in your workplace. |

The development and currency of quality CPGs to promote optimal and consistent health care is time-consuming and requires substantial resources. In the last few years some organisations have looked to guideline adaptation as a way of reducing duplication, saving resources, ensuring currency and increasing utilisation of EBP by taking advantage of good-quality existing guidelines developed by others. The ADAPTE Collaboration has developed a systematic approach for the adaptation of practice guidelines which have been developed for use in one cultural and organisational context, so that they can be used in a different cultural and organisational context.

STOP AND THINK

Think about a clinical policy or guideline from your work area.

- Would you consider this a good-quality policy or guideline?
- If not, how could it be improved?

Implementing EBP: issues, strategies and using audit for implementation

Establishing what is EBP is not the same as carrying it out. It is the implementation that creates the challenge for practitioners. In order to implement EBP, we must first establish what current practice is. This can best be achieved by measuring it against what the evidence advocates should be done according to a meta-analysis or metasynthesis of the research evidence, by undertaking a process of **clinical audit**. Clinical audit is about clinical effectiveness, since the evidence against which current practice is measured is what has been established as being effective from the research evidence published in the literature. The ongoing goal of clinical audit is about improving the quality of health care provided. Importantly, clinical audit can also be used as a clinical risk management/mitigation strategy. Clinical risk is defined as 'an action or inaction on the part of the organisation result[ing] in a potential or actual adverse health impact on consumers of health care' (Australian Centre for Evidence Based Aged Care 2009).

Clinical audit is a process that provides a systematic framework for establishing care standards based on best evidence. It is a practical way to compare day-to-day practice with best evidence care standards and it can identify areas of care that require improvement.

Clinical audit: A process that provides a systematic framework for establishing care standards based on best evidence. It can identify areas of care that require improvement.

Clinical audit can identify the areas of needed practice change in sufficient detail that it can also be used as an implementation tool for instigating and then evaluating the improvements. Clinical audit can also provide evidence that the care currently being provided is of a quality standard and thereby gives positive feedback, which is just as important as identifying what improvements need to be made. According to Prasad and Reddy (2004, p. 112), clinical audit is 'essential for achieving and maintaining professional credibility, and necessary for defending decisions, policies and action on a scientific rather than an intuitive basis'.

The starting point for clinical audit is evidence-based guidelines from which statements can be converted into audit indicators. An indicator is a broad statement of good practice based on the best available evidence. The next step is to determine what criteria are necessary in order to achieve best practice as encapsulated by the indicator. The criteria provide the more detailed and practical information on how to meet the indicator. Criteria refer to the resources (structure) that you need, the actions (process) that must be undertaken, and the results (outcomes) you intend to achieve (Morrell & Harvey 2003, p. 28). Structure criteria are the resources in the system that are necessary for the successful achievement of the indicator: a consideration of staffing levels and skill mix, requirements for knowledge and expertise, organisational arrangements and the provision of equipment and physical space, and existing policies, assessment tools, procedures or protocols. Process criteria are the actions and decisions taken by staff in conjunction with those for whom the care is being provided in order to achieve the specified indicator: assessment, planning, intervening, evaluation and documentation. It is one thing to have policies—process is what you do with them. Outcome criteria are what you expect to achieve by meeting the structure and process criteria. They describe the desired results from the perspective of the recipient of the service or care, and they measure adherence or compliance with EBP as encapsulated in the indicator derived from the recommendation in the evidence-based guideline. Outcome criteria are typically expressed in terms such as physical or behavioural response to an intervention, reported health status or level of knowledge and satisfaction. All these criteria need to be measurable (Morrell & Harvey 2003).

In a guideline about oral and dental hygiene in older people living in residential care facilities, a recommendation statement that advocates an assessment of oral health using the Oral Health Assessment Tool (OHAT) can be converted into an indicator affirming that residents will have their oral health assessed using the OHAT within two days of being admitted to the facility. The structure, process and outcome criteria necessary to meet this indicator can then be identified. Table 16.2 demonstrates how the indicator and criteria can be set out in the form of an audit tool.

Each of these structure and process criteria has an associated/defined audit activity, such as checking whether the registered nurses have attended the education sessions about oral health assessment. This check is made then measured against the targeted outcome. In this example, for instance, a check of the number of nurses who had attended the education sessions may reveal that only 80 per cent compliance had been reached. It then needs to be established why the expected outcome as a measure of adherence to the indicator of EBP in this clinical area has not been achieved. Once the reason has been identified, a strategy to

TABLE 16.2   Audit indicator

AUDIT INDICATOR		
Residents will have their oral health assessed within two days of being admitted to the residential aged care facility using the Oral Health Assessment Tool (OHAT).		
STRUCTURE	**PROCESS**	**OUTCOME**
S1–1 OHAT is available.	P1–1 Registered nurses access assessment tool and undertake assessment.	O1–1 Oral health assessments are undertaken and documented for 100% of residents within two days of being admitted to the residential care facility.
S2–2 Education program targeted to registered nurses about oral health assessment is available in the residential care facility.	P2–2 Registered nurses are able to attend education sessions.	O2–2 100% of registered nurses working in the residential care facility have attended education session on oral health assessment.
S3–3 The residential care facility has developed (or has) competencies for registered nurses in oral health assessment.	P3–3 Registered nurses have their competency to undertake oral health assessments measured.	O3–3 100% of registered nurses working in the residential care facility are competent to undertake oral health assessment.

Source: Adapted from Morrell and Harvey (2003, pp. 181–2)

rectify this gap can be decided and then implemented. For instance, in this example it may be that registered nurses working overnight have not attended the education because the sessions are held only during the day. Scheduling education at a more appropriate time for night duty staff, training a night staff member to provide the education at night, or organising some 'paid' education time for night staff during the day when they are not working, are all examples of strategies or interventions that could be put into place to improve compliance with the requirements of EBP in this clinical area. A staff member, for example the clinical educator, would be given or take on the responsibility of implementing the strategy within an expected time-frame; then a repeat audit would be done to determine whether there has been improvement in adherence to the required evidence-based indicator.

Feedback to all key stakeholders is an essential component of effective clinical auditing. A systematic review on audit and feedback (Jamtvedt *et al.* 2006, p. 2) concluded that the 'relative effectiveness of audit and feedback is likely to be greater when baseline adherence to recommended practice is low and when feedback is delivered more intensively'.

The advantage of using clinical audit as a means of determining adherence to EBP is that it is not just a measure of what is currently happening, but an implementation tool which highlights gaps in enough detail that strategies for improvement can be identified then implemented. There is no point offering education if the obstacle to implementation is documentation.

Deirdre Fetherstonhaugh, Rhonda Nay and Margaret Winbolt

According to Solomons and Spross (2011), Asadoorian *et al.* (2010) and Callahan *et al.* (2014), barriers to EBP being translated into practice typically include:

- lack of time
- lack of organisational support
- resistance to change
- inability to understand and appraise research
- lack of access to the internet or inability to navigate it
- lack of relevant research evidence.

Ideally, addressing these barriers requires an 'all of organisation' approach. If the systems, including documentation, value task completion at the expense of clients and staff, accessing evidence and implementing change will be seen as privileges rather than an expectation of the health care environment. Similarly, when education and research are not built into role expectations, they will be neglected. Most staff still do not have well-developed skills in accessing and appraising evidence. Processes and structures that support training, access to the internet and implementation of evidence into practice, at least to the same extent as training in clinical 'problems' and new equipment, will demonstrate to staff that EBP is significant and not just rhetoric.

We found that building research discussions into current practice, rather than making it something separate that staff have to 'go to', can embed it more in everyday practice. For example, case conferences and handover can be simply the handing over of tasks and information—or they can be an opportunity for discussions about what the best available research evidence offers.

Any change will meet with some resistance. But Thompson and Learmonth (2002, pp. 214–15) offer some examples of helpful strategies. These include:

- identifying all groups involved in, influenced by or able to influence the change
- assessing the characteristics of the proposed change that might influence its acceptance
- assessing readiness and enabling factors for this change
- identifying possible external barriers to this change.

Contemporary leadership is essential. The change literature from diverse fields demonstrates how essential a component leadership is to an organisation's ability to implement EBP (Raffel *et al.* 2013; Pryse *et al.* 2014; Kim & Yoon 2015). If change is simply imposed and staff feel devalued, they will resist. Transformational leadership, on the other hand, can excite staff about change and indeed grow leaders at every level. Nay and Fetherstonhaugh (2007) report from their research that facilitation is vital, and we would support this contention. Such facilitators are often termed 'local champions' as they keep staff enthused and committed. Some health facilities have formal relationships with universities and this can assist the implementation of EBP, provided clinical staff feel that they have ownership of the process and do not see it as simply the university's project that will stop if the link with the university is broken.

Summary

EBP is shown to be much more than just reading the research. As Nay and Fetherstonhaugh (2007, p. 461) suggest, 'EBP involves much more than locating, analyzing, and appraising the best evidence available about the effectiveness of an intervention'. We argue here that there is a need to increase the extent to which practitioners use EBP rather than experience, tradition or relying on unappraised research papers. Barriers to implementation are common in all health professions and settings. Lack of time is always cited as a major barrier, as is the difficulty practitioners have in appraising research. We acknowledge that practitioners usually do not have time to conduct systematic reviews, develop guidelines and work through all of the steps involved in EBP. But many areas of practice now have guidelines based on the best available evidence, and we encourage practitioners to become expert in finding and appraising these guidelines. The time wasted across the health sector when every organisation, and sometimes every unit within an organisation, develops its own guidelines could be much better spent implementing evidence-based guidelines already in existence. We have provided examples to assist guideline appraisal and offered strategies for implementation. Finally, we show the significance of transformational leadership in translating evidence into practice and transforming task and disease-based environments into EBP environments.

Practice exercises

1   Think about a situation from your experience where some change was proposed. What barriers do you recall to that change? What strategies were used to overcome the barriers? Can you think of others that may have been more successful?

2   Develop a presentation to explain to your colleagues how EBP differs from research-based practice. Convince them of why EBP is beneficial to an organisation, health professionals and clients.

Further reading

Australian Centre for Evidence Based Aged Care (2009). *Strengthening care outcomes for residents with evidence (SCORE) summary report May 2009.* <www.health.vic.gov.au/agedcare/downloads/score/score_summary_report_may_09.pdf>.

Daly, J., Jackson, D. & Nay, R. (2014). Visionary leadership for a 'greying' health care system. In R. Nay, S. Garratt & D. Fetherstonhaugh (eds), *Older people: issues and innovations in care*, 4th edn. Elsevier: Sydney, 489–501.

Dawes, M., Davies, P., Gray, A., Mant, J., Seers, K. & Snowball, R. (2005). *Evidence-based practice: a primer for health care professionals*, 2nd edn. London: Elsevier.

Deirdre Fetherstonhaugh, Rhonda Nay and Margaret Winbolt

DiCenso, A., Guyatt, G. & Ciliska, D. (2005). *Evidence-based nursing: a guide to clinical practice*. St Louis: Elsevier Mosby.

Dyer, K. & das Nair, R. (2012). Why don't healthcare professionals talk about sex? A systematic review of recent qualitative studies conducted in the United Kingdom. *Journal of Sex Medicine*, published online 31/7/12. <http://onlinelibrary.wiley.com/doi/10.1111/j.1743-6109.2012.02856.x/pdf>.

Haesler, E., Bauer, M. & Nay, R. (2010). Factors associated with constructive nursing staff–family relationships in the care of older adults in the institutional setting: an update to a systematic review. *International Journal of Evidence-Based Healthcare*, 8(2), 45–74.

Kim, S. & Yoon, G. (2015). An innovation-driven culture in local government: do senior managers' transformational leadership and the climate for creativity matter? *Public Personnel Management*, 44(2), 147–68.

Morrell, C. & Harvey, G. (2003). *The clinical audit handbook*. London: Elsevier Science.

Nay, R. & Fetherstonhaugh, D. (2007). Evidence-based practice: limitations and successful implementation. *Annals of the New York Academy of Sciences*, 1114, 456–63.

Ryan, R., Santesso, N., Hill, S., Lowe, D., Kaufman, C. & Grimshaw, J. (2011). *Consumer-oriented interventions for evidence-based prescribing and medicines use: an overview of systematic reviews*. Cochrane Database of Systematic Reviews, Issue 5, Art. No. CD007768. DOI: 10.1002/14651858.CD007768.pub2.

Sackett, D.L., Richardson, W.S., Rosenberg, W. & Haymes, R.B. (1997). *Evidence-based medicine: how to practice and teach EBM*. London: Churchill Livingstone.

Vlayen, J., Aertgeerts, B., Hannes, K., Sermeus, W. & Ramaekers, D. (2005). A systematic review of appraisal tools for clinical practice guidelines: multiple similarities and one common deficit. *International Journal for Quality in Health Care*, 17(3), 235–42.

Websites

www.g-i-n.net/document-store/working-groups-documents/adaptation/adapte-resource-toolkit-guideline-adaptation-2-0.pdf

> This guideline adaptation resource toolkit was developed by the ADAPTE Collaboration.

www.cochrane.org

> The Cochrane Collaboration website provides access to systematic reviews of health care interventions.

www.nice.org.uk

> The National Institute for Health and Clinical Excellence in the UK is responsible for providing national guidance on the promotion of good health and the prevention and treatment of ill health in the areas of public health, health technologies and clinical practice.

www.nhmrc.gov.au/guidelines/health_guidelines.htm

> The National Health and Medical Research Council website lists guidelines and provides access to them.

www.agreecollaboration.org/intr

> This website provides information on the appraisal of guidelines, research and evaluation collaboration.

www.york.ac.uk/inst/crd

> The Centre for Reviews and Dissemination is a department of the University of York and is part of the National Institute for Health Research. The Centre undertakes high-quality systematic reviews that evaluate the effects of health and social care interventions and the delivery and organisation of health care.

17

Evidence-based Practice
in Therapeutic Health Care

MEGAN DAVIDSON AND ROSS ILES

Chapter objectives

In this chapter you will learn:

- what evidence-based practice is
- about a five-step approach to evidence-based practice
- to discuss evidence hierarchies and evidence quality
- to apply the evidence to current practice
- to provide a case study for a therapy question
- to provide a case study for a diagnostic question

Key terms

Clinical practice guidelines
Evidence-based practice
PEDro (Physiotherapy Evidence Database)
Randomised controlled trial
Systematic review

Introduction

Evidence-based practice (EBP) is a concept whose modern genesis can be found in the words of Archie Cochrane, a British epidemiologist (1909–88), who said, referring to the profession of medicine, 'It is surely a great criticism of our profession that we have not organised a critical summary, by specialty or sub-specialty, adapted periodically, of all relevant randomized controlled trials' (Cochrane 1979, p. 8). The legacy of Cochrane's criticism is the Cochrane Collaboration, a worldwide multidisciplinary organisation established some years after his death, which is dedicated to doing precisely what he said was needed. The technology of the systematic review (see Chapter 19) has transformed health care practice from care based largely on expert opinion and tradition to one in which the question 'what is the evidence?' informs practice decisions. Critical summaries (systematic reviews and clinical practice guidelines) now provide practitioners with readily accessible access to research evidence. The availability of these documents on the web means that patients have almost as much access to the 'critical summaries' as their doctor or therapist.

Although definitions of EBP abound, it is commonly agreed that EBP is the use of best research evidence, along with clinical expertise, available resources and patient's preferences, to determine the optimal assessment, treatment or management option in a specific situation (see also Chapters 15, 16, 18, 19).

The underlying assumption of EBP is that if health care is based on evidence about what is most effective, the quality of care will be better than if it is not. Sackett's widely adopted five-step approach to EBP (Table 17.1) provides a practical framework for teaching and practising EBP (Sackett *et al.* 2000).

TABLE 17.1　The five steps of EBP

EBP STEP	KNOWLEDGE AND SKILL REQUIRED
1　ASK an answerable clinical question	Recognise a knowledge gap and formulate a structured question that defines the problem, the intervention and the outcomes of interest
2　ACQUIRE the best available evidence	Know evidence sources and types, and search databases
3　APPRAISE the evidence	Critically appraise the evidence to determine its validity and clinical importance
4　APPLY the evidence	Integrate the evidence with clinical expertise and patient preferences
5　ASSESS the process	Reflect on Steps 1–4 and identify ways to improve efficiency

Source: Based on Sackett *et al.* (2000) and Del Mar *et al.* (2004). Reproduced from Iles & Davidson (2006), with permission from Wiley-Blackwell.

Evidence hierarchies and evidence quality

Step 2 of the EBP process is to acquire the best available evidence. A brief encounter with an electronic database such as PubMed or even Google Scholar is enough to reveal that there is a mountain of research 'out there'. Without a system to organise the available research, the evidence you need may as well be a needle in a vast electronic haystack. Developing a clearly answerable clinical question (Step 1) to guide your search is the first way to organise your way through the maze of available research papers. However, even the best questions may result in a mountain of evidence. Since time is a barrier to EBP for many practitioners (Scurlock-Evans *et al.* 2014), some system is needed to identify which papers should be read, or what evidence is most important or credible.

How much confidence you can have in the results of research will depend at least in part on the research design. For a question about therapy effectiveness, you are more likely to use a well-designed **randomised controlled trial** (RCT) to inform practice than a single case study, because you can be more confident that the outcomes are actually due to the intervention and can be generalised to patients who are like those included in the study (see Chapters 12, 15). By classifying studies according to the research design, it can be easier to identify evidence that has greater capacity to inform and change practice.

The Centre for Evidence Based Medicine (CEBM) and the National Health and Medical Research Council (NHMRC) provide a hierarchy (levels) of evidence showing the relationship between the research design and the level of confidence that it conveys. The higher the level of evidence, the greater the confidence we can have in applying that evidence to clinical practice. Across all research designs, a **systematic review** represents the highest level of evidence and various forms of case study the lowest. Depending on whether the clinical question is about therapy efficacy, diagnostic accuracy or clinical prognosis, the levels in between will look slightly different. Research design alone does not guarantee research quality. **Clinical practice guidelines** generally take into account both the research design and the quality of the research in arriving at a recommendation for clinical practice. Systematic reviews also frequently summarise the strength of evidence based on research design and quality.

An evidence hierarchy allows you to use a top-down approach to the evidence. If you can locate a relevant, well-conducted and reasonably recent systematic review you may not need to search any further. A well-performed systematic review will have gathered, critically appraised and summarised all the relevant research with a minimum of bias, providing the reader with results that can be incorporated into practice with a high degree of confidence (see Chapter 19).

If no systematic reviews are available on the topic, the next level of evidence should be sought to answer the question. In the case of therapy efficacy, this would be to examine relevant RCTs (see Chapter 15). If this level of evidence is not available, the next highest is sought and so on. How much influence the evidence should have when making clinical decisions depends on the level and quality of the evidence. This requires the reader to critically evaluate the evidence (Step 3) to determine its quality and therefore the extent to which it is

Randomised controlled trial: A clinical trial where participants are randomly assigned to groups in order to receive different interventions. This randomisation removes many of the effects that may bias the true result.

Systematic review: A comprehensive identification and synthesis of the available literature on a specified topic.

Clinical practice guidelines: Systematically developed statements which assist the health professional and the patient to make decisions about what is the appropriate health care in specific circumstances.

valid or believable. All evidence should be assessed (critically appraised) to determine the extent to which the results are free from bias. This can be a time-consuming process, and not all physiotherapists have the ability or confidence to appraise research (Scurlock-Evans *et al.* 2014). A database such as PEDro (Physiotherapy Evidence Database), where individual studies have been critically evaluated and carry a quality rating, provides physiotherapists who are short of time or expertise with a valuable resource (see also Chapters 15, 19). However, even if the research report has not been pre-appraised, there are a number of tools that can assist in quality appraisal of research, including the quality scale used by PEDro (see the box 'Quality appraisal tools').

QUALITY APPRAISAL TOOLS

- CEBM has critical appraisal tools for systematic reviews, RCTs and diagnostic studies.
- The Critical Appraisal Skills Program (CASP) of the NHS in the UK provides a number of tools for various study designs.
- The PEDro scale.
- The International Centre for Allied Health Evidence at the University of South Australia (see the Websites section at the end of the chapter).

Current practice

The process of locating, appraising and applying the research evidence is no different between medical practitioners, nurses, dentists, physiotherapists, speech therapists, podiatrists, social workers or any other health professional. However, the types of questions that are of primary concern to the different disciplines are diverse, and the body of evidence available to answer questions varies enormously. For the profession of physiotherapy, a relatively large body of relevant research evidence is available and has been collected, appraised and made available as **PEDro**. PEDro contains (as at November 2015) over 31,000 clinical practice guidelines, systematic reviews and clinical trials of direct relevance to the discipline of physiotherapy.

Most health practitioners are now trained in the basics of EBP in their pre-qualification courses. Many therapists who graduated before this was the case have acquired the skill by taking short postgrad courses or by self-directed learning. Surveys of EBP-related attitudes, knowledge and skills indicate that, while attitudes are generally positive, there is considerable variation in the self-reported knowledge and skills, confidence and competence in EBP within and between health professions (Scurlock-Evans *et al.* 2014; Upton & Upton 2006; Upton *et al.* 2012; Weng *et al.* 2013; Wilkinson *et al.* 2012). Younger, more recently graduated practitioners are often found to have better self-rated knowledge and skills. Many health professionals have some learning to do to optimise their practice.

PEDro (Physiotherapy Evidence Database): This collects, appraises and makes available a relatively large body of physiotherapy research evidence.

Barriers to EBP are typically identified as lack of time, high workload pressures, and less than optimal levels of knowledge or skills. Without sufficient knowledge and skills in locating, appraising and applying the best available research evidence, physiotherapists continue to rely on other sources, such as personal experience, colleagues and short courses (Scurlock-Evans *et al.* 2014).

STOP AND THINK

Self-rate your competence on these aspects of EBP on a 0–10 scale where 0 means 'not competent' and 10 means 'very competent':

- asking an answerable clinical question
- acquiring the best available evidence
- appraising the evidence
- applying the evidence to practice.

Are there one or more aspects that you have rated lower than others? Is this important for your practice? What is your plan to improve your knowledge and skills?

Therapy case study

Danny, a physiotherapist who graduated a couple of years ago, is working in the outpatient department at a metropolitan hospital where chronic musculoskeletal conditions are common. He has diagnosed his patient with Achilles tendinopathy (AT); he generally treats this condition with an eccentric exercise (EE) program with good outcomes. Danny's patient says he has read about a treatment for AT called shock wave therapy, and wonders whether that would be a useful treatment for him. Danny is not sure how effective shock wave therapy is in treating AT or whether EE will give his patient a better outcome.

Recalling his undergraduate training in the five-step approach to EBP and using his textbook from the course (Herbert *et al.* 2011), Danny sets out to determine whether eccentric exercise or shock wave therapy is the better treatment option for his patient.

Step 1: Ask an answerable question

Danny knows that formulating the question well will help find the answer. An answerable question defines the problem or patient group, an intervention, a comparison intervention and an outcome. Danny decides to use the PICO format (Population, Intervention, Comparison, Outcome; see Chapter 19) to structure his question. Danny writes his question as: 'For people with chronic AT, is extracorporeal shock wave therapy (ESWT) or EE more effective in reducing pain and improving function?'

Step 2: Acquire the evidence

Danny decides the first place to look is the Cochrane Library, as it is a source of high-quality systematic reviews and the most likely place to find Level 1 evidence. The Cochrane Library contains the full text of reviews conducted under the aegis of the Cochrane Collaboration, but also identifies reviews published elsewhere. He enters Achilles tendin* in the first search box, using the * as a truncator to find records using either tendinitis or tendinopathy. This yields four Cochrane reviews (Fig 17.1). The first two reviews are not relevant. The third title is only a protocol for a review which won't include shock wave therapy. The fourth review, 'Interventions for treating acute and chronic Achilles tendinitis' (McLauchlan & Handoll 2011), is relevant but has been withdrawn because it is out of date and includes studies only up to 2000.

FIGURE 17.1   Cochrane Library advanced search screen

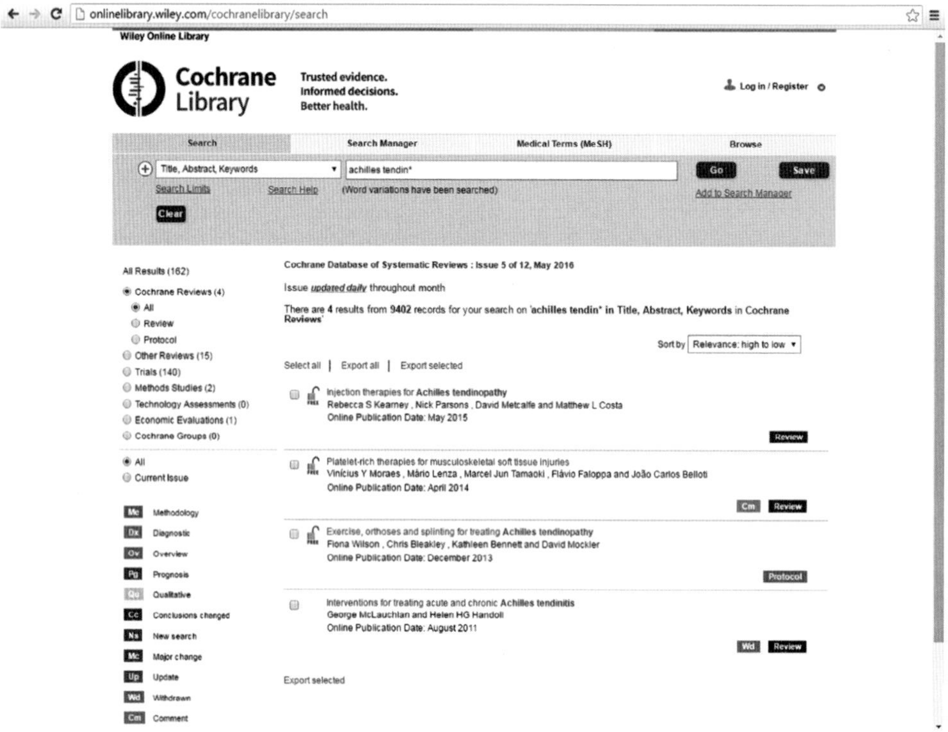

The search of the Cochrane Library also identifies fifteen non-Cochrane reviews. A quick scan of the titles reveals a review of ESWT on chronic AT (Al-Abbad & Simon 2013). The Cochrane Library provides a structured abstract and quality appraisal of this review, which showed that the review was of a reasonable quality. While the review authors concluded that there was 'satisfactory evidence' for the effectiveness of ESWT, the appraisal of the review concluded that the findings are of uncertain reliability because only four of the six included studies were RCTs (highest level of evidence), only two of those four showed a benefit in favour of ESWT, and there was no meta-analysis performed. Danny sees he can sort the reviews by date to have the latest reviews appear first, and notes two fairly recent reviews of EE (Malliaras *et al.* 2013; Habets & van Cingel 2015) and the more general 'Treatment for insertional Achilles tendinopathy' (Wiegerinck *et al.* 2013), which do not yet have a provisional abstract. Danny pastes the titles into Google Scholar and finds the first review (Al-Abbad & Simon 2013) is behind a paywall, but he can access the full text of the other three reviews.

Danny decides the next step is to search the Physiotherapy Evidence Database (PEDro). He knows this is a useful source of pre-appraised evidence that rates clinical trials on a 10-point quality scale. He wants to see if PEDro identifies any systematic reviews not found in Cochrane, and to locate any clinical trials that have made a direct comparison of EE and ESWT. He goes to the PEDro website (Figure 17.2) and enters 'achilles tendin*' in the title/abstract search box; this yields sixty results. He repeats the search, this time selecting 'electrotherapies, heat and cold' from the therapy drop-down menu. Danny is not sure whether AT would be classified as 'lower leg or knee' or 'foot and ankle' in the body part box so he decides to leave it blank. This search returns twenty-five records, including a very recent systematic review that he did not find in the Cochrane database (Mani-Babu *et al.* 2015). The brief abstract says that although the evidence for ESWT is limited, the reviewers conclude that there is moderate evidence that ESWT is more effective in the short term than EE for problems at the tendon insertion, and equivalent for problems at the midportion of the tendon, and that combining ESWT and EE may be better again. Unlike the earlier review of ESWT, this one has performed a meta-analysis. Danny decides to obtain the full text of this review, published in the *American Journal of Sports Medicine*. He opens Google Scholar, pastes in the article title and finds that this article is available online but behind a paywall and will cost $US36 to purchase. Frustrated that he is not able to affordably access the best evidence to answer his question, Danny decides to raise the issue at the next practice meeting to explore other pathways to access journal articles, such as via professional association memberships, or university library access for alumni.

FIGURE 17.2 PEDro advanced search screen

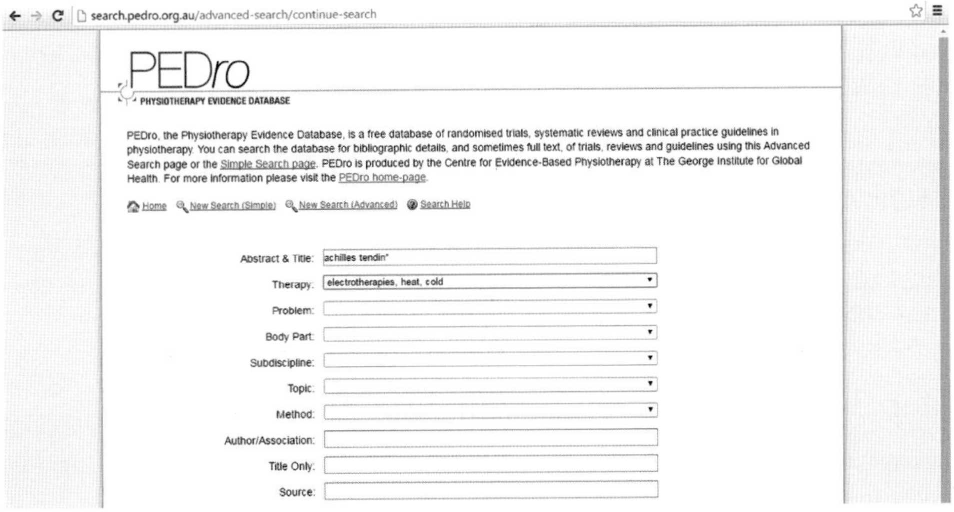

Source: Centre for Evidence-Based Physiotherapy, Musculoskeletal Division,
The George Institute for Global Health, www.pedro.org.au

Megan Davidson and Ross Iles

Danny's PEDro search also locates a recent review of EE (Frizziero *et al.* 2014) that the Cochrane search did not show. He retrieves the full text (without having to pay anything) by copying and pasting the title into Google Scholar. Danny notes that his PEDro search also lists a number of relevant RCTs. The best-quality (9/10) study (Rasmussen *et al.* 2008) shows that ESWT had better outcomes than sham ESWT at four, eight and twelve weeks. There were three good-quality trials (8/10) comparing eccentric exercise and ESWT. In the earliest trial (Rompe *et al.* 2007), ESWT was equal to EE, and both were superior to wait-and-see in people with chronic non-insertional AT. In the next trial (Rompe *et al.* 2008), ESWT was superior to EE in people with chronic insertional AT. In the latest trial (Rompe *et al.* 2009), a combination of EE and ESWT was superior to EE alone in people with chronic non-insertional AT. Danny finds full text copies of all four trials by pasting the titles into Google Scholar. He notes that the size of the treatment effect (the average difference in outcome between the groups) in the 2009 study was 13.5 points on the 100-point VISA-A scale and 1.5 points on a 10-point pain scale.

At this point Danny stops to consider the evidence. There are two systematic reviews of ESWT for AT (Al-Abbad & Simon 2013; Mani-Babu *et al.* 2015), but both articles are behind paywalls. However, the available abstracts show that both reviews conclude there is some benefit from ESWT, and that it may be superior to EE alone. However, these conclusions are from a fairly limited evidence base (and he suspects might be largely based on the three trials by the Rompe group). The review by Frizziero and colleagues (2014) described the three trials by Rompe and another trial that compared another intervention to EE and ESWT combined. The reviews by Habets & van Cingel (2015) and Malliaris *et al.* (2013) were focused on EE and included two and one of the Rompe trials respectively. The Wiegerinck *et al.* (2013) review identified two of the Rompe trials and another pre/post study by the same group. Danny concludes that the evidence comparing EE and ESWT appears to be limited to three good-quality trials by the same research team. For chronic non-insertional AT, one trial found both EE and ESWT to be better than wait-and-see and one found that EE and ESWT combined were superior to EE alone. For chronic insertional AT, one trial found that ESWT was better than EE.

STOP AND THINK

- The Cochrane Library also contains RCTs—why did Danny prefer to search for these types of studies in the PEDro database rather than Cochrane?
- Why is the RCT considered the gold standard test of treatment efficacy?

Step 3: Appraise the evidence

By targeting pre-appraised sources of evidence, Danny has been able to rely on the appraisal from experts in the area. This has saved him valuable time. However, he has not been able to access either of the recent systematic reviews of ESWT and no pre-appraisal was available for those reviews.

Step 4: Apply the evidence

Danny's patient has non-insertional AT so he looks more closely at the two relevant trials and finds that the participants were not like his patient in that they had at least six months of failed non-operative management including 'physiotherapy' (although it isn't clear if this might have included EE, and previous EE was not excluded).

Danny shares what he has found with his patient. He explains that there is good evidence to support the use of EE as an effective treatment for AT. ESWT is a newer treatment and there are two trials, both of good quality, comparing EE and ESWT, one of which found that they were both better than doing nothing, and the other suggesting that the two treatments combined achieve better outcomes than EE alone. However, the participants in the trials were different from him so Danny can't be sure about the effect in this particular case. The patient agrees to a trial of EE. Danny says he will raise the issue of whether or not the practice should buy an ESWT device at the next practice meeting.

Step 5: Assess the process

Danny reflects on the process of searching and is confident that between Cochrane and PEDro he probably found the most recent and relevant research. He found the structured abstracts in the Cochrane database to be useful summaries of the systematic reviews, but these were not always available. The PEDro database does not provide any analysis of systematic reviews but provides a quality rating of clinical trials. Danny decides that next time he might begin his search with PEDro. He is not sure how to improve his access to publications that are behind paywalls, and resolves to explore this issue at the next team meeting.

Diagnosis case study

Donna, a physiotherapist who graduated a couple of years ago, is working in a private practice that has a strong relationship with various sports clubs and sees quite a lot of sports-related knee injuries. The practice runs a regular professional development program; as part of this, Donna has been asked to prepare a session on diagnostic tests for anterior cruciate ligament (ACL) injuries.

Recalling her undergraduate training in the five-step approach to EBP and using her textbook from the course (Herbert *et al.* 2011), Donna sets out to provide the practice with the best evidence available relating to clinical tests for ACL injuries.

Step 1: Ask an answerable question

Like Danny, Donna knows that formulating the question well will help find the answer. An answerable question defines the problem or patient group, an intervention, co-intervention and an outcome. In this case, the problem is ACL injury, the intervention is the diagnostic test, and the outcome is the test accuracy. Donna is familiar with common tests of ACL integrity

(Lachman, anterior drawer, and pivot shift tests), but in case there are other tests that she does not know about Donna writes her question as, 'What is the diagnostic accuracy of tests for identifying injuries to the anterior cruciate ligament of the knee?'

Step 2: Acquire the evidence

Donna knows that good, recent systematic reviews of original studies are the type of publication at the top of the hierarchy of evidence and will provide the best snapshot of the evidence in the least time. She also knows that an evidence-based clinical practice guideline (CPG) might be worth looking for.

Donna's first thought is to search PEDro, but she is unsure whether this database includes research relating to diagnostic tests. She determines also to search PubMed, which is a freely available version of Medline. Although she knows that she might miss something on the other major databases, such as Embase and Cinahl, her time is limited and she does not have ready access to those databases.

Donna goes to the PEDro website and searches for 'Anterior cruciate ligament'; this yields 232 articles. On PEDro CPGs are listed first, followed by systematic reviews then clinical trials. Donna does not have time to screen 232 articles, but she knows that CPGs usually cover assessment as well as treatment. The first listed practice guideline is recent (American Academy of Orthopaedic Surgeons, 2014) and endorsed by a number of peak professional bodies in the USA. She clicks on the link to obtain the quick reference guide for this guideline.

The guideline summary makes a strong recommendation for the diagnostic utility of obtaining a good history and performing a physical examination. Accurate diagnosis of the injury will allow an appropriate conservative management plan to be devised or, for conditions that are not amenable to conservative management, an appropriate referral to be made. The guideline recommends a minimum physical exam that includes Lachman's test. Donna would like to see a systematic review with meta-analysis that quantifies test characteristics such as sensitivity and specificity for each of the available tests for ACL injury. She tries to find this information in the full version of the guidelines, but finds only a brief summary of the information she is looking for.

Donna next searches PubMed, the freely accessible version of Medline (Figure 17.3). She chooses the 'Advanced' search option, and searches the title/abstract fields for 'Anterior Cruciate Ligament AND Diagnosis', which yields 727 hits. She filters this yield by selecting 'Systematic Review', 'human' and 'English', leaving sixteen references which she sorts by relevance. Two of these (Benjaminse et al. 2006; Solomon et al. 2001) appear directly relevant but are quite old. Donna tries the PubMed Clinical Queries site (Fig 17.3), searching 'anterior cruciate ligament injuries' category 'diagnosis' and scope 'narrow'. She notes two fairly recent relevant reviews (Van Eck et al. 2013; Leblanc et al. 2015). The Leblanc article is behind a paywall, and the abstract gives only the pooled sensitivity values for the Lachman and pivot shift tests. The review included eight studies and looked at the Lachman, pivot shift and anterior drawer tests compared to a gold standard of MRI or arthroscopy. The Van Eck article is also behind

FIGURE 17.3   PubMed advanced search screen

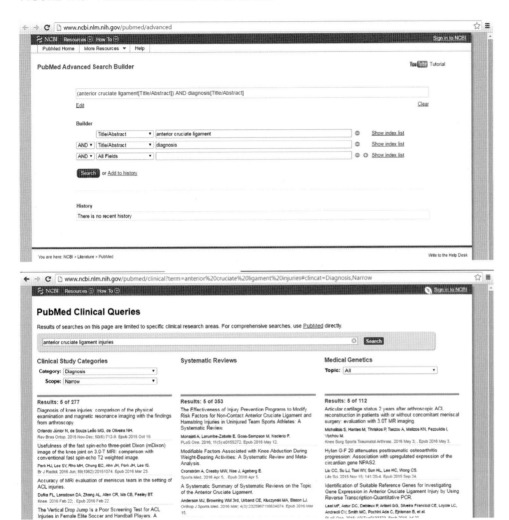

Source: National Center for Biotechnology Information, US National Library of Medicine

a paywall. The abstract reveals that the review included twenty studies and only looked at diagnosis of acute, complete ACL ruptures. The Lachman test was overall 81 per cent sensitive and specific, compared to 38 per cent and 81 per cent for the anterior drawer test. Donna is frustrated by her inability to access the articles cost-effectively, as they cost almost $US40 each to purchase. However, all three sources identify the Lachman test as the most useful.

Donna finds that she can access the older review by Benjaminse and colleagues (2006). The review covers the Lachman, anterior drawer and pivot shift tests and includes twenty-eight individual studies. Having obtained the relevant article, Donna knows that she now needs to evaluate the quality of the review before she decides if she can use it with confidence to inform clinical practice.

Megan Davidson and Ross Iles

Step 3: Appraise the evidence

In her copy of Herbert *et al.* (2011), Donna sees that she can use three questions to appraise a systematic review.

1   Was it clear which studies were to be reviewed?

   a   Is there a list of inclusion and exclusion criteria that defines the patients or population?

2   Were most relevant studies reviewed?

   a   Were key databases searched with sensitive search strategies?

   b   Was the search conducted recently?

3   Was the quality of the reviewed studies taken into account?

   a   Was there a minimum quality for studies to be included?

   b   Was quality evaluated with a scale or checklist and were the quality assessments taken into account in drawing conclusions?

She creates a table (Table 17.2) and reads the article with a view to finding this information and noting relevant results. Donna concludes that despite the problem of the overall low quality of the reviewed studies, they may still be of some use to inform clinical practice. She knows that biased studies are likely to overestimate estimates of test accuracy. From the article, Donna extracts only the results relating to performance of the test without

TABLE 17.2   Quality appraisal of the Benjaminse review

WAS IT CLEAR WHICH STUDIES WERE TO BE REVIEWED?	WERE MOST RELEVANT STUDIES REVIEWED?	WAS THE QUALITY OF THE REVIEWED STUDIES TAKEN INTO ACCOUNT?
Yes: human; at least one test for ACL rupture; arthroscopy, arthrotomy or MRI gold standard; 2 × 2 table could be constructed	Yes: Medline, Embase and Cinahl to April 2005 plus reference checking and personal contacts	No. All studies were included. Quality evaluated independently by two authors using Cochrane Methods Group approach. Only three studies had independent, blind comparison of index and reference tests and only three studies avoided work-up or verification bias. Pooled sensitivity and specificity was weighted only by sample size

TABLE 17.3 Extracted results for whole group and subgroups, without anaesthesia, from the Benjaminse review

	SENSITIVITY	SPECIFICITY	LR+	LR-
Whole group data				
Anterior drawer	55 (52–58)	92 (90–94)	7.3 (3.5–15.2)	0.5 (0.4–0.6)
Lachman	85 (83–87)	94 (92–95)	10.2 (4.6–22.7)	0.2 (0.1–0.3)
Pivot shift	24 (21–27)	98 (96–99)	8.5 (4.7–15.5)	0.9 (0.8–1.0)
Acute subgroup group data				
Anterior drawer	49 (43–55)	58 (39–76)	1.4 (0.5–4.4)	0.7 (0.5–1.0)
Lachman	94 (91–96)	97 (93–99)	9.4 (0.4–210)	0.1 (0.0–1.1)
Pivot shift	32 (25–38)	100 (48–100)	1.3 (0.1–23.7)	1.0 (0.7–1.3)
Chronic subgroup group data				
Anterior drawer	92 (88–95)	91 (87–94)	8.9 (5.3–15.2)	0.1 (0.0–0.5)
Lachman	95 (91–97)	90 (87–94)	7.1 (1.2–40.2)	0.2 (0.1–0.7)
Pivot shift	40 (29–52)	97 (95–99)	7.7 (1.7–36.4)	0.8 (0.4–1.4)

anaesthesia, as this is what is relevant to physiotherapy practice. The review presents pooled estimates for the whole group and for acute and chronic subgroups for each of the three ACL tests (Table 17.3). She notes that while the estimates for the whole group are based on more than 1000 subjects for each test, the numbers used to calculate the acute subgroup estimates are quite small, only twenty-seven for specificity of the pivot shift, and only seventy-seven for the anterior drawer test. This has made the 95 per cent confidence intervals for those estimates quite large.

Step 4: Apply the evidence

Donna notes that the reviewers conclude that the Lachman and pivot shift tests are recommended over the anterior drawer. This information is more or less confirmed by the information presented in the abstracts of the more recent reviews (Van Eck *et al.* 2013; Leblanc *et al.* 2015) and appears to be in line with the comprehensive AAOS guidelines.

Donna is therefore confident that the Lachman test is a useful clinical test for acute and chronic ACL tears. It has high sensitivity and specificity and this means that most positive test results will be true positives, and most negative test results true negatives. The pivot shift test is very specific in chronic injuries, but the estimate of specificity in acute injuries has a very large confidence band (from 48–100 per cent), so she decides this test is most useful as a follow-up test to the Lachman in the assessment of chronic injuries.

Using the guideline, the systematic review and an article from the *Australian Journal of Physiotherapy* (Davidson 2002) on the interpretation of diagnostic tests, Donna draws the following conclusion: 'Where the patient history suggests an ACL injury may have occurred (i.e. sporting injury, audible "snap" or "pop", a sense of instability of the knee and swelling following the injury), a positive Lachman test is strongly suggestive of an ACL tear. In chronic injuries, a positive pivot shift test is strongly suggestive of an ACL tear.' Donna suspects that both tests might not be necessary and calculates the pre- and post-test probabilities of an ACL tear. She determines that she would be 50 per cent confident in her diagnosis given a patient history suggestive of an acute ACL injury. She calculates that if the Lachman test was positive, using the positive LR of 9.4, she would then be 90 per cent confident of the diagnosis.[1] If the condition was chronic, a subsequent positive pivot shift test would increase her confidence to 99 per cent.[2] Donna thinks that in fact the second test is not essential.

Step 5: Assess the process

Donna feels she used her time effectively in answering her clinical question using the best available evidence. The next time she has a clinical query regarding diagnostic accuracy, she is confident she can efficiently perform the steps required to make the best use of the available evidence. She continues to be frustrated at finding key articles behind paywalls.

STOP AND THINK

- What test or tests do you use most often in your practice?
- Can you find a systematic review of the evidence for the accuracy of these tests?

Summary

By following a step-wise approach to locating, appraising and applying the best research evidence, therapists are likely to arrive at conclusions regarding treatment that ultimately lead to better outcomes for their patients. EBP does not aim to base clinical decisions purely on research, but to ensure that the characteristics of the patient and the expertise of the therapist are combined with the most up-to-date and clinically relevant knowledge to guide treatment.

While there may be a very large body of research for some questions, several mechanisms can streamline the process of accessing them. Understanding what type of research design will provide the highest level of evidence can significantly shorten the search for research articles. Knowledge of databases containing pre-appraised literature can mean that therapists need to spend less time determining the quality of the research.

Finally, the best way to make the process more efficient is to practise. Honing EBP-based skills can be just as important as developing clinical techniques, as greater confidence will lead to the ability to effectively work around barriers such as access to full versions of articles. Physiotherapists recognise the importance of EBP but find the process of searching for and appraising the best evidence time-consuming. If Danny and Donna continue to answer their own clinical questions using the step-wise approach, not only are their patients likely to experience better outcomes, but time will become less of a barrier to practising evidence-based physiotherapy.

Practice exercises

1   What question regarding the effectiveness of therapy do you want to answer? Write that question in the PICO format.

   P—Population: what group of people are you interested in?

   I—Intervention: what therapy do you want to know about?

   C—Comparison: what do you want to compare the therapy to?

   O—Outcome: what do you expect to be the result of applying the therapy?

2   Using the terms from your research question above, search the Cochrane Library and PEDro for evidence to answer your question.

3   Are there any clinical guidelines that will help answer your question(s)? These can be found in PEDro.

4   Is there any pre-appraised evidence that answers your question(s)? This can be found in PEDro and the Cochrane Library.

Notes

1   Pre-test probability of 50% converts to pre-test odds of 1 (odds = p/(1–p)), multiplied by the +LR of 9.4 gives a post-test odds of 9.4, which converts to a post-test probability of 90% (p = odds/(1–odds)).

2   Pre-test probability of 90% converts to pre-test odds of 9 (odds = 0.90/(1–.90)), multiplied by the +LR of 7.7 gives a post-test odds of 69.3, which converts to a post-test probability of 99% (p = 69.3/70.3).

Megan Davidson and Ross Iles

Further reading

Herbert, R., Jamtvedt, G., Mead, J. & Birger Hagen, K. (2011). *Practical evidence-based physiotherapy*, 2nd edn. Edinburgh: Elsevier Butterworth Heinemann.

Hoffmann, T., Bennett, S. & Del Mar, C. (2010). *Evidence-based practice across the health professions*. Sydney: Elsevier Churchill Livingstone.

Websites

www.cebm.net

> The Centre for Evidence Based Medicine is an excellent source of information and tools to help with critical appraisal.

www.pedro.org.au

> The Physiotherapy Evidence Database contains clinical practice guidelines, systematic reviews and clinical trials. Clinical trials in the PEDro database have been critically appraised using the PEDro scale.

www.thecochranelibrary.com/view/0/index.html

> All residents of Australia and New Zealand have access to the Cochrane Library.

www.ncbi.nlm.nih.gov/pubmed

> PubMed (Public Medline) Database is a freely available database containing millions of citations that may or may not have links to full text content.

www.nzgg.org.nz

> The New Zealand Guidelines Group provides access to a range of practice guidelines and practice tools including patient information brochures.

www.unisa.edu.au/cahe/

> The International Centre for Allied Health Evidence at the University of South Australia has a range of online resources to support clinicians, researchers, students and consumers.

18

Metasynthesis in Health Care Research

TERESE BONDAS, ELISABETH O.C. HALL AND ANITA WIKBERG

Chapter objectives

In this chapter you will learn:

- what metasynthesis is and its history
- how metasynthesis applies to research in health care
- how to design and conduct a metasynthesis study

Key terms

Effect size

Line of argument

Meta-data analysis

Meta-ethnography

Meta-method analysis

Meta research

Meta-study

Metasummary

Metasynthesis

Meta-theory

Qualitative research

Qualitative research synthesis

Reciprocal translation

Refutational translation

Introduction

Metasynthesis is a generic term for review approaches to qualitative studies in a field of interest (Thorne *et al.* 2004). Barroso and colleagues (2003, p. 154) give the following definition: 'Qualitative meta-synthesis refers to both an interpretive product and the analytic processes, by which the findings of studies are aggregated, integrated, summarized, or otherwise put together.' Sandelowski and Barroso (2007) further explain that metasynthesis is an interpretive integration of qualitative findings that are themselves interpretive syntheses of data, including phenomenologies, ethnographies, grounded theories, and other integrated and coherent descriptions or explanations of phenomena, events or cases. Metasynthesis means integration that is more than the sum of the parts, in that a novel interpretation of findings is offered. The goal is to achieve an integrative interpretation of findings that is more substantive than those resulting from individual studies. Thus metasynthesis research evokes both ontological questions (what is knowledge?) and epistemological questions (how to arrive at knowledge?) (see Chapter 1).

Research related to the insider perspectives in health care (Mantzoukas 2009) and in nursing (Beck 2013) has increased. This research is largely qualitative and often relies on open-ended interviews; it is a science of words, compared to quantitative research which is a science of numbers (Denzin 2008; Liamputtong 2013; see Chapter 1). This verbal scientific knowledge is not always used to develop evidence-based care. Nevertheless, the interest in metasynthesis indicates a paradigmatic crisis in the health disciplines and points to a new developmental phase of qualitative research (Bondas & Hall 2007a; Paterson 2013). Generally, in social and health care research, there is interest in new methodological approaches that engage novice as well as seasoned researchers (Thorne *et al.* 2004) and are appropriate to verbal as well as visual methodologies (Guillemin 2004; Liamputtong & Rumbold 2008; Guillemin & Drew 2010).

Beginning in the late 1980s, pleas went out for integrating qualitative nursing research studies (Estabrooks *et al.* 1994; Jensen & Allen 1996; Kirkevold 1997; Sandelowski *et al.* 1997; Schreiber *et al.* 1997). The search for unifying qualitative knowledge has since become important to further an evidence-based practice (EBP), spark critical discussion and add to theoretical development (Sandelowski & Barroso 2007; Hannes & Lockwood 2011). In this century, the number of metasynthesis studies has increased enormously (see Hannes & Macaitis 2012; France *et al.* 2014). A terminology has slowly emerged and is becoming established in methodological as well as empirical metasynthesis studies. There are, however, different views of terminology and applications in methodological articles and textbooks. Some of them will be mentioned here.

The metasynthesis development in health research started with **meta-ethnography** (Noblit & Hare 1988), continued in nursing science with meta-study including **meta-data analysis**, **meta-method analysis** and **meta-theory** analysis to create a metasynthesis (Paterson *et al.* 2001) and went further with **metasummary** (Sandelowski and Barroso 2007) (see also Chapter 6). Metasynthesis as an approach is outlined in several studies

---

Metasynthesis: A generic term that represents qualitative review approaches to previous qualitative studies in a field of interest.

Meta-ethnography: An approach that enables a rigorous procedure for deriving substantive interpretations about any set of ethnographic or interpretive studies.

Meta-data analysis: Analysis of processed data from selected qualitative research studies.

Meta-method analysis: The study of research methods to determine the way qualitative methods are interpreted and implemented. Underlying methodological assumptions and trends and their meaning for the research finding are studied.

Meta-theory: Part of a meta-study: determining the link between the theoretical perspective that frames each primary study and the methods, findings and conclusions of the research.

(Beck 2002a, b; Britten *et al.* 2002; Finfgeld 2003; McCormick *et al.* 2003; Bondas & Hall 2007a, b; Major & Savin-Badin 2010; Hannes & Lockwood 2012; Paterson 2013). Drawing on Bondas and Hall's (2007b) division of studies in (1) health, illness and suffering, (2) care and support and (3) parenting, newborn and child care, we provide some examples from recent metasynthesis studies and their employed methodology (Table 18.1).

Metasummary: Aggregation of reports of primary qualitative studies containing findings in the form of topical or thematic summaries or surveys of data, which are not interpretive syntheses of data.

TABLE 18.1   Examples from metasynthesis studies and their employed methodology

RESEARCH AREAS	EXAMPLES OF METASYNTHESIS STUDIES	EMPLOYED METHODOLOGY
Health and illness	Flemming 2009, 2010	Dixon-Woods *et al.* 2006b
	Malpass *et al.* 2009	Noblit & Hare 1988
	Duggleby *et al.* 2012	Sandelowski & Barroso 2007
	Lundgren *et al.* 2012	Noblit & Hare 1988
	Vaismoradi *et al.* 2016	Noblit & Hare 1988
Care and support	Gomersall *et al.* 2011	Paterson *et al.* 2001
	Goethals *et al.* 2012	Noblit & Hare 1988
	Walsh & Devane 2012	Joanna Briggs Institute 2008c
	Uhrenfeldt *et al.* 2013	Sandelowski & Barroso 2007
	Franzel *et al.* 2013	Noblit & Hare 1988
Parenting, newborn, child and adolescent care	Aagaard & Hall 2008	Noblit & Hare 1988
	Reid *et al.* 2009	Noblit & Hare 1988
	Wikberg & Bondas 2010	Noblit & Hare 1988
	Beck 2011	Noblit & Hare 1988
	Fegran *et al.* 2014	Sandelowski & Barroso 2007
	Eri *et al.* 2015	Noblit & Hare 1988
	Lee *et al.* 2015	Paterson *et al.* 2001
Reviews of metasynthesis studies	Finfgeld 2003	Thematic analysis
	Bondas & Hall 2007a, b	Paterson *et al.* 2001
	Dixon-Woods *et al.* 2006b	Noblit & Hare 1988
	Hannes & Macaitis 2012	Review
	Finfgeld-Connett 2014	Content analysis
	France *et al.* 2014	Systematic review

Metasynthesis will now be outlined through the questions of 'what', 'why' and 'how'.

The 'what' of metasynthesis

Meta- is a prefix meaning among, along with, of a higher or second-order kind, and often denoting change. The aim of metasynthesis is critical analysis and synthesis resulting in a deepened understanding and development of new or modified theories, thus creating a

Terese Bondas, Elisabeth O.C. Hall and Anita Wikberg

knowledge base from qualitative studies for EBP. The research process in metasynthesis is akin to qualitative empirical studies, with some exceptions primarily related to data and sampling. Previous research publications in a topic are the primary and only data, making metasynthesis meaningful only if there are enough studies in the topic area. In other words, primary researchers are limited in their topic choice only by their creativity, while metasynthesists study topics that are found in the literature.

Metasynthesis research may be compared to other review types such as integrative reviews, systematic reviews, meta-analysis and secondary analysis, but it aggregates, interprets and synthesises only qualitative findings; integrative and systematic reviews include both quantitative and qualitative research (Kirkevold 1997; Sandelowski *et al.* 2007, 2012; Gough *et al.* 2012; Whittemore *et al.* 2014). The main idea is to record the progress in a given domain, identify the gaps and weak points that remain, and thus plot future interventions or summarise evidence regarding a specific clinical problem. Meta-analysis is a summary of quantitative research of similar methodology, using statistics to transform findings of studies with related hypotheses into a metric, calculating magnitude of effect to estimate this effect of interventions or relationships (Glass *et al.* 1981; Whittemore *et al.* 2014). Mixed methods have developed in recent years, combining meta-analysis of quantitative studies and metasynthesis of qualitative studies, such as critical interpretive synthesis (Dixon-Woods *et al.* 2006a). In secondary analysis (Thorne 1994, 1998; Heaton 2004, 2008; Long-Sutehall *et al.* 2010), researchers return to their own or other primary data and ask new questions to get a new perspective on the topic.

Metasynthesising in nursing science has several roots (Bondas & Hall 2007a), which can be traced to sociology and ethnography through meta-theorising discussions (Ritzer 1990; Zhao 1991) and Noblit and Hare's meta-ethnography (1988). Actually, meta-ethnography is the most common methodological choice in metasynthesis research in nursing science (Thorne *et al.* 2004; Bondas & Hall 2007b). One root emanates from the critique of qualitative research in nursing science and another goes back to meta-analysis. Approaches to metasynthesis have many similar charateristics but differ depending on epistemology, analytical approach, techniques and synthesis output (Zimmer 2006; Ludvigsen *et al.* 2013). Table 18.2 offers examples of metasynthesis methods and their key characteristics from Noblit and Hare's meta-ethnography in 1988 and since.

TABLE 18.2 Metasynthesis methodologies and their key characteristics

AUTHOR(S), YEAR DEVELOPED	NAME OF SYNTHESIS METHOD	KEY CHARACTERISTIC OF METHOD
Noblit & Hare 1988	Meta-ethnography	Translating study findings into each other and interpreting the results in a synthesis
Kearney 1998a, b, 2001b	Formal grounded theory	Middle-range theory is developed using theoretical sampling and constant comparison from substantive theories but is restricted to grounded theory findings

AUTHOR(S), YEAR DEVELOPED	NAME OF SYNTHESIS METHOD	KEY CHARACTERISTIC OF METHOD
Paterson *et al.* 2001	Meta-study	A social construction of interpretations of findings, methods and theories in primary studies. The key concepts are meta-theory, meta-method, meta-findings
Dixon-Woods *et al.* 2006b	Critical interpretive synthesis	Large sample that draws on both qualitative (following Noblit & Hare 1988) and quantitative reports to present a comprehensive, interpretive narrative
Sandelowski & Barroso 2007	Qualitative research synthesis study	Integrates findings in primary qualitative studies into metasummaries and metasynthesis through effect sizes, narratives and visual displays
Thomas & Harden 2008	Thematic synthesis	Coding text of findings, developing descriptive themes, generating analytical themes (inspired by grounded theory and earlier metasynthesis methods)
Major & Savin-Baden 2010	Qualitative research synthesis	Developing a conceptual translation, a reinterpretation of findings in primary qualitative reports

STOP AND THINK

Several terms have been used for metasynthesis. List them and try to figure out what they mean and how they differ from each other.

The 'why' of metasynthesis

The motives for metasynthesis research in health sciences are twofold.

- Will this knowledge make a difference in the life of people that it may concern?
- Will the findings of the study develop knowledge that furthers the development of the discipline?

Some answers are given in the next section.

Terese Bondas, Elisabeth O.C. Hall and Anita Wikberg

Development of evidence-based health care

The number of qualitative studies related to health, illness and care is increasing. The publications, however, have often been widely scattered. The significance of a metasynthesis lies in its potential to present condensed knowledge in an area of interest, and thus its potential to strengthen research-based care in the field and make it easier to use in evidence-based health care. There is a need to gather what is known for the benefit of health care, and for qualitative research findings to have a stronger impact on decision-making in health policies (Finfgeld 2003). The question is to communicate the findings in a meaningful way and in relevant media so that they are accessible and interesting to practitioners. Thus, conclusions drawn need to have meaning outside the context of the study (Finfgeld-Connett 2010). Metasynthesis makes a difference for qualitative studies because they often cannot be generalised outside their own context.

Deepening the knowledge and understanding

Metasynthesis encompasses strategies for both critique and evaluation of previous research, and strong incentives for generating new theory. Metasynthesis, similar to any qualitative methodology, may be inductive (generating theory on different levels), deductive (based on an explicit theoretical perspective) or abductive (a rhythmic movement between theory and practice) (Råholm 2012; Bondas 2013). The aim is a new, integrated and more complete interpretation of findings that offers deeper and broader understanding than the findings from individual studies. 'Push the level of theory' is a phrase that contains the message for metasynthesis (Schreiber *et al.* 1997, p. 315). Over the past two decades, more than twenty methods of metasynthesis have been developed (Paterson 2013). The importance of the question of disciplinary development in a **meta-study** is emphasised (Noblit & Hare 1988; Paterson *et al.* 2001; Thorne *et al.* 2002; Sandelowski & Barroso 2007). The studies may include comparison and consideration of the implication of context, theory and method, and a philosophical perspective that furthers the development of the actual substance and the growth of the discipline. All synthesis of multiple qualitative studies includes interpretation. Synthesis means, according to Noblit and Hare (1988), giving meaning to a set of studies, and thus it is a true kind of qualitative research. **Meta research** allows organisation in a comprehensive bibliography as well (Paterson *et al.* 2001). The findings of meta research could thus provide an interesting basis for new research questions, especially for deepening the possibilities of cross-disciplinary research. As well, there is a strong ethical reason to choose meta-studies when vulnerable themes are involved that have already gained research attention, especially when there seem to be conflicting findings (Thorne 1998). Finfgeld-Connett (2014) writes that metasyntheses are often analysed into new categories prematurely and suggests that categories should be compared to each other to maximise meaning, for example into a metaphor or a model, which could improve their use in clinical care, policy-making and theory generation.

Meta-study: A systematic interpretive research approach that involves a tripartite analysis of data, method and theory, then a metasynthesis of an existing body of qualitative research and creative interpretation of the primary research to produce new and expanded understandings.

Meta research: Critical analysis and synthesis resulting in a deepened interpretive understanding and development of new or modified theory, thus creating a qualitative knowledge base for evidence-based care.

STOP AND THINK

Why have metasynthesis methods been developed? What is their goal? Which arguments are in favour and which are against using metasynthesis for EBP?

The 'how' of metasynthesis

There are several different metasynthesis methods and there is ongoing development in the field. A metasynthesis always includes searching for studies to answer a specific question, quality evaluation of the studies, breaking up data (the different parts of the reported studies), looking at the whole of each study and data in order to undertake aggregation, analysis, synthesis and interpretation.

As seen in Table 18.2, there are plenty of methods to choose from when considering a metasynthesis study. In this section, we present two of them in depth: Noblit and Hare's (N&H) meta-ethnography because it is the most common, and Sandelowski and Barroso's (S&B) **qualitative research synthesis** study (QRSS) because, together with experiences of our own metasynthesis, it most rigorously furthers phases from meta-ethnography. We illustrate the methods with examples from Wikberg and Bondas (2010) to give readers a picture of the complexity of a metasynthesis study.

Noblit and Hare developed their meta-ethnography approach in 1988, primarily to synthesise ethnographies. However, the approach enables a rigorous procedure for deriving substantive interpretations about any set of interpretive or descriptive studies. Meta-ethnography holds the two premises that interpretive explanation is essentially translation and that a metasynthesis is a **reciprocal translation** of studies. These premises make it possible to retain the uniqueness of the primary findings even when synthesised, as well as presenting meta-ethnography as a whole that is more than the parts alone imply. The process is described in seven phases (Noblit & Hare 1988; Britten *et al.* 2002; France *et al.* 2014):

- getting started
- deciding what is relevant to the initial interest
- reading the studies
- determining how studies are related
- translating the studies into one another
- synthesising translations
- expressing the synthesis.

Through a series of studies on HIV among women, Sandelowski and Barroso developed the qualitative research synthesis with methodological scrutiny of every step. They introduced the term 'metasummary' for aggregation of issues from the included reports, which do not aim

Qualitative research synthesis: This is both an interpretive product (the synthesis itself) and the methods and techniques used to create that product.

Reciprocal translation: In meta-ethnography, studies can be combined such that one study can be presented in terms of another. The accounts are then directly comparable as 'reciprocal' translations and analogous ones.

for interpretive syntheses of data but still are interesting enough to present (Sandelowski & Barroso 2003, 2007). The techniques involve the extraction and reduction of data and the calculation of effect sizes, which may serve as a foundation for the metasynthesis (for effect size see Chapter 26). The phases of their QRSS studies (Sandelowski 2007; Sandelowski & Barroso 2007) concern:

- conceiving the qualitative research synthesis study
- deciding the target of the study
- appraising included reports
- developing metasummaries
- performing targeted comparison using imported concepts and reciprocal translations
- forming the metasynthesis
- presenting the syntheses
- transforming the findings for use in practice.

Several phases of Noblit and Hare's and Sandelowski and Barroso's methodologies overlap, and this is the main reason why we chose to present them together.

Getting started: conceiving the synthesis

An old proverb says, 'Well planned is half done'. This is certainly true for metasynthesis research, and Sandelowski and Barroso (2007) do not hesitate to emphasise the importance of a start that is well thought through. Noblit and Hare (1988, p. 27) add, 'this phase is finding something that is worthy of the synthesis effort', something that requires a deeper understanding when combining what we know with what we don't yet know. Either we need to be acquainted with the studies in the field of interest, or the aim needs to be changed alongside the study (Finfgeld-Connett 2014; Ludvigsen *et al.* 2016) This first phase is about conceiving the synthesis study, which according to Sandelowski and Barroso (2007) needs time and reflection. Researchers have to:

- get acquainted with the research process
- define a significant research problem
- formulate a research purpose
- consider the resources available to the group
- decide the target of the study
- consider inclusion and exclusion criteria
- develop a working definition of the topic.

The last point is extremely important: it is easily underestimated and doing so might cause unnecessary problems in the procedure of the study. The working definition is subject to change but needs to be focused from the beginning in order to proceed with the literature search. We consider the working definition as analogous to what Noblit and Hare (1988, p. 26) refer to as 'identifying an intellectual interest that qualitative research might inform'.

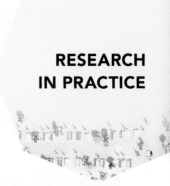

**RESEARCH
IN PRACTICE**

INTERCULTURAL CARING IN MATERNITY CARE SEARCH

The aim in Wikberg and Bondas' (2010) metasynthesis was to explore and describe intercultural caring (Wikberg & Eriksson 2008) in maternity care research from a patient perspective. The theoretical perspective of the study was the theory of caritative caring developed by the Finnish nurse theorist Katie Eriksson. This reflective process of ontology and epistemology, of assumptions and theoretical contexts in the first phase of the study assisted the researchers to acknowledge what was important to focus on and why. Methodological reflections made the researchers choose Noblit and Hare's meta-ethnography because its design corresponded with their intellectual and interpretive interest. Early reflection on the method helped them understand how to create knowledge of the topic and how to keep the focus.

Deciding what is relevant to the initial interest: the target of the study

The literature search follows the conceiving of the study, a part of the metasynthesis in which today's researchers engage intensely. They often present a flowchart that shows the search process (e.g. Jones 2004, p. 274).

MeSH (Medical Subject Headings)-terms or CINAHL Subject Headings can be checked for finding good search words (www.nlm.nih.gov/pubs/factsheets/mesh.html or http://support.ebsco.com/knowledge_base/detail.php?id=5172 or http://support.ebsco.com/knowledge_base/detail.php?id=4568).

Previous metasynthesis and meta-analysis studies, as well as systematic reviews on the topic, are relevant to search for. Exhausted searching of health and social science literature requires a range of search strategies and techniques such as citation searching, reference list checking and contact with experts and librarians (Papapioannou *et al.* 2009; Booth *et al.* 2012). Havill and colleagues (2014) describe how their team managed the literature search through separating the search in topic-specific text-word search strings. Sandelowski and Barroso focus more on the meaning of the validity of the search, which needs to be exhaustive, than do Noblit and Hare. Based on the working definition, researchers should set parameters to use in the electronic search, and they are advised several times to use a 'berry-picking' strategy to search sources in reference lists, footnotes and journals relevant to the target area. No study of relevance has to be left behind. Sample size alone does not predict the sophistication of findings (Finfgeld-Connett 2014), and therefore needs to be decided in relation to each metasynthesis study and its aim. Finfgeld-Connett (2014) even recommends a randomised selection of a sample or narrowing the aim and research question. Enough time should be allotted to search in databases with the help of a librarian, to search 'cited citations' or 'similar titles' in elected databases, to read journals specific to interest, and to hand-search in reference lists, thematic issues of journals and known web pages. Author searches may be performed, both as back- as well as forward-tracking of references (Sandelowski & Barroso 2007).

Terese Bondas, Elisabeth O.C. Hall and Anita Wikberg

Noblit and Hare call this phase 'deciding what is relevant to the initial interest'. They argue for a justified reason for doing a huge search. Is it relevant to synthesise all ethnographies on a certain topic? Accordingly, 'the answer to this question seems to dictate gross generalizations that an interpretive meta-ethnography would find unacceptable' (Noblit & Hare 1988, p. 27). To do an exhaustive search is, from an ethnographic point of view, fruitless. More importantly, according to Noblit and Hare, the search needs to consider what is credible and of interest for the readers of the study and for the researchers themselves. However, it seems today that journals ask for exhaustive literature searches and a flowchart—either the metasynthesis follows Noblit and Hare's now twenty-five-year-old methodology or it doesn't. Requests for validity have changed. As seen below, Wikberg and Bondas (2010), who use Noblit and Hare's methodology, describe their search process with scrutiny.

RESEARCH IN PRACTICE

SYSTEMATIC LITERATURE SEARCH

Wikberg and Bondas (2010) write that this phase of deciding the target involved a search for previous metasynthesis studies on the topic, followed by a literature search and the establishment of inclusion and exclusion criteria. They found six metasynthesis studies on maternal care, four studies on caring but only one on intercultural caring, and that one had a nurse perspective. A systematic literature search was done on several occasions during the course of the study. Inclusion criteria were scientific qualitative empirical articles in languages understood by the researchers (English, German, Finnish, Swedish, Norwegian and Danish). The substantive inclusion criterion was intercultural caring in the context of maternity care from the perspective of patients from all ethnic groups. The time criterion was also decided. If there were several perspectives, such as nurses', students'

or relatives', or if it was a qualitative and quantitative study, it had to be possible to separate the results. Theoretical and review articles were excluded because they would have been difficult to compare with empirical studies. Dissertations and Master's theses and research reports were excluded because it is difficult to get hold of them. Doctoral studies are often published as articles and the review process with Master's theses is not the same as with articles. The literature was searched electronically on web pages, in databases and reference lists, through author names and journal names. The database search included Cinahl and Medline and several full-text databases completed by manual searches. A combination of keywords (caring, transcultural, maternity) was used. Choosing studies proceeded from hits (>3,000,000) to titles (>10,000) to abstracts (500–1000) to full text (119), and finally to included studies (40).

Reading the studies: appraising included reports

In this phase (reading and appraising the reports), the researchers spend time reading the included studies over and over again to form metaphors—the expression Noblit and Hare (1988) use for categories and themes—to know how each contributes to the overall aim of the study. Noblit and Hare do not mention appraisal but they emphasise that researchers should appreciate the studies: 'Meta-ethnography … requires extensive attention to the details in the accounts, and what they tell you about your substantive concerns' (p. 28).

Using Sandelowski and Barroso's (2007) methodology, this phase involves both repeated reading and critical appraisal. 'Appraisal' refers to two elements: appreciation and evaluation. 'Appreciation' means to understand what is said and found in the report, to pay attention to details. 'Evaluation' involves what is and what is not in a report and the reviewers' judgment on the usefulness of the study. There are several appraisal tools to choose from (see e.g. Walsh & Downe 2006; Tong *et al.* 2007; Dixon-Woods *et al.* 2007b; Sandelowski & Barroso 2007; Joanna Briggs Institute 2008a, b; CASP 2013). We suggest that researchers get acquainted with some of them, then choose one that is comfortable to use and not too lengthy. Also, do not underestimate your own ability to form judgments about the quality of a study, as doing this is similar to many peer review processes. Appraisal checklists are not always easy to operate. The reviewers also have to rely on their own judgments. Meta-study and critical interpretive synthesis—two more subjective idealist approaches—look to the content and utility of findings rather than methodology in order to establish quality (Barnett-Page & Thomas 2009). Noblit and Hare (1988) originally discussed quality in terms of quality of the metaphor, but recent use of this method has used amended versions of CASP (the Critical Appraisal Skills Program tool), yet has only referred to studies being excluded on the basis of lack of relevance or methodological weakness. In summary, it is evident that the issue of quality appraisal varies and is still in development.

A CHECKLIST FOR APPRECIATION AND EVALUATION

Wikberg and Bondas (2010) used Sandelowski and Barroso's (2007, pp. 75–131) appraisal ideas as a checklist for appreciation and evaluation. The studies were checked for aim and research questions, result of literature review, perspective and assumptions, methods, findings and ethical considerations. The findings had to be congruent with the study's aim and described method. A short summary was done on the content of all forty included articles, to get a manageable picture of the whole. The text that answered the aim in each article was underlined and codes that later were clustered together to become themes or metaphors were written in the margins. Close readings of the summaries showed that eleven of the studies were published in the USA or Canada, ten in the UK, eight in Australia, eight in Scandinavian countries and one each in Japan, Israel and South Africa. Most articles were published in nursing journals and a few were in medical, public health and psychology journals. More than 1160 women from more than fifty cultures were represented in the articles. The samples varied from five to 388. Interviews were the most common data-collecting method and ethnography, content analysis, grounded theory and thematic analysis were used as analysing methods. The context in all the studies was prenatal, birth or postnatal care, or a combination of these.

RESEARCH IN PRACTICE

Terese Bondas, Elisabeth O.C. Hall and Anita Wikberg

Developing metasummaries

A special feature of the Sandelowski and Barroso methodology is the emphasis on numbers and counting. Developing metasummaries refers to addressing the manifest content in findings throughout primary studies. Metasummaries are powerful rhetorical devices that illuminate the labour put down in qualitative work. By extracting, grouping and abstracting findings, researchers calculate the frequency and approximate effect size of findings, thus adding to study validity. Calculating effect sizes offers reviewers a big picture of the findings, stimulates the testing of hypothesis and helps make analytic or idiographic contextual generalisations (Sandelowski & Barroso 2007). The idea is to take the number of primary studies containing a theme and divide that number by the total number of primary studies included in the studies. If the same sample is used in several studies, they can only be counted as one sample. Table 18.3 shows the principle of this calculation using a metasynthesis of four studies. The approximate effect size of Theme 1 is 75 per cent if three-quarters of all studies contribute to that theme. Fegran and colleagues (2014, p. 127) calculated effect sizes in their metasynthesis about adolescents' and young adults' experiences of transition. The authors found that data were relatively equally distributed across the subthemes regardless of the methodological approach of the primary studies.

TABLE 18.3   An example of the principle for showing approximate effect size of themes in a metasynthesis

	THEME 1	THEME 2	THEME 3	THEME 4
Primary study 1	x		x	
Primary study 2	x	x	x	x
Primary study 3	x	x	x	x
Primary study 4		x	x	
Approximate effect size	75%	75%	100%	50%

Determining how studies are related: targeted comparison

The next phase focuses on how the studies are related, putting together and determining relationships between them. Noblit and Hare (1988) suggest that researchers create a list of the key metaphors, phrases, ideas and/or concepts and their relations used in each account, and juxtapose them. At the end of this phase, an initial assumption about the relationship between the studies is often reached. It is vital that researchers be explicit about any assumption made. There are at least three ways to order the studies.

- The studies can be combined such that one study can be presented in terms of another. The accounts are then directly comparable as reciprocal or analogous translations. Analogous translations are the most common finding.

- The studies can be set against one another such that the grounds for one study's refutation of another become visible. The accounts stand in relative opposition to each other and are essentially **refutational** or oppositional. Synthesising refutations is a procedure that sensitises researchers to the assumptions guiding the involved studies. The primary studies construct interpretations under very different rules; any variations may be due to these rules. Refutations may be driven by dogma, and refutations of such dogma may be dogmatic in themselves. If the descriptions are reasonable but the interpretations are ideological, then multiple interpretations are recommended (Noblit & Hare 1988). Refutational accounts (also called deviant or disconfirming cases) are particularly important because synthesists naturally look for similarities (Booth *et al.* 2013).

- The studies can be tied to each other by noting how one study informs and goes beyond another. The studies taken together then represent a **line of argument**. The guiding question is what can be said about the whole based on selective studies of the part.

Sandelowski and Barroso (2007) have similar thoughts and see the translations as ways of doing a constant targeted comparison using imported (borrowed from other disciplines) concepts that confirm, extend or refute each other.

Translating the studies into one another: forming the qualitative metasynthesis

A couple of phases are described together here because they interrelate. Translations are unique because they protect the particular, respect holism and enable comparison. An adequate translation maintains the central metaphors and/or concepts of each account in their relation to other key metaphors or concepts in that account. It also compares both the metaphors or concepts and their interactions with those in the other accounts. A metaphor is adequate when it achieves the explanation without redundancy, ambiguity and contradiction (Noblit & Hare 1988). An ideal metaphor is 'economic, cogent, apparent, broad and credible' (Finfgeld-Connett 2014, p. 1586). Paterson (2007, p. 76) states that 'key metaphors are words, phrases, ideas, concepts or categories that encapsulate research findings'. Dam and Hall (2016) use 'compass' as a metaphor for how children of mentally ill parents navigate their daily life.

Sandelowski and Barroso (2007) warn against re-presentation of findings in metasynthesis research. Metasyntheses are conducted with the intention of being useful in practice, to present evidence for practice. The experiences lived or told in the primary sources are, however, retold by the research participants then reinterpreted by the reviewers. Along the path, the research participants' experiences have been transformed. The problem for the reviewers is to get the researchers'—not the research participants'—interpretations right because the participants' descriptions have already been transformed by the researchers. What the reviewers should come up with, therefore, is not the reality through a mere reorganisation or recategorisation of existing findings. Rather, reviewers should place the findings into context and articulate relationships between phenomena or themes (Finfgeld-Connett 2014). This is to achieve 'a lived border of reality and representation' (Gubrium & Holstein, cited in Sandelowski 2006, p. 12).

Refutational: In meta-ethnography, studies can be set against one another such that the grounds for one study's refutation of another become visible. The accounts stand in relative opposition to each other and so are essentially 'refutational' or oppositional.

Line of argument: In meta-ethnography, studies can be tied to one another by noting just how one study informs and goes beyond another. The guiding question is what can be said about the whole based on selective studies of the part.

Terese Bondas, Elisabeth O.C. Hall and Anita Wikberg

Expressing and presenting the metasynthesis

In expressing and presenting the metasynthesis, researchers have to choose their audience and what and how they want to publish. Narrative accounts and visual displays are ways of presenting. Narrative accounts presented in thematic sentences make the findings accessible and usable in clinical practice (Sandelowski & Leeman 2012). Visual displays are powerful rhetorical devices. Sandelowski and Barroso (2007) call on reviewers to be creative and spend just as much time constructing visual devices as writing narrative text. Their handbook includes a handful of figures (see also visual displays in Reid *et al.* 2009; Uhrenfeldt *et al.* 2013; Leeman *et al.* 2015; Dam & Hall 2016).

RESEARCH IN PRACTICE

PRESENTING FINDINGS IN REFUTATIONAL METAPHORS

Wikberg and Bondas (2010) expressed their metasynthesis by writing an article and presenting it at international conferences. The findings were presented in refutational metaphors. There was also an overarching metaphor, which had three aspects. First, the names of the metaphors were given and the content described, then quotations were used from as many different studies as possible to validate the content. Quotations were mostly original expressions from participants but were occasionally descriptions from the authors of the original study. The metaphors were:

- caring versus non-caring

- language and communication problems versus information and choice
- access to medical and technological care versus incompetence
- acculturation: preserving the original culture versus adapting to a new culture
- professional caring relationship versus family and community involvement
- caring is important for well-being and health versus conflicts cause interrupted care
- vulnerable women with painful memories versus racism
- 'Alice in Wonderland' as an overarching metaphor that captured all the studies.

STOP AND THINK

Reflect on the method phases in your metasynthesis study and try to answer the following questions.

- What does it mean to create a working definition when starting a metasynthesis study?
- How can a librarian assist in searching the literature?
- What does it mean to translate studies into each other?
- What is the difference between a metasummary and a metasynthesis?

Validity of a metasynthesis

For Noblit and Hare (1988), evaluation of a meta-ethnography relates to whether it clarifies and resolves rather than observes inconsistencies or tensions between material synthesised, whether a progressive problem shifts results, and whether the synthesis is consistent, parsimonious, elegant, fruitful and useful. Over the years the demands on validity of metasynthesis reports have been tightened. Sandelowski and Barroso (2007, pp. 227–34) call on reviewers to consider their take on validity from the time they conceive the study, because validity relates to the truth of the study. There are multiple versions of truth—for Sandelowski and Barroso, truth is socially constructed. For them, optimising validity in a metasynthesis study is enhanced through descriptive, interpretive, theoretical, pragmatic and negotiated consensual validity. The meaning of these terms is shown in Table 18.4.

TABLE 18.4   Ways of optimising validity

Descriptive validity	Identification of all relevant research reports Accurate characterisation of each report
Interpretive validity	Full and fair representation of the primary researchers' understanding or point of view
Theoretical validity	Credibility of the reviewers' interpretation of the primary researchers' finding
Pragmatic validity	Utility and transferability of knowledge Applicability, timeliness and translatability for practice of evidence synthesis
Negotiated consensual validity	Intra- and inter-reviewer negotiations and explications of judgments 'Think aloud' strategies

Source: Sandelowski and Barroso (2007)

STOP AND THINK

During a metasynthesis study, researchers need to keep asking the following validity questions (see Paterson *et al.* 2001; Bondas & Hall 2007a; Sandelowski & Barroso 2007).

- Has it, as completely as possible, integrated, beyond aggregating, the research in this field within the disciplines of health sciences?
- Has it generated new or expanded knowledge, an alternative perspective on the phenomenon?
- Has it illuminated the implications of the contexts, methods and theories that have influenced the body of research?
- Has previous research been ethically analysed?
- Has a cultural multilingual approach facilitated understanding?
- Is a plan made for research reports to reach policy-makers, citizens and scholars?
- Has it enlarged human science knowledge for the benefit of patients and their families?

Terese Bondas, Elisabeth O.C. Hall and Anita Wikberg

Summary

In this chapter we have introduced metasynthesis as a qualitative research approach and several methods in development. The goal when choosing metasynthesis is to achieve an integrative interpretation of previous qualitative research that is more substantive than the findings from individual studies. We argue that metasynthesis research in health science research can make a difference in the life of people that it may concern; it can develop EBP in health care, and the findings of the metasynthesis study may further the development of the discipline.

An example of a metasynthesis study by Wikberg and Bondas (2010) on intercultural maternity care is provided to help readers plan a metasynthesis study. Metasynthesis research may be compared to other review types such as integrative reviews, systematic reviews, meta-analysis and secondary analysis, but metasynthesis is the type of review that aggregates and synthesises qualitative findings only. The development of metasynthesis started with meta-ethnography by Noblit and Hare in 1988, then continued with meta-study including meta-data analysis, meta-method analysis and meta-theory analysis to create metasynthesis (Paterson *et al.* 2001), and further with metasummary to qualitative research synthesis (Sandelowski & Barroso 2007).

The validity of a metasynthesis study depends on whether it clarifies and resolves rather than observes inconsistencies or tensions between material synthesised, and whether a progressive shift results. We agree with Noblit and Hare's view of a valid metasynthesis as consistent, parsimonious, elegant, fruitful and useful. And, finally, we argue that the metasynthesist needs to ask if their metasynthesis study enlarges human science knowledge.

ARGUMENTS FOR USING METASYNTHESIS
- Addresses the information explosion and knowledge fragmentation.
- Identifies gaps and omissions in a given body of research or within a single article.
- Provides ways to advance theory.
- Sparks dialogue and debate.
- Adds a depth dimension to qualitative studies, sometimes referred to as 'little islands of knowledge never to be revisited' (Sandelowski & Barroso 2007, p. 53).
- Aids development of EBP and policy. Qualitative research is endangered if not linked (Sandelowski & Barroso 2007, p. 3).
- Cost-effective approach.

ARGUMENTS FOR NOT USING METASYNTHESIS

- Restricted to what is already available in the literature that serves as data.
- Too much variety among qualitative methods for synthesis to be meaningful.
- The researcher lacks access to primary data.
- Context is stripped.
- Uses participants' and researchers' work without permission.

See also Bondas and Hall (2007b), Sandelowski and Barroso (2007), Major and Savin-Baden (2010).

Practice exercise

1 Reflect on the arguments for using or not using metasynthesis in the research area and write down the arguments for your metasynthesis study.

Further reading

Atkins, S., Lewin, S., Smith, H., Engel, M., Fretheim, A. & Volmink, J. (2008). Conducting a meta ethnography of qualitative literature: lessons learnt. *BMC Medical Research Methodology*, 8(21). DOI: 10.1186/1471-2288-8-21.

Campbell, R., Pound, P., Morgan, M., Britten, N., Pill, R., Yardley, L., Pope, C. & Donovan, J. (2011). Evaluating meta-ethnography: systematic analysis and synthesis of qualitative research. *Health Technology Assessment*, 15(43). <www.hta.ac.uk/fullmono/mon1543.pdf>.

CASP. (2013). *Qualitative checklist*. Critical Appraisal Skills Programme. http://media.wix.com/ugd/dded87_29c5b002d99342f788c6ac670e49f274.pdf.

Dixon-Woods, M., Sutton, A., Shaw, R., Miller, T., Smith, J., Young, B., Bonas, S., Booth, A. & Jones, D. (2007). Appraising qualitative research for inclusion in systematic reviews: a quantitative and qualitative comparison of three methods. *Journal of Health Service & Research Policy*, 12(1), 42–7.

Finfgeld-Connett, D. (2010). Generalizability and transferability of meta-synthesis research findings. *Journal of Advanced Nursing*, 66(2), 246–54.

Finlayson, K.W. & Dixon, A. (2008). Qualitative meta-synthesis: a guide for the novice. *Nurse Researcher*, 15(2), 59–71.

Hansen, H.P., Draborg, E. & Kristensen, F.B. (2011). Exploring qualitative research synthesis: the role of patients' perspectives in health policy design and decision making. *Patient*, 4(3), 143–52.

Paterson, B.L., Dubouloz, C., Chevrier, J., Ashe, B., King, J. & Moldoveanu, M. (2009). Conducting qualitative metasynthesis research: insights from a metasynthesis project. *International Journal of Qualitative Methods*, 8(3), 22–33.

Sandelowski, M. & Barroso, J. (2002). Finding the findings in qualitative studies. *Journal of Nursing Scholarship*, 34(3), 213–20.

Terese Bondas, Elisabeth O.C. Hall and Anita Wikberg

Sandelowski, M. & Barroso, J. (2003). Creating meta-summaries of qualitative findings. *Nursing Research*, 52(4), 226–31.

Stige, B., Malterud, K. & Midtgarden, T. (2009). Toward an agenda for evaluation of qualitative research. *Qualitative Health Research*, 19(10), 1504–16.

Websites

www.cochrane-handbook.org

> Homepage of the Cochrane Collaboration (see J. Noyes, J. Popay, A. Pearson, K. Hannes & A. Booth, on behalf of the Cochrane Qualitative Research Methods Group (2011), Ch. 20: Qualitative research and Cochrane reviews).

> Evidence from qualitative studies can play an important role in adding value to systematic reviews for policy, practice and consumer decision-making in Cochrane reviews. The synthesis of qualitative research is an area of debate and evolution. The Cochrane Qualitative Methods Group provides a forum for discussion and further development of methodology in this area.

19

Everything You Wanted to Know about Systematic Reviews

NORA SHIELDS

Chapter objectives

In this chapter you will learn:

- about the advantages of systematic reviews and their implications for health professionals
- about the constituent parts of a systematic review, including the setting of the research question, search strategies, assessing risk of bias, data extraction and data synthesis
- practical advice and assistance about how to conduct a systematic review
- the limitations inherent in systematic reviews and their implications for the conclusions that can be drawn from a review

Key terms

Data extraction

Data synthesis

Electronic databases

Inclusion/exclusion criteria

Meta-analysis

Narrative review

PICO concept

PRISMA statement

Risk of bias

Search strategy

Systematic review

Introduction

A **systematic review** is a comprehensive identification and synthesis of the available literature on a specified topic (Centre for Reviews and Dissemination 2009). This method can be used to review the literature in any area of health. It is often used to synthesise the results of randomised controlled trials (RCTs) (see Chapter 15), but the method can also include research from many types of study designs including diagnostic tests and observational studies (Higgins & Green 2011; see Chapters 11, 12). All systematic reviews adhere to a strict scientific protocol with well-described methods.

A systematic review is a useful process to collate previous literature in an area, either to answer a clinical question or to identify areas for future research. One of the key advantages of systematic reviews is that they can make it easier for researchers and practitioners to cope with the volume of literature available to review, by quickly identifying the relevant information and by excluding literature that is not relevant (Higgins & Green 2011). They are particularly useful for health professionals, as they summarise the key information in an area, allowing clinicians to read one paper that provides data from any number of other papers. High-quality systematic reviews can provide reliable evidence with which to aid clinical decision-making and inform the development of clinical practice guidelines (Shamseer *et al.* 2014; see also Chapters 15, 16, 17).

Systematic reviews are different from **narrative reviews** in that they provide an objective or scientific summary of the literature rather than a subjective or opinion-based summary. In a systematic review, literature is treated like data (see Chapter 2).

Bias related to selective reporting is a problem in clinical research, including clinical trials and review papers (Shamseer *et al.* 2014). With narrative reviews there is a high risk of researcher bias, that is, the author might review only a small amount of the literature or present only one side of the argument because their beliefs can influence how they appraise the literature. There is also a risk that the breadth and depth of the literature reviewed is reduced or that the reviewer has decided to include some material but not other (Shamseer *et al.* 2014). This **risk of bias** can be minimised in a systematic review because the methods used are transparent and can be replicated in the same way as an empirical research study. The systematic review process recognises that we are likely to bias the results of a review unless we follow clearly defined rules.

Systematic reviews follow a strict protocol to make sure that as much of the relevant research base as possible has been considered (Moher & Tricco 2008). The review protocol—how you are going to review the literature—is decided in advance (*a priori*). This helps reduce the biases associated with your selection of the literature you review. The method to be used at each stage of the protocol is defined and reported. The original studies included in a systematic review are appraised and synthesised in a rigorous and valid way and the results are presented in context with other relevant studies.

Systematic reviews can reveal 'new' evidence, particularly when they include a **meta-analysis** (see Chapter 17). Small studies are often unable to provide a final conclusion on a research question because of a lack of power. However, when a number of studies are combined (using predetermined set criteria), their results added together can reveal new information. A meta-analysis is a statistical technique that combines the results of similar studies (for example, a group of RCTs or a group of comparative studies) into a single result that provides an estimate of the overall effect (Higgins & Green 2011). See Chapter 25 for statistical analysis in quantitative research.

A step-by-step guide to conducting a systematic review

This chapter outlines a six-step approach to conducting a systematic review.

Step 1: Set an answerable question for your review.

Step 2: Decide on a strategy that comprehensively searches for evidence.

Step 3: Define **inclusion and exclusion criteria**.

Step 4: Assess the risk of bias of individual studies.

Step 5: Extract standardised data from each report.

Step 6: Summarise or synthesise the findings of your review.

Systematic reviews are usually completed by two or more reviewers. The method for each step of the review process should be determined at the start and is not normally changed once the protocol has been agreed. Any decisions made after this should be fully justified and agreed on by all the reviewers.

Step 1: Set an answerable question for your review

You might assume this is the easiest part of the review process. It is very important to spend some time thinking about the research or clinical question you want to answer in your review, since the question you set will decide how you approach every other step in the process.

A useful process to start you off is to develop a **PICO concept** or logic grid (Moher & Tricco 2008). PICO stands for:

- Population
- Intervention or indicator
- Comparator or control
- Outcome

A well-thought-out review question will comprise these four elements.

Your review question should indicate your research population—the relevant participants in the research study—for example adults or children, but it is better to be even more specific, for example adults with multiple sclerosis or children with developmental coordination disorder.

The intervention or indicator is likely to be the entity you are most interested in. For example, it might be a treatment technique such as intravenous antibiotics, or a diagnostic test such as amniocentesis, or a construct such as quality of life.

Inclusion/exclusion criteria: Inclusion and exclusion criteria are the rules set *a priori* (before the review is completed) that determine which studies are selected for inclusion in the systematic review and which studies are omitted from the review.

PICO concept: Population, Intervention or indicator, Comparator or control, and Outcome.

Nora Shields

The comparator or control is what you are comparing the intervention or indicator with, or the main alternative to the indicator or intervention you are proposing. This might be usual care or a placebo in the case of a clinical intervention, or another population, for example comparing children with spina bifida to children with typical development.

The review question also needs to state what outcome you are interested in. There might be only one such outcome, for example length of hospital stay, or many outcomes, for example pain and mobility.

In some cases, a fifth component is added to your review question—research design. This element is included if you are limiting the review of the literature to a particular type of study design, such as RCTs or economic evaluations.

STOP AND THINK

What research or clinical question do you want to answer in your review? Write it down.

Does your review question contain all four PICO elements?

Do the studies to be included in your review need to be of a particular type? If so, is this included in your research question?

Has a previous review been published on this topic? How would you check this?

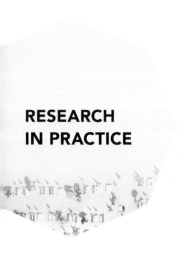

RESEARCH IN PRACTICE

The following examples are provided to help you set an answerable question for your own systematic review.

EXAMPLE OF A REVIEW QUESTION ABOUT INTERVENTIONS

Do pre-operative non-surgical and non-pharmacological interventions for hip and knee osteoarthritis provide benefit to people with hip or knee osteoarthritis before and after joint replacement? (Wallis & Taylor 2011)

EXAMPLE OF A REVIEW QUESTION ABOUT OUTCOME MEASUREMENTS

What are the psychometric properties of patient-related outcome measures used in clinical studies of patients with proximal humeral fractures? (van de Water et al. 2011)

EXAMPLE OF A REVIEW QUESTION ABOUT INCIDENCE OR PREVALENCE OF A CONDITION

What percentage of people return to sport following rehabilitation after anterior cruciate ligament reconstruction surgery? (Ardern et al. 2011)

EXAMPLE OF A REVIEW QUESTION ABOUT AETIOLOGY OR RISK FACTORS FOR A CONDITION

What are the perceived barriers and facilitators to physical activity among children with disability? (Shields et al. 2012)

EXAMPLE OF A REVIEW QUESTION ABOUT ECONOMICS

Is there a difference in cost for patients admitted to adult inpatient rehabilitation, compared to rehabilitation in another setting? (Brusco et al. 2014)

STOP AND THINK

To figure out if your review question is too broad or too narrow, try 'scoping' the electronic databases to get a feel for the extent of the literature in the area. This consists of running some basic searches to get an idea of how much literature might exist. There is a section later in this chapter which will help you set up a simple **search strategy**. Scoping the literature will help you decide whether to focus your question if there is a large amount of literature (for example, fifty to 100 published studies that might be included) or broaden your question if the literature base is small (for example, one to three published studies that might be included).

Search strategy: This is the process by which the potential literature to be included in the systematic review is identified.

Step 2: Decide on a strategy that comprehensively searches for evidence

The easiest and most common way to find relevant literature for your review is by searching **electronic databases** (Higgins & Green 2011). This can be supplemented by searching through the key journals relevant to your research question and by using citation tracking of key papers or leading researchers via the web, through electronic databases, or by contacting experts in the field. The best search strategies are those that combine these methods to locate literature (Greenhalgh & Peacock 2005; see Chapter 17).

Electronic databases: These include general medical databases, discipline-specific databases and other speciality databases. These databases catalogue published health-related literature including journal articles, textbooks and reports.

STOP AND THINK

Introduce yourself to your local health sciences librarian. Librarians are a terrific resource for helping you to locate literature and find your way around electronic databases and library systems.

Which electronic databases to choose

There are many electronic databases available for you to search for literature. A good place to start is to search either the general medical databases such as PubMed, Embase, Cochrane or Medline or the general allied health databases such as Cinahl, Amed or Psychinfo.

The next step is to search discipline-specific databases such as PEDro (physiotherapy) (see Chapter 17), OT seeker (occupational therapy), ERIC (education) or other speciality databases such as AustSportMed and Sportdiscus, DARE (database of abstracts of reviews of effects), or the Campbell database (education, criminal justice and social welfare).

Finally, you can supplement your electronic searches by using the following methods.

1   *Manual searching.* Read through the reference lists at the end of the articles you include in your review, to help identify any additional references that did not come up in your electronic searches.

2   *Web of Science.* This database is useful for citation tracking backwards and forwards. It provides a list of all references cited by a particular article (this is the same information

you get when you search manually), but it also provides a list of articles that have subsequently cited that paper (forward citation tracking).

3   *Google Scholar.* This database performs a function similar to the Web of Science in that you can track articles that have referenced a paper since publication.

4   *Contact key authors in the area.* Contacting the leading researchers in an area can help to validate the articles you have sourced. If you have missed any major papers they will be able to let you know very quickly as they are the people most knowledgeable in that area. They can also tell you about the current research that is being done in the area.

5   *Related articles feature on PubMed.* This can be a useful feature to identify papers that are similar to those you have included in your review.

6   *Manual search of key journals.* Most disciplines will have a key journal(s) in that area. Often it is important to hand-search electronic or hard copies of these journals to identify relevant studies in the area, particularly more recent studies that have not yet been indexed on the electronic databases.

7   *Clinical trials registers.* Most journals are moving to the point where they will only publish clinical studies that were preregistered with a relevant clinical trial register. Examples of clinical trial registers are the Australian New Zealand Clinical Trials Registry and the WHO International Clinical Trials Registry Platform.

STOP AND THINK

Before using an electronic database, make sure you create a personal account on that database so that you can save and edit your searches. When you have completed your searching, you can create an alert so that you receive an email when new items added to the database relate to your search strategy.

How to select keywords or search terms

The PICO concept or logic grid used in Step 1 can also be used to help select your key search terms. When choosing your search keywords you need to identify MeSH terms and free text terms. MeSH (Medical Subject Headings) terms are controlled terms or phrases used by databases or libraries in the life sciences to describe the content of journal articles, books and other documents and to index them in catalogues. For example, 'Exercise', 'Occupational Therapy' and 'Elbow joint' are all MeSH terms. It is important to know how a database or library defines these terms so that you can identify the literature most relevant to your review question. For example, 'Exercise' is defined as 'physical activity which is usually regular and done with the intention of improving or maintaining physical fitness or health'. It is used to catalogue articles about aerobic exercise, for example. Compare this to 'Physical Exertion', which is defined as 'the expenditure of energy during physical activity' and used to catalogue articles about exercise exertion, perceived exertion or physical effort. The choice of whether to use both 'Exercise' and 'Physical Exertion' in your search strategy will depend on your particular research question.

Free text terms are any other terms that can be used to describe your key concepts but that are not MeSH terms. It is important to include your MeSH terms in your free text search, as errors are often made when cataloguing the electronic databases (see Table 19.1).

STOP AND THINK

For each element of your review question, write a list of the key terms used by professionals in your discipline to describe those elements.

Are alternate terms used by professionals in related disciplines?

Are alternate terms used by professionals in other parts of the world?

Before running your final searches, it is worthwhile checking if the key words you select identify the correct types of literature. If a term returns a large amount of unrelated literature, you might want to consider excluding it from your search strategy. Remember that your search terms are like the key to a lock—if you have the wrong key it won't open the lock; if you use the wrong search terms, you won't identify the literature you need.

EXAMPLE OF A SEARCH STRATEGY

You have decided your review question is: 'What effect does participation in a progressive resistance exercise program, compared with usual care, have on the body structure and function, activity limitation and participation restriction of people with Down syndrome?'

Your PICO concept terms are:

- P: people with Down syndrome
- I: progressive resistance exercise
- C: usual care
- O: body structure and function, activity limitation and participation restriction.

For each concept you need to write out all other terms and words used for that concept, for example:

- P: Down syndrome, Trisomy 21, intellectual disability

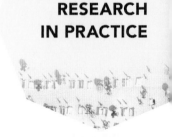

RESEARCH IN PRACTICE

TABLE 19.1   An example of a search strategy

	POPULATION		INTERVENTION	
AND →	MeSH	Free text terms	MeSH	Free text terms
OR ↓	Down syndrome	Down syndrome	Exercise	Progressive resistance training
	Mental retardation	Mental retardation	Physical therapy	Strength training
		Trisomy 21	Rehabilitation	Exercise
		Intellectual disability		Physical therapy
				Rehabilitation
				Physical training

Nora Shields

- I: progressive resistance exercise, strength training, rehabilitation, physical therapy.

  For each concept, check the corresponding MeSH terms:

- P: Down syndrome, mental retardation

- I: exercise, physical therapy, rehabilitation.

  Now you are ready to finalise your concept grid.

  Your final search strategy would look like this.

1   exp Down syndrome/ OR exp Mental Retardation/ (these are MeSH terms)

2   (Down syndrome OR Mental$ Retard$ OR Intellectual$ Disab$ OR Trisomy 21).ti,ab. (these are free text terms)

3   1 OR 2 (this combines MeSH terms and free text term searches for the same concept)

4   exp exercise/ OR exp Physical Therapy/ OR exp Rehabilitation

5   (exercise$ OR Physical Therapy OR Rehabilitation OR progressive resistance training OR strength training OR physiotherapy OR physical training).ti,ab

6   4 OR 5

7   3 AND 6 (this combines the two concepts in your PICO system).

Note:

'exp' tells the database to use the 'explode' function. This means it will search for items in that subject heading and any subheadings.

$ is an example of a truncation symbol. Truncation is a searching technique in which a word ending is replaced by a symbol. This allows you to search different forms of a word simultaneously. For example, disab$ allows you to search for disability and disabilities simultaneously. Different databases use different truncation symbols (e.g. * or ?), so use the help function in each database to check which symbol you need.

ti,ab tells the database to search for these terms in either the title or the abstract of an article.

STOP AND THINK

It can be easy to get confused by the mechanics of searching and to worry about whether you need to use the advanced functions the databases offer (e.g. filters or limits). The simplest search strategies are often the best. If you do find you are getting addled by the mechanics of searching, it is best to speak to the librarian. They are the experts in this area and are always happy to help.

What to do with your search yields

Use a bibliographic software package such as EndNote, RefWorks, or Mendeley to download all yields from the databases you have searched. Usually, you can download the search yields directly from the databases. In some instances, you will need to download a filter for that database to your bibliographic management software first; for example, filters for the PEDro databases are freely available on the PEDro website (see Websites section at the end of the chapter; see also Chapter 17).

It is important to document each stage of the process, so make sure you note the number of items identified in each database or search strategy. Remember to keep a copy of the final search yield for future reference. When you start to exclude items based on title and abstract, do so using a copy of your final search yield.

Continue to document the final strategies employed and note all changes and amendments from the protocol.

Step 3: Define the inclusion and exclusion criteria

How to decide on your inclusion/exclusion criteria

Not every item identified by your search strategy will be relevant to your review question. Therefore you need a way of deciding what is relevant to your review question (inclusion criteria) and what can be left out (exclusion criteria). This step in the process lets you select the articles that will help you answer your review question (Centre for Reviews and Dissemination 2009).

Your inclusion and exclusion criteria should flow logically from your review question. An easy way to decide on your criteria is to use the PICO concept grid again. Ask yourself:

- P: Who should the included studies be about?
- I: What intervention(s) should the included studies have investigated?
- C: What should the intervention be compared to?
- O: What are the outcomes I am interested in?

EXAMPLE OF INCLUSION/EXCLUSION CRITERIA

Let us return to our review question: 'What effect does participation in a progressive resistance exercise program, compared with usual care, have on the body structure and function, activity limitation and participation restriction of people with Down syndrome?'

- **P**: people with Down syndrome
- **I**: a progressive resistance exercise program of minimum six weeks duration
- **C**: a control or 'usual care' group
- **O**: all outcomes—impairments, functional activities, quality of life, social participation.

  Studies will be included in our review if they investigated:

- people with Down syndrome

- a strengthening program, which was six weeks minimum in duration, compared the intervention with a control group or a 'usual care' group such as usual physiotherapy, participation in their usual physical activity.

  Studies will be excluded if:

- they include people with other forms of intellectual or physical disabilities such as cerebral palsy
- they involved a single exercise training session
- full details of the intensity of the exercise program are not included
- there was no comparison group (it was a single group study).

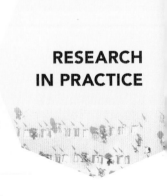

RESEARCH IN PRACTICE

Nora Shields

The method by which the inclusion and exclusion criteria are applied is also important. It is always best for at least two assessors to decide independently whether a study meets the inclusion criteria. If they disagree, then they can use a consensus method to make a final decision on whether to include a study. This decision is based on a discussion of their reasons for including or excluding a study. Having two reviewers undertake the task helps ensure that studies are not missed by chance. If the consensus method fails to produce a decision, it is possible to ask a third reviewer to adjudicate.

Step 4: Assess the risk of bias of the included studies

Why assess the risk of bias?

Assessing the risk of bias (or quality) of the included studies is an integral component of any systematic review (Shamseer *et al.* 2014). As systematic reviews are generally written to assist health care professionals in answering a clinical question, you want to include only the best possible evidence to help them make their decisions. Therefore an additional inclusion criterion can be valuable—that only articles that meet particular design or 'quality' features (e.g. randomisation) are included in the review. Assessing the risk of bias of studies will help you determine whether a study meets any set criterion.

The assessment of risk of bias can guide the interpretation of the review findings and help determine the strength of inferences we can make from the results (Shamseer *et al.* 2014). Considering the risk of bias of the included studies is helpful when interpreting heterogeneous data and helps you decide if the internal validity of the studies has affected the reported outcome(s). When interpreting the data, we might also place more emphasis on the studies with a low risk of bias compared with those with a high risk of bias. Finally, assessing the risk of bias can help guide future research by determining the limitations of previous research studies and making recommendations for how future studies might eliminate possible sources of bias.

What is risk of bias?

Risk of bias is the degree to which a study has employed measures to minimise bias. We assess internal validity, or the degree to which the results are likely to approximate the truth and external validity, or the extent to which the effects observed in a study can be applied outside the study.

How to assess the risk of bias

Assessing the risk of bias of studies included in a systematic review is a standardised process, so that we appraise all studies equally. Start by choosing a method to assess risk of bias, such as a scale, checklist or individual components (Shamseer *et al.* 2014). If you choose to assess the risk of bias using a scale, it is best to select one with strong psychometric properties (one that is valid and reliable). Which scale you select depends on the research design of the studies you are assessing. If your inclusion criteria specified a particular study design (e.g. RCTs), then the scale you choose needs to reflect that criterion. An example is the PEDro scale for assessing the risk of bias of RCTs.

An approach to assessing the risk of bias in your systematic review is to identify the features of the study that you plan to assess, and say how you are going to assess these features. For example, randomisation, concealed allocation, blinding, and loss to follow-up are common markers of the validity of RCTs (Cochrane Risk of Bias tool). This approach is usually necessary when your review includes studies with a non-randomised design (Shamseer *et al.* 2014).

Risk of bias assessment is completed at the same time as **data extraction** (see Step 5) and should be carried out by two reviewers. The reviewers normally assess the included studies independently of each other, to reduce the risk of reviewer bias. They then compare their assessments. If disagreements arise, these should be resolved by consensus (see Step 3). If agreement cannot be reached, a third reviewer should be called on to adjudicate.

You also need to document the process for assessing risk of bias. It is best to use a standard form and keep a record of the process, including, for example, the number of items on which there was initial agreement. These data can be used to calculate a kappa squared statistic, which gives an indication of the level of agreement between the reviewers.

Data extraction: The process by which information that will help answer the review question, such as data on study characteristics and findings, is obtained from the studies included in the systematic review.

STOP AND THINK

Assessing the risk of bias tells us about the quality of individual pieces of evidence from each included study, that is the degree to which an individual study reduced potential sources of bias. This process tells us about the risk of bias 'within studies'.

- How do we assess the strength of 'the body of evidence' (the risk of bias between studies)?

The GRADE system (Grading of Recommendations on Assessment, Development and Evaluation) is used in systematic reviews to assess the quality (or strength) of a body of evidence overall. It can help make a decision about the strength of subsequent clinical recommendations.

The quality of a body of evidence might be described as high (further research is unlikely to change our confidence in the estimate of effect), moderate (further research is likely to have an impact on our confidence in the estimate of effect and may change the estimate), low (further research is very likely to have an impact on our confidence in the estimate of effect and is likely to change the estimate) or very low (very uncertain about the estimate of effect) (Shamseer *et al.* 2014).

A series of articles outlining the GRADE system was published in 2008 in the *British Medical Journal* (see Guyatt *et al.* 2008a, b, c, d: Schünemann *et al.* 2008).

Step 5: Extract standardised data from each report

Data extraction is the process by which you obtain the information you need to answer your review question from what was reported in the included articles. As with the previous steps, it is important to have a standardised process for extracting data and minimising error. This can be done by designing a good data extraction form and by having two reviewers extract the data independently of each other. At a minimum, one reviewer can extract the data if the extraction is then checked by a second reviewer (Higgins & Green 2011).

What to include in your data extraction form

You need to be careful that your data extraction form is balanced in the amount of data you intend to extract. If you extract too much data, then the process might be wasteful; include too little detail and you may have to re-extract data later. The key thing to keep in mind is that the information extracted should be related to the research questions posed.

Data extraction forms are often very similar in structure, so if you develop a good data extraction form for one review, you will be able to adapt it for subsequent reviews. An example of a data extraction form can be found on the Cochrane Effective Practice and Organisation of Care Group website (http://epoc.cochrane.org/epoc-specific-resources-review-authors).

Step 6: Synthesise the findings of your review

How to synthesise your data

Data synthesis: This involves summarising and collating the findings of the individual studies included in the systematic review. It can include descriptive analysis or more formal quantitative analysis, including meta-analysis.

Now that you have located all the studies you want to include in your review, and have extracted all the data, how do you go about collating the data and summarising the results? This is referred to as **data synthesis**. It is probably easiest to start with a descriptive analysis of your data.

Descriptive analysis is where you provide information about the study characteristics that gives context for the population data and the environment within which the study was conducted. Tables are the easiest way to collate descriptive data and to identify trends in the data. For example, a table can summarise the key elements of the study under the headings sample size, participant details (sex, age, height, weight, employment or schooling characteristics), intervention details (frequency, intensity, duration, equipment used, personnel involved) and outcome measures. This type of data analysis will help you judge whether the characteristics of the included studies allow for generalisation of the results (see Chapters 25, 26). It will also help to identify restrictions and omissions in the results.

Quantitative data analysis can also be completed by calculating effect sizes and performing a meta-analysis. Before deciding to perform a meta-analysis, it is important to determine whether data from the included studies are clinically and statistically homogeneous and whether you have all the data you need. The descriptive data analysis will help you identify clinical homogeneity (e.g. were the participants of similar age, were similar outcome measures used, was the intervention similar across studies). There are statistical methods of identifying statistical homogeneity (see Chapter 25). While a meta-analysis may be appropriate in a systematic review, not all good systematic reviews need to contain meta-analyses. If a meta-analysis is appropriate, then you need to decide which comparisons should be made and which outcome measures will be used.

Meta-analysis can be useful when there is a large body of smaller studies in an area. Combining their data can increase the power of the analysis and therefore improve the precision of the estimate of effect. This reduces the uncertainty across several independent studies and can 'reveal' new information. Meta-analysis is based on lots of assumptions, and the variation between studies (clinical heterogeneity) might make the results meaningless. Larger studies can have a proportionally greater effect, depending on the model used to conduct the meta-analysis. You can download statistical software called RevMan from the Cochrane Informatics and Knowledge Management department website (http://tech. cochrane.org/revman) that can be used to complete meta-analyses.

How to write your review

Now that you have completed all the major steps involved in performing a systematic review, it is time to write up your work for publication. A key resource to follow while writing your review is the **PRISMA statement** (Preferred Reporting Items for Systematic Reviews and Meta-Analyses). This is an evidence-based set of guidelines on what to include in a report of a systematic review and/or meta-analysis. A copy of the statement can be downloaded free from the PRISMA website. The PRISMA statement should be used in conjunction with the PRISMA Explanation and Elaboration document (Shamseer *et al.* 2014), which explains the meaning and rationale for each item on the checklist and includes useful examples.

More detailed advice on how to present and write up your research findings is provided in Chapter 26.

PRISMA statement: The PRISMA statement (Preferred Reporting Items for Systematic Reviews and Meta-Analyses) is an evidence-based set of twenty-seven items for reporting in systematic reviews and meta-analyses.

STOP AND THINK

You can register your systematic review protocol with PROSPERO (www.crd.york.ac.uk/PROSPERO/), an international database of prospectively registered systematic reviews in health and social care developed and implemented by the Centre for Reviews and Dissemination. Prospective registration of systematic reviews provides transparency in the review process by safeguarding against bias (e.g. publication bias or reporting bias) and avoiding duplication.

Summary

A systematic review is a comprehensive identification and synthesis of all relevant studies on a review question. It is conducted according to an explicit and reproducible method to minimise the risk of reviewer bias. Systematic reviews help health professionals cope with large volumes of literature by summarising it and providing more reliable evidence that can aid clinical decision-making. They are also used by researchers to identify gaps and strengths in the current literature, assisting research design.

Nora Shields

The method of conducting a systematic review should be transparent, easily replicated and scientifically rigorous. The process comprises setting an answerable clinical question, searching for relevant information, deciding which studies should be included and excluded, assessing the risk of bias of the included studies, extracting relevant data and synthesising the findings of the review.

Practice exercises

What clinical question do you wish to answer? Write it down, and develop a protocol for a systematic review that would help you answer it. Your protocol should include the following:

1   an answerable review question
2   a list of the electronic databases you intend searching, plus the methods you would use to supplement your search strategy
3   a list of your inclusion and exclusion criteria
4   a method for assessing the risk of bias of individual studies
5   a data extraction form for the review
6   a plan for how you intend to synthesise the data.

Further reading

Centre for Reviews and Dissemination (2009). *CRD's guidance for undertaking reviews in Health Care*. University of York. www.york.ac.uk/inst/crd/SysRev/!SSL!/WebHelp/SysRev3.htm.

Higgins, J.P.T. & Green, S. (2011). *Cochrane handbook for systematic reviews of interventions*, Version 5.1.0 [updated March 2011]. www.cochrane-handbook.org.

Websites

www.campbellcollaboration.org
       The Campbell database.
www.anzctr.org.au
       The Australian New Zealand Clinical Trials Registry.
www.who.int/ictrp/en
       WHO International Clinical Trials Registry Platform.
www.nlm.nih.gov/mesh
       MeSH headings.

www.pedro.org.au/english/downloads/pedro-scale/

>   PEDro scale.

www.cochranelibrary.com/

>   The Cochrane Library is a collection of databases containing high-quality independent evidence to inform decision-making in health care. This library gives you immediate access to several hundred systematic reviews covering all aspects of health care. It should be your first stop in reviewing the literature to answer a clinical question—Cochrane reviews are the highest level of evidence on which to base clinical management decisions.

www.york.ac.uk/inst/crd/SysRev/!SSL!/WebHelp/SysRev3.htm

>   An excellent resource to help you write your systematic review is the Centre for Reviews and Dissemination report, *CRD's guidance for undertaking reviews in health care* (2009). A copy of the report is available free at this website. It includes a list of information requirements for data extraction.

http://epoc.cochrane.org/epoc-specific-resources-review-authors

>   This is the Cochrane Effective Practice and Organisation of Care Group website. It gives an example of a data extraction form.

www.prisma-statement.org/

>   The PRISMA statement is a very useful guide when writing or critically appraising systematic reviews and meta-analyses. It can be downloaded from this website.

www.crd.york.ac.uk/PROSPERO/

>   PROSPERO is an international database of prospectively registered systematic reviews in health and social care developed and implemented by the Centre for Reviews and Dissemination.

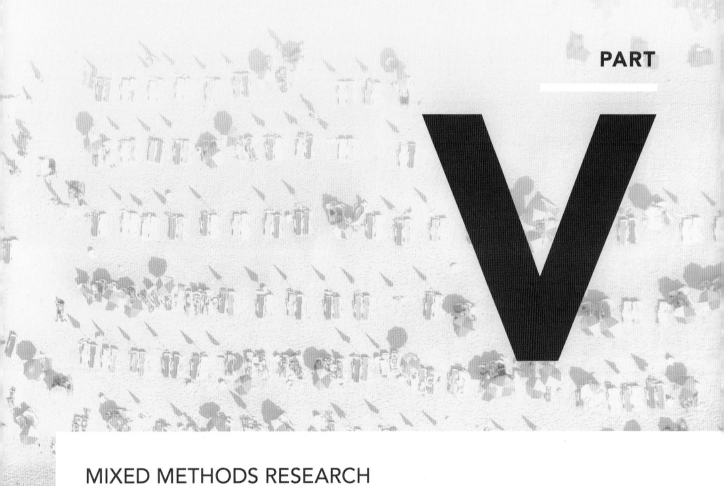

MIXED METHODS RESEARCH

20   Integrated Methods in Health Research   361

21   The Use of Mixed Methods in Health Research   375

22   Collaborative Participatory Research with Disadvantaged Communities   397

20

Integrated Methods in Health Research

CAROL GRBICH

Chapter objectives

In this chapter you will learn:

- about the issues and practicalities regarding the integration or mixing of methods in health research from three perspectives
- about ontological (theoretical) and epistemological (design and data collection) integration
- how to integrate and interpret the results of data analysis

Key terms

Concurrent design

Constructivism

Epistemology

Ontology

Positivism

Pragmatism

Q^2 or Q squared

Sequential design

Transformative

Triangulation

Introduction

Within both qualitative styles alone and quantitative styles alone, it is possible to use multiple approaches for data collection, data analysis and data interpretation, but it is the combining of quantitative and qualitative approaches (**Q² or Q squared**) that is currently of greatest interest (see also Chapters 1, 21). The first question you, as a researcher, need to ask yourself before considering a Q² approach is 'Does my question have both qualitative and quantitative components?' A typical question with a Q² possibility might be 'What is the impact of (x) on the attitudes of (y) towards (z)?' Here it would be useful to get an overall sense of the impact of some change or existing issue on a large group by perhaps using a survey (see Chapter 13) then, to find out more detail, adding face-to-face interviews (see Chapter 4) or focus groups (see Chapter 5) to clarify the in-depth individual views of a smaller sample of this group.

Another indicator that an integrated approach could be useful would be the presence of the potential to measure relationships between variables in addition to gaining the views of a group of people. For example, 'What are the effects of the latest safe sex campaign on the perceptions and behaviours of young males and young females?' Here the question can be broken down into more than one component. For example, 'Are males and females different in terms of behaviours following exposure to a safe sex campaign?', which forms the quantitative component where relationships between variables could be measured, and 'What are the effects of the images and information of the campaign on young males and females in terms of their perceptions regarding safe sex?', which forms the qualitative component to be collected through interviews or focus groups. Implicit in this are the questions 'Why are there differences between males and females?' (if these are found) and 'How could a better campaign be constructed?' (if the current one was ineffective).

Integrated approaches

The integration of theoretical ideas, data collection techniques and/or data analytic techniques is generally used to provide answers to more complex questions, to enable the inclusion of a broad overview of larger numbers of people, or to measure relationships between variables in a situation where rich in-depth information is required.

Other reasons for attempting integration include bringing together two or more sets of data to illuminate different aspects of a research question, a process called **triangulation**: the clarification of one set of results by or from another, and the extension or development of one set of results into another set.

Integrated approaches offer many advantages to the researcher. For example, you can attempt to answer more complex research questions with greater certainty. You can explore the detail of individual experiences behind the statistics and, conversely, statistics can provide an overview and a context for narratives. The approaches help in the development of particular measures or questions. They can track changes over time and allow one data set to feed into the development of another. They can foster the mix of a range of traditional designs as well

Q² or Q squared: The combination of quantitative and qualitative approaches in a research study. It is the concept used in mixed methods research design.

Triangulation: The clarification of one set of results by or from another, and the extension or development of one set of results into another set.

as encourage the development of innovative mixes to provide better answers to research questions while enhancing the generalisability of the results.

However, there are also disadvantages or weaknesses in these approaches. For example, the study will be larger; it may take longer or require a larger research team to carry it out effectively. Greater skills are needed to successfully design, undertake, analyse and interpret integrated data sets. One paradigm (see definitions below and Chapter 1) may dominate and be treated appropriately, while the other may be glossed over in terms of design, data collection, analysis and interpretation. Last, different weightings of paradigms and techniques need appropriate clarification and justification, or the validity of both may be severely compromised (see Chapter 21).

We will examine in more detail the three major issues—ontology, epistemology and the integration and interpretation of multiple data sets—so you can see what is involved.

Ontological integration

In research, the word **ontology** refers to the theoretical underpinnings of different paradigms or methodological approaches. Both quantitative and qualitative approaches come from different paradigms—usually defined as agreed-upon sets of assumptions or collections of underpinning beliefs about the twin natures of reality and knowledge— and these paradigms guide the research to be undertaken (see Chapter 1). The quantitative paradigm (often termed **positivism**) is characterised by a focus on development and implementation of research instruments, 'objective' (distant, non-involved) researchers, deduction (the formation of hypotheses for testing from observable empirical facts), confirmation and explanation of facts as a result of theory and hypothesis-testing, the use of statistical analysis, and an assumption that the results found can be widely generalised and easily replicated. The qualitative paradigm (often termed **constructivism** or interpretivism) is characterised by 'subjective' researchers who are the research instruments and whose biases contribute to the construction of perspectives, by induction (creating explanations from diverse observations) or discovery, and by theory or concept development to interpret findings (see Chapter 1).

Those favouring Q^2 approaches have suggested that one way to bypass the complexities of these two differing paradigms and to circumvent the pitfalls inherent in combining the two is to adopt the philosophical position of **pragmatism** (Teddlie & Tashakkori 2003; Johnson & Onwuegbuzie 2006; see also Chapter 1). Pragmatism was originally a set of values developed by Charles Pierce, George Herbert Mead, William James and John Dewey in the late nineteenth and early twentieth centuries to enable us to make a connection between the nature of knowledge and the techniques or methods we use to gain knowledge.

Put simply, pragmatism refers to the connection between knowledge and the methods by which this knowledge is gained. In more detail, pragmatism seeks the middle ground in areas that have previously been polarised, as have quantitative and qualitative approaches, particularly in terms of their subjective and objective positions. According to pragmatist positions, knowledge of the world can be obtained by observation, experience and experimentation. In this manner,

Ontology: The study of the nature of things.

Positivism: Where information is derived from a logical interpretation of what can be seen in the world.

Constructivism: People are viewed as constructing knowledge through life experiences.

Pragmatism: The belief that if it works then it must reflect truth.

the focus becomes the research question that requires answers by whatever mix of data collection approaches appear to be most useful. Humans are viewed as interacting with the physical world to create meaning and knowledge, which leads to the development of theories that can be tested on the grounds of how well they can be applied. Each notion or theory or concept can be interpreted in terms of actions and outcomes in the real world, and seen as a contribution to a dynamic and changing set of 'truths' or theories. Within the limits of change, these results are seen as providing some predictability. Thus the meanings or outcomes of a research study provide a path to be followed in order to produce new explanations or to confirm existing ones. There is an underlying assumption that where problems are uncovered, solutions do exist and they can be trialled and evaluated in an ongoing fashion. Morgan (2007) sees the following terminology shift as one way of integrating quantitative and qualitative within a pragmatic paradigm: induction and deduction become 'abduction' (allowing you to move backwards and forwards between induction and deduction, from one set of results to another); subjectivity and objectivity become 'intersubjectivity' (which accepts that there is a real world but adds that we all have individual interpretations of this world); and context and generality become 'transferability' (where you decide how much of your results are likely to be applicable to a similar setting or situation).

Another paradigm, **transformative** (Mertens 2010), has emerged recently. In orientation and like pragmatism, multiple realities are seen as being shaped by cultural, social, economic and political influences, and knowledge is viewed as historically and socially situated. However, the emphasis here is on two other aspects: that the issues of power between researcher and researched must be properly addressed and that all research must include the ethical human rights agenda of social justice, must be for the betterment of humankind, and must provide a basis for action and social change.

> **Transformative:** The belief that behaviour can be changed through knowledge gained.

STOP AND THINK

You have decided to investigate the issue of youth homelessness. If you think that changes may be needed in this field, which paradigm (pragmatist or transformative) could provide the major underpinning for your design? Why? How would this affect your design?

Epistemological integration

> **Epistemology:** The study of beliefs and the nature of knowledge.

Epistemology is related to the methods used to gain knowledge (see Chapter 1). Putting together quantitative and qualitative approaches in terms of design is simpler than arguing over the differences in paradigms, and relies largely on your creativity. However, there are areas of decision-making you will need to address. The first is your research question(s), which will need to be suitable for integrated approaches. The second is whether one approach is to be dominant or both are to be equal, as this will determine the final weighting of your results and interpretation. The third decision relates to issues of time: should you collect your data sets at the same time (concurrent) or at different times (sequential)?

Sampling

The inclusion of both probability and non-probability sampling strategies has opened up options for you as a Q^2 researcher. The usual probability approaches (random, stratified, systematic, cluster and multiple approaches) are joined by the non-probability approaches (maximum variation, homogeneous, typical case, intensity, extreme, snowballing, convenience, opportunistic and multiple approaches) to provide a wide variety of options within the sequential, concurrent and multilevel designs that can be designed from these two options (see also Chapter 1). It has been suggested by Collins and colleagues (2007) that the size of your sample needs to match your method or data collection technique so that your focus groups have six to twelve participants, your ethnography has a defined culture of whatever number is involved, for example six street youths or 250 people in a tribal group, and your correlational and causal comparative studies have at least sixty (one-tailed hypothesis) to over eighty (two-tailed hypothesis), depending on the desired proportion of the total population available.

Design

There are two major design orientations and one emergent one at your disposal.

Sequential designs

In **sequential design**, one data set follows another and extends or explores the findings from the first set. For example, you could undertake a qualitative study to explore a particular issue or phenomenon and you could create hypotheses from those results that you could test using a survey or experimental design. Alternatively, you could develop a short questionnaire survey to elicit key issues that can then be explored in depth using qualitative approaches of interviewing and observation. Synthesis of the two sets of results is needed to clarify the dual outcomes and to utilise the increased validity these two approaches provide. You can see here that the questions for the second part of the study evolve from the results of the first part (see also Chapter 21).

> **Sequential design:** One data set follows another and extends or explores the findings from the first set.

Research example: sequential design quantitative to qualitative

A simple sequential investigation into the role of information in online investment (Williamson 2008) addressed the research question, 'What is the role of information in online investment in Australia?'

The quantitative component involved a broad-based survey overview (predominantly using six-point rating scales) of the behaviour patterns and habits of 520 investors, accessed through two online companies, the Commonwealth Bank and Sanford Online, who put the survey questionnaire up on their websites. Of the respondents, 200 offered to be interviewed and twenty-nine were chosen to create a geographically representative sample Australia-wide. Interviews were face to face, lasting up to two hours and pursuing in greater depth both the original question areas and the outcomes of the wider survey, compared with each individual's survey profile.

There was considerable value in combining the two methods, especially as both were treated separately and with respect to the differing ontological, epistemological and data-analytic orientations. The equal balance allowed one set of data to feed into another and to complement the original survey finding by providing depth of explanation.

Research example: sequential design qualitative to quantitative to qualitative

Baluch and Davies (2008) have used a three-way sequential design—qualitative to quantitative to qualitative—in a longitudinal study examining the poverty dynamics and trajectories in rural Bangladesh following particular government interventions of microfinance in 1994, new agricultural technologies in 1996–97 and the introduction of educational transfers in 2000 and 2003. They used three sequential phases.

Phase 1 involved the collection of qualitative data by 116 focus groups in eleven districts to examine perceptions of change regarding the interventions for 'poor' and 'better-off' groups of men and women.

Phase 2 involved a quantitative household survey of 2152 households to compare with an earlier brief survey undertaken by other researchers that had measured the initial impact of the interventions.

Phase 3 involved the collection of 293 qualitative life history interviews in order to understand the processes and institutional contexts that influence livelihood trajectories.

The combination of data collection techniques in a sequential manner enabled a better understanding of the changing profiles of risk and opportunities that the poor in Bangladesh face and how these profiles shape the dynamics of poverty much more clearly. The patterns and trends thus exposed have implications for policy.

Combining the two data sets helped to compensate for the blind spots that often eventuate from a single approach, and strengthened the overall research process.

STOP AND THINK

What might be the disadvantages of initially undertaking a survey with closed-ended questions (Yes/No or rating scales) rather than first using open-ended qualitative interview questions in your research design?

Concurrent/parallel/triangulation designs

Concurrent design: Qualitative and quantitative data sets are collected at the same time and their results compared.

In a **concurrent design** your questions would tend to be framed from the start and you could consider using multiple reference points where intact but separate data sets are collected concurrently. For example, you could use dual sites with the same sampling approach but with different designs (one quantitative, one qualitative), then use the synthesised results to build up a complex picture (see also Chapter 21). Within the concurrent approach, an internal integration or merging or synergy of data collection approaches occurs. This involves processes where aspects of the usually separate techniques intermingle. For example, using both focused (limited response) quantitative and open-ended (qualitative) questions in the same survey allows immediate comparisons and a more holistic view of the questions to be addressed. It also allows you to follow up responses on the spot. Another possibility involves asking why your participants have chosen a particular course of action, then counting the responses and presenting these as a percentage of the total, then establishing variables and measuring relationships between them.

CONCURRENT DESIGN

The Sakai Virtual Research Environment is an open-source virtual collaboration environment developed by a consortium of research-intensive universities to encourage collaborative research (Procter *et al.* 2008). This modular environment (Sakai) can be set up either as a virtual learning or a virtual research environment. Access is controlled and email lists, chat room and 'work sites' are provided. The site collects usage data through log data that provides the user's address and password, their type of Web browser and the page from which they were referred. In addition, the database tables stored inside the virtual research environment provide a record of the 'click stream' showing individual actors chatting, editing pages, viewing documents and so on. In this evaluation, quantitative data was collected over time to identify patterns and trends regarding the amount of time spent in a particular arena. To identify differences between individual participants and projects, the 'who', 'what' and 'where' patterns of use and trends were treated as rudimentary qualitative data to create 'user stories' from within the database of use. These were expanded to semi-structured interviews both on- and offline where participants were asked to comment on and make sense of graphs of their own activity online at the Sakai site.

Using reduced quantitative data as the focus for qualitative enquiry was very illuminating, especially when, as part of the evaluation, we involved participants in 'sense-making', that is, explaining their own profile data graphs.

MULTILEVEL CONCURRENT DESIGN

A triangulation approach can often be seen in multisite research. In an investigation of strategic scanning in organisations (Audet & d'Amboise 2001), four organisations were selected for cross-case comparison along two polar dimensions: performance of the firm and level of uncertainty in the firm's environment. Two of the firms selected had high levels of uncertainty—one with a high and the other with a lower performance level, and the remaining two had low levels of uncertainty and either a high or lower performance level. Data comprised semi-structured interviews in all sites with different levels of staff. Interview schedules comprised closed- and open-ended questions relating to the variables that had been identified. Within-case analysis was followed by cross-case analysis of firms with similar performance levels.

The advantage of a detailed research design is that it allows for greater flexibility, but when the diversity of sites is too great the study can head off in unexpected directions that are hard to control in terms of variables.

RESEARCH IN PRACTICE

New and innovative approaches

At present, most data collected are still within the survey/interview/observation/document analysis framework in multiple data sets, with the documents traditionally being written communications or transcriptions, but looking to the field of media images should alert you to what is being attempted in this field. Gamberini and Spagnolli (2003) have brought together both qualitative and quantitative data sets under the heading of an exploration of human–computer interactions, encompassing the digital, physical, real and artificial aspects of this through three triangulated data sets. The first set involves the split screen technique, which allows a synchronised visualisation of different environments on the same screen, in this case the real and the virtual environments a participant is involved in on screen. Individual interaction with a computer can be seen on one-half of the screen, while the other half details the depth view of what is actually happening as the individual interacts with the program. This process can be undertaken by one individual or multiple users by splitting the monitor into further blocks of two-screen displays. The second option is the action indicator augmented display, which picks up the faster individual interactions with the computer interface, particularly quick hand movements on buttons, which are reflected in arrows at the bottom of the screen. The third is the pentagram, which allows transcription of multiple sequences of events in their own time-line. Although these approaches can be used as tools to provide a single conclusion, they can also provide individual or multimedia displays in their own right, allowing the reader to observe all the data collected.

As new and innovative approaches are developed by researchers, it becomes harder to confine these within the boundaries of standard definitions. The example below is one that exhibits both concurrent and sequential approaches in a complex multilevel design.

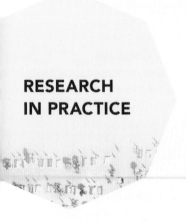

**RESEARCH
IN PRACTICE**

MULTILEVEL CONCURRENT AND SEQUENTIAL DESIGN

Thurston et al. (2008) combined epidemiological, survey and qualitative methods in a longitudinal study to evaluate domestic violence interventions in emergency care settings in Canada. The focus was on accessing the factors that influence uptake and maintenance of the intervention at the micro (individual management, staff and patient), meso (organisational and collective) and macro (extra-oganisational) levels.

Data were collected by:

- observation of the five emergency departments and three urgent care sectors (repeated over several hours) observing environment, employees, patterns and procedures, case meetings and committee meetings

- 105 open-ended interviews with nursing staff and managers in seven hospitals over two phases

- a review of five years of de-identified patient notes

- a review of relevant media coverage over six years

- a review of site-specific documents, meeting minutes, annual reports etc.
- a brief questionnaire survey of female residents in shelters for abused women in the city of Calgary
- ten ethnographic interviews with five different types of health care professionals were conducted to follow up the themes identified in the second item, regarding the nature of their work.

This study has the multiple characteristics of different levels and styles of data collected over time in phases with sequential follow-up.

Further debate is needed on the issue of methodological congruence and method triangulation so that researchers have some guidelines on what will be acceptable as 'sound'.

Although validity of findings in mixed methods is still contentious, two instruments have recently been developed: one is the Instrument Development and Construct Validation (IDCV) tool (Onwuegbuzie *et al.* 2010) and the other is the Validation Framework (VF) (Leech *et al.* 2010) The former is a ten-phase tool covering an interdisciplinary literature review, instrument development and evaluation, and construct validation process and product, while the latter provides a five-element approach for foundational elements and construct validity in qualitative, quantitative, mixed, inferential, historical and consequential data elements. These developments have led Denzin (2010) to comment on the dangers of the moves in mixed methods of quantifying qualitative data by quantitative researchers with minimal training in qualitative research.

STOP AND THINK

- What are the dangers of integrated methods becoming overquantified?
- Why would this be a problem, particularly for qualitative data?
- How could you, as a researcher, avoid overquantification?

Analysis, display, interpretation and synthesis of results

Bryman (2007) has identified three major groupings of barriers faced by researchers who have attempted to conduct mixed method research:

- intrinsic differences between qualitative and quantitative in terms of theory, data sets and the additional time taken to gather these and to merge analyses
- institutional differences of audience, publication, discipline and funding agencies
- researcher preference or comfort zone in a particular style.

Of these, the merging of analyses in the first point appeared to be the most confronting. So let us see if we can attempt to break down this barrier. The choices in terms of data management are to treat the data sets as separate and to analyse and display them separately. Alternatively, you can analyse them separately but integrate them in terms of display, taking care to weight the display appropriately. The third option is to integrate your data sets in some way and present an amalgam for display.

Separate data sets

The difficulties surrounding presentation of qualitative and quantitative approaches lie in the management of a very large results section requiring a comprehensive drawing together of the findings in a summary so that readers can make sense of the diversity presented. In a study of the usefulness of written asthma plans in general practice (Sulaiman *et al.* 2011), the researchers decided to present their results separately. The quantitative (survey questionnaire) data were summarised in detailed tables and the longitudinal qualitative data (focus groups and interviews) followed in a separate section, demonstrated in quotes and case studies. Equal weight was given to both sets of data and sufficient information was provided that readers could see the links and differences.

Combined data sets

In contrast to the separation of data sets, it may be preferable to amalgamate the findings in such a way that a neat display of graphical information occurs, followed by a few carefully chosen qualitative quotes that serve to display the homogeneity (or diversity) of the data gathered. The use of matrices can bring together variables, themes and cases, as can lists, network diagrams and graphical displays. Wacjman and Martin (2002) studied managers in six companies. A questionnaire was completed by a random sample of 470 managers, and interviews were held with eighteen to twenty-six managers from each company. The data are presented equally, with the quantitative survey results displayed in an extensive single table and the career narratives of 136 managers divided into male and female responses and presented as substantial quotes and commentary. The totality of this approach may well be neater and more powerful in capturing readers' attention through the juxtaposition of different perspectives presented side by side, but it may also result in the complexity of the findings being 'dumbed down' and those findings that are not matched by the other data set somehow dropping off the radar screen.

Integrated data sets

It has been suggested (Dixon-Woods *et al.* 2005) that several approaches might be appropriate in the transformation and integration of data. The two main ones—integrative and interpretive syntheses—are detailed below.

Integrative synthesis

This synthesis is used where the major tool is summarising—collating the key concepts under categories. For example, in a study of doctor–patient interaction the key categories derived from both data sets might be doctor–patient interactive style, financial constraints, time constraints and so on. These concepts have already been determined through data analysis and do not need further development at this stage. A theoretical interpretation or model of communication styles can then be used to reflect on the aggregated emphasis now displayed by the data. Integrative synthesis can be undertaken using a variety of summarising approaches:

- content analysis (a summary of the major content of your data sets by categorising and determining frequency; see Chapter 23)

- thematic analysis (summarising your findings via the identification of recurrent themes, although it is useful to know if the generation of these themes has been data- or theory-driven; see Chapter 23)

- case survey (summarising the overview of a large number of cases by coding data via a set of closed questions for quantitative analysis; see Chapter 13)

- qualitative comparative analysis, useful for smaller numbers of cases with Q^2 data (via the construction of a table showing logically possible combinations of pairs of independent and corresponding outcome variables).

These examples have been minimised to the most relevant few.

Interpretive synthesis

This synthesis is grounded in the data collected. It seeks to develop explanatory concepts and theories from data groups that have been analysed but minimally conceptualised. This can be done using:

- narrative form (recounting and describing using data juxtaposition and the creation of interpretive fames; see Chapter 6)

- grounded theory (using the constant comparison of data sets and creating grids for cross-case comparisons. Concepts are clustered into categories and axial coding is undertaken for the generation of theoretical explanations; see Chapter 8)

- meta-ethnography involving reciprocal, translational analysis (where metaphors, themes and concepts from each data set are translated into the other sets, contradictions are identified, and lines of argument are developed from the separate data sets; see Chapter 18)

- meta-study (carefully critiquing how the theories and methods have impacted on the data collected)

- realist approach (a theory-directed approach to analysis of all findings from all sources)

- matrix synthesis (clustering the data into categories and codes in matrices for cross-case comparison).

Carol Grbich

The processes of integrating data in this way are still subject to the major question, 'Should we attempt to integrate data that have been collected qualitatively or quantitatively within very different paradigms and traditions?' This leads to other questions, such as, 'Should we even attempt to "quantitise" qualitative data or "qualitise" quantitative data?' and 'Which approach should be treated to these processes first?', 'How should we read the results of integrated studies?', 'Are we reading too much into minimalist quantitative data and losing too much of the rich detail of qualitative data in these processes?' The lack of transparent detail of process and outcome in health research means that we too often have inadequate information on which to judge these processes.

Summary

The advent of the third paradigm, the Q^2 approach, is an exciting one. The development of pragmatic and transformative paradigms as underpinnings allows considerable flexibility with regard to design and analysis of collected data. The advantages of using an integrated Q^2 approach lie in increasing the numbers of methods and techniques of data collection that can be applied to a particular question, enabling more aspects of the problem to be investigated and more complete answers to be achieved. The disadvantages lie in the use of a wide range of data collection techniques that may look at such different aspects of the question that comparison becomes impossible, the achievement of minimal data analysis such that only homogenous results are achieved and complexities are overlooked or smoothed down, and inadequate transparency of the processes of integrating results so that it is not evident how the different data sets were treated, understood or interpreted.

Practice exercises

1   Construct a research question that you think will be suitable for a mixed methods approach and divide it into two questions: one that would enable you to collect qualitative data and one that would enable you to collect quantitative data.

2   Take the following research question and identify which qualitative and quantitative data collection techniques would be most appropriate. Justify your choice. 'How are the current waiting times in the emergency outpatient clinic viewed by staff and patients?'

3   You have collected some quantitative data and some qualitative data in an integrated methods study where you have been observing primary health care in action. Your data sets comprise:

- observations of twenty family practices and 1000 patient visits to forty GPs in a city environment
- medical case notes for each patient
- patient questionnaires after each visit
- billing data for each patient
- a practice environment checklist
- ethnographic field notes.

You then undertake descriptive statistics on the survey and billing data, concentrating on percentages. You also undertake thematic analysis of your interviews and field notes, content analysis of the case notes, and thematic and content analysis of visits and the practice environment. Explain how these various sets of data could be brought together for display and indicate which approach you think would be the most effective.

4   The concept of pragmatism has been briefly outlined in this chapter. Google 'pragmatism' and see what else the original research theorists who introduced this word have to say about it. How do their views differ from those briefly outlined in this chapter?

Further reading

Brewer, J. & Hunter, A. (2006). *Foundations of multimethod research*. Thousand Oaks, CA: Sage.

Creswell, J. (2013). *Research design: qualitative, quantitative and mixed method approaches*, 3rd edn. Thousand Oaks, CA: Sage.

Creswell, J.W. (2015). *A concise introduction to mixed methods research*. Thousand Oaks, CA: Sage.

Creswell, J.W. & Plano Clark, V.L. (2011). *Designing and conducting mixed methods research*, 2nd edn. Thousand Oaks, CA: Sage.

Creswell, J., Fetters, M. & Ivankova, N. (2004). Designing a mixed methods study in primary care. *Annals of Family Medicine*, 2, 7–12. This article evaluates five mixed methods studies in primary care and develops three models for designing such investigations.

Curry, L. & Nunez-Smith, M. (2015). *Mixed methods in health sciences research*. Thousand Oaks, CA: Sage.

Dixon-Woods, M. (2005). Synthesising qualitative and quantitative evidence: a review of possible methods. *Journal of Health Service Research and Policy*, 10(1), 45–53.

Kelle, U. (2001). Sociological explanations between micro and macro and the integration of qualitative and quantitative methods. *Forum: Qualitative Social Research*, 2(1) February. <www.qualitative-research.net/fqs-texte/1-01/1-01kelle-e.htm>. Kelle presents three versions of triangulation design: triangulation as mutual validation, triangulation as the integration of different perspectives on the investigated phenomenon, and triangulation in its original trigonometrical meaning.

Teddlie, C. & Tashakkori, A. (eds) (2003). *Handbook of mixed methods in social and behavioral research*. Thousand Oaks, CA: Sage. This book covers issues and controversies, cultural issues, transformational and emancipatory research, research design, sampling and data collection strategies, analysing, writing and reading and their applications across such disciplines as organisational research, psychological research, the health sciences, sociology and nursing.

Websites

http://mra.e-contentmanagement.com

The website of the *International Journal of Multiple Research Approaches*.

http://mmr.sagepub.com

The website of the *Journal of Mixed Methods Research*.

21

The Use of Mixed Methods in Health Research

ANN TAKET

Chapter objectives

In this chapter you will learn:

- what is meant by 'mixed methods'
- about the different types of mixed methods
- what uses mixed methods have in health research
- about the advantages and disadvantages of mixed methods
- approaches to the critical appraisal of mixed methods studies
- about the challenges in using mixed methods

Key terms

Critical appraisal

Epistemology

Mixed methods

Ontology

Pragmatism

Triangulation

Introduction

At the outset, it is important to recognise that there is little consistency in the use of the term **mixed methods**; the term can be and has been used in a multiplicity of ways. It is not that some of these uses are 'right' and the others 'wrong', but that there are many different ways in which the term can be productively used when discussing the design or implementation of research. Multiple uses of the term only present a difficulty if we do not scrutinise how each author uses the term (see also Chapters 1, 20).

The use of mixed methods has proliferated, with a growth in journal articles and books, even specific journals devoted to mixed methods research. This chapter considers mixed methods in relation to health research, research carried out with the general purpose of understanding how to promote health more effectively and improve the care and cure of those who are ill. A particular focus for this chapter is research in public health and health promotion.

STOP AND THINK

- What does the term 'mixed methods' mean to you?
- Take a couple of minutes to jot down your thoughts. Keep them for later.

Different types of mixed methods

The term 'mixed methods' can be understood in a number of different ways. First of all, it can simply refer to a number of different types of methods being used within a single study. Often it is used to refer to mixing qualitative and quantitative methods (see Chapters 1, 20), but it can also refer to mixing different types of qualitative method within a study. Second, it may refer to mixing that occurs at different stages in the research process, for example in data collection or data analysis or indeed in both these stages. Third, different modes or ways of mixing methods within a single study need to be considered. Sometimes a research study is divided into a number of stages, carried out sequentially, so a qualitative stage may be followed by a quantitative stage or vice versa; for example, a qualitative component such as focus groups may be used to help define and pilot a structured survey schedule. Sometimes the mixing is parallel—a qualitative component in a study runs alongside a quantitative one, without interaction, answering different research questions. Or the mixing may be a 'blend'—two or more interacting strands, answering the same research question(s) (see Chapter 20). In the following sections, I elaborate on these with some examples.

The range of situations in which mixed methods can be used is extremely wide. Focusing particularly on health research, Table 21.1 presents some of the most common purposes for which a mixed design may be particularly helpful, and gives examples of studies. The list of purposes in this table is illustrative rather than exhaustive.

TABLE 21.1 Examples of different purposes for the use of mixed methods

PURPOSE	EXPLANATION	EXAMPLES
Understanding health and quality of life	Contrasting findings from qualitative and quantitative approaches can help deepen our understanding of important health outcomes and/or how best to measure or assess them.	Barclay *et al.* 2015 Dunning *et al.* 2008 Johansson *et al.* 2012 John 2012
Understanding health-related behaviour and its relationships with health and health-related outcomes	Contrasting findings from qualitative and quantitative approaches can help tease out the complex interaction of different factors in accounting for health-related behaviour, and help in exploring the role of factors like appropriateness, accessibility and acceptability.	Bull 2014 Sinha *et al.* 2007 Wagner *et al.* 2012 Zierold *et al.* 2015 See also the case study in this chapter
Designing and developing interventions*	Use of qualitative methods alongside quantitative outcome measures can help to understand how an intervention works, enabling researchers to refine intervention design, often within the early stages of intervention. Formative evaluations often use mixed methods.	Bussing *et al.* 2014 Coa *et al.* 2015 Hopkinson & Richardson 2015 Piedra *et al.* 2012
Evaluating interventions*	Use of qualitative methods alongside quantitative outcome measures can help to understand which parts of the intervention were important in enabling different outcomes to be achieved or, alternatively, help to understand failure to achieve outcomes. Use of mixed methods can aid in achieving greater understanding. Process evaluations often use mixed methods.	Bailey & Kerlin 2015 Celik *et al.* 2012 Griffiths *et al.* 2015 Merrill *et al.* 2012
Improving research design	Use of qualitative methods provides a way of improving aspects of a quantitative design. This can apply at different stages, e.g. defining specific hypotheses to test, designing a sampling strategy, designing recruitment strategies, designing survey instruments.	Donovan *et al.* 2002 Kenaszchuk *et al.* 2012 O'Leary *et al.* 2015 Ross *et al.* 2012 Weaver & Kaiser 2015

*To be understood as encompassing a spectrum from simple interventions right through to complex system-wide interventions.

Ann Taket

Why use mixed methods?

The simplest, and arguably most important, answer to this question is that the use of mixed methods can enable researchers to tackle questions that would be difficult or even impossible to tackle with a single-method design (see Chapter 1). For example, while the randomised controlled trial (RCT) might be the preferred design for testing hypotheses about the outcomes from particular interventions (see Chapter 15), understanding the processes behind those outcomes requires the use of qualitative methods (see chapters in Part II). Another example is provided by the value of **triangulation** of different methods of data collection and/or different methods of analysis in teasing out answers to complex questions on health-related behaviours (see Chapters 1, 20). O'Cathain and colleagues (2007) present an interesting analysis of studies funded by a single commissioner in England between 1994 and 2004. They found that 18 per cent (119 out of 647) of the studies commissioned were mixed methods, and that the main stated reason for using mixed methods research was to answer a wider range of questions than quantitative methods alone would permit.

> Triangulation: The use of multiple methods, researchers, data sources or theories in a research project.

But the necessity of a mixed approach is not the only reason for choosing mixed methods. Another potential reason for their use is promoting choice and empowerment for research participants: offering the choice of how to provide their data (e.g. self-completion schedule versus one-to-one interview versus group interview) can be personally empowering for participants, acting to reinforce their autonomy in choosing how and whether to participate. Providing this kind of choice may assist in reaching different subgroups within the population of interest, thereby enabling research participation whereas, for example, offering only a self-completion questionnaire at once excludes those with low reading and writing ability.

STOP AND THINK

- Review what you wrote in response to the first 'Stop and think' exercise.
- How has your understanding of the terms 'mixed methods' changed?

Critical appraisal of mixed methods studies

The growth of concern with the critical appraisal of research evidence and the use of systematic literature reviews and various forms of rapid evidence review has led to the development of a wide range of **critical appraisal** tools that can be used to assess the methodological quality of individual studies using different research designs (see Chapters 20, 27). As use of mixed methods grows, so does focus on the question of how mixed methods studies can be critically appraised. A number of rather different approaches have resulted. One approach proposes that the qualitative and quantitative components need to be treated separately, arguing that this is necessary as they are based on different paradigms (e.g. Sale & Brazil 2004). Another approach does not agree that methods are strictly paradigm-specific, and argues that some common criteria can be identified, although the means for measuring these

> Critical appraisal: The systematic examination of a research study to assess its strengths, weaknesses and trustworthiness, as well as its value and relevance in different contexts.

may differ according to methodological approach (e.g. Bryman *et al.* 2008), and otherwise a combination should be used. Some argue that it is particularly important that the design and the integration between methods receive specific assessment (e.g. Caracelli & Riggin 1994), and that appraising a mixed methods study requires examining the justification for a mixed methods approach, the transparency of the design as well as the sampling and data collection and analysis of individual components (e.g. Caracelli & Riggin 1994; Creswell *et al.* 2004; Creswell 2013). For an example of a study which illustrates how the question of integration of methods can be approached, see Franz *et al.* (2013). A useful review of different approaches to critical appraisal of mixed methods studies can be found in Heyvaert *et al.* (2013).

In what follows, some different approaches to critical appraisal are presented and discussed in order of their level of complexity. The first of these focuses on research design and execution. Two different examples are presented (see Table 21.2).

TABLE 21.2   Guidance for critical appraisal of mixed methods studies

THREE QUESTIONS (ADAPTED FROM CRESWELL & PLANO-CLARK 2011)	SIX ELEMENTS (ADAPTED FROM O'CATHAIN *ET AL.* 2008, p. 97)
1 Were rigorous mixed methods used? 2 Is the mixed research purpose statement, research question, type of mixed methods design, and data analyses presented clearly and comprehensively? 3 Do the study's author(s) present information regarding challenges that may have arisen during the study (e.g. unequal sample sizes, how participants were selected, the steps taken throughout the study)?	1 The justification for using a mixed methods approach to answer the research question(s). 2 The design in terms of the purpose, priority and sequence of methods. 3 Each method in terms of sampling, data collection and analysis. 4 Where integration has occurred, how it has occurred and who has participated in it. 5 Any limitation of one method associated with the presence of another method. 6 Any insights gained from mixing or integrating methods.

The first is that of Creswell and Plano Clark (2011), in which, once it is determined that a study is mixed methods, three questions guide appraisal. Second, there is GRAMMS (Good Reporting of A Mixed Methods Study) guidance offered by O'Cathain and colleagues (2008). GRAMMS was produced as part of their study of the quality of mixed methods studies from 1994 to 2004 funded by the Department of Health in England. The GRAMMS guidance consists of six elements that must be presented in detail. As can be seen in both examples, the questions posed or areas that must be covered are presented in very broad terms. The other types of critical appraisal approaches attempt to provide further guidance in terms of specific criteria or standards.

Moving up in terms of complexity, or alternatively providing more specific detail about some aspects of what is to be included in a high-quality study, a program of research in Canada has resulted in the production and testing of the Mixed Methods Appraisal Tool (MMAT) checklist (Pluye *et al.* 2009; Pace *et al.* 2012). This is a rather different kind of tool, having been produced specifically for use in a new form of systematic literature review—the mixed studies review, which includes qualitative, quantitative and mixed methods studies. The MMAT checklist has sections for qualitative, RCTs, quantitative non-randomised, quantitative descriptive and mixed methods. For a mixed methods study, the questions for appropriate qualitative and quantitative components must also be applied. Table 21.3 reproduces the MMAT checklist. Pace and colleagues (2012) describe the reliability and efficiency of the MMAT tested in the course of a systematic mixed studies review that examined the benefits of participatory research. Pluye and colleagues (2009) explain a scoring system that can be used with the MMAT. Each of the relevant items in Table 21.3 is scored 1 if the criterion is satisfied and 0 if it is not, then the overall 'quality score' is calculated by expressing the number of criteria satisfied as a percentage of the number of relevant criteria for that study. Pluye and colleagues emphasise that it may be necessary to use supplementary documentation and contact with the authors to gain enough information to fully appraise a study.

In contrast, a slightly different direction has been taken in a number of interconnected contributions originating in the USA. Teddlie and Tashakkori (2009) present a schema with two domains, each associated with a number of criteria (Table 21.4). Collins and colleagues (2012) argue that there are two further levels of criteria that should be addressed. The first relates to the clarity of the researchers' philosophical assumptions and stances in relation to all components, claims, actions and uses in a mixed research study, as well as their clear articulation for scrutiny. The second criterion relates to the perspectives, values and standards of the relevant communities of practice, requiring clear identification and articulation in dialogue, both reflective and actual. Collins *et al.* (2012) delineate what they call the 'holistic and synergistic legitimation research process', a detailed treatment of which is beyond the space restrictions of this chapter.

Yet another approach proceeds by examining the question of 'validity' for mixed methods studies. Dellinger and Leech (2007) introduce the notion of a validation framework to provide guidance in this area. For mixed methods, elements of construction validation are drawn from Teddlie and Tashakkori's schema, plus a third domain of legitimation (used as an alternative term for validity because of the latter's association with a positivist research paradigm), with nine associated criteria (or types of legitimation) drawn from Onwuegbuzie and Johnson's typology (2006). Four further elements, with associated appraisal questions, are present to complete the framework (see Table 21.5). Dellinger and Leech describe how the framework can be used in many different ways at different stages of planning or execution of a study as well as for appraising studies. As they note, some elements of construction validation (elements 3 and 4 above), are not totally under the researchers' control, and will change over time. An application of the validation framework to three studies in the fields of education, health care and counselling can be found in Leech *et al.* (2010), and a very useful discussion of guidelines for writing up reports and papers on mixed methods studies in Leech *et al.* (2011). There is considerable overlap in some of the areas of the four additional elements in the validation framework and the additional two levels of criteria distinguished in Collins and colleagues' legitimation process discussed above.

TABLE 21.3 MMAT checklist

TYPES OF MIXED METHODS STUDY COMPONENTS OR PRIMARY STUDIES METHODOLOGICAL QUALITY CRITERIA	RESPONSES			
	YES	NO	CAN'T TELL	COMMENTS
Screening questions (for all types)				
• Are there clear qualitative and quantitative research questions (or objectives), or a clear mixed methods question (or objective)?*				
• Do the collected data allow the research question to be addressed (objective)? For example, consider whether the follow-up period is long enough for the outcome to occur (for longitudinal studies or study components).				
Further quality appraisal may be not feasible when the answer is 'No' or 'Can't tell' to one or both screening questions.				
1 Qualitative	1.1 Are the sources of qualitative data (archives, documents, informants, observations) relevant to address the research question (objective)?				
	1.2 Is the process for analysing qualitative data relevant to address the research question (objective)?				
	1.3 Is appropriate consideration given to how findings relate to the context, e.g. the setting in which the data were collected?				
	1.4 Is appropriate consideration given to how findings relate to researchers' influence, e.g. through their interactions with participants?				

(continued)

TABLE 21.3 MMAT checklist (continued)

TYPES OF MIXED METHODS STUDY COMPONENTS OR PRIMARY STUDIES		RESPONSES			
METHODOLOGICAL QUALITY CRITERIA		YES	NO	CAN'T TELL	COMMENTS
2 Quantitative randomised controlled (trials)	2.1 Is there a clear description of the randomisation (or an appropriate sequence generation)?				
	2.2 Is there a clear description of the allocation concealment (or blinding when applicable)?				
	2.3 Are there complete outcome data (80% or above)?				
	2.4 Is there low withdrawal/drop-out (below 20%)?				
3 Quantitative non-randomised	3.1 Are participants (organisations) recruited in a way that minimised selection bias?				
	3.2 Are measurements appropriate (clear origin, or validity known, or standard instrument; and absence of contamination between groups when appropriate) regarding the exposure/intervention and outcomes?				
	3.3 In the groups being compared (exposed vs non-exposed; with intervention vs without; cases vs controls), are the participants comparable, or do researchers take into account (control for) the difference between these groups?				
	3.4 Are there complete outcome data (80% or above), and, when applicable, an acceptable response rate (60% or above), or an acceptable follow-up rate for cohort studies (depending on the duration of follow-up)?				

4 Quantitative descriptive	4.1 Is the sampling strategy relevant to address the quantitative research question (quantitative aspect of the mixed methods question)?			
	4.2 Is the sample representative of the population under study?			
	4.3 Are measurements appropriate (clear origin, or validity known, or standard instrument)?			
	4.4 Is there an acceptable response rate (60% or above)?			
5 Mixed methods	5.1 Is the mixed methods research design relevant to address the qualitative and quantitative research questions (or objectives), or the qualitative and quantitative aspects of the mixed methods question (or objective)?			
	5.2 Is the integration of qualitative and quantitative data (or results) relevant to address the research question (objective)?*			
	5.3 Is appropriate consideration given to the limitations associated with this integration, e.g. the divergence of qualitative and quantitative data (or results) in a triangulation design?			
	Criteria for the qualitative component (1.1–1.4), and appropriate criteria for the quantitative component (2.1–2.4, or 3.1–3.4, or 4.1–4.4) must be also applied.			

*This item is not considered a double-barrelled question since, in mixed methods research, qualitative and quantitative data may be integrated, and/or qualitative findings and quantitative results can be integrated.

Source: Pace et al. (2012, pp. 51–2, Appendix A)

Ann Taket

TABLE 21.4   Assessing design quality and interpretive rigour

DESIGN QUALITY	INTERPRETIVE RIGOUR
1 Design suitability: to what degree are the methods suitable to responding to the research question(s) and to what degree are the different strands, and how they are mixed, appropriate?	1 Interpretive consistency: to what degree are the inferences and findings aligned in terms of type, scope and intensity?
2 Design fidelity: to what degree are the different components such as sampling, data collection and data analysis executed with rigour and quality?	2 Theoretical consistency: to what degree are inferences consistent with theory and the extant knowledge base?
3 Within-design consistency: do the components and strands fit together in a logical and appropriate manner?	3 Interpretive agreement: to what degree are the inferences and conclusions likely to be reached by other scholars and to what degree are the inferences aligned to the participants' constructions?
4 Analytic adequacy: to what extent do the analysis procedures address the research question(s) and are analytic strategies executed successfully?	4 Interpretive distinctiveness: to what degree are the inferences credible in contrast to other plausible interpretations of the findings?
	5 Integrative efficacy: to what degree are the inferences integrated, leading to meaningful meta-inferences; to what degree are the inconsistencies between inferences viewed as credible and theoretically validated?
	6 Interpretive correspondence: to what degree are the inferences per approach aligned to the inquiry's purpose and research question; to what degree do the meta-inferences address the mixing purpose of the inquiry?

Source: Adapted from Teddlie & Tashakkori (2009, pp. 301–2)

TABLE 21.5   Additional elements in the validation framework approach

1 Foundational element	a What preconceptions, prelogic, biases, prior knowledge and/or theories are (un)acknowledged by the researcher as relates to the meaning of the data? b Is the review of literature appropriate for the purpose of the study? c What is the quality of the review of literature (e.g. evaluation and synthesis of literature is appropriate. Does the review inform the purpose, design, measurement, analysis and inferences? Is it comprehensive, relevant, thorough, etc.)? d Does the review confirm or disconfirm grounded theory?
2 Translation fidelity/ inferential consistency audit	a Do the inferences follow from the links between the theories/lived experience, research literature, purpose, design, measurement and analysis? b Are meta-inferences consistent with these elements? c How well does the chosen methodological approach maximise the available information necessary to achieve the purpose of the study? d Is there a better approach, given the theory, research literature, purpose, design, measurement and analysis?
3 Utilisation/historical element	a How often, by whom and in what ways have findings/measures been utilised? b How appropriate were the uses of the findings/measures? c What, if anything, worthwhile does this contribute to the meaning of data?
4 Consequential element	a What are or have been the consequences of use of the findings/measures? b Are/were those consequences socially/politically acceptable? c What, if anything, worthwhile do the consequences contribute to the meaning of data?

Source: Adapted from Dellinger & Leech (2007)

Ann Taket

STOP AND THINK

Thinking about your knowledge of critical appraisal and your knowledge of different types of mixed methods study:

- In what circumstances does critical appraisal for these studies require the development of new appraisal tools?
- In what circumstances can the tools for appraisal of qualitative and quantitative studies be sufficient?

A case study: exploring reasons why women do not use breast screening

In this section, I consider a mixed methods study, drawn from my own research. This is a very simple example of such a study, where data collection and analysis contained both qualitative and quantitative components; it can be regarded as a blended study in the terms discussed earlier. In this study, the use of mixed methods turned out to be crucial in understanding women's behaviour in using or not using breast screening. Here the focus is on only some of the results, illustrating the usefulness of mixed methods in this case.

Background

The study was commissioned in 2004 by the Department of Public Health in south-east London, against a background of concern about low local uptake of breast screening for the target group of women aged fifty to sixty-four. Average uptake was just over 60 per cent for the area as a whole and as low as 54 per cent in some parts; this fell below government targets, at the time of a minimum acceptable level of uptake of 70 per cent. The area is characterised by high levels of deprivation, with pockets of relative affluence within its urban inner-city setting. It is a culturally and ethnically diverse area: in some parts of the area, half or more of the local population is black or minority ethnic. Around 130 languages are spoken across the area (Barter-Godfrey & Taket 2007).

Study recruitment

Between July and December 2004, a sample of 306 women aged fifty to sixty-four was recruited opportunistically from a variety of community sources, including voluntary groups, community sector organisations and faith groups. Women were offered the choice of how they would like to give their views: group interview, individual interview (face-to-face or telephone), or self-completed questionnaire (see Chapter 13). The majority (85 per cent) chose to complete the questionnaire themselves and return it by post. Of the 15 per cent who chose to have the questionnaire administered, the majority chose to do this over the telephone; their answers were noted by the researcher taking the call.

Information about the study was presented in English and other relevant languages (Bengali, Arabic, Somali, Turkish, Vietnamese, Albanian, Cantonese, French, Spanish, Portuguese), and questionnaires were produced in English and French (no demand for other languages was expressed). The use of a variety of recruitment mechanisms ensured that the sample contained women from all the major ethnic communities in the area, and diversity in the sample in terms of other socio-demographic characteristics. Women were offered £20 in vouchers for their participation in the study. Ethics clearance for the study was gained from London South Bank University Research Ethics Committee. Participation in the study was entirely voluntary and respondents were assured of confidentiality. No ethical issues arose during the study.

Designing the study

Funds available for the research, as well as the requested timetable for completion, constrained our choice of study design. In particular, they ruled out a totally qualitative design (see chapters in Part II) and a sequential mixed methods design with a qualitative stage preceding a larger quantitative survey (see Chapter 20). The decision was therefore made to use a single schedule that was largely structured, for both interviews and self-completion. Themes of interest were initially established by considering the research problem of low uptake of breast screening, using themes already identified in research literature and from an advisory group of relevant professionals. Specific structured questions were selected for each theme; these are discussed in the next section.

The schedule explored the health issues that are important for women, their knowledge and beliefs in relation to breast cancer and their use or non-use of breast cancer screening. Information about socio-demographic characteristics and aspects of daily life (living situation, work, caring responsibilities) was also collected. Asking about daily life was intended to provide some insight into the daily burden of our sample, in terms of themes of responsibilities and isolation. Most of the questions were structured with a set of responses to choose from, one of which was always 'Other', with space to specify further. There were three open questions, placed carefully within the schedule, which provided the main qualitative strand within the study; these are discussed below.

The schedule underwent several stages of piloting before finalisation. Using a small availability sample of women in the right age group, living or working in south London, we tested the acceptability of question topics. Items that were acceptable to the group included asking direct questions about attending and rejecting breast screening. There was a preference for providing alternative answers to choose from rather than being expected to articulate their own reasons for behaviour choice, especially when behaviour did not conform to health promotion messages. Time and resource constraints led us to be highly selective about the questions included in order to keep the instrument to no more than four sides of A4 in its self-completion form. We considered that this restriction in length would also maximise the likelihood of women completing the questionnaire, and improve rates of response. See also Chapter 13.

The qualitative strand

The qualitative strand of the study focused on the comments supplied by respondents against selection of the category 'Other' in the closed questions, and answers to the three open questions. The first of these was on the first page of the schedule, before any mention of breast cancer or breast cancer screening (these questions appeared on the second page, not visible initially). This first open question asked women, 'What are your main health concerns?' Note that the study was presented under the title 'Women and Health'. This was in order to appeal to the broadest possible section of the target population. We were concerned about the possibility that non-attenders who distance themselves from breast screening and those who do not identify with breast cancer would deselect themselves from the sample if the research was presented as a breast cancer or breast screening study. This was borne out by the lack of reference to breast cancer in the open 'Health Concerns' section and the small proportion of the sample who held strong beliefs opposing mammography and rejecting breast screening.

The second qualitative section was designed to elicit further information about our respondents' health concerns, this time more indirectly, through two open questions that formed the two closing sections of the schedule. Under the heading of improving local health services we asked, 'What are your suggestions for improving health care service provision, for you and women like you?' Then, finally, under the heading 'Any Other Comments', we asked, 'Is there anything else you would like to say about looking after your health or health care provision for women over 50?'

The quantitative strand

The quantitative strand of the study focused on the answers to structured questions. These explored a number of different areas. First of these were women's daily life, their health and health-related behaviour, concerns about specific health issues (diabetes, breast cancer, heart disease, osteoporosis), exploring in particular notions of candidacy. 'Candidacy' refers to an individual's personal conception of their being 'a candidate for' developing a particular disease, and explains the causes and prevention of disease in terms of an individual's beliefs about who is affected by it and who is not (Davison *et al.* 1991, 1992). The second major section related to breast cancer screening, where questions explored past behaviour in some detail (including reasons for attendance and non-attendance), convenience of appointments and, finally, future intentions. A third major section explored sources of health advice/information and health service provision, attitudes to looking after their own health, views about health service communications (relevance and clarity), and asked about attitudes to breast cancer screening in terms of three different dimensions (whether screening was important, reasonable, reassuring).

STOP AND THINK

Identify a health topic you are interested in.

- Draft two open-ended questions regarding this topic.
- Draft two closed structured questions relating to this topic (draw on the research literature relating to the topic if you wish, just as the case study does in relation to the notion of candidacy).

Analysis and interpretation of data

An SPSS database (version 11) was created for use in analysing the data (see Chapter 25). Reponses to the open-ended questions were coded thematically on the basis of the researchers reading about a third of the sample and noting emerging themes (see Chapter 23). Themed responses were included as separate variables in the database with dichotomous coding: theme raised or theme not raised. Some 'flags' were also included in the database, to record issues that were not overtly included in the schedule, such as mental health, literacy and menopause. The flag system was used to identify which participants had included narratives supplementary to the direct questions about breast cancer and breast screening, for later use in qualitative analysis.

All the questionnaires and interviews were coded prior to data entry, using the coding schedule. Any items in the data set that were not obviously allocated to one particular code were discussed between the researchers and coded by consensus about what would best represent the participant's responses. Quantitative data were subject to a range of descriptive and simple inferential statistical analysis and a limited amount of multivariate analysis (see Chapter 25). Moving between analysis of qualitative data and quantitative data helped illuminate our understanding of women's behaviours in relation to breast cancer screening.

Breast cancer and breast screening: not a major health concern for our sample

One very important finding from the study came in response to our first open question: 'What are your main health concerns?' At this stage, only 4 per cent of our sample mentioned anything that we could link to breast cancer or breast screening, as one of their main health concerns. In other words, for our sample, other concerns were more important. This question was deliberately placed before any specific breast screening questions were introduced into the schedule, since we wanted to get some idea of women's specific concerns before introducing the topic of breast cancer or breast screening. Instead, women talked about a chronic medical or physical condition (60 per cent of the sample), an acute medical or physical condition (27 per cent), psychological issues (19 per cent), pain, including pain management (17 per cent), ageing/deterioration (11 per cent), weight loss or maintenance (10 per cent), maintaining good health (9 per cent), menopause (9 per cent), provision of services (6 per cent), concerns not about self (2 per cent). Other issues (not groupable!) were mentioned by 11 per cent of the sample. Twenty-three of our sample (7.5 per cent) did not report any health concerns.

Comments and concerns about breast screening and, to a lesser extent breast cancer, were made in the undirected open sections at the end of the schedule by 26 per cent of the sample. However, these are mostly comments that supplement the options provided in the screening uptake section of the questionnaire and appear to be prompted by the presence of questions about breast screening, hence the increase from 4 per cent of women raising the issue at the start of the questionnaire to 26 per cent raising the issue at the end. This strongly suggests that breast cancer and breast screening are not high priorities for concern for the women in the sample. Women in our sample did not spend time worrying about breast cancer. They had

Ann Taket

plenty of other matters of greater concern. We doubt whether we would have identified this without the blended design, where the first open question invited women to speak about 'their main health concerns' rather than being led by mention of particular topics. As a contrast, an international study (NOP World 2005), carried out at roughly the same time, gives a very different impression. This study, a quantitative one, asked, 'Thinking now about breast cancer, how concerned, if at all, would you say you are about getting it?' In the UK sample, the percentage answering 'Very' or 'Quite' concerned was 71 per cent for women aged forty-five to fifty-four, and 69 per cent for women aged fifty-five to sixty-four. This different form of questioning gives quite a different impression of women's concerns; arguably the higher response is led by the question, which invites an expression of concern.

Our finding about the low level of concern with breast cancer at once begins to make the low levels of screening uptake in the population more understandable.

STOP AND THINK

Using the questions you have formulated for your health topic, experiment with changing the order in which the questions are asked. For each ordering of questions you investigate, ask the questions to a cooperative friend/fellow student, jot down or record their replies and at the end ask for their comments on the questions and the ordering.

- What did you find out about the effects of the order of questions for your health topic?

Understanding breast screening behaviour: rational and personally justifiable

Moving backwards and forwards between the data in the qualitative and quantitative strands of the study enabled us to conclude that the decision to attend or decline screening is rational and personally justifiable, engaging factors linked to emotions and attitude. A few examples are presented here in terms of three patterns of screening behaviour identified in the sample: those who adhere to, reject or are ambivalent towards the screening program.

The adherence group is made up of those who always attend screening, the largest group in our sample, 78 per cent. Our sample was not representative of the population at large in terms of screening behaviour, and this is perhaps not at all surprising; other research in inner cities suggests that literacy, participation and concerns about health are important issues, so people who are non-participative, have difficulties with English language notices or are unconcerned about health issues are less likely to screen (Lai Fong Chiu 2002; Pfeffer 2004) and similarly are less likely to join a health research study such as this. The rejection group is those who have never been to breast screening and have no intention of attending in the future (6 per cent). The third group, which we labelled the 'ambivalent', were those who sometimes attend, sometimes decline (16 per cent). Notice that our study design, achieving a total sample of 306, contained enough women in the rejection and ambivalent groups to allow meaningful analysis in those groups. A smaller, purely qualitative study would have been unlikely to achieve this, since no access to an accurate sampling frame that identified women by their screening behaviour was possible.

The adherers were women who always go to screening—they adhere fully to the screening program— and simply receiving the invitation is enough to encourage them to attend:

I had the appointment so I went. It was just a thing you do, like having your eyes tested.

The second group, the rejecters, simply reject the breast screening program outright, have never been to screening and have no intention of ever going:

I have never attended screening and would rather not know as nature knows best. In my opinion it is best to leave things alone regardless what the experts say.

I do not like the idea of six lots of four x-rays on my breasts by the time I am 65 years old.

Breast screening is likely to lead to minor problems being treated with major surgery.

To a certain extent, some of the issues the women raise can be approached as misconceptions, for example concerns about the radiation, which can be changed through health promotion over time. But, for raising uptake at the point of the next invitation, this would be the group least amenable to change.

The third group was those whose behaviour was changeable: sometimes attending, sometimes not. Inconvenience was the most commonly reported reason for not attending an appointment (31 per cent of those who have declined breast screening at least once). Other options, such as 'something came up' (8 per cent), and 'I was unwell that day' (10 per cent), also indicated that the appointment was untimely rather than unwelcome. Inconvenience as a reason to miss breast screening appointments was a prolonged state rather than a reflection of the specific day or time of day offered for the appointment. This can be seen as a reflection of the pressures and demands in the woman's life at the time of the invitation. Less than half of those who missed inconvenient appointments rescheduled them. In the context of other demands competing for the time and resources of these women, perceived inconvenience can de-prioritise attending screening to the point of missing appointments.

Experiencing or expecting pain is associated with the decision to decline screening; 16 per cent of women who decline screening reported doing so to avoid pain:

I now do not want to go because the last screening I had was so painful.

Twenty-one per cent of women who declined screening reported doing so to avoid anxiety:

I find it quite traumatic going to screening and have to work myself up to it.

Fourteen per cent reported doing so to avoid embarrassment, with 10 per cent feeling uncomfortable getting undressed:

I feel unable to go as I hate my weight. Silly excuse … but it affects me badly.

Put this with the role of anticipated regret and worry, and we found that many of the women in our sample are emotionally involved with mammography. They attend screening or avoid it in ways that look after their emotional well-being, aside from their potential physical health.

Ann Taket

Positive attitude and perceived personal importance of breast screening were the most important variables in our study. These were the variables that were predictive of consistent attendance compared to inconsistent attendance, and consistent declining compared to attendance. At point of invitation, some women are switched off by their own beliefs about screening, whereas others almost automatically attend. For some women, attitude is shaped by previous negative experiences, to the point where they no longer feel that it is reasonable for them to attend. These women may be motivated to return, they have attended before and may be persuaded that the pain or anxiety is worth it, especially to avoid anticipated regret. One implication is that we may need to focus on changing their attitude towards the value of screening. For others, their attitude towards screening is generally positive but not strong enough to convert it into behaviour, either because there are too many other demands competing for priority or because they never quite get around to it, and so far they have not knowingly suffered for that decision. These women may be persuaded by encouraging them to see attendance as important, given their overall positive attitude.

Thus, once we examine the details of women's reasoning when they receive the invitation to screening, we find their behaviour perfectly reasonable in response to their particular circumstances at the time. The concept of the decisional balance, an individual weighing up the pros and cons of competing behaviour choices, drawn from the trans-theoretic model (Velicer *et al.* 1998), proved useful in understanding women's screening behaviour.

STOP AND THINK

Thinking about your chosen health topic, what are two different qualitative methods that could be used to research it? Think about in-depth interviews, focus groups, observation, narrative research, ethnography (see chapters in Part II in this volume).

- Which of these methods might be most appropriate for different socio-demographic groups?

Challenges and terrors of mixing methods

The case study illustrates the value of mixed methods within a relatively small and contained study. The qualitative data aided our interpretation of the quantitative findings and vice versa, producing a richer understanding of the complexity of factors underlying low uptake rates for breast screening in the population studied, and providing a number of different insights into the action that could be taken to improve these (see also Chapter 1).

In this final section, the challenges of using mixed methods are explored. In some cases, the literature presents these issues in such stark and terrifying terms as to imply that they are to be avoided at all costs (together with the use of mixed methods) rather than merely as challenges to be addressed!

The first concern that is sometimes raised is the danger of epistemological confusion. Different methods rest on quite different assumptions about how the world is (**ontology**) and how we can come to gain knowledge of that world (**epistemology**) (see Chapters 1, 20). Some argue that there is a danger in using methods in a single study that rely on different epistemologies. For example, Sale and colleagues (2002) would see this as forbidden in certain circumstances. A different position is offered here, namely that this does not matter, provided that the differences are acknowledged and brought into play when results are discussed and interpretations made. We can label this a position characterised by theoretical pluralism, underpinned by **pragmatism** (in the sense explained so fluently by the US philosopher Richard Rorty) (Rorty 1989; see also Chapters 1, 20). Some would argue that this position amounts to wanting to have our cake and eat it, but is that not a desirable position? The notion that we have to choose a single theoretical position and not deviate from it conveys a kind of rigidity that is no longer expected even within the hard sciences—consider the wave/particle duality accepted in terms of theories of light, Heisenberg's uncertainty principle, chaos and complexity theory, to name but a few. For more detailed exposition of this stance, see the editorial by Johnson (2008), who labels this a dialectical approach. For an excellent case study of some of the difficulties that can arise when the researchers in a team come from different epistemological traditions, see Lunde *et al.* (2013).

Mixed methods research is often regarded as multiplying the work involved, with consequent implications for resources, not only in terms of finance but in terms of finding researchers with the necessary range of skills, particularly since the tendency in the past has been for individuals to focus on either qualitative or quantitative methods in their research careers. Of course, this can be overcome by the use of teams, so perhaps it is merely that mixed methods research makes studies carried out by a lone researcher rarer (although it still does not remove them entirely). Mixed methods research is not necessarily extremely expensive, as the case study shows. There is, however, a need to consider how a broader training in research methods could be encouraged for individuals. This is a matter that is beginning to receive attention.

One final question is whether it is harder to get mixed methods research published. This connects to the related challenge of publishing qualitative research. Journals still tend to specialise in either qualitative or quantitative research. Mixed methods studies, owing to their relative rareness, are arguably harder to get through referees, as there may be a shortage of referees with the relevant experience. The growth of specialist journals for mixed methods research, such as the *Journal of Mixed Methods Research* (first published in 2007) and the *International Journal of Multiple Research Approaches* (first published in 2006), provides a partial answer but does not satisfy those of us who would rather see our research published in health journals to reach our intended audiences. There is also the question of word length. On purely practical grounds, it is far harder to summarise a complex mixed methods design in the same word length that a simpler non-mixed design would take. To satisfy the demands of peer reviewers, the description of method may take so many words as to prohibit the discussion of the results to any great extent!

Ontology: The study of the nature of being, existence or reality in general.

Epistemology: This is concerned with the nature of knowledge and how knowledge is obtained.

Pragmatism: Argues that reality exists not only as natural and physical realities but also as psychological and social realities, which include subjective experience and thought, language and culture.

Ann Taket

STOP AND THINK

- Thinking about your personal experience of research, what are your terrors and challenges in thinking about doing mixed methods research?
- How might you overcome these?

In conclusion or inconclusion?

I make no apology for the pun in this heading. It is difficult to offer hard-and-fast conclusions about the use of mixed methods in health research. There are too many unknowns, which the preceding section has alluded to.

My position is that, increasingly, those of us in the fields of health research, especially public health and health promotion, will need to become passionate practitioners of mixed methods research in order to answer the complex questions that need to be addressed if we are to successfully design and implement programs to address health inequities in the diverse communities that we serve. However, there are often difficulties in achieving the funding necessary for the extent of such research. Competitive research funding still disadvantages qualitative and mixed methods designs, perhaps not as much as twenty or even ten years ago, but still clearly evident. Within universities, where the drivers are winning the highest category of research funding and publishing in the most highly regarded journals (not usually read by practitioners), this may militate against mixed methods research. On the other hand, I see a positive development in the growth of practitioner-based and community-based research, with the concomitant advantages of ownership and relevance. So perhaps the most fertile base for growth in mixed methods research is within communities of practice.

Summary

The term 'mixed methods' can refer to different types of methods being used within a single study; often it is used to refer to mixing qualitative and quantitative methods. But it can also refer to mixing different types of qualitative method within a study, or to mixing that occurs at different stages in the research process, for example in data collection or data analysis or in both these stages. There are also different modes or ways of mixing methods within a single study—sequential, parallel or blended.

There are various situations in which different types of mixed method may be appropriate. Each has advantages and disadvantages, along with the challenges (or fears) that mixed methods evoke. The chapter considers the potential reasons for mixing different types of qualitative method and the development of critical appraisal tools for use with these studies. Some of the issues involved in using mixed methods in health research are illustrated by means of a case study of research carried out by the author.

Practice exercises

1   Read the following article: R.A. Laws, S.E. Kirby, G.P.P. Davies, A.M. Williams, U.W. Jayasinghe, C.L. Amoroso & M.F. Harris (2008). 'Should I and can I': a mixed methods study of clinician beliefs and attitudes in the management of lifestyle risk factors in primary health care. *BMC Health Services Research*, 8.

Discuss the following questions.

(a)   What type(s) of mixed methods are being used?

(b)   What advantages did the use of mixed methods give?

(c)   What disadvantages did its use give?

2   Read the following article: M. Stewart, E. Makwarimba, A. Barnfather, N. Letourneau & A. Neufeld (2008). Researching reducing health disparities: mixed methods approaches. *Social Science & Medicine*, 66(6), 1406–17.

Discuss the following questions.

(a)   What type(s) of mixed methods are being used?

(b)   What advantages did the use of mixed methods give?

(c)   What disadvantages did its use give?

3   Compare and contrast the use of mixed methods in the two articles.

4   Using one of the critical appraisal approaches for mixed methods studies introduced in the chapter, compare the two articles.

5   You are approached by a community group to help produce a report about community views on local health services. The community group serves a population diverse in ethnicity, religion, educational achievement and income. Outline how you might use mixed methods to do this, and the advantages and disadvantages of your proposed design.

Ann Taket

Further reading

Creswell, J.W. (2015). *A concise introduction to mixed methods research*. Thousand Oaks, CA: Sage.

Creswell, J.W. & Plano Clark, V.L. (2011). *Designing and conducting mixed methods research*, 2nd edn. Thousand Oaks, CA: Sage.

Curry, L. & Nunez-Smith, M. (2015). *Mixed methods in health sciences research*. Thousand Oaks, CA: Sage.

Greene, J.C. (2007). *Mixed methods in social inquiry*. San Francisco: Jossey-Bass.

Hall, B. & Howard, K. (2008). A synergistic approach: conducting mixed methods research with typological and systemic design considerations. *Journal of Mixed Methods Research*, 2(3), 248–69.

Johnson, B. (2008). Editorial. Living with tensions: the dialectic approach. *Journal of Mixed Methods Research*, 2(3), 203–7.

Mendlinger, S. & Cwikel, J. (2008). Spiraling between qualitative and quantitative data on women's health behaviors: a double helix model for mixed methods. *Qualitative Health Research*, 18(2), 280–93.

Teddlie, C. & Tashakkori, A. (2009). *Foundations of mixed methods research: integrating quantitative and qualitative approaches in the social and behavioral sciences*. Thousand Oaks, CA: Sage.

Websites

http://mra.e-contentmanagement.com

International Journal of Multiple Research Approaches.

http://mmr.sagepub.com

Journal of Mixed Methods Research.

http://qhr.sagepub.com

Qualitative Health Research.

These are three important journals for reporting mixed methods research.

22

Collaborative Participatory Research with Disadvantaged Communities

ANKE VAN DER STERREN, PETER WAPLES-CROWE AND PRISCILLA PYETT

Chapter objectives

In this chapter you will learn:

- to understand the key features of collaborative participatory approaches for research with disadvantaged communities
- when and why to use collaborative and participatory approaches
- details of the method in practice
- how to use collaborative participatory research in an Indigenous health context

Key terms

Collaborative participatory research

Community

Indigenous people

Participatory action research

Project agreement or memorandum of understanding

Steering committee or advisory group

Introduction

In this chapter we will discuss the use of a collaborative participatory approach for research, particularly with disadvantaged communities. Readers might have come across terms such as 'collaborative', 'participatory' or 'community-based' research, as well as 'participatory action research' or 'action research'. Each of these approaches promotes the active involvement in research by people who have been conventionally the 'subject' of the research. Such research approaches do not seek to discover widely generalisable findings, but rather to generate understandings specific to particular contexts, and to produce actions and outcomes that are relevant and of benefit to local communities.

The term 'action research' was first coined by Kurt Lewin (1946/1988) in the late 1940s in the USA, and this approach has been widely used in organisational development, workplace relations and education. Participatory research was developed a little later in what were then known as 'Third World' settings by people such as Paulo Freire (1972) in South America. In recent decades, participatory action research and collaborative approaches to research are increasingly used by practitioners in health and welfare, who recognise the importance of consumer or patient involvement in the production of knowledge, for example in developing patient care plans, conducting a community needs analysis or assisting people living with chronic illness (de Koning & Martin 1996; Koch *et al.* 2002; Stringer & Genat 2004; Wadsworth 2010; Higginbottom & Liamputtong 2015).

Participatory action research

Participatory action research (PAR) involves a repetitive cycle of observing, reflecting, planning and acting (see Figure 22.1). This process is sometimes depicted as a spiral or helix to show that the process occurs repeatedly over time. A PAR project must involve not only research or enquiry and the participation of community members, but also action to improve their situation. Furthermore, the research and action generated from it is ongoing, with continuous evaluation and modification of the action. Many resources are available that

Participatory action research: A method where informants become co-researchers and the researcher becomes a participant, using their research expertise to assist the informants in self-research.

FIGURE 22.1   The action research cycle

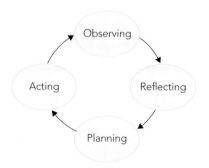

describe PAR in greater detail, as well as its application in various contexts (Carr & Kemmis 1986; Hart & Bond 1995; Bray *et al.* 2000; Stringer & Genat 2004; Chevalier & Buckles 2013; Higginbottom & Liamputtong 2015).

EXAMPLES OF PAR

Women living with multiple sclerosis in South Australia

This project sought to understand the experiences of living with chronic illness. The researcher initially established and participated in a discussion group comprising eight women living with MS, and four nursing consultants. This group met for ten sessions over six months. The format of the sessions enabled the sharing of expertise and experiences; in the initial sessions nurses provided information about incontinence, while subsequent sessions opened up opportunities for the women to share their experiences of incontinence or any other matters they wished to raise. Analysis of the themes arising from the group sessions was ongoing, and feedback of each session was given to participants at the beginning of each of the sessions that followed. The women were then involved, both individually and collectively, in developing, planning and implementing actions to address each of the issues raised in the group. Subsequent additional discussion groups were established; the authors note that the use of PAR principles allowed for the development of distinctive group dynamics and outcomes (Koch & Kralik 2001; Koch *et al.* 2002).

Prevention of schistosomiasis among schoolchildren in Tanzania

This project sought to investigate sustainable ways to prevent schistosomiasis (a tropical skin disease) by targeting schoolchildren, among whom infection is high. As a result of an initial screening and treatment program, several school- and community-based activities were developed. Teachers, children, parents and the broader community became involved in the development and evaluation of health promotion activities. Schoolchildren were trained to conduct household sanitation surveys and were involved in redesigning and readministering modified household surveys. Reflection by participants on the findings of the screenings and household surveys, and evaluations of health promotion activities, led to further activity, including the development of a curriculum for schistosomiasis education in schools (Freudenthal *et al.* 2006).

RESEARCH IN PRACTICE

Health workers in an urban Aboriginal Medical Service

Bill Genat and colleagues undertook a PAR project with Aboriginal health workers (AHWs) and some non-Indigenous health workers in an urban Aboriginal Medical Service (AMS). At the heart of the research process were two focus groups with these health workers. One group decided they wanted to get better at their work and to focus on best practice. They reviewed practices such as home visits, ways to encourage clients to maintain medication schedules and so on. Working collaboratively in the groups, the health workers developed protocols for these practices, implemented the protocols in the field, then reviewed and refined the protocols in subsequent focus group meetings. The other group decided to focus on increasing the status of AHWs through organisational policy within the AMS. Working collectively, they developed policy recommendations and pursued them with management. The health workers were acknowledged as co-authors of the book that describes this project. These processes constituted the typical action–reflection cycles within an action research project and they were participatory (Genat 2006).

Anke van der Sterren, Peter Waples-Crowe and Priscilla Pyett

Collaborative participatory research

The practicalities involved in conducting research in most developed countries means that ongoing action and evaluation are rarely incorporated into the research process. The reality is that funding for community-based research projects generally comes from governments or other organisations whose accountability structures result in inflexible timelines. This inflexibility does not allow the luxury of true action research projects where ongoing reflection enables the repetition of the research activity towards a solution.

We have found that our own research practice can be better described through the use of the term **collaborative participatory research** (CPR), a term that highlights the importance of collaboration and participation. This model recognises that the researcher has certain technical expertise, and that community leaders and community members have knowledge of their community needs and perspectives. Importantly, this approach involves a transfer of knowledge, including knowledge of how to undertake research with community organisations (Nyden & Wiewel 1992). Actions or outcomes that are useful and relevant to the participants, and an ongoing reflection process to continually improve these outcomes, are still desirable but may not be achievable.

Collaborative participatory research: CPR involves a transfer of knowledge between researchers, community leaders and community members, including knowledge of how to undertake research with community organisations.

> **KEY FEATURES OF CPR**
> - Research is conducted for and with communities, not on or about communities.
> - Research takes time to build relationships of mutual trust.
> - Researchers are accountable to the community.
> - Benefits of the research are decided by the community.
> - Community members are involved in planning and carrying out the research, in analysing, reporting and acting on the findings.
> - The knowledge and experience of community members are valued.
> - Researchers respect community members' interests, values and perspectives.
> - Research is a two-way partnership of knowledge and skills exchange.
> - Researchers build community capacity by sharing knowledge of how to do research.
> - The research process is empowering.
> - The research is solution-focused.
> - Researchers are committed to social change through practical or policy outcomes.

Twin goals: empowerment and change

Rather than being a method of health and social research, CPR is more an approach to research that has explicit political goals. The first is to empower people through their involvement in the research process and the production of knowledge about their situation, and to enable them to identify those aspects of their situation that they would like to see improve. Involvement in the research process may occur at a number of levels: setting the research agenda, guiding and monitoring the research process, being part of the research team in designing the project, collecting and analysing data, and writing up the findings. In CPR, the location of power in all stages of the research process ideally lies with the research participants. They become agents, stakeholders and co-researchers, and the role of the researcher ranges from director to facilitator or catalyst for action (Stringer 1999; Stringer & Genat 2004). Because of its potential for empowerment and capacity-building, the process of a CPR project is as important as the outcome. Indeed, capacity-building is one of the intended outcomes of CPR.

The second goal of CPR is to carry out research that will bring about changes and improvements in the lives of the participants. As such, it is an approach that seeks to address structural inequality and social injustice. CPR has been used in research with oppressed, marginalised or disadvantaged communities in many contexts, such as people living in poverty in developing countries, refugees, illicit drug users, sex workers and people living with HIV/AIDS (Warr & Pyett 1999; Maher *et al.* 2002; Coupland *et al.* 2004; Liamputtong 2007, 2010, 2013; see also Chapter 1). CPR aims to produce tangible outcomes for the communities involved. These may be changes in knowledge, attitudes or behaviour, changes to policy or practice, or improvements to service delivery or in the material circumstances of people's lives (Higginbottom & Liamputtong 2015).

EXAMPLES OF CPR IN DEVELOPED AND DEVELOPING COUNTRIES

In Australia

A collaborative partnership was established to develop and evaluate a program for overdose management for people using injecting drugs. The local drug user group initiated the program, and was directly involved in providing comprehensive overdose management training, alongside the prescription and supply of naloxone (that acts to reverse opioid overdose). Other partners included the local alcohol and other drugs peak body, health and emergency service providers, the Australian Capital Territory government, and a number of research institutions. All partners shared a commitment to reducing harms among people injecting drugs, and specifically to reducing deaths from opioid overdose. A consultative group was established to provide expert guidance to the project, including guiding the development and implementation of the evaluation. This collaborative project showed that naloxone could be provided safely and effectively, and this has impacted on policy change to improve health outcomes for people using opioids in the Australian Capital Territory (Lenton *et al.* 2014).

In Tanzania

Researchers in Mwanza, Tanzania, used CPR to develop appropriate methods, monitoring and feedback processes for conducting a large-scale randomised control clinical trial. They held community workshops with study participants (women working in food and recreational facilities), and managers and project workers in community-based clinics that offered reproductive health services. These workshops enabled the researchers

RESEARCH IN PRACTICE

to build a shared understanding with participants of appropriate community structures and approaches for the research trial. They established a Community Advisory Committee based on the guidance given through the workshops. The committee worked closely with the researchers to determine appropriate clinical procedures, mobilisation activities and referral mechanisms for sexually transmitted infection contact tracing and HIV/AIDS-related care. It also served as a mechanism through which the project could be monitored and adverse effects reported and dealt with. CPR also enabled the research team to implement location-specific targeted interventions related to the trial (Vallely *et al.* 2007; Shagi *et al.* 2008).

Why use CPR with disadvantaged communities?

With the increasing realisation that health problems are related to social inequalities, health researchers need to engage with disadvantaged and marginalised groups (Liamputtong 2007, 2010, 2013; Higginbottom & Liamputtong 2015). If we are to understand more about the circumstances of people's lives and the pathways to better health and well-being, we need to conduct our research in such a way that it can give people a voice. However, access to marginalised groups is often extremely difficult, particularly when compared to some of the more common subjects of health research, such as the relatively 'captive' populations that can be recruited from schools, hospitals, clinical settings and general households (Liamputtong 2007). In addition, the researcher may meet with resistance, since people who are disadvantaged and marginalised often have good reason to mistrust people such as researchers, who represent authority. There is also a high likelihood that the researcher will encounter problems with language, literacy, cultural difference or comprehension (Liamputtong 2010, 2013). Finally, locating members of marginalised communities for follow-up research is also more difficult.

Since the Ottawa Charter (WHO 1986), strategies for health research that emphasise participation have been gaining attention and respectability in both industrialised and less industrialised and resource-poor countries. Such participation, particularly with its combination of insider and outsider knowledge, has the potential to increase the validity, relevance and cost-effectiveness of the research, and to improve longer-term outcomes (de Koning & Martin 1996; Stringer & Genat 2004). The validity and legitimacy of a CPR approach are grounded in the honesty and reflexivity of the research process in declaring agendas, carrying out the research and implementing its goals, and in the honesty, clarity and detailed reporting of the process and context of the research (Hagey 1997; Waterman 1998). CPR is thus becoming increasingly important in the health field (de Koning & Martin 1996; Stringer & Genat 2004; Israel *et al.* 2005, 2012; Minkler & Wallestein 2008).

Ideally, a community group working with a researcher identifies a problem or situation that they want to change, and participates collaboratively in the planning and process of research, the interpretation of results and the development and application of any intervention for change. However, community groups rarely have sufficient resources to carry out research on their own, while budget cutbacks in university, health service and community settings in Australia, as in other industrialised societies, increase the need for more cooperation as a way of using limited resources more effectively. The different perspectives of researchers, health professionals and community representatives on the same health problem or social issue can lead to more productive and rigorous research, more relevant and creative problem-solving, more culturally appropriate interventions and more effective social change.

Collaborative participatory approaches to research are generally used with smaller communities, particular those experiencing disadvantage. **Community** can refer to a geographic community or a community of 'interest' or 'identity'. A geographic community might be as large as the population of Australia or as small as a neighbourhood or a suburban street. A community of interest or identity may be a group with a shared history or cultural affinity such as age, gender, religion, ethnicity or sexual orientation, or it may be a group that shares an experience of disadvantage such as poverty or homelessness, or a group who are stigmatised by their behaviour, such as sex workers, injecting drug users or people with mental health problems. Any of these communities or population groups may have shared experiences of disadvantage, but we also need to be aware that there may be a diversity of interests, values and aspirations within groups.

> **Community:** This can refer to any group of people living in geographic proximity or sharing an interest, a history or a cultural affinity.

People living in geographic communities are relatively easy to locate, access and describe, but groups of people or communities that are linked by shared identity, history or interests are often described as hard to reach for the purposes of research or health promotion. They are also hard to define or put a boundary around, so it is difficult to draw a representative sample for a research project. Developing collaborative relationships with community representatives of such hard-to-reach populations is crucial to planning research that will include a broader representation of the relevant population (Liamputtong 2007, 2013).

Research with marginalised and disadvantaged populations requires a high degree of reflective practice, one that is responsive to the social context of the research (Pyett & VicHealth Koori Health Research and Community Development Unit 2002; Liamputtong 2007, 2013). We have to ensure that not only do our actual research processes not cause harm to the groups we are researching, but that the research is not used to further marginalise these already vulnerable people (Liamputtong 2007, 2013; Pyett *et al.* 2008). CPR involves the community in determining what they see as the benefits from the research.

STOP AND THINK

As researchers, we all bring to our projects a particular world-view that is shaped by aspects such as our background, upbringing and education. This in turn shapes all stages of our research, from the approaches that we choose, to the ways we interact with participants and the ways in which we interpret our findings. Thinking about this is particularly important when doing CPR and when working with groups or communities where we are 'outsiders' (i.e. not members of the researched community).

Choose an example from one of the 'Research in practice' boxes, and put yourself in the shoes of the researcher.

Anke van der Sterren, Peter Waples-Crowe and Priscilla Pyett

- What aspects of your background and your world-view might impact on how you do this project?
- Think about aspects such as your gender, ethnic background, education, marital status and health status.
- Think about how these might impact on the research approaches you choose, how you would interact with participants, and how you interpret the findings.

CPR in practice

The key to CPR is the respectful engagement of participating communities throughout all stages of the research process: research design, data collection, data analysis, communication and dissemination, and action and evaluation. Here we discuss how the community can be engaged at each of these stages, and some of the issues involved in such engagement.

Research design

A long lead-up time that pays attention to relationship-building and appropriate planning of the research is essential to the success of any CPR project (see 'Research in practice' below). The participating community should be involved in developing aims, objectives and appropriate methods for data collection and analysis, and deciding on processes for monitoring the project, feedback and dissemination of findings. Such participation can be built through appropriate community engagement and consultation, through the development of a memorandum of understanding or project agreement, and through the establishment of an advisory group.

RESEARCH IN PRACTICE

THE IMPORTANCE OF A LONG TIME-FRAME

Successful collaborations are often preceded by lengthy periods of consultation and time for the partners to get to know one another. For example, in the Victorian Blood Borne Virus and Injecting Drug Use (BBV/IDU) Training Project (see pp. 413–414), the partners knew each other from previous working relationships over several years; the project took twelve months planning and development (Waples-Crowe & Pyett 2005). Similarly, Wand and Eades (2008) report that consultation with health workers began over a year before a student research project in Aboriginal mental health began. Finally, in the Talking About The Smokes project (see p. 413), many of the researchers had good long-term connections with Aboriginal communities, including those involved in the project.

However, you should be aware that some researchers can find it quite challenging to spend the time required to develop relationships, trust and strategies that will facilitate collaboration (Mayo et al. 2009).

Community engagement and consultation

Ideally, in CPR, the research is community-initiated. But in practice, it is more often the case that a researcher approaches a community with an idea for a research project or the offer of partnering with the community to conduct research that will be of benefit to it. What is most important about the early stages of engaging with a community is that the researcher communicates openly, listens respectfully and responds clearly. The researcher may have previous experience of working with the community or with other community groups, or they may be initiating their first community partnership. It is the researcher's responsibility to be as well informed as is reasonably possible about the community, its organisational structures and relationships, its history and culture, its strength and resilience, as well as its needs and circumstances of disadvantage.

We have written elsewhere about the importance of time in building relationships of mutual trust (Waples-Crowe & Pyett 2005; Pyett *et al.* 2009). Trust can only develop over time; this early stage of engagement requires a significant investment of the researcher's time and a demonstration of their commitment to listen to and learn from the community.

Part of the initial engagement will be to establish what level of involvement and responsibility the community wishes to have. We need to be aware that people will have competing time commitments such as paid employment, family responsibilities, child care, household maintenance and educational pursuits, and they may not have the confidence, interest, time or energy for research. Sometimes an underresourced and time-poor community might welcome a researcher who is prepared to do most of the work so long as the community is kept fully informed of the process and outcomes of the research. Where possible, however, a greater level of community involvement will enrich the process, increasing the validity and relevance of the findings while also building community capacity.

Initial consultation should include explanations of the need to obtain both funding and ethics approval, and the possibility that these applications may involve long delays or be ultimately unsuccessful. The researcher needs to balance the need for negotiation with communities before applying for funding. against the risks of disappointing communities if the funding is not obtained. Since the capacity of communities to participate in research may be limited by lack of skills, resources, time, interest or commitment to the project, we need to build funding and resources into the project to support community participation. These may include skill-building, back-filling organisations for staff involvement in the project, or providing child-minding facilities. Employing community members as part of the research team is a valuable way of facilitating a two-way knowledge exchange.

Developing a project agreement

A **project agreement or memorandum of understanding** (MOU) can be drawn up to clarify the roles, responsibilities and expectations of the researcher and the community partners on particular matters such as ownership of data, outcomes and publications. While MOUs are seldom legally binding, this process is important for the collaborating partners to develop an

Project agreement or MOU: This is drawn up to clarify the roles, responsibilities and expectations of the researcher and the community partners on issues such as ownership of data, outcomes and publications.

understanding of each other's values and expectations. The MOU is a useful document to refer to and possibly to amend as the project develops. It is important to have a process for monitoring and enforcing the principles of the MOU if one of the partners is not adhering to it.

Researchers can be uncertain where to begin and who to consult (Wand & Eades 2008). As we have argued elsewhere, it is important to identify key stakeholders and consult with them about others who should be included (Pyett *et al.* 2009). A community organisation may have a clear structure and protocols identifying who should be consulted, such as a director, board of management, executive officers or community liaison personnel. Some communities may not be represented by organisations, but there may be identifiable spokespersons or community elders. Representation is complex and not easily understood by outsiders. As already mentioned, group members are likely to have diverse as well as shared interests and values. This is where relationships are important. Health professionals or welfare workers may be able to identify key community members, but although existing networks can help you get started it is also necessary to consult more broadly. Establishing a steering committee or advisory group can help in identifying who should be consulted and how the community should be represented.

Steering committees or advisory groups

Steering committee or advisory group: Provides advice and guidance on all matters pertaining to the community with whom and for whom the research is being conducted.

Researchers using CPR often establish a **steering committee or advisory group** to provide advice and guidance on all matters pertaining to the community with whom and for whom they are conducting the research (Higginbottom & Liamputtong 2015). This is the group to whom researchers or health professionals must refer if they are to accurately identify the group's needs, interests and priorities, and the group who must finally judge and decide whether the research has described their situation or met their needs. It should include key stakeholders and experts in particular topics or cultural aspects. These people may be community elders, relevant service providers or health specialists, or people with other relevant technical expertise. Membership may change over the duration of the research as advice may be needed on different aspects of the project. It is a good idea to build in some project funding to reimburse members for their time and travel costs and to provide refreshments during meetings.

Data collection and analysis

We need to be mindful that academic language can be alienating (Pyett *et al.* 2008, 2009) and we should communicate in ways best suited to the communities we are working with. We find that community groups are more comfortable with more familiar terms such as 'information-gathering' rather than 'data collection', and 'understanding what we have found out' rather than 'analysis and interpretation'.

While both quantitative and qualitative methods can be used in CPR, quantitative data collection is often more difficult in community-based contexts. Sample sizes are usually small, which means that data analysis may be limited to simple descriptive statistics. Qualitative methods, which rely on face-to-face interaction and enable more in-depth exploration of issues, are often more appealing and accessible to community groups (see Liamputtong 2007, 2010, 2013; Chapter 1 and chapters in Part II).

Working with communities to do CPR means that we need to be flexible and open to learning from our community partners. Involving community members in data collection and analysis is not only important for showing respect for their experience and contribution but also because the validity and relevance of the findings will be enhanced by the breadth of their understanding and through the sharing of insider and outsider knowledge (Stringer & Genat 2004; Liamputtong 2013).

Maintaining confidentiality can be problematic when working in small communities. People in the community may recognise research participants or communities mentioned in reports even when names and all obvious identifying characteristics have been removed. It is often hard to maintain confidentiality within the research team when community members are also researchers, and special strategies may need to be developed to protect the confidentiality of participants. For example, standard protocols may need to be adjusted so that names and potentially identifying characteristics are removed from transcripts before other members of the research team have access to the raw data.

STOP AND THINK

A common method in CPR is to train and work with peer-researchers who come from the same community as the participants. For example: for a research project involving people who use injecting drugs, you might train current or former drug users to conduct the interviews; for a project involving homeless youth, you might train a number of young homeless people to collect data.

What would be the benefits and risks of working with peer researchers who come from disadvantaged or marginalised communities?

DATA ANALYSIS

One of us was involved in a project working with members of a consumer advocacy group, in which we conducted a number of focus groups with women who had all participated in a similar health screening process. We noticed that in all the groups, younger women seemed less interested in the discussions than older women. We were not sure if the younger women had fewer concerns about the program or whether the older women were dominating the discussion and inadvertently intimidating the younger ones. So we organised an extra focus group for younger women. In that focus group all the young women had plenty to say. While their experiences were not dissimilar to those of the older women, we realised that in the mixed age groups the younger women did not want to be seen to share the attitudes or values of the older women.

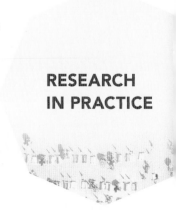

RESEARCH IN PRACTICE

Anke van der Sterren, Peter Waples-Crowe and Priscilla Pyett

Communication and dissemination

In CPR, it is important that the research findings are reported in a way that is appropriate to the community. This may include community reports, community forums, posters, videos or more innovative formats such as a dance performance (see 'Research in practice' below; Liamputtong 2007, 2010, 2013). It is essential to write clearly, using lay language and avoiding academic jargon or medical terms. Community members and advisory groups should be given plenty of opportunity to read and provide feedback on any publications or other outcomes of the project.

Because we are collaborating with our community participants as co-researchers, we need to include them as co-authors in any publications, even if they do not actually do the writing. Most people in any community other than the academic community do not like writing and are more comfortable with verbal communication. Neither providing access to a community for research purposes nor conducting interviews or administering surveys actually constitutes authorship for academic purposes, but in CPR the community members provide far more input. They contribute valuable knowledge about the community, their ideas shape the planning and implementation of the project, their understanding informs the interpretation of data—in these ways they deserve co-authorship. It is also important to acknowledge the support of community organisations, boards of management and advisory groups as well as funding bodies (Pyett *et al.* 2008).

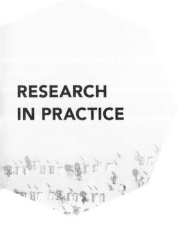

RESEARCH IN PRACTICE

DANCE AS DISSEMINATION

One of the most innovative examples of feedback about a research process that we have come across involved a dance performance. Staff of the Aboriginal Community Controlled Health Organisation (ACCHO) and members of the university research team participated in a performance by the local Indigenous men's cultural dance group to illustrate the value of CPR in an applied research setting. The performance was an innovative, culturally appropriate way of disseminating the finding that by working together the ACCHO and the university researchers had improved well-being for community members and contributed to greater harmony within the community. The community set the research agenda and the university researchers facilitated the development of appropriate social health programs and increased the capacity of the community to administer and run those programs. Participants have reported increases in self-esteem, resilience, self-reflection and problem-solving abilities. The programs have expanded from a Men's Group to include a Women's Group, a Youth Group, a diversionary program for court-referred men, and the Indigenous men's dance group, which has performed commercially and aspires to professional status (Mayo *et al.* 2009).

Action and evaluation

We recognise that it is not always possible to achieve the outcomes recommended through the process of CPR, nor do we always have the time or resources to evaluate outcomes even when they are implemented. Nevertheless, CPR is solution-focused and the goal is to bring about changes for the benefit of the participating communities. Outcomes can be policy-directed or practice-based; they may be health promotion resources, material resources, training and workshops or community forums. The researcher or the community may wish to use the evidence collected for advocacy or service improvement. The process of CPR is an outcome in itself through its potential for community empowerment and providing training for community researchers. There may be unintended consequences from the way the researcher engages with a community. With a CPR approach, it is essential to have some flexibility in order to respond to issues that arise, even though they might be strictly outside the scope of the research.

Actions and outcomes may be limited by the agenda of the funding body, or by the capacity and resources available within the community to carry out the actions they desire. Alternatively, senior management or board members may disagree with the recommended actions. A process for managing disagreements should be developed early in the project-planning phase and written into the project agreement or MOU.

LIMITATIONS IMPOSED BY A FUNDING BODY

Two of us were involved in a project that was funded by a government department and conducted by a community-controlled organisation. Our task was to carry out a research and awareness-raising project around alcohol and pregnancy in an Indigenous community. The community-controlled advisory group recommended setting the research on alcohol within a holistic approach that is compatible with Indigenous views of health, and using the findings to develop training for Aboriginal health workers. Representatives of the government department insisted that the funding was allocated specifically for alcohol research and drew our attention to the funding agreement, which required a resource kit to be developed. We were accountable to the Indigenous community but constrained by the funding requirements. Fortunately, we were able to negotiate a compromise where we developed a holistic resource kit and the government department funded a number of regional and metropolitan training sessions that were conducted every time the kit was launched in an Aboriginal organisation.

RESEARCH IN PRACTICE

A community context: Indigenous health research in Australia

It is unfortunately well known that in Australia today the greatest inequalities in health and life expectancy are between Indigenous[1] and non-Indigenous populations. The health status of Aboriginal and Torres Strait Islander people is poorer than the rest of the population in relation to almost every disease or condition for which information is available, and across the entire life cycle. According to the latest reports from the Australian Institute of Health

Anke van der Sterren, Peter Waples-Crowe and Priscilla Pyett

and Welfare (2015a), Indigenous Australians have a life expectancy that is around ten years lower than that of non-Indigenous Australians (p. 761), they are three times more likely than non-Indigenous Australians to have diabetes (p. 328) and almost seven times more likely to commence treatment for end-stage renal disease (p. 363). They are almost four times as likely to be unemployed (AIHW 2015b, p. 34) and are significantly less likely to have completed Year 12 or a Certificate III or above (p. 30). Perhaps the most disturbing statistic is that they are thirteen times more likely than non-Indigenous Australians to be in prison (AIHW 2015a, p. 1462). As the Australian federal government has acknowledged in its response to the annual 'Closing the Gap Report' policy, there has been varied progress on health and well-being targets, and many of these statistics have changed little in recent decades (Commonwealth of Australia 2016).

These gross disparities are the consequences of multiple social, economic, political and historical factors that we can only touch on briefly here. As noted by the Council for Aboriginal Reconciliation (1994, p. 19), the 'history of control and exclusion has had a deep and lasting spiritual and psychological impact on Aboriginal and Torres Strait Islander peoples and communities'. This has had 'continuing intergenerational impact' and 'Indigenous Australians continue to be excluded from social and economic opportunities both through individual discrimination and through systematic factors' (Chirgwin & D'Antoine 2016).

Why CPR is appropriate in this context

A collaborative and participatory approach to research is appropriate to an Indigenous world-view of health and well-being that ties individual health to spiritual and social well-being and to the well-being of their entire community. The National Aboriginal Health Strategy Working Party (1989, p. x) defines health as 'not just the physical well-being of the individual, but the social, emotional, and cultural well-being of the whole community'. For Aboriginal peoples, health is 'not merely a matter of the provision of doctors, hospitals, medicines or the absence of disease and incapacity' but 'a matter of determining all aspects of their life, including control over their physical environment, of dignity, of community self-esteem, and of justice' (p. ix). CPR enables communities to apply these holistic understandings of health, and to promote community well-being by building self-esteem and community capacity in health.

Collaborative approaches that promote active indigenous participation in research are necessary to further the process of self-determination. **Indigenous people** have a particularly troubled history with researchers, who have often been part of the colonisation, oppression and ongoing surveillance of indigenous populations in Australia, New Zealand, Canada and North America. Research is still considered a dirty word in most Aboriginal and Torres Strait Islander communities because it is seen historically as taking knowledge without any benefit to the communities that are researched (Smith 1999; Humphery 2001; Liamputtong 2010,

Indigenous people: The original inhabitants of countries that have been colonised by other cultural groups. Indigenous peoples are often marginalised from the mainstream political and social systems of these countries, and are widely recognised as disadvantaged across a range of social, political and health indicators.

2013). A great deal of anthropological and other medical and social science research has been undertaken since colonisation, but it has rarely led to improvement in the lives of Indigenous people, as is reflected in the continuing gap in health outcomes across Australia. Indigenous people have often been neglected in the research process, treated as subjects rather than active agents (Smith 1999; Humphery 2001; Liamputtong 2010, 2013). A systematic review of Australian Indigenous child health, development and well-being epidemiological studies conducted in 2006 found that only 28.6 per cent of 217 studies identified reported involvement of Indigenous people in the research process (other than as participants) (Priest *et al.* 2009). It is this kind of finding that explains why many Aboriginal and Torres Strait Islander communities feel neglected in the research process.

Recognition of the rights of Indigenous peoples to self-determination, together with increasing numbers of Indigenous researchers, have resulted in calls for respectful, reciprocal and equal relationships between researchers and Indigenous communities (National Aboriginal and Torres Strait Islander Health Council 2003; NHMRC 2003). In recent years, many researchers (both Indigenous and non-Indigenous) with the help of Indigenous communities have been trying to address the imbalance from research being 'done to' communities to research being 'done with' or 'done by' communities. For example, the Lowitja Institute has developed a number of resources, including *Researching Indigenous health: a practical guide for researchers* (Laycock *et al.* 2011), and the Cooperative Research Centre for Aboriginal Health (currently known as the Lowitja Institue CRC) has developed an Indigenous Research Reform Agenda (Henry *et al.* 2002a, b; Matthews *et al.* 2002; <www.lowitja.org.au>). Publications like the NHMRC's *Values and ethics: guidelines for ethical conduct in Aboriginal and Torres Strait Islander health research* (2003) and *Keeping research on track* (2005) provide advice for researchers and Indigenous communities on culturally respectful and ethical research practice. Several researchers in Aboriginal and Torres Strait Islander health have used their experiences to develop and publish principles of effective and culturally respectful health research (Waples-Crowe & Pyett 2005; Pyett *et al.* 2009; Jamieson *et al.* 2012; Kelly *et al.* 2012). CPR demonstrates several of the core values espoused by these documents: respect for the knowledge that community leaders and community members bring to the research partnership; responsibility in that researchers are accountable to the communities they research with; reciprocity through capacity-building and feedback of research findings to the communities; and relationships of equality between the researcher(s) and the communities involved in the research.

Awareness of and respect for cultural issues, cultural diversity and cultural safety are essential to ethical research with Indigenous communities (Ramsden 1990; Coffin *et al.* 2008). It is the researcher's responsibility to become educated about the history and culture of the local community and to ensure that the research process is culturally secure and adopts appropriate methods (Liamputtong 2010, 2013).

Anke van der Sterren, Peter Waples-Crowe and Priscilla Pyett

STOP AND THINK

The NHMRC has developed specific guidelines for ethical research with Aboriginal and Torres Strait Islander people.

- Should specific ethics guidelines be developed for other disadvantaged research populations?
- Why or why not?

Applying CPR in an Indigenous context

While the broad principles of CPR outlined in the previous sections are equally relevant in the Indigenous health research context, consideration needs to be given to the socio-cultural context, and in particular how the power relations resulting from colonisation influence the way in which relationships are developed and research is undertaken. For instance, Indigenous cultures are extremely diverse, and have been impacted by colonisation in diverse ways. Colonisation has forced Indigenous people to adapt; the culture has changed, not disappeared. Some people still live a very traditional life, but many have been dislocated from their traditional homelands and have been influenced by the dominant European culture. More than three-quarters of Indigenous Australians live in major cities and regional areas, while only 21 per cent live in remote or very remote areas (AIHW 2015b). When approaching an Indigenous community or population group about research, time must be taken to get to know the particular history and culture of the group that researchers will be working with, rather than assuming that all Indigenous communities are the same.

Getting to know the Indigenous community means developing an understanding of which organisations or groups are appropriate to be approached and involved in the research. In Aboriginal health research, this may mean developing relationships with Aboriginal community-controlled health organisations (ACCHOs), or Aboriginal Medical Services, as they are called in some states and territories. Local Aboriginal health organisations are usually members of regional or state-level peak bodies which may also wish to be involved in the research. Aboriginal health organisations are incorporated, community-controlled services committed to a holistic approach to health care, to responding to the needs of the community and to community participation in decision-making. Aboriginal health workers are integral to service delivery in these organisations, although in many states of Australia they also work in mainstream (non-Aboriginal) health organisations. Other Aboriginal community-controlled organisations may also be appropriate to be involved in the research, depending on the research topic, for example Aboriginal housing boards, legal services, child care agencies and family violence services. As community-controlled spaces, ACCHOs are central components of self-determination within Aboriginal communities and thus are logical partners in CPR.

The diversity of Indigenous communities throughout Australia means that it is impossible to provide definitive guidelines for undertaking CPR in these contexts. Instead, we will give two examples that illustrate some of the principles and complexities of CPR in this context. We draw on one of these projects to offer some practical steps for successful collaboration between mainstream and Indigenous organisations.

CPR IN INDIGENOUS SETTINGS

The Talking About The Smokes Project

The Talking About The Smokes Project was a national project that involved surveying a representative sample of 2522 Aboriginal and Torres Strait Islander adults to assess the impact of tobacco control policies in Australia. Daily smoking rates among Aboriginal and Torres Strait Islander people are 2.6 times higher than among other Australians, and smoking is a significant cause of morbidity and mortality in these communities. The project implemented a community-based CPR approach to conduct surveys in thirty-five locations.

The research involved formal consultation, negotiation and partnership between the Menzies School of Health Research and the National Aboriginal Community Controlled Health Organisation (NACCHO). The principles guiding the partnership and the project were laid out in an MOU. The project included researchers from non-government organisations, two state affiliate organisations of NACCHO, and researchers representing NACCHO. A Project Reference Group (PRG) was also established, with representation from NACCHO state affiliate organisations. Deliberate processes were therefore in place to involve community representatives in all stages of the project. NACCHO provided advice on conducting the research in an ethical and responsible manner, and communication with and coordination of the participating Aboriginal Community Controlled Health Services (ACCHSs).

Importantly, the ACCHSs were key partners in the research process and were resourced to engage local community members to conduct the surveys in their own communities. Project workers provided these research assistants with training in data collection methods, and provided ongoing support to them throughout the project.

Findings of each of the two waves of data collection were reported back to the community in a brief plain-language document. These findings were used by many of the communities to immediately impact on smoking cessation services and programs. The findings of the project more broadly have been reported in academic papers (with members of the PRG included as co-authors), and are impacting on local and national policy and practice around tobacco control in Aboriginal and Torres Strait Islander communities (Couzos *et al.* 2015).

RESEARCH IN PRACTICE

The Victorian Blood Borne Virus and Injecting Drug Use Training Project

The initial idea for this project was born from discussions between workers from one Indigenous and two mainstream organisations who had worked together on a number of projects over several years. The aim of the project was to provide Aboriginal workers throughout Victoria with current information about blood-borne viruses (BBV) and to begin discussion on the emerging issues associated with injecting drug use (IDU) in Aboriginal communities. The training would also aim to break down stigma about IDU and improve the services available to Indigenous users. Funding was provided by what was then known as the Office of Aboriginal and Torres Strait Islander Health (OATSIH).

An MOU was drawn up and signed by senior executives in all three organisations, which supported the collaborative arrangements and time necessary for relationship-building and developing mutual understanding. At this stage two further

>>

organisations (one mainstream and one Indigenous) were invited to join the project and participate in the planning and delivery of the training.

The five partner organisations attended a two-day cross-cultural awareness and skill-sharing workshop. This was an important two-way learning experience where the mainstream workers learnt about Indigenous history, values and perspectives and the Indigenous workers learnt how mainstream organisations dealt with the sensitive issues associated with BBV/IDU.

Three training sessions were designed and a resource kit developed. Each of the partners brought unique skills that were recognised and valued by other partners in planning and implementing the program. The training targeted Aboriginal drug and alcohol workers, hospital liaison workers, mental health workers and workers in cultural and spiritual well-being. The training was successful in increasing workers' understanding of people with hepatitis C and HIV/AIDS and in reducing some of the stigma associated with IDU. The mainstream and Indigenous organisations learnt to respect and trust each other and all were confident of ongoing collaboration (Waples-Crowe & Pyett 2005).

Identifying elements of a successful collaboration

OATSIH became interested in why the BBV/IDU training project succeeded with such a sensitive topic and as a collaboration between three mainstream and two Indigenous organisations, when many similar partnership projects have failed because relationships have broken down. OATSIH funded a further study to identify the factors that facilitated such a successful collaboration; two of us were involved in that project (Waples-Crowe & Pyett 2005). We identified ten steps to guide successful collaboration between mainstream and Indigenous organisations. In disseminating these findings we have sought feedback and added two further steps that were integral to the BBV/IDU project but were not identified by the participants themselves.

**STEPS TO GUIDE SUCCESSFUL COLLABORATION
BETWEEN MAINSTREAM AND INDIGENOUS PARTNERS**

1 The project should be community-initiated.

2 A long time-frame is necessary for developing relationships and planning the project.

3 Mainstream organisations need to take responsibility for getting educated about the Indigenous community rather than expecting the Indigenous organisation to explain everything to them.

4 Mainstream organisations need to undertake cultural awareness training for their staff before engaging with Indigenous community organisations.

5 Mainstream and Indigenous partners need to value each other's skills, experience, values and perspectives.

6 Building trust takes time and mainstream organisations need to work within the time-frame of the Indigenous community.

7 It is important to identify all the key partners and formalise partnerships through project agreements or MOUs.

8 Good planning is essential and must involve all partners.

9 The project needs to produce an outcome that is seen as useful to the participants.

10 Supportive work environments are essential and require the support of senior management.

11 Ongoing communication and feedback are important at all times throughout the project.

12 Individuals in both mainstream and community organisations need to show leadership in order to support their co-workers and community members through the collaborative process.

Source: Adapted from Waples-Crowe & Pyett (2005)

Summary

The principal benefits of CPR are that it is inclusive, and that it builds confidence, capacity and trust. A collaborative participatory approach to research facilitates social change for the benefit of participating communities. It is therefore particularly important that researchers collaborate with marginalised and disadvantaged groups, who have every reason not to trust, who have experienced exploitation and have few opportunities to have their perspective seen or heard. As health researchers, we have a responsibility to give something back to the communities we research. This can be achieved by sharing our findings and validating their experiences but also, through collaboration, by increasing the skills and the confidence of people with whom we are researching.

In this chapter we have learnt the importance and value of including disadvantaged communities in the planning, implementation and dissemination of research that affects them. We have seen that CPR is particularly valuable for research with Indigenous communities. We have learnt the importance of time spent in building relationships of mutual trust in order to carry out research that will be relevant and beneficial to the collaborating partners, and we have been introduced to some practical guidelines for undertaking CPR.

Anke van der Sterren, Peter Waples-Crowe and Priscilla Pyett

Practice exercises

1   What is the name of the traditional owners of the land you live on? What are some of the Aboriginal and Torres Strait Islander organisations in your local area? They could be in health, housing, social services, child care, land councils, etc. It is important for non-Indigenous people to get some knowledge of the Aboriginal and Torres Strait Islander group they intend to research; doing so will make approaching community organisations a lot easier.

2   Imagine you are working with Aboriginal and Torres Strait Islander patients/ clients and you recognise a health issue or service gap that could be researched. How will you involve Aboriginal and Torres Strait Islander people in planning your project? What organisations would you approach? What steps would you take to discuss how Aboriginal and Torres Strait Islander people want to be involved in the project?

3   Draw up an MOU or project agreement. Devise a template for a project agreement or MOU between yourself (or your organisation) and a community group or organisation. What are the important things that would need to be included?

4   Look again at the Talking About The Smokes Project. Applying the steps outlined in the box, can you identify the CPR strategies that made the project a success? Can you think of anything else the research team could have done to improve their process in a culturally appropriate and ethical manner?

Note

1   We use the terms 'Indigenous', 'Aboriginal and Torres Strait Islander' and 'Aboriginal' interchangeably to refer to all Aboriginal and Torres Strait Islander peoples and communities in Australia. We recognise that communities have different preferences for the way they are named and described but we are unable to refer to individual tribal groups in this chapter.

Further reading

Hart, E. & Bond, M. (1995). *Action research for health and social care: a guide to practice.* Buckingham, UK: Open University Press.

Israel, B.A., Eng, E., Schultz, A.J., Parker, E.A. (eds) (2012). *Methods for community-based participatory research for health*, 2nd edn. San Francisco: Jossey-Bass.

Laycock, A. with Walker, D., Harrison, N. & Brands, J. (2011). *Researching indigenous health: a practical guide for researchers.* Melbourne: Lowitja Institute.

NHMRC (2003). *Values and ethics: guidelines for ethical conduct in Aboriginal and Torres Strait Islander health research.* Canberra: NHMRC. <www.nhmrc.gov.au/_files_nhmrc/publications/attachments/e52.pdf>.

NHMRC (2005). *Keeping research on track: a guide for Aboriginal and Torres Strait Islander peoples about health research ethics.* Canberra: Australian Government Publishing Service. <www.nhmrc.gov.au/guidelines/publications/e65>.

Nyden, P.W., Figert, A., Shibley, M. & Burrows, D. (1997). *Building community: Social science in action.* Thousand Oaks, CA: Pine Forge Press.

Smith, L.T. (1999). *Decolonizing methodologies: research and Indigenous peoples.* Dunedin, NZ: University of Otago Press.

Stringer, E. & Genat, W. (2004). *Action research in health.* New Jersey: Pearson.

Websites

Methodology

www.communityresearchcanada.ca

> A Canadian Centre for Community Based Research focused on strengthening communities through social research.

www.luc.edu/curl

> A website from Loyola University in Chicago that has developed CPR relationships with many community organisations.

Indigenous health

www.healthinfonet.ecu.edu.au

> The Australian Health Information Network offers information on Australian Indigenous people's health, health practice and health policy.

www.lowitja.org.au

> The website for the Lowitja Institute, a research body bringing together Aboriginal organisations, academic institutions and government agencies to facilitate collaborative research into Aboriginal and Torres Strait Islander health (incorporates the Cooperative Research Centre for Aboriginal Health).

www.naccho.org.au

> The website for the National Aboriginal Community Controlled Health Organisation (NACCHO), the national representative body for Aboriginal community-controlled health services. The website provides details of its programs and activities, as well as links to the state and territory affiliates.

Anke van der Sterren, Peter Waples-Crowe and Priscilla Pyett

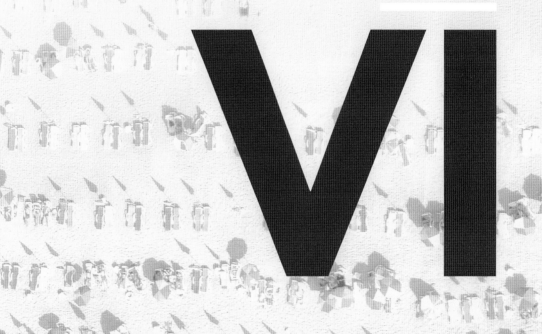

VI

MAKING SENSE OF AND PRESENTING DATA

23

Making Sense of Qualitative Data

PRANEE LIAMPUTTONG AND TANYA SERRY

Chapter objectives

In this chapter you will learn:

- about the fundamental premises and generic concepts of qualitative data
- about the use of coding strategies
- how to perform content analysis
- how to perform thematic analysis

Key terms

Axial coding

Code

Coding

Content analysis

Data analysis

Data display

Data reduction

Descriptive/open coding

Focused coding

Selective coding

Thematic analysis

Introduction

> Analysis takes you step by step from the raw data … to clear and convincing answers to your research question. Your analysis is strengthened by what you have initially built into your design—the richness, the thoroughness, the balance, the nuance and detail—that allows you to prepare a report that is vivid and convincing, based on what your [participants] have said (Rubin & Rubin 2012, p. 190).

The analysis of qualitative data is a rich experience that requires the researcher to combine creative and reflective thinking alongside systematic and rigorous standards of empirical enquiry. The process of qualitative analysis is data-based and highly data-driven (Bogdan & Biklen 2007). There are several analytical approaches available to the qualitative researcher that will help to turn data, which are often voluminous, into 'a clear, understandable, insightful, trustworthy and even original analysis' (Gibbs 2008, p. 1). In this chapter we will focus on two more commonly used approaches: content analysis and thematic analysis.

Principles regarding qualitative data analysis

Data analysis: The way that researchers make sense of their data. In qualitative research it means looking for patterns of ideas or themes, whereas in quantitative research data are analysed by counting various response alternatives.

Attempting **data analysis** may seem daunting to the novice qualitative researcher. In fact, data analysis in qualitative research is an ongoing, cyclical process that occurs from the very beginning of the research (Miles & Huberman 1994; Miles *et al.* 2013; Liamputtong 2013). Researchers need to treat data analysis as an integral component of the research design, the literature review, the formation of theory, data collection, the ordering of data and the writing process (Northcutt & McCoy 2004; Gibbs 2008; Bryman 2016). In this way, analytical decisions are made from the initial stages of reviewing literature through to data collection, organisation, conclusion drawing and verification. In essence, data analysis continues throughout every step of the research process (Braun & Clarke 2013; Grbich 2013; Liamputtong 2013; Corbin & Strauss 2015), such that the process is a 'continuous, iterative enterprise' (Miles & Huberman 1994, p. 12) between the existing data that have been analysed and newly collected data, in order to complete, challenge or resolve issues and queries that arise.

Accordingly, data analysis in qualitative research is not a discrete operation. The interactive and iterative nature of qualitative research also allows data analysis to inform and guide upcoming data collection within the one research project (Miles *et al.* 2013; Bryman 2016). In turn, data analysis should be an ongoing, lively and cumulative enterprise that contributes to the energising process of fieldwork. Many qualitative researchers advise interweaving data collection and analysis from the beginning (Mason 2002; Gibbs 2008; Carpenter & Suto 2008; Bryman 2016). All these matters have significant ramifications for how we undertake our data analysis.

A common question of the novice qualitative researcher centres on sample size and when to stop collecting data. Data saturation can partly address this perplexing question. Data saturation occurs when regularities emerge from your analysis; more information will not offer you any new understanding (Padgett 2012; Liamputtong 2013). At this point, if well-supported conclusions can be drawn via detailed analysis, further data collection is not needed. It is not possible to determine exactly how long this will take before commencing data collection, though the reflective nature of qualitative research does allow further sampling to occur until saturation is reached (Bryman 2016; Chapters 1, 6, 8, 9).

Traditions of qualitative data analysis

Grbich (2013, p. 25) outlines a broad, two-step plan for data analysis that provides a useful framework, regardless of the analytical approach being used. Phase 1 involves 'preliminary data analysis' (2013, p 21), which she describes as a means of highlighting emerging issues by keeping track of key information from the data collection process. For example, she suggests that researchers systematically record identifying facts and features from each participant or case using a 'face sheet' (p. 22). This can be followed up by the researcher noting points such as emerging themes, issues of interest and future data collection goals. Phase 2 analysis or 'post data collection' (2007, p. 31) explores data at an increasingly sophisticated or deeper level. In this phase, the researcher has a number of options for analysing data depending on the nature of the enquiry and the approach used. Figure 23.1 represents these phases.

FIGURE 23.1 The two phases of data analysis

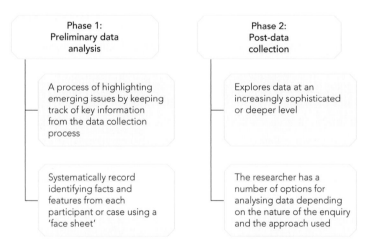

Source: Grbich (2013)

For the Phase 2 analysis, researchers typically use a 'block and file' approach in which the data are segmented and categorised into manageable chunks, or 'conceptual mapping' whereby a diagrammatic approach is used to organise data. Frequently, both processes are applied to the data during the analysis phase (Grbich 2007). Techniques used in post-data collection analysis serve to prepare researchers to draw and verify conclusions that ultimately form the outcomes of their research.

The cyclical nature of qualitative data analysis

To demonstrate the continuous nature of qualitative data analysis, along with applying Grbich's two-phase model (2007, 2013), we have used Miles and Huberman's Components of Data Analysis: Interactive Model (1994) as a generic framework for conducting qualitative data analysis. Figure 23.2 displays our version of their model. We describe each component below, with the exception of data collection (see chapters in Part II for discussions about qualitative data collection methods).

FIGURE 23.2   Components of data analysis: interactive model

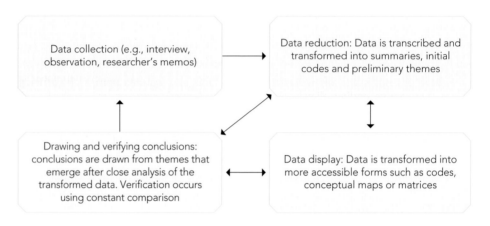

Source: Adapted from Miles & Huberman (1994, p. 12)

Data reduction occurs when raw data are transcribed and transformed into summaries, initial codes and preliminary themes. Data reduction forms the preliminary phase of analysis. The process requires analytical choices to be made throughout, which form the foundations for deeper levels of analysis. As such, data reduction is a critical component of the entire analytical framework. It is also a fluid process since initial analytical choices are likely to be modified, transformed or collapsed with other themes that emerge. Miles and colleagues (2013) emphasise that data reduction is not a quantitative process. Rather, it is a series of analytical decisions made about the data in which the 'anticipatory' phase should start occurring even before data collection has formally commenced.

Data display is defined by Miles and Huberman (1994, p. 11) as an 'organised, compressed assembly of information that permits conclusion drawing'. For example, data display can take place when rather cumbersome transcripts and observation descriptions are transformed into more accessible forms such as codes, conceptual maps, matrices or even graphs.

Conclusions are drawn from the data, based on themes and regularities that emerge. Tentative conclusions typically surface as data are collected and analysed but, as Miles and Huberman (1994, p 1) recommend, 'openness and skepticism' are important qualities that the researcher should maintain until sufficient data are collected and analysed and conclusions can be verified.

Coding

Coding is central to qualitative research and is typically the starting point for most forms of qualitative analysis (Bryman 2016). Saldaña (2009, p. 3) defines a **code** as 'a word or short phrase that symbolically assigns a summative, salient essence-capturing and/or evocative attribute for a portion of language-based or visual data'. In essence, coding is the first step that allows researchers to move beyond tangible data to make analytical interpretations. According to Charmaz (2006, p. 43), coding is 'the process of defining what the data are about' so that researchers can delve into their data and search for meaning (p. 46). When coding, researchers name chunks of data with 'a label that simultaneously categorizes, summarizes, and accounts for each piece of data'. These codes ultimately form the foundation for categories and themes that are drawn from the data.

The process of coding the data should be dynamic and reflective rather than linear and discrete. This active coding allows researchers to repeatedly interact with their data and to ask many different questions about it. Coding may lead the researchers into areas they have not previously considered. In doing so, new or expanded research questions may arise (Charmaz 2014).

While coding, writing marginal notes or memos on the data or transcripts will allow researchers to maintain their attention to detail (Saldaña 2009). These marginal notes can also assist colleagues or other researchers who wish to see how the researchers code their transcripts. Often, later on, marginal notes are used in the coding cycle. As the researchers read through the transcripts again and again, new codes may be added; this can be easily done in the marginal notes. Bryman (2016) points out that the marginal notes the researchers write on the transcripts will gradually be refined into codes.

There are useful strategies or steps for qualitative researchers to follow (Miles & Huberman 1994; Mason 2002; Saldaña 2009; Liamputtong 2013; Miles *et al.* 2013; Charmaz 2014). Minichiello and colleagues (2008, p. 268) suggest that when experienced researchers develop codes, a common strategy is to ask, 'What is this thing (or things) I have before me?' As an example from our own work, we initially set out to explore the perspectives of both parents and teachers regarding children with reading difficulty who were receiving intervention. As our coding progressed, we began to ask further questions of the codes such that we developed an additional line of enquiry that explored how parents and teachers differed in their causal attributions for the child's reading difficulty.

Flick (2006, p. 300) suggests the following list of basic questions that qualitative researchers may use as coding strategies (Table 23.1). He also suggests that researchers should examine the text regularly and repeatedly with these questions so that they will be able to disclose the text.

The process of coding is a labour-intensive task that requires many readings of transcripts and other data to complete the progressively more sophisticated levels of coding. It is usual for novice researchers to feel unskilful, clumsy or simply overwhelmed at the beginning of the coding process. More often, the researcher may not feel confident about assigning code names and searching for meanings. However, confidence will gradually increase with their continued efforts with data analysis. Holton (2007, p. 276) points out that 'as coding progresses, patterns begin to emerge. Pattern recognition gives the researchers confidence in the coding process and in their own innate creativity.'

Code: A label or short phrase which symbolically provides a 'salient essence' that captures the meaning in the data or the text.

Pranee Liamputtong and Tanya Serry

TABLE 23.1   Basic questions to use as coding strategies

What?	What is the concern here? Which course of events is mentioned?
Who?	Who are the persons involved? What roles do they have? How do they interact?
How?	Which aspects of the event are mentioned (or omitted)?
When? How long? Where?	Referring to time, course, and location: When does it happen? How long does it take? Where did the incident occur?
How much? How strong?	Referring to intensity: How often is the issue emphasised?
Why?	Which reasons are provided or can be constructed?
What for?	What is the intention here? What is the purpose?
By which?	Referring to means, tactics, and strategies for achieving the aim: What is the main tactic here? How are things accomplished?

What can be coded?

There are several schemes that researchers may use to develop codes from their data. We have found the following suggestions, compiled from Miles and Huberman (1994, p. 61), Bogdan and Biklen (2007, pp. 174–8) and Gibbs (2007, pp. 47–8), to be particularly useful:

- *setting and context*: general information on surroundings that allows the researchers to place the study in a larger context

- *definition of the situation*: how individuals understand, perceive or define the setting or the topics on which the study is based

- *perspectives*: ways of thinking about the things that are shared by the participants, such as how things are done here

- *ways of thinking about people and objects*: understandings of each other, of outsiders, of objects in their world, but more detailed than the perspectives

- *process*: sequence of events, flows, transitions, turning points and changes over time

- *activities*: regularly occurring types of behaviour

- *actions*: what people do or say

- *events*: specific activities, particularly the events that occur infrequently

- *conditions or constraints*: the causes of actions and things that constrain the actions

- *consequences*: types of consequences of the actions or behaviour

- *strategies*: ways of accomplishing things, i.e. people's strategies, tactics, methods, techniques for meeting their needs

- *relationship and social structure*: unofficially defined patterns such as cliques, coalitions, romances, friendships, enmities

- *meanings*: the verbal expressions of the participants that 'define and direct action'.

According to Gibbs (2007), those meanings are at the core of most qualitative analysis (see also Chapter 1). Meanings include how people see their world and the symbols they use to understand their situation. Meanings direct the actions of the participants. We rely heavily on this schema to code in our own work.

The suggestions provided above will assist researchers in thinking about categories in which codes will be developed. It is unlikely that all of these aspects will be relevant in any one study. In fact, Creswell (2013) recommends that researchers should carefully consider and scrutinise code segments used to represent their data and construct emerging themes, rather than adhere solely to the schemes presented above. In turn, the researcher is afforded greater ownership of their analysis with codes that may reveal:

- data that the researchers may expect to elicit before the study
- surprising data that the researchers have not expected to discover
- data that is crucial for the construction of theory, or unusual to the researchers, the readers and even the participants themselves.

CODING

Read the following excerpt from a transcript with a parent about her son, now ten years old, who has a learning difficulty. Consider the options for coding at a descriptive and focused level.

Jamie's very young for his year. My husband and I were very reluctant whether we should send him to kinder when he turned three or hold him back. And a lot of people said to us, because he's a very social child, he should be right. So we put him through. We got to the second year of kinder and the kindergarten teachers were starting to introduce words on cards and simple books for the children to take home. And we found already then that Jamie was struggling. He couldn't do it. And I had already brought up with the kindergarten teacher 'Should I send Jamie to school?' Coz the way he was interpreting information and that, it just wasn't getting through to him.

Descriptive codes could include the following:
- age of child relative to peers
- shared parenting decision-making
- reluctance about sending child to kinder
- social skills of child

RESEARCH IN PRACTICE

- people said 'he'd be fine'
- child struggled at kinder
- child had difficulty interpreting information
- struggled with reading word cards
- parent seeking advice from kinder teacher
- parent worried about child going to school.

Are there any other descriptive codes you might include? Would you consider noting any memos from this excerpt?

Using the codes listed above, focused coding could proceed as follows:
- parental decision-making processes
- child attributes used in decision-making regarding kindergarten readiness
- parental concerns about school readiness.

Are there other focused codes you might draw from the descriptive codes listed earlier?

Steps and strategies for coding

Our suggestions are paraphrased from Bryman (2016, pp. 581–3) in conjunction with a conceptual framework developed from the work of various qualitative researchers (Miles & Huberman 1994; Liamputtong 2013; Miles *et al.* 2013; Charmaz 2014; Corbin & Strauss 2015). This conceptual framework is discussed below and presented in Figure 23.3. It will lead you through the increasingly deeper and more abstract levels of coding that will allow you to formulate theories and/or key theses arising from your data. See also Chapter 8 for coding in grounded theory research.

FIGURE 23.3   A conceptual framework for the practice of coding

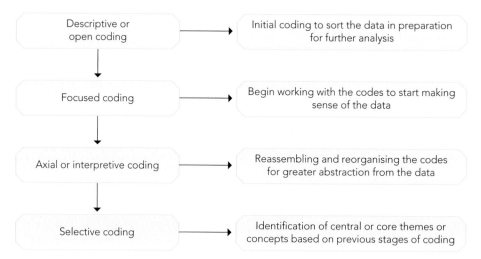

1 Descriptive or open coding

Descriptive or open coding: Often the first step in coding in qualitative data analysis, where the aim is to sort and organise the data so that further analysis can take place.

Coding commences at a **descriptive** (Miles & Huberman 1994; Miles *et al.* 2013) or **open** level (Corbin & Strauss 2015), in which the central aim is to sort and organise the data so that further analysis can take place (Liamputtong 2013). This initial phase of coding stays close to the data (Charmaz 2014) and allows you to develop an understanding of the different categories within the data.

- Commence coding as soon as possible, well before your data collection is complete. As with the practice in grounded theory research, it is wise to start coding while data are still being collected. This will permit you to have a better understanding of the data, to follow up ambiguous data and to help with theoretical sampling. Additionally, it may reduce the feeling of being overwhelmed with too much data, which usually happens when the researchers commence data analysis after all the data are collected.

- Read through the initial set of transcripts, field notes or documents without making any notes or attempting to interpret the data. After reading through the data, you may wish to write down a few notes or keep a reflective journal about what appears to be particularly interesting or significant.

2 Focused coding

Focused coding (Charmaz 2014) follows descriptive or open coding. This is when you begin working with the codes themselves in order to start making sense of the data. Focused coding may involve synthesising the codes and determining relationships between various events or phenomena.

- Read through the data again. This time you should start making notes or memos about significant observations or categories that emerge. Make as many of these as possible. This is also coding. Initially, your notes or memos may be very basic. You may use key words expressed by the participants or you may give names to themes in the data. A combination of both is often used.

- It may be useful to generate an index of terms or names that may assist you to interpret and theorise about the data.

- Review the codes. If you have two or more words or phrases that refer to the same issue, delete one of them. Look closely to see if the developed codes are relevant to concepts and categories in the existing literature. See if there are any connections between the codes or if there is evidence that may suggest one thing that tends to be associated with or caused by something else.

> **Focused coding:** A step that follows descriptive or open coding, when researchers begin working with the codes themselves in order to start making sense of the data.

3 Axial coding or interpretive coding

You are now moving towards a greater level of abstraction from the data. The task at this level of coding will be to evaluate the codes further to determine what needs to be reassembled or reorganised. This may involve processes such as breaking codes into smaller categories or collapsing more than one code into a single category. This interpretation and comparison of coded data is known as the constant comparison method (Flick 2006; Marshall *et al.* 2007). At this point, coding relies more on inferential analysis to make sense of the emerging patterns or themes. **Axial coding** (Corbin & Strauss 2015) essentially refers to drawing data back together once they have been sorted in the initial phase of coding.

> **Axial coding:** The task of further evaluating the codes to determine what needs to be reassembled or reorganised.

4 Selective coding

Corbin and Strauss (2015) argue that **selective coding** necessitates a level of analysis beyond axial coding, whereby a central or core theme is identified using the previous levels of analysis. At this point, you can begin formulating propositions (Miles *et al.* 2013) by drawing conclusions, making causal connections and developing theoretical constructs. These will need to be verified in order to test their plausibility and conformability (Miles *et al.* 2013). Otherwise, as these authors point out, you run the risk of writing interesting narrative that may lack scientific rigour.

It is important that you consider more general theoretical understandings in relation to codes and data. By the time you reach this point, you should be able to construct some general theoretical notions or concepts about your data. Attempting to outline connections between concepts and categories that you are generating is a useful strategy to employ at this time. You could also examine how these tentative concepts and linkages relate to the existing literature.

> **Selective coding:** A level of analysis where researchers can begin formulating propositions by drawing conclusions, making causal connections and developing theoretical constructs.

Pranee Liamputtong and Tanya Serry

Further points to consider about coding

- In the early stages of your analysis, it is likely that you will generate a large number of codes. You will soon find that some codes will be useful, while others will not. It is important to be inventive and imaginative at the beginning. Your codes can be tidied up, reorganised and reassembled as you work through the hierarchy of steps in coding.
- Recognise that any piece of data can be coded in more than one way or in multiple coding categories.
- The process of coding requires you to be rigorous and thorough while maintaining a flexible and receptive approach to the data.
- Codes allow for easy organisation and retrieval of data from a large body of information.

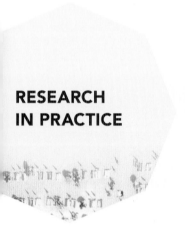

RESEARCH IN PRACTICE

EXAMPLES OF CODES

To demonstrate some codes we developed regarding experiences of parents whose children are struggling to learn to read at school, we have provided some examples taken from our analysis of interview data.

When asking parents to describe the process by which their child was allocated additional help with reading, one parent said:

> We only got it I believe [because] my husband and I sourced all that we did, and I went armed with more things, and follow-up reports from the speech pathologist.

We coded this text in an umbrella category at the level of focused coding as 'access to additional help at school' and a subcategory or descriptive code that we called 'needing to advocate for help'. From our data, we found that we needed to contrast this descriptive code with 'readily available help'.

Similarly, when parents were asked what they thought might have been influential for their child's difficulty in learning to read, one of our descriptive codes was 'parent unsure why'. Here are some comments coded accordingly:

> And it's err … I hadn't expected it would happen to us coz I had done all those pre-reading kind of things …

> I have absolutely no problem with how he was taught. It was really that for some unknown reason, it just didn't seem to be coming together.

> Honestly, at this point I'm at a loss to see why it's happened. I mean we've read to them and you know, we've spoken to our kids from when they were very young.

Types of data analysis

In the following sections, we describe two different types of qualitative data analysis: content analysis and thematic analysis. Both approaches are widely used, often within the one data set. Content analysis is the least complicated form of qualitative analysis but may not be appropriate for many qualitative research projects. Thematic analysis emphasises the power of words and meaning inherent in those words. There are other kinds of data analysis in qualitative research and we encourage you to read further (see Liamputtong 2013; Chapters 6, 8, 9).

Content analysis

Content analysis, according to Bryman (2016, p. 285), is an analytical approach that attempts to 'quantify content in terms of predetermined categories and in a systematic and replicable manner'. Although qualitative research does not typically work with numbers or counting, in practice, data analysis sometimes makes use of some underlying counting elements, particularly when judgments about qualities need to be made.

An essential goal of qualitative content analysis requires codes to be identified before they are searched for in the data. The practice of content analysis, Daly and colleagues (2007) suggest, requires the researchers to know what they want to look for in the text. Accordingly, Silverman (2010) suggests that content analysis involves developing categories or a consistent set of codes, seeking them out from the data then systematically recording or counting the number of times the categories occur. In this way, the researchers can gauge what content is contained within the data.

Furthermore, Grbich (2013) suggests that content analysis is also useful in examining textual data unobtrusively in order to check the patterns and trends of words used, their frequency and relationships. This approach is popularly used for the analysis of published material such as newspapers and magazines, policy documents, visual images, public records, medical records, speeches and interview transcripts (see Chapters 4, 5). We performed a content analysis when looking for theoretical perspectives held by educators involved with supporting young children with reading difficulty. Based on individual interviews that we collected, we searched for particular words that we had identified as critical to our research query. As a result, we were able to propose some novel conclusions from our data (Serry *et al.* 2014).

We demonstrate content analysis in a study by Shugg and Liamputtong (2002), who examined how the media portray women's health issues in Australian society. Two leading daily newspapers in Melbourne were chosen as sources of articles. A simple statistical analysis was used. They found that the predominant issues in the women's health articles were children/motherhood and pregnancy. In all, 157 (33.4 per cent) articles of 470 women's health articles related to children/motherhood. The second most frequent subject was pregnancy, with 107 articles (22.77 per cent). There was a large gap between these two and the remaining categories, the next being court rulings/damages with fifty-seven articles (12.13 per cent). Table 23.2 presents a selected list of the topic areas.

Content analysis: A form of data analysis used by both qualitative and quantitative researchers in which codes are identified before searching for their occurrence in the data.

TABLE 23.2   Frequency of women's health articles by topics

CATEGORIES	FREQUENCY	PERCENTAGE
Children/motherhood	157	33.4
Pregnancy	107	22.7
Court rulings/damages	57	12.13
Sexual violence/abuse	34	7.23

Pranee Liamputtong and Tanya Serry

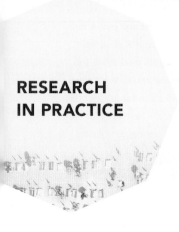

RESEARCH IN PRACTICE

CONTENT ANALYSIS

We provide an example from our own research (Serry *et al.* 2014) in which we used content analysis as a small but influential part of our overall data analysis. As part of our investigation exploring how teachers collaborate with their non-teaching colleagues regarding children with learning difficulty, in the individual interviews we noticed differences between the groups in the use of key terminology and jargon. Since we were exploring collaboration, we considered that this variability might be significant enough to explore further. We performed a simple form of content analysis on our interview data where we simply searched for the terminology in question from the texts across all participants. At the outset we did not expect that terminology variability was going to be significant. However, based on our content analysis, we were able to develop a central theme related to the entire study. To demonstrate, we interviewed twenty-five school-based staff of varied backgrounds about their views, practices and experience in helping struggling readers (Serry 2010). When discussing children's difficulty decoding and deciphering written text, 92 per cent of our sample generated terminology related to 'sounds' and 'sound knowledge', whereas only 12 per cent initiated the use of terminology related to the more theoretically sound concepts of phonology. Further, we found that the 12 per cent of participants came from a specific subgroup of staff from particular professional disciplines. On the surface, such a dichotomy of terminology use may seem minor. Nevertheless, at a theoretical level, terms related to sounds cannot be used interchangeably. This particular content analysis in our research made a valuable contribution when understanding reasons why collaborative processes between classroom-based and various specialists did not always run as planned.

Thematic analysis

> [D]iscovering themes is the basis of much social science research. Without thematic categories, investigators have nothing to describe, nothing to compare, and nothing to explain (Ryan & Bernard 2003, pp. 85–6).

Qualitative researchers believe that words are more powerful than numbers (Liamputtong 2013). Hence, content analysis may not be appropriate for most qualitative research. A more common type of analysis in qualitative research is thematic analysis, sometimes called interpretive thematic analysis (Ryan & Bernard 2003; Braun & Clarke 2006; Liamputtong 2013; Bryman 2016). **Thematic analysis** is 'a method for identifying, analysing and reporting patterns (themes) within the data' (Braun & Clarke 2006, p. 79) and is perceived 'as a foundational method for qualitative analysis' (p. 78).

Thematic analysis: The identification of themes through careful reading and rereading of the data.

The techniques used for analysing data in thematic analysis and grounded theory are broadly similar (see Chapter 8 for data analysis in grounded theory research). There are two main steps. First, you need to read carefully through each transcript. Then, as part of a collective set, you must examine the transcript and make sense of what is being said by the participants as a group (Minichiello *et al.* 2008). Thematic analysis 'involves searching across a data set—be that a number of interviews or focus groups, or a range of texts—to find repeated patterns of meaning' (Braun & Clarke 2006, p. 86). Coding plays a major part in thematic analysis, whereby the researcher needs to perform the various levels of coding in order to deconstruct data and find links between the various codes. Axial coding is the step that will allow you to connect the different codes that you have identified in the initial coding. It is 'a way of organising the data together by making connections between a major category and its sub-category' (Minichiello *et al.* 2008, p. 280). This allows the researchers to find themes in the data (see Figure 23.4).

The steps proposed by Braun and Clarke (2006, p. 87) are given in Figure 23.4.

FIGURE 23.4   Steps for thematic analysis

Make yourself familiar with your data	
Transcribe the data yourself	Read and reread the data and write down your initial impressions and ideas

Start to generate initial codes, as suggested above

Look for themes by collating codes into tentative themes

Gather all data that is related to each potential theme

Revise the themes you have developed	
Check if the themes work in relation to the codes you have extracted and the entire data set	You may also find it useful to develop a thematic 'map' of the analysis

Define the name your themes
It is also important to carry out an ongoing analysis to refine the themes so that clear definitions and names for each theme can be generated

RESEARCH IN PRACTICE

WOMEN WITH HIV/AIDS IN CENTRAL THAILAND

We would like to show the way themes were found in a study on the experience of living with HIV/AIDS for women in Central Thailand (Liamputtong *et al.* 2009). One woman remarked on her experience:

> People in community tend to see this disease as *rok mua* [promiscuous disease]. As women, we can have only one partner or one husband. But, for those who have HIV/AIDS, people tend to see them as having too many partners and this is not good. They are seen as *pu ying mai dee* [bad women]. And they will be *rang kiat* [discriminated against] more than men who have HIV/AIDS. Men who live with this disease are not seen as bad as the women are. If you are women and have HIV/AIDS, it is worse for you.

From this short transcript of one woman, we may develop the following codes:

- gender and HIV/AIDS
- HIV/AIDS and discrimination
- HIV/AIDS as promiscuous disease
- HIV/AIDS and bad women
- women and stigma
- gender inequality and HIV/AIDS.

As an illustration, we think the main theme of these codes could be termed 'gender and the stigmatised discourse'. The theme comes from the researchers' understanding of the woman's story. She did not use the word 'stigma' at all, but what she said implied stigma; it is clear from this short transcript that women living with HIV/AIDS are more stigmatised than men living with it. This example is only simple and is based on one short transcript. Once we analyse more transcripts, as Minichiello and colleagues (2008) suggest, and find that several other women speak similarly, the theme will become confirmed. However, this theme may change, as there may be other issues emerging from the data. See also Chapters 6, 8, 9.

STOP AND THINK

Google a recent newspaper report about domestic violence, use of the drug 'ice', bullying in the workplace or any other health or social sciences area. Read it carefully and answer the questions.

- What do you think would be the report's main theme?
- What would be your conclusion about this report?

Summary

> It's right to say that qualitative data analysis is a craft—one that carries its own disciplines. There are many ways of getting analysis 'right'—precise, trustworthy, compelling, credible— and they cannot be wholly predicted in advance (Miles & Huberman 1994, p. 309).

As Miles and Huberman suggest, there are many ways that researchers can transform qualitative data, which are often voluminous, more meaningfully. At the beginning, qualitative researchers are likely to feel overwhelmed with the volume and breadth of the data and ambivalent about the analysis. It is only with exposure and experience that the task becomes not only easier but very rewarding. It is essential to state here that qualitative data analysis is also socially constructed. It means that how researchers analyse their data depends on their theoretical understanding on which the research is based, and their intentions about the research outcomes. Each researcher must make decisions about what works for them—what one qualitative researcher does may be different from others. Hence, making sense of qualitative research data can be a diverse endeavour.

Practice exercises

Conduct a data analysis of the transcript sample given below, by doing the following.

1   Conduct initial coding from the transcript portion.

2   From this initial coding, perform a content analysis—what categories have you come up with? How many times does each category appear in the interview?

3   From this initial coding, attempt a thematic analysis—what themes emerge from the text?

4   Look for a missing or hidden agenda within the text—what do you think is not said in the text? What might be the reason for the missing text? You need select only one or two of these exercises to practise your analytical skills.

Researcher What was your sense of you ever finishing school and even going to university as you got a little bit further on in school?

Participant Yeah. I think before I realised, before I was diagnosed I felt like I was, there was something wrong with me and I would come home from school and I'd be very upset and I'd tell my dad, 'Uh oh, Dad. I think I'm dumb. I'm not like the other kids. I think I'm really dumb.' So that was something that I really struggled with in those early years. I think I probably did feel a sense of relief when I did find out that it, there was something wrong [dyslexia] and it didn't have anything to do with my intelligence. Yeah. I guess, I never, I don't think I ever seriously contemplated not finishing school, but I feel, I definitely think if I hadn't have gotten that intervention early on I – I definitely wouldn't have finished school. And I think once I got sort of, you know, Year 11 and Year 12 or even earlier, I definitely wanted to go to Uni. Yeah. I really enjoyed being academic. I really enjoyed writing essays. I really enjoyed reading. It's something that I've really enjoyed, so I really like the challenge. So I wasn't quite sure what I wanted to do, but it definitely involved Uni.

Researcher Okay. What do you think got you to the point of actually getting to University?

Participant I don't know. I guess just having support from my dad especially. Having my tutor for so long; I was so lucky that I was able to have so much help. Also, certain teachers around me who would give me positive feedback, telling me when I was doing well and not just seeing me as a slow reader. I guess those sort of little things kind of helped me build my self-confidence and know that I actually was pretty capable.

Further reading

Braun, V. & Clarke, V. (2006). Using thematic analysis in psychology. *Qualitative Research in Psychology*, 3, 77–101.

Bryman, A. (2016). *Social research methods*, 5th edn. Oxford: Oxford University Press.

Corbin, J. & Strauss, A. (2015). *Basics of qualitative research: techniques and procedures for developing grounded theory*, 4th edn. Thousand Oaks, CA: Sage.

Elo, S. & Kyngäs, H. (2008). The qualitative content analysis process. *Journal of Advanced Nursing*, 62(1), 107–15.

Gibbs, G.R. (2007). *Analyzing qualitative data*. London: Sage.

Grbich, C. (2013). *Qualitative data analysis: an introduction*, 2nd edn. London: Sage.

Guest, G., MacQueen, K.M. & Namey, E.E. (2012). *Applied thematic analysis*. Thousand Oaks, CA: Sage.

Liamputtong, P. (2013). *Qualitative research methods*, 4th edn. Melbourne: Oxford University Press.

Miles, M.B. & Huberman, A.M. (1994). *Qualitative data analysis*, 2nd edn. Los Angeles: Sage.

Miles, M.B., Huberman, A.M. & Saldaña, J. (2013). *Qualitative data analysis*, 3rd edn. Los Angeles: Sage.

Ryan, G.W. & Bernard, H.R. (2003). Techniques to identify themes. *Field Methods*, 15(1), 85–109.

Saldaña, J. (2009). *Coding in qualitative data analysis*. Thousand Oaks, CA: Sage.

Thorne, S. (2000). Data analysis in qualitative research. *Evidence-Based Nursing*, 3, 68–70.

Williamson, T. & Long, A.F. (2005). Qualitative data analysis using data displays. *Nurse Researcher*, 12(3), 7–19.

Websites

www.nova.edu/ssss/QR/QR3-1/carney.html

> This website leads you to a paper on a method of categorising, coding and sorting/manipulating qualitative (descriptive) data using the capabilities of a commonly used word processor, WordPerfect®.

https://www.youtube.com/watch?v=7X7VuQxPfpk

https://www.youtube.com/watch?v=DRL4PF2u9XA

https://www.youtube.com/watch?v=59GsjhPolPs

> These three clips contain many similar themes yet present a slightly different angle on doing qualitative data analysis.

24

Computer-Assisted Qualitative Data Analysis (CAQDAS)

TANYA SERRY AND PRANEE LIAMPUTTONG

Chapter objectives

In this chapter you will learn:

- what computer-assisted qualitative data analysis is and, importantly, what it is not
- about the functions of CAQDAS
- about the benefits and cautions of CAQDAS
- how to optimise the use of CAQDAS in qualitative research

Key terms

CAQDAS

Qualitative data analysis

Theory-builders in CAQDAS

Introduction

Qualitative data analysis: An analysis that looks for patterns of ideas or themes that emerge from qualitative data.

CAQDAS: Specifically designed software programs that can assist in the data analysis of qualitative data.

Computers are now a regular and expected feature of our lives. There was much excitement when software programs were first developed to assist with research, then gained increasing prominence in both data collection and data analysis. These days, we expect computer-assisted options to be available for our research and there is an increasing literature about using computer-assisted qualitative data analysis software (CAQDAS) (see Woods *et al.* 2015). This chapter will describe the conceptual features of CAQDAS and consider the advantages as well as potential disadvantages of this genre of computer-assisted research software in **qualitative data analysis**.

Computer-assisted qualitative data analysis software (CAQDAS), a term first coined by Lee and Fielding (1991), refers to specifically designed software programs (of which there are many) that can take over a substantial amount of the manual and organisational labour that permits you to analyse your qualitative data (see Chapters 6, 7, 8, 9, 23). In this chapter we will briefly discuss some of the key functions available via CAQDAS. We will also describe how we have adopted this software in our own research, along with the circumstances when we have decided not to use it. We do not present a step-by-step approach to using computer programs (see Gibbs 2008, Ch. 8; Bryman 2016, Ch. 25 for such detail), nor do we promote any one CAQDAS over another. Although Bryman (2016) refers to the fact that there is no one stand-out product, with regard to CAQDAS options, we will present evidence later in this chapter about what CAQDAS programs researchers tend to use.

What is CAQDAS?

Throughout this chapter we have adopted the acronym CAQDAS since it is widely used (Rademaker *et al.* 2012; Gapp *et al.* 2013). However, you may find the equivalent terms Qualitative Data Analysis Software or QDAS in certain publications (e.g. Bazeley 2012; Woods *et al.* 2015). Computer-assisted qualitative data analysis software can take over a substantial amount of the manual labour involved with analysing your data. In this way, it is time-efficient and provides order to what may often seem like an overwhelming amount of data. Any standard CAQDAS program can search, organise, sort and annotate your data. More recently developed CAQDAS programs can store and manage audio and visual data, including directly transcribing from multimedia and social media uploads (see Woods *et al.* 2015, p. 5) and have a well-established capacity to store and manage textual data (e.g. interview transcripts, memos, journal entries and field notes). As such, computer-assisted qualitative data analysis programs can be a valuable asset to your research experience.

In addition, CAQDAS is being promoted as a valuable tool for managing literature to complete tasks such as literature reviews and research projects involving document analyses. Along with Woods *et al.* (2015), we were unable to find supporting peer-reviewed literature on using CAQDAS for these purposes. Woods and colleagues (2015, p. 15) suggest that maybe 'researchers are using QDAS for this purpose but not reporting it'. However, a quick Google search results in a range of blog posts, YouTube clips and university training sessions advocating for and describing how CAQDAS can support the process of managing large volumes of literature (e.g. Cabrall 2012; Turner 2016).

As with any software, the program is only as good as the user (García-Horta & Guerra-Ramos 2009; Rademaker *et al.* 2012) since 'the researcher is the instrument of data analysis' (Jacelon & O'Dell 2005, p. 217). Although many of the physical, administrative and clerical tasks involved in qualitative research can be efficiently managed by this software, the rigour of organising, processing and interpreting data remains the province of the researcher (see Chapter 1). For example, Bryman (2016, p. 602) suggests that the computer 'takes over the physical task of writing marginal codes, making photocopies of transcripts or field notes, cutting out all chunks of text relating to a code, and pasting them together'. CAQDAS programs can relieve the qualitative researcher from the stereotypical notion that sticky tape, scissors and an empty lounge room floor are all you need for cutting up and reorganising vast amounts of paper in order to work with your data (Jacelon & O'Dell 2005, p. 217; Woods *et al.* 2015).

It is important to emphasise that although many researchers limit their use of CAQDAS to data management, a variety of programs can also be used to support theory-building by visualising the various relationships that have been coded in your data. We describe specific functions throughout this chapter.

STOP AND THINK

If you are already a qualitative researcher, have you used a CAQDAS program?

If yes, what prompted you to do this? What advice would you give the novice CAQDAS user?

What, if any, reservations do you have about using a CAQDAS program?

WHAT CAQDAS CAN DO

It can facilitate your qualitative research activity by:

- efficiently managing and organising your data as a sophisticated database
- allowing easy retrieval of data such as codes, text content and even specific words or phrases within texts
- supporting theory-building (not available in all CAQDAS programs)
- facilitating multiple researchers to work on a single project or data set without fear of losing or interfering with previous analyses
- acting as a valuable adjunct to the qualitative research process.

What CAQDAS is not

Statements such as 'I use a particular CAQDAS to "analyse" data' reflect a misinterpretation of how CAQDAS is and is not used. CAQDAS can undoubtedly be a valuable adjunct, assisting researchers to code, categorise, locate, organise and retrieve data or text more quickly than a manual search would. But it cannot interpret or collapse codes and analyse data on its own (Jacelon & O'Dell 2005; Gibbs 2008; Bryman 2016). Generating ideas, codes and conceptual thinking remains the role of the researcher (Gibbs 2008; García-Horta & Guerra-Ramos 2009)—the actual analytic ideas must be generated by the researcher. As such, we caution against comments such as 'using a CAQDAS to analyse data' because experienced qualitative researchers and reviewers will be alerted to the fact that this reflects a lack of knowledge about the nature of data analysis in qualitative research (see Chapter 23). CAQDAS has a range of tools for producing reports, summaries and visual representations of codes and categories, but the interpretation of these is generated by you, the researcher. Importantly, there is nothing superior about using CAQDAS for your research (MacMillan & Koenig 2004).

One of the other risks we have found when using CAQDAS is an incorrect assumption that coding equates with analytical reasoning, particularly when the coding is well ordered. We assert that in much qualitative research coding (manually or using CAQDAS) is an early step in the analytical process and should be seen as a precursor to the construction of your categories and themes (see Chapter 23). Another important caution is to avoid the trap described by Cisneros Puebla (2003)—over-reliance on the computer technology, which risks the quality of your own analytical process of critical and reflexive thinking.

WHAT CAQDAS CAN'T DO

CAQDAS has limitations. It cannot:

- process and interpret your coding
- analyse your data
- generate analytical reports
- be a substitute for the reasoning and intellectual rigour required of the researcher.

**RESEARCH
IN PRACTICE**

USING CAQDAS TO SUPPORT CONTENT AND THEMATIC ANALYSES

CAQDAS programs can be applied to both content and thematic analyses and to a number of theoretical positions (e.g. phenomenology, narrative analyses, ethnography and discourse analyses). In a study exploring who uses CAQDAS and for what main purposes across 763 articles, Woods *et al.* (2015) report that the overwhelming data types used between 1994 and 2013 were interview data (73.3 per cent) and focus group data (23.5 per cent). It is worth noting that

72 per cent of the 763 articles audited in Woods *et al.* (2015) were in journals related to the health sciences including medicine and general health care, public health, nursing, mental health, nutrition and health education. They also note that at least one-third of the 763 articles used more than one data type in a single study. For example, the 'search' functions of NVivo 11 facilitated efficient and accurate of content analysis following a series of interviews with university students who had a chronic and significant reading difficulty. By searching for a particular word or phrase such as 'dyslexia', aspects such as frequency of use or subgroups more likely to use certain terms can quickly be identified. Being able to search for the target word or phrase with or without surrounding text was a great asset.

Thematic analysis, which involves seeking key concepts, categories and themes that reflect repeated patterns of meaning from the data (see Chapter 23) can also be ably supported by CAQDAS. For example, hierarchical coding is a standard process when analysing data qualitatively; a CAQDAS user would input their codes accordingly and develop a coding schema. A valuable resource when conducting thematic analyses with CAQDAS was being able to easily and efficiently see or print out this hierarchy on a regular basis (often daily) as the coding hierarchy was modified through progressive data analysis and conceptualisation. The ability to retrieve and review particular quotes and/or codes using CAQDAS assists with validation of increasingly more conceptual coding and abstraction in a time-efficient way. The process of constant comparison, a necessary component of any qualitative analysis, is facilitated by the use of CAQDAS.

CAQDAS program options

There have been several computer packages that qualitative researchers have used (see website references and comments on various CAQDAS programs at the end of this chapter). Before the early 1990s, Ethnograph was the best-known and most widely used software. Since then, other programs have been developed. NUD*IST (Non-numerical Unstructured Data Indexing Searching and Theorizing) became very popular in the 1990s, and was developed into QSR NUD*IST Vivo, referred to as NVivo (Bryman 2016). Many researchers have used the program for their qualitative research (see Bazeley 2007; Lewins & Silver 2007.) At present, NVivo 11 (NVIVO: The #1 software for qualitative data analysis) is the most recent version from the QSR team.

In 2008, Gibbs reported that three CAQDAS programs were most commonly used by qualitative researchers. These were Atlas.ti (now in version 7), MAXqda (now in version 12) and NVivo (now in version 11). More recently, Woods *et al.* (2015) have pointed out that 99.6 per cent of articles using CAQDAS published between 1994 and 2013 utilised Atlas.ti and NVivo to support their research. Although they have many features in common, it is worth taking care when selecting a CAQDAS program to ensure it meets your specific needs. CAQDAS programs:

- can transfer text and display it in a visual display
- are able to construct code lists as a hierarchy
- permit researchers to retrieve texts that have been coded, with or without surrounding text

- allow the examination of coded texts in the context of the original data
- permit the writing of memos that can be linked to codes and data
- can accommodate research teams to work on the one data set.

CHOOSING THE RIGHT CAQDAS FOR YOUR PROJECT
- Familiarise yourself with the CAQDAS packages and make your choice based on knowing that the program will be adaptable for what you need it to do. For example, if you are using media clips, your choice of CAQDAS may be restricted. It certainly appears that as CAQDAS programs are updated, features such as visual displays and collaborative analyses are added.
- Become as familiar as you can with the various functions and features of the program.
- Sometimes, the best way to learn any software package is to simply start using it. In this case it is wise to assume that on your first few attempts at using CAQDAS with your data, you may not be using the program to capacity. You may also find you need to stop and restart. Factor this time into your research schedule. The long-term benefits of optimal use of your CAQDAS should be worth the short-term loss of time.
- Check what support options are available for the CAQDAS. Making sure that there are options such as a user-friendly HELP function or access to 'live' technical support can ease the transition into using CAQD in your research.
- Find colleagues, friends or chat rooms that use the CAQDAS you have chosen. We have found that sharing and despairing (at times) can be extremely useful. We have also come across a number of blogs dedicated to CAQDAS, including the Researchophile site as well as those hosted by the CAQDAS program developers.
- If possible, attend a workshop or training session to help you get started with your CAQDAS.

CAQDAS functions: general features

As a starting point, we present a list of ways that CAQDAS can support your qualitative research. We have compiled this list from our own experience and reading widely. It comprises three key sections that depict the general features of CAQDAS: storage features, code-and-retrieve features, and assistance with analysis of data. The first component primarily reflects the clerical aspects of any CAQDAS.

Steps and strategies for storing and managing your data:

- entering storing data (including transcripts, journal entries, memos and field notes)
- using CAQDAS to revise your data as needed

- organising storage of all data, typically with back-up function.

Code-and-retrieve features:

- coding—linking ideas and/or or concepts to named codes

- recording your memos—in order to support the conceptual leaps made from your raw data (Birks *et al.* 2008)

- retrieval functions—the ability to locate particular segments of data for closer inspection, including searching for codes, words, combinations of codes and Boolean searches (Weitzman & Miles 1995)

- linking your data to other relevant segments to form categories, clusters, sets, attribute features and themes.

Assisting with analysis:

- performing content analyses

- displaying data visually, such as a graph, matrix or model

- assistance with theory-building

- assistance with the process of drawing conclusions

- reflecting the transparency of your research.

Most of the well-known CAQDAS programs are based on the code-and-retrieve theme (Woods *et al.* 2015; Bryman 2016). They enable researchers to code texts while working at the computer and to quickly and easily retrieve the coded text. For example, Bryman (2016, p. 606) says that when he used CAQDAS in his work on the Disney Project he carried out the following steps:

1   he read through the interviews both in printed form and in the Document viewer

2   he then developed some codes that were relevant to the documents

3   he went back into the document and coded them using NVivo.

USING CAQDAS TO CODE-AND-RETRIEVE

We provide an example from our own research experience as new users of CAQDAS (see Figure 24.1), as a way of tracking our journey developing familiarity and skill with CAQDAS.

In our research exploring perceptions of parents and educators regarding children with reading difficulty, we undertook a series of steps using CAQDAS. It is important to note that planning the steps shown in Figure 24.1 did not occur at the outset. In many ways, the process of coding and categorising was itself one of trial and error, to ensure that the data would be optimally managed by our CAQDAS. This flexibility is productive and valuable for both novice and experienced qualitative researchers.

Despite using CAQDAS, we still had to read and reread transcripts, develop our codes and reflect constantly on our data. Nevertheless, the use of CAQDAS assisted immensely with coding efficiency, visual analysis of data and retrieving coded material in a timely and economical way.

RESEARCH IN PRACTICE

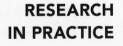

Tanya Serry and Pranee Liamputtong

FIGURE 24.1   The planning steps using CAQDAS

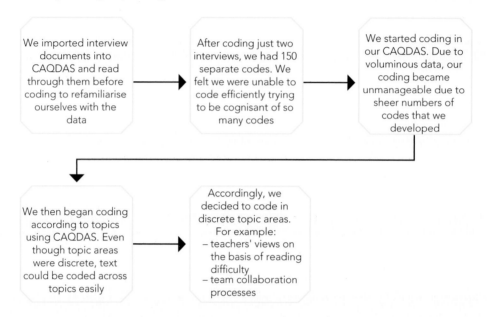

Since CAQDAS allows for automatic linking of data, we made use of functions such as highlighting coded text or using coding stripes to show us what lines were coded and the frequency of various codes. We were constantly engaged in reviewing and exploring all of our codes. Using CAQDAS, it was easy to view this on an entire screen. We also generated a coding report which we printed and kept alongside as coding continued. To examine the test within a particular code, we started retrieving. Retrieved text let us examine how our participants spoke about a particular theme. Using CAQDAS, it was easy to select information for display. Tools such as these allow for easy display of coded text.

We were able to move beyond our original codes to develop more refined categories.

Retrieved data

For example, we retrieved items that we coded as 'developmental co-morbidities' in a broad category exploring what educators believed underpinned severe reading difficulty. The steps to retrieve the data are quick and easy. Here are the comments that we coded accordingly. Note that the CAQDAS we used automatically told us the percentage of the transcript that each statement made. It also told us who made each comment and provided a hyperlink back to the statement in the original transcript. Pseudonyms have been used to protect anonymity.

Soula: 0.55% coverage

> … little lass that I've got at the moment, she's had a lot of other difficulties. She's got vision difficulties, speech delay. She's very immature.

Jenna: 0.50% coverage

> The children that are presenting with severe difficulty have got other learning issues already identified that have already been recognised.

Fiona: 0.43% coverage

> … if they've got other issues like it might be sight, hearing, developmental delay, a few things like that …

Although we have not demonstrated it here, we were able to use the retrieval function further to determine whether factors such as the number of years that participants had been teaching or what their original professional discipline was influenced the nature of our participants' responses

STOP AND THINK

- Do you think that CAQDAS could be applied to your own research data? Can you explain why, or why not?
- Who and what is available to support your readiness to undertake using CAQDAS?

Although CAQDAS has been primarily used as a code-and-retrieve tool (Woods *et al.* 2015), both Gibbs (2007) and Seale (2005) mention that more recent programs have also attempted to provide researchers with analytic procedures that support the generation and testing of theory. These programs offer different facilities, such as conceptual mapping, to help researchers examine relationships between codes and categories from text. Often these facilities are referred to as **theory-builders** (Seale 2005, p. 202). Importantly, this capacity does not mean that the program can build theory on its own. Rather, the CAQDAS will have various in-built tools that help researchers to make comparisons and develop some theoretical ideas.

For example, models that display relationships between codes and memos can assist your conceptual theory-building (Gibbs 2002). Certain CAQDAS programs will create models drawn from the stored data according to your instructions. For example, we have created a model, based on our data, that maps the views of a particular subset of educators in our cohort regarding issues they raised about a particular intervention to help struggling readers (Figure 24.2). We were attempting to analyse what this subset of educators thought about this particular intervention.

Theory-builders: Programs that assist researchers to examine relationships in the text and facilitate the building of conceptual understanding about the data.

FIGURE 24.2 A model created from our CAQDAS, used to support theory-building

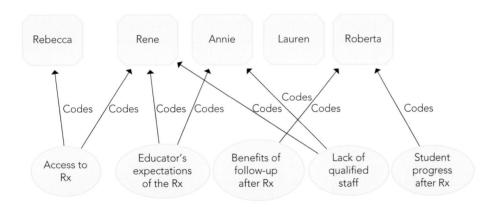

Rx is an abbreviation for the treatment program referred to by our participants

We created models exploring other subsets of educators from our study and were able to begin to build theory on factors that influenced various groups of educators' views about the treatment. We found the visual representation of the models using our CAQDAS was powerful in the process of theory-building, providing leverage for us to ask further questions of our data.

Tanya Serry and Pranee Liamputtong

Although more recent versions of CAQDAS can include functions to help build models and theory, Woods *et al.* (2015) point out that researchers have used this capacity far less frequently than using CAQDAS for data storage, analysis and management.

Benefits of CAQDAS

CAQDAS offers a highly efficient data management system for storing, coding, organising, sorting and retrieving data. As we mentioned earlier, more recent programs now have the facility to manage data well beyond word-processed documents. Such features widen the scope of who may find CAQDAS useful to their research. We were recently involved in a training program for new or aspiring users of a recent version of NVivo. It was interesting to note the breadth of research fields represented at the workshop. People working in areas such as art history, tourism, advertising, economics and law were present.

It is essential that users of CAQDAS programs have realistic expectations of their program. Although this seems obvious, we want to emphasise this point. The benefits of any program are only as good as the user's analytical thinking, expertise with the program, and decision-making. We encourage anybody who is contemplating using CAQDAS to gain as much familiarity and skill as possible with their chosen program before launching into serious use. For example, Tanya attended a training workshop and sought input from colleagues who were already familiar with the NVivo range before applying CAQDAS to her own data.

Tanya has found the capacity of recent CAQDAS programs to manage documents such as published articles, policy statement and newspaper clips particularly useful. For example, Tanya now imports relevant published articles and newspaper clippings into her NVivo program and codes these in the same way as she codes interview data. This feature greatly assists the interpretation of her data and the efficiency of writing up results is greatly enhanced because everything is stored and accessed in the one location.

Cautions about CAQDAS

Although many CAQDAS users maintain that the computer packages have helped them with data analysis, a number of authors report reservations about the use of CAQDAS. For example, both Fielding and Lee (1998) and Gibbs (2007) argue that there is a sense of being distant from the data when using CAQDAS, and that those who use paper-based analysis feel they are closer to the words of their participants. This may be because many of the early CAQDAS programs did not make it easy for researchers to move back and forth between the data to examine the context of coded or retrieved text. Recent programs have allowed for this this facility, but many researchers still wish to be closer to their data—CAQDAS will limit that closeness.

As we pointed out earlier, CAQDAS does not, and cannot, assist with decisions about coding or the interpretation of findings. Computer programs cannot develop propositions from the data or tell researchers that there are different theories they can apply. Any theoretical framework and analytic approach that researchers use has to be introduced by the researchers themselves.

Another reservation is that the code-and-retrieve process of CAQDAS may result in a fragmentation of the textual materials (Weaver & Atkinson 1995; Gibbs 2008). Hence the narrative flow of the data may be diminished (Bryman 2016). Context is crucial in qualitative research (Liamputtong 2013; Bryman 2016; see Chapter 1 and chapters in Part I). Decontexualisation of the data may also occur, because of the fragmentation process of coding text into chunks that are then retrieved and grouped into related fragments (Buston 1997; Fielding & Lee 1998).

CAQDAS programs may not be suitable for certain types of qualitative data. From their experience, Catterall and MacLaren (1997) argue that CAQDAS needs to be used with specific mindfulness for focus group data because the code-and-retrieve function may result in a loss of the communication and interaction process, which is essential in the focus group method (see Chapter 5). For some data analysis, particularly grounded theory (see Chapter 8), the use of computer packages for data analysis may be problematic (Glaser 2003) and should be adopted with particular care. This is because, as Holton (2007, p. 287) makes clear, 'the coding process in classic grounded theory is not a discrete phase but rather an intricate and integral activity woven into and throughout the research process'.

Some qualitative researchers (see Stanley & Temple 1995; La Pelle 2004; Ryan 2004), argue that the coding and retrieval features can be done through powerful word-processing software such as the Microsoft Word 'Find' function. By implication, this means that researchers may not need to go through a lengthy period of becoming familiar with the operations of CAQDAS. La Pelle (2004, p. 86) says she has found that the built-in functions of Microsoft Word 'serve admirably for many qualitative research projects' and they do not require programming skill. She often prefers to use Word to do many basic data analysis functions.

Pranee has used Microsoft Word to analyse text from key informant interviews, focus groups, document reviews and open-ended survey questions, among other sources of data. She uses Word functions such as Table, Table Sort, Insert File, Find/Replace, and Insert Comment to do this work. Projects have ranged in size from short simple tasks to complex multiyear research endeavours that involved more than 200 interviews, more than 2000 pages of transcribed texts and more than 200 codes.

CAQDAS: to use or not to use

Many students and researchers have considered whether they should use CAQDAS programs to assist with data management and analysis. We have suggested several concerns that many qualitative researchers have discussed. However, Bryman (2016) offers this advice: if you have a small number of cases, it may not be worth the time and effort to master new software.

It may also be too expensive for your personal purchase. But if you have a free access or a site licence to the CAQDAS, you may like to try. If you plan to use it in future research, it may be worthwhile taking the time to learn. Learning new software gives you useful skills that you can make use of in the future. Many of our own postgraduate students take this position.

Our own thoughts are that computers can be very useful as adjuncts to qualitative research; CAQDAS can provide efficiencies and order in data analysis process. Nevertheless, we also argue that computer programs are not always required, nor do they solve many of the central problems of qualitative research. Pranee remains more ambivalent about the role of technology in helping qualitative researchers analyse their data, on the grounds that computer packages cannot do this for us with the thoroughness that we require. Holton (2007, p. 287) says it clearly: 'Experienced classic grounded theorists continue to await a "package" that can replicate the complex capabilities of the human brain for conceptualization of latent patterns of social behaviour'. Pranee does not really use any computer package to do her data analysis. Although she has done CAQDAS training and agrees that it can be useful for many research projects, Pranee prefers to work closely with her data by using coloured pens and highlighters, and word-processing to cut and paste the data (see also Chapter 23). In contrast, Tanya has used CAQDAS more routinely, but remains deeply aware of the importance of the foundational thinking and the critical reflection that is required to conduct rigorous and valuable qualitative research.

Summary

In this chapter, we have discussed issues relating to the use of CAQDAS and suggested that CAQDAS can be useful for many qualitative research projects. There are many commercial and free internet-based CAQDAS programs that researchers may wish to explore and use. Despite the many benefits of CAQDAS, there are some cautions that must be considered; in particular, that the CAQDAS program assists with your data analysis but cannot do the in-depth analysis and interpretation for you.

Practice exercises

1   In the qualitative studies referenced below, some researchers have chosen to use CAQDAS while others have not. Read one from each group of articles and take careful note of the following issues.

   (a) How was data storage and management described?

   (b) How was the code-and-retrieve process managed?

   (c) Do you think that CAQDAS was beneficial or justified when it was used? Why or why not?

(d) Do you think the use of manual coding and retrieving was justified? Why or why not?

(e) Would you have done anything differently if you were one of the authors? Justify your responses.

Papers using CAQDAS

Erickson, S. & Serry, T.A. (2016). Comparing alternate learning pathways within a problem-based learning speech-language pathology curriculum. *International Journal of Speech-Language Pathology*, 18(1), 97–107. doi: 10.3109/17549507.2015.1089936

Hopkins, T., Clegg, J. & Stackhouse, J. (2015). Young offenders' perspectives on their literacy and communication skills. *International Journal of Language & Communication Disorders*. doi: 10.1111/1460-6984.12188

Klauda, S.L. & Wigfield, A. (2012). Relations of perceived parent and friend support for recreational reading with children's reading motivations. *Journal of Literacy Research*, 44(1), 3–44.

Williamson, P., Koro-Ljungberg, M.E. & Bussing, R. (2009). Analysis of critical incidents and shifting perspectives: transitions in illness careers among adolescents with ADHD. *Qualitative Health Research*, 19, 352–65.

Papers not using CAQDAS

Lasser, J. & Corley, K. (2008). Constructing normalcy: a qualitative study of parenting children with Asperger's Disorder. *Educational Psychology in Practice*, 24(4), 335–46.

Bailey, R.L, Stoner, J.B., Angell, M.E. & Fetzer, A. (2008). School-based speech-language pathologists' perspectives on dysphagia management in the schools. *Language, Speech & Hearing Services in Schools*, 39(4), 441–50.

2   Review one of the freely available CAQDAS programs (see below) and consider the following.

(a) How was data storage and management described?

(b) How was the code-and-retrieve process managed?

(c) Are there any options to seek Help?

(d) Would you consider using this particular program? Why or why not?

Software options

Table 24.1 lists a range of commercially available and freely downloadable CAQDAS options. The associated websites were the latest releases at the time of publication of this book. It is likely that there will be updates as programs are revised, refined and enhanced. While all CAQDAS programs offer the ability to store, code, organise and retrieve data, some programs are differentiated by functions that may be of particular value for some researchers. For example, functions may include the capacity to upload social media as a data source, the ability to manage data from virtually alphabetic or character-based language or the availability of a number of languages at the interface. We have listed the CAQDAS programs alphabetically because we do not advocate the use of any specific CAQDAS. Websites for the various programs are informative, with many offering online tutorials and a free trial period.

TABLE 24.1 Commercially or freely available CAQDAS options

COMMERCIALLY AVAILABLE CAQDAS EXAMPLES	WEB-BASED CAQDAS EXAMPLES
AQUAD 7	Dedoose (supported by a monthly fee)
Atlas.ti	Transana (supported through licence purchase)
Ethnograph 6.0.1.0	
HyperResearch™. HYPERTranscribe™ is required for transcription. Both programs can be bought together as HYPERBundle	**FREE WEB-BASED CAQDAS EXAMPLES**
MAXQDA	Coding Analysis Toolkit (CAT)
NVivo 11	R Qualitative Data Analysis *(RQDA)
QUALRUS	Text Analysis Markup System
QDA Miner v4	WEFT Qualitative Data Analysis

Further reading

Bazeley, P. (2012). Regulating qualitative coding using QDAS? *Sociological Methodology*, 42(1), 77–8.

Bazeley, P. & Jackson, K. (2013). *Qualitative data analysis with NVivo*, 2nd edn. London: Sage.

Bryman, A. (2016). *Social research methods*, 5th edn. Oxford: Oxford University Press.

Jacelon, C.S. & O'Dell, K.K. (2005). Analyzing qualitative data. *Urologic Nursing*, 25(3), 217.

La Pelle, N. (2004). Simplifying qualitative data analysis using general purposes software tools. *Field Methods*, 16(1), 85–108.

MacMillan, K. & Koenig, T. (2004). The wow factor preconceptions and expectations for data analysis software in qualitative research. *Social Science Computer Review*, 22(2), 179–86.

Websites

http://qrtips.com/

This site offers techniques and tips for qualitative researchers.

www.surrey.ac.uk/sociology/research/researchcentres/caqdas/

This site offers practical support, training and information in the use of a range of software programs designed to assist qualitative data analysis.

25

Data Analysis in Quantitative Research

JANE PIERSON

Chapter objectives

In this chapter you will learn:

- about the purpose of data analysis in quantitative health research
- about considerations in selecting data analysis procedures
- about the use of procedures to examine differences between two or more measures of central tendency
- about the use of procedures to examine relationships between two or more sets of measures

Key terms

ANOVA

Chi-square test

Correlation coefficient

Degrees of freedom

Descriptive statistics

Inferential statistics

MANOVA

Multiple regression analysis

Statistical significance

t-test

Introduction

Descriptive

statistics: These include

measures of central

tendency such as means,

median (50th percentile)

or mode (most frequently

occurring score), and

measures of dispersion

(e.g. the standard deviation

and the range).

Analysis of data that comes from quantitative research studies typically involves the use of statistical procedures. Thus, statistics are of key importance in health research (and in related fields such as evaluation of health programs and services). Statistics are, therefore, of importance in the application of health research evidence to health practice. A key reason for this is that statistical procedures allow for the determination of whether an effect that is found in a study is real. Whether or not an effect can be considered to be statistically significant (i.e. real) is an important consideration in deciding whether evidence drawn from a quantitative study (or studies) should be used to inform practice.

Quantitative health research involves the measurement of health phenomena (see chapters in Part III). The resulting data are commonly summarised and analysed using statistics. **Descriptive statistics** include measures of central tendency (e.g. the mean and the median), and measures of dispersion (e.g. the standard deviation and the range). **Inferential statistics** include a variety of procedures that are commonly referred to as 'statistical tests'. While inferential statistics differ from each other in terms of their specific characteristics, they all have essentially the same purpose, which is to determine whether or not an outcome of a research study is statistically significant (see also Chapter 26). Inferential statistics include procedures which are used to estimate the likely value of population parameters from values for a sample, and which can also be used to determine the statistical significance of effects. In this chapter discussion will, however, be limited to statistical tests.

Inferential statistics: These

include various procedures

commonly referred to as

statistical tests.

Statistics in health research

Statistical

significance: Whether

or not an outcome is

statistically significant can

be established by using a

statistical test to decide

whether the outcome is

likely to be due to chance,

or to be real.

Whether or not an outcome has **statistical significance** can be established by using a statistical test to determine the likelihood of the outcome occurring by chance. To appreciate what is meant by chance in this context, consider the (hypothetical) study summarised in Table 25.1. This study was a randomised controlled trial (RCT; see Chapter 15) that examined the effectiveness of a new drug in lowering blood pressure (BP) in those who suffer from hypertension (high blood pressure).

In this study, participants were randomly assigned to one of two groups—treatment or control—with twenty-four participants per group. Before the commencement of the treatment phase of the trial, each participant's BP was measured and the mean diastolic BP was calculated for each group. While it could be expected that the means would be similar

TABLE 25.1   Mean diastolic BP and standard deviation (in brackets), pre- and post-treatment

GROUP	TREATMENT	CONTROL (PLACEBO)
Pre-treatment BP (mmHg)	100.25 (8.76)	98.04 (8.94)
Post-treatment BP (mmHg)	86.25 (7.97)	96.17 (9.09)

before the treatment phase began, it would not be expected that they would be exactly the same (at least, this would not happen very often). This is because individuals differ from each other and there are different individuals in the groups. However, random assignment to groups means that they should be effectively equivalent to each other, so any difference between them before treatment is by chance. While the means for the two groups at the conclusion of the treatment phase are, again, not the same as each other, the difference between them now reflects both chance and any effect (i.e. action) of the drug. See also Chapter 15.

A statistical test allows the establishment of the probability of obtaining an effect (which in this case can be thought of as the difference between the group's means after treatment) by chance. If this probability is relatively high, it is concluded that the effect is due to chance. If, however, this probability is low, it is concluded that the effect is real, that is, it is statistically significant. (In this example a real effect is one that is due to the drug being effective in lowering diastolic BP.) The probability of getting an effect by chance is considered to be low if it is equal to or less than a criterion probability value. While this value (the alpha level) may be one of a range of values, it is conventionally set at 0.05 (which corresponds to a probability of occurrence by chance of five times in 100). So, if a statistical test determines that the probability of getting an effect by chance is equal to or less than 0.05, it can be concluded that the effect is statistically significant (real). If the probability of getting the effect by chance is greater than 0.05, it is concluded that the effect is not statistically significant (due to chance).

Conducting a statistical test involves calculating the value(s) of a statistic, which can be thought of as standing for the effect(s). The probability of obtaining the calculated value of the statistic by chance is then determined. If this probability is equal to or less than the alpha level, the effect is deemed to be statistically significant. If the probability is higher than the alpha level, the effect is deemed not to be statistically significant. See also Chapter 26, which deals with reading statistical data.

STOP AND THINK

Although a research study may find a statistically significant effect, it needs to be considered whether this is enough on its own to warrant the use of the evidence from the study to inform practice. The size of the effect (the effect size) is of key importance in deciding if evidence should be applied to practice. That is, it is necessary to consider whether an effect is large enough to be considered to have clinical or practical significance or importance. This is usually conceptualised in terms of the effect being large enough to correspond to a meaningful (positive) change in people's health status. To illustrate, consider a clinical trial of a new intervention for reducing the body weight of those who are overweight or obese. This study found that the intervention produced an effect, which was a mean loss of body weight of 3.4 kg, and this effect was statistically significant.

Do you think that a mean body weight loss of 3.4 kg could be considered to be clinically/practically significant/important?

Jane Pierson

Choosing statistical tests

As there is a variety of statistical tests that can be employed in the analysis of quantitative data, decisions about which statistical test is appropriate are often viewed as being somewhat complex. In practice, however, there are just two key criteria that need to be considered when choosing a statistical test or other inferential statistical procedure: the characteristics of the study design, and the characteristics of the study data.

Design characteristics

The first study characteristic that needs to be considered when choosing an inferential statistical procedure is whether the study is experimental or quasi-experimental, or correlational. Broadly speaking, experimental and quasi-experimental studies look for differences in values or scores between two or more groups or conditions or situations or time-points, while correlational studies look for associations or relationships between categories, or between two or more sets of values or scores. Experimental studies (e.g. RCTs) involve random assignment into groups, while in quasi-experimental studies the groups are naturally occurring or are formed on the basis of participants' pre-existing characteristics. Some (but not all) studies where the same participants are observed under two or more conditions or in two or more situations or at two or more time-points (within subjects or repeated measures designs), can be considered as special cases of experimental designs, as each participant serves as their own control.

For both experimental and quasi-experimental studies, the design characteristics that need to be considered when choosing a statistical test are as follows: the number of independent variables, the number of levels of each independent variable; whether observations are repeated or not across the levels of each independent variable, and the number of dependent variables. In practice, all this comes down to considering how many groups/conditions/situations/time-points, are to be compared with each other, whether the values or scores that are to be compared come from the same participants (or from matched pairs) or from different participants, and how many variables were quantified (measured). For correlational designs, the study design characteristic that needs to be considered when selecting inferential statistical procedures is the number of variables (the number of sets of categories or values or scores). See chapters in Part III.

Data characteristics

The characteristic of the study data that is most important in the choice of statistical test or other inferential statistical procedure is the data type. There are four types of data that are typically distinguished from each other: nominal, ordinal, interval and ratio (see Chapters 11, 13). The type of data is itself related to the properties of the scale that was used to collect the data. Thus, the points on a nominal scale can be thought of as corresponding to categories that are different from each other but can't be ordered with respect to each other (e.g. the response categories 'Yes', 'No', 'Don't know'). The points on an ordinal scale can be thought of as corresponding to categories that can be put in order with respect to each other, but the intervals between each of the points are not necessarily equal to each other (e.g. a rating scale with points corresponding to 'Strongly disagree', 'Disagree', 'Neutral', 'Agree', 'Strongly agree'). On an interval scale, the intervals between each of the scale points are equal to each other but the scale does not have an absolute zero, which is a point that corresponds to the absence of what is quantified (measured) by the scale (e.g. the Celsius and Fahrenheit temperature scales). A ratio scale has both equality of intervals and an absolute zero (e.g. scales for measuring weight).

For interval and ratio data, another data characteristic that needs to be considered, when deciding on the appropriate statistical test, is normality, which is assessed in terms of the extent to which the distribution of the values or scores (the distribution of the study data) approximates that of the normal distribution. It may also be necessary to take other data characteristics, such as homogeneity of variance, into account.

Example of choosing a statistical test

The study that is summarised in Table 25.1 can serve as an example of the use of the criteria outlined above for choosing statistical tests. This study used an experimental design. There are two groups to be compared with each other, and the scores that are to be compared come from different participants. One characteristic (diastolic BP) has been measured. Thus there is one independent variable (group), which has two levels (treatment and control) and, as there are different participants in the two groups, measures are not repeated across the levels of the independent variable. There is one dependent variable (diastolic BP). The data are ratio in type (as blood pressure is measured using a ratio scale), and the distribution of the scores approximates that of the normal distribution. The specifics of the study design, together with the data characteristics, indicate that an independent t-test is the appropriate statistical test for data analysis. The conduct of t-tests is discussed in the next section.

Conducting statistical tests

Experimental and quasi-experimental designs

There are a number of statistical tests that can be used with these designs. These include the t-test, analysis of variance (and of covariance), and multivariate analysis of variance (and of covariance).

The t-test

A **t-test** is used to compare two means with each other, to establish if there is a statistically significant difference between them. There are several versions of the t-test, including the one-sample t-test, used to compare a mean for a single set of values or scores with another mean, and the two-sample t-test, used when the means of two sets of values or scores are to be compared with each other. As the latter is the most commonly encountered t-test in health

t-test: A t-test is used to compare two means with each other, to establish if there is a statistically significant difference between them.

research, the following discussion will be limited to it. Two-sample t-tests are appropriate when there is one independent variable with two levels and one dependent variable, when the data are interval or ratio in type and approximately normally distributed. When the two sets of values or scores come from different participants, an independent t-test (unpaired t-test) is used. When the two sets of values or scores come from the same participants or from matched pairs of participants, a related t-test (paired-samples t-test) is used.

A two-sample t-test is conducted by calculating a value of the t-test statistic that stands for the effect, which is the mean difference (the difference between the means for the two groups, or the difference between the means for the two conditions/situations/time-points). The probability of obtaining the calculated value of t (and therefore the effect) by chance, with the applicable **degrees of freedom** (df)1 is then determined. If this probability is equal to or less than the alpha level set for the test, then the t value (and therefore the effect) is deemed to be statistically significant. If the probability is greater than the alpha level, then the t value (and therefore the effect) is deemed to be not statistically significant. As the conduct of the two subtypes of two-sample t-tests is essentially the same, only the conduct of the independent t-test is described below.

The study summarised in Table 25.1 has one independent variable with two levels, and one dependent variable. The data are ratio in type and approximately normally distributed. The two sets of measures of BP come from different participants. An independent t-test is therefore applicable. For the post-treatment data summarised in Table 25.1, the calculated value of t is 4.02. With 46 degrees of freedom, the probability of getting this t value by chance is 0.0002. As this value is lower than the alpha level (0.05) set for the test, this t value, and therefore the effect (the mean difference), is statistically significant.

Strictly speaking, the distribution of the data should be approximately normal for t-tests to be used. This is because the value of t (which is calculated using the data) will be distorted if the distributions of values or scores is non-normal. However, so-called parametric tests, including the t-test, and the various types of analysis of variance (see below), are regarded as being robust to violations of the assumption of normality and therefore the calculated value of the statistic is little affected, unless the deviation from normality is extreme (Maxwell & Delaney 2004; Elliot & Woodward 2006). Therefore t-tests can be used for most interval and ratio data.

When the non-normality of the data is such that t-tests would be inappropriate, a non-parametric equivalent can be used. Non-parametric statistics are sometimes called distribution-free statistics, because they do not have assumptions about the characteristics of the distribution of the values or scores. There are two non-parametric statistical tests that are equivalent to (two-sample) t-tests. The Mann-Whitney U-test is used when different participants provide the two sets of values or scores, and the Wilcoxon signed-rank test is used when the two sets of values or scores come from the same participants (or from matched pairs of participants). The conduct of these tests is essentially equivalent to that of the corresponding parametric t-tests. These non-parametric statistical tests are also used when the data are ordinal, and two medians are to be compared with each other. While detailed discussion

Degrees of freedom: Values associated with a test statistic that represent the number of scores that are free to vary. These values are used in determining the statistical significance of a test statistic.

of these and other non-parametric statistics is beyond the scope of this chapter, there are a number of texts that provide such discussion (see Siegel & Castellan 1988; Gibbons 1993).

STOP AND THINK

A T-TEST FOR A DRIVING PERFORMANCE STUDY

In a study that examined the effects of alcohol on driving performance, it was planned to test people's driving performance in a driving simulator while they were sober and when they were under the influence of alcohol (had a blood alcohol level greater than 0.05 g/100 mL). It was planned to use a related t-test to compare the means for the group of participants for these two conditions: sober, and under the influence. However, before this could be done, a design problem needed to be dealt with, so that the means could be validly compared. It was likely that participants' driving performance in the simulator would improve with practice, and therefore they would perform better in their second testing session than in their first.

- What do you think could be done to ensure that the order of testing was not confounded with the two conditions? That is, what could be done to 'untangle' the variable of interest, which was state (with two levels that corresponded to the two conditions: sober/under the influence), from the potentially confounding variable, which was testing session (first session/second session)?

Analysis of variance

An **analysis of variance** (ANOVA) is used to compare the means of three or more sets of values or scores, to determine if there are statistically significant differences between them. An ANOVA can be used when the data are interval or ratio in type and reasonably normally distributed. As there are a number of types of ANOVA, the decision about which one is appropriate depends on the study design. When there is one independent variable (factor) with three or more levels, and one dependent variable (measure), a one-way ANOVA is appropriate. When the three or more sets of values or scores come from different participants (i.e. measures are not repeated across the levels of the independent variable) the independent variable is termed a between-subjects factor, and the one-way ANOVA for independent groups is used. When the three or more sets of values or scores come from the same participants, the independent variable is termed a within-subjects factor and the design is referred to as a 'within-subjects (repeated-measures) design'. For such designs, a one-way ANOVA for repeated measures is used.

> ANOVA: An ANOVA is used to compare the means of three or more sets of values or scores to determine if there are statistically significant differences between them.

A one-way ANOVA is conducted by calculating a value of the F statistic that stands for the effect, which can be thought of as the set of differences between the means (for the three or more groups, or the three or more conditions/situations/time-points). Thus a single ANOVA simultaneously compares all of the means with each other. The probability of obtaining the calculated value of F (and therefore the effect) by chance, with the applicable degrees of freedom[2] is then determined. If this probability is equal to or less than the alpha level set for the test, then the value of F (and therefore the effect) is statistically significant. If the probability is greater than the alpha level, then the value of F (and therefore the effect) is not statistically significant. Therefore a statistically significant value of F indicates that there is at least one statistically significant difference between the means. However, the test does not allow for a decision to be made as to which of the mean differences are statistically significant. To determine which of the differences are likely to be statistically significant, follow-up tests (post-hoc tests) are required (Grove 2007).

As the processes involved in the conduct of the two types of one-way ANOVA are essentially the same, only an example of the application of the one-way ANOVA for independent groups is given here. The (hypothetical) study summarised in Table 25.2 compared three different diet plans, each of which aimed to produce weight loss, in those who are overweight. There were thirty participants in each group. The data shown in Table 25.2 relate to the amount of weight lost by participants, over a two-month period.

This study has one independent variable (one between-subjects factor): Group (which has three levels: plan A, plan B and plan C) and one dependent variable: body weight loss. The data are ratio in type and approximately normally distributed. The sets of measures of body weight loss come from different participants. A one-way ANOVA for independent groups is therefore appropriate. For the data summarised in Table 25.2, the calculated value of F is 3.81. With (2, 87) degrees of freedom, the probability of getting this value of F by chance is 0.026. As this probability is lower than the alpha level (0.05) set for the test, this value of F (and therefore the effect) is statistically significant. Table 25.2 shows that the mean for plan A was significantly higher than the means for plans B and C, which were similar to each other. It is therefore likely that the mean for plan A is significantly different from those for both plans B and C. However, a post-hoc procedure would be needed to confirm this.

TABLE 25.2   Mean amount of weight loss (and standard deviation) for plan A, plan B and plan C participants

GROUP	PLAN A	PLAN B	PLAN C
Body weight loss (kg)	8.12 (2.38)	6.75 (1.97)	6.87 (2.01)

As discussed above (in the context of the t-test), the distortion of the value of F, due to non-normality of the data, is only of consequence when the departure from normality is very marked. It is also relatively robust to another assumption about the data, that is, homogeneity of variance (Maxwell & Delaney 2004). Therefore the ANOVA can be used for most interval or ratio data. When the non-normality of the data is such that an ANOVA would be inappropriate, a non-parametric equivalent can be used. The Kruskal-Wallis test is used when different participants provide the three or more sets of values or scores. The Friedman test is used when the three or more sets of values or scores come from the same participants. These non-parametric statistics are also used when the data are ordinal and three or more medians are to be compared with each other. Detailed discussion of these non-parametric tests is provided in Siegel and Castellan (1988) and Gibbons (1993).

When there are two or more independent variables (factors) and one dependent variable (measure), the data are interval/ratio in type and reasonably normally distributed, a factorial ANOVA is used. Each factor can have two or more levels. Measures on each factor can be non-repeated or repeated and therefore designs can be fully independent, fully within subjects, or mixed (repeated measures on one or more factors and non-repeated measures on one or more of the other factors).

The (hypothetical) study summarised in Table 25.3 investigated the effectiveness of a new therapy in reducing asthma symptomology for people diagnosed with allergic asthma and people diagnosed with idiopathic asthma. The therapy was administered at two times of day, 8 a.m. and 8 p.m. Thus there are two factors: Type of Asthma, which has two levels (allergic and idiopathic) and Time of Day, which also has two levels (a.m. and p.m.). Forty-eight asthmatic participants were divided into two groups on the basis of whether their asthma was allergic or idiopathic. Members of each group were then randomly assigned to one of the two administration times, with twelve participants in each of the resulting four groups. After one month of therapy, peak flow volumes were measured for each participant (higher peak flow represents a lower degree of asthma symptomology). As there are two independent variables (factors), the data are ratio in type and approximately normally distributed, and there are different participants in each of the groups, a factorial ANOVA (for independent groups) is applicable.

TABLE 25.3 Mean peak flow volume (L/min) and standard deviation (in brackets)

TYPE OF ASTHMA	ALLERGIC	IDIOPATHIC
a.m. administration	468.33 (63.94)	424.17 (44.81)
p.m. administration	426.67 (44.99)	478.33 (56.22)

A factorial ANOVA yields a number of values of F (and the probability of obtaining each of these by chance, with the corresponding degrees of freedom). These values of F correspond to the main effect for each factor and to the interaction(s) between factors. In the context of the study summarised in Table 25.3, the main effect for Type of Asthma corresponds to the difference between the overall means for allergic and idiopathic, and the main effect for Time of Day corresponds to the difference between the overall means for a.m. and p.m. Thus the overall mean for allergic asthma is 447.50 and the overall mean for idiopathic asthma is 451.25, the overall mean for a.m. is 446.25 and the overall mean for p.m. is 452.50. The means that correspond to the interaction effect are those shown in Table 25.3. In this study, neither of the main effects was significant (i.e. there was no statistically significant difference between the overall means for Type of Asthma or for Time of Day). There was, however, a statistically significant interaction between Type of Asthma and Time of Day. Thus for allergic asthma, a.m. administration was more effective than was p.m. administration; for idiopathic asthma, p.m. administration was more effective than was a.m. administration. Note that interactions can take on a number of patterns or forms, according to which of the means differ from each other.

A modified version of ANOVA, namely analysis of covariance (ANCOVA), is used when a (continuous) extraneous variable is systematically confounded with the levels of the independent variable(s). A confounding variable of this kind is referred to as a 'covariate'. Such a situation is not uncommon when quasi-experimental designs are used. To appreciate the nature of this situation, consider the following (hypothetical) study. This study aims to compare the level of strain (as measured by the Carer-strain Index) experienced by people who are acting as a carer for a person with one of three different medical conditions: severely disabling osteoarthritis, cancer, or dementia. Thus the independent variable of interest is the care-recipient's medical condition. The confounding variable is the carer's health status (as measured by the MOS SF 36). Hence there are apparent differences in the health status of participants in the three groups. Those caring for a person with cancer have, on average, poorer health status than do those caring for a person with osteoarthritis, and those caring for a person with dementia have, on average, the poorest health status. As it has been established through previous research that there is a degree of relationship between these two variables, such that level of carer strain (irrespective of the health condition(s) experienced by the care-recipient) increases with declines in the health status of the carer, any differences in carer strain in this study may be due only to the differences in health status of the three carer groups, or due to both differences in health status and differences in the nature of the care-recipient's condition. To allow the group means for carer strain to be compared, to look for differences that are attributable to the differences in the nature of the care-recipient's condition, an ANCOVA is needed.

In simple terms, an ANCOVA identifies, and puts to one side, differences between the groups that are due to the covariate. It therefore adjusts for any influence of the covariate, and allows for the examination of differences between the groups that are due to the variable of interest. In the example study described above, the variable of interest is the care-recipient's medical condition. The ANCOVA removes the effects of the covariate (the carer's health status) and allows the groups to be compared, to look for differences that are due to the differences in the medical condition of the care-recipient.

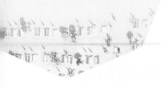

RESEARCH IN PRACTICE

REDUCING CHILDHOOD OBESITY

I have recently been part of a team that evaluated the effectiveness of two programs, each of which aimed to reduce the levels of obesity among program participants, who were children. For each of the programs, measurements were made of participants' height and weight at each of three time-points: immediately before the program, immediately after the conclusion of the program, and at a follow-up six months after the conclusion of the program. The height and weight values were used to calculate the body mass index (BMI) for each participant, at each of the three time-points. It was originally planned to use a repeated-measures ANOVA to compare the mean BMI at the three time-points, for each of the programs. However, there were too few participants for whom data was available at the six-month follow-up to allow for meaningful comparison of the data for all three time-points. Therefore related t-tests were used to compare the mean BMI for before the program, with mean BMI immediately after program conclusion.

Multivariate analysis of variance

Multivariate analysis of variance (MANOVA) is used when there are two or more dependent variables (measures), each of which is measured on an interval or ratio scale, where the set of values or scores for each is reasonably normally distributed and there is correlation between the sets of values or scores. A MANOVA can be applied to designs where there is/are one or more independent variables, each with two or more levels.

A MANOVA determines if there are significant differences between the groups, in terms of scores on a 'new' dependent variable, which can be thought of as an amalgam of the scores (for each participant) on the two or more dependent variables. If the groups are shown to differ significantly by the MANOVA, separate ANOVAs (one for each dependent variable) are then used. These tests are used to determine if the groups are significantly different for only one of the dependent variables, or for some or all of the dependent variables. When there are two or more dependent variables and one or more covariates (as described above), a multivariate analysis of covariance (MANCOVA) is usually used. Further consideration of MANOVA and MANCOVA is beyond the scope of this chapter. Likewise, profile analysis, which is recommended as an alternative to MANOVA when there are two or more dependent variables and repeated measures on one or more of the independent variables, will not be covered here. Further discussion of these procedures can be found in a number of texts (e.g. Tabachnick & Fidell 2012).

> **MANOVA:** This is used when there are two or more dependent variables, each of which is measured on an interval or ratio scale.

A RESEARCH STUDENT'S DILEMMA

For her thesis project, Elaine Tsang examined self-perceived quality of life among older Chinese people living in Melbourne, Australia. She recruited older Chinese people into two groups: those who were living in the general community, and those who were living in a Chinese-specific aged care facility. The study used a mixed methods approach. Participants were interviewed and measures were made of a number of characteristics that are likely to be associated with quality of life. These measures included the MOS SF 36, the Geriatric Depression Scale and a life satisfaction index. Each participant also completed a questionnaire that collected basic demographic information, including age (in years). Elaine had intended to compare the measures for the two groups, but when she examined the demographic data she realised that such comparison would be problematic. This was because the people living in the aged care facility were older, on average, than were the people who were living in the community. She knew that previous research had shown that quality of life declines with advancing age, and realised that this meant that any differences between the groups could be due to the difference in average age of the two groups, rather than to differences in the measures that related to self-perceived quality of life. Elaine was concerned about this problem, until she consulted several statistics texts. She learnt from them that she could use analysis of covariance (specifically, multivariate analysis of covariance) to analyse her data. This analysis would adjust for the age difference between the two groups, and allow her to compare the two groups on the measures that related to quality of life. For more discussion of the methods used in this study, see Tsang *et al.* (2003).

RESEARCH IN PRACTICE

Jane Pierson

Correlational designs

For correlational designs, there are a number of statistical procedures that researchers can use. These include chi-square tests, correlation coefficients and multiple regression.

Chi-square tests

There are two types of **chi-square test**, which are used when the data are nominal in type and the data therefore consist of frequency counts for categories. These are the one-way chi-square test, which is sometimes called the goodness of fit test, and the two-way chi-square test, which is sometimes referred to as the test of independence. While the one-way chi-square test has some applications in health research, it will not be considered further here. The two-way chi-square test is referred to as being a test of independence, because it determines whether two variables are independent of each other, or whether there is a relationship or association between the two variables that is statistically significant. The data analysed by a two-way chi-square are arranged in a contingency table, which shows the frequency counts (the observed frequencies) for a number of categories. Such a contingency table is shown in Table 25.4.

TABLE 25.4   Number of female and male participants in each response category

	YES	NO
Females	55	45
Males	38	62

The table summarises participants' responses to two of a number of questions on a (hypothetical) survey. The first question asked participants to specify their gender. Responses were recorded using a nominal scale, which had two points: male and female. The second question asked participants whether they had visited a general practitioner (GP) in the preceding six months. Again responses were recorded using a nominal scale with the points yes and no. On the basis of their responses, participants were classified into one of four categories. The table shows that there does appear to be some degree of association between the variable Gender and the variable GP Visits. Thus more females say yes than no, while more males say no than yes. In other words, more females than males report having visited a GP. As there are two variables and the data are nominal in type, a two-way chi-square test is appropriate.

The two-way chi-square test compares the observed frequencies for the categories with the expected (on the basis of chance) frequencies for these categories. It is conducted by calculating a value of the chi-square statistic, which stands for the effect (the association between the two variables). The probability of obtaining the calculated value of chi-square (and therefore the effect) by chance, with the applicable degrees of freedom,[3] is then determined. If this probability is equal to or less than the alpha level set for the test, then the chi square value (and therefore the effect) is statistically significant. If the probability is greater than the alpha level, then the chi-square value (and therefore the effect) is not statistically significant.

For the data summarised in Table 25.4, the calculated value of chi-square is 5.81. With 1 df, the probability of getting this chi-square value by chance is 0.016. As this probability is lower than the alpha level (0.05) set for the test, this chi-square value, and therefore the effect (the association between gender and GP visits), is deemed to be statistically significant. Thus it can be concluded that there is a statistically significant difference between males and females in GP visits, such that more females than males reported having visited a GP in the preceding six months.

For designs where the two-way chi-square test applies, it is possible for each variable to have any number of levels (points on the scale/categories). Hence a contingency table can have an unlimited number of both rows and columns. In practice, however, there are limits on these numbers. This is partly because a prerequisite for the use of the chi-square test is that no more than 50 per cent of the expected frequencies can be less than five. As the expected frequencies are based on the observed frequencies, this essentially limits the number of categories. A multivariate analysis (based on chi-square) can be used to examine associations between three or more variables. This procedure (multi-way frequency analysis) is yet to come into common use in health research. Discussion of this analysis is provided by Tabachnick and Fidell (2012).

STOP AND THINK

Some of the other questions on the hypothetical survey (referred to above in the context of chi-square) were about participants' age and their opinions about the health care system. One question asked participants about their age in terms of which of two categories they fitted into: under forty years of age/forty years of age and over. Another question asked about whether the health care system generally met their health-related needs.

In the paper that reports the survey, one of the research questions being addressed is expressed as follows: Is there a difference between the two age groups in terms of their opinion about the health care system (i.e. whether they think the health care system generally meets their health-related needs). The outcome of a chi-square test is also reported; it is stated that the chi-square value is statistically significant and that there is therefore an association between age and opinion.

Given the way the research question was phrased, how can this description of the outcome of the chi-square test serve to answer it?

Correlation coefficents

Correlation coefficients summarise the degree of relationship (correlation) between variables. In the case of bivariate correlation, these variables correspond to two sets of values or scores for one group of participants. The value of a correlation coefficient ranges from +1 (a perfect positive correlation), through 0 (no correlation), to –1 (a perfect negative correlation). There are a number of correlation coefficients, two of which are commonly encountered in health research.

Correlation coefficents: These are used to summarise the degree of relationship (correlation) between variables.

Jane Pierson

These are the Pearson correlation coefficient and the Spearman correlation coefficient. The former is used when data (for both variables) are interval or ratio. The latter is a non-parametric statistic that is used when the data are ordinal or where one variable is ordinal scale and one is interval or ratio (in which case, the higher-level scale is reduced to an ordinal scale). While these correlation coefficients are descriptive statistics, they can also function as inferential statistics (i.e. as statistical tests, effectively), as it is possible to establish the probability of obtaining the value of the coefficient by chance. It is therefore possible to decide if the effect that the coefficient summarises (the correlation between the two variables) is statistically significant (real) or due to chance. As the use of the two coefficients for this purpose is essentially the same, only one example, using the Spearman coefficient, is given here.

The data shown in Table 25.5 are (hypothetical) data from a study that assessed basic life support (BLS) knowledge, and BLS performance, for a group of twelve health care professionals who had recently completed BLS training. Both knowledge and performance were measured on a 5-point scale, where 1 equated to very poor and 5 equated to very good. As there are two variables and the data are best characterised as ordinal, a Spearman correlation coefficient is the appropriate statistic. The table shows that there appears to be some degree of positive correlation between the two sets of scores. The calculated value of the Spearman correlation coefficient for these data is 0.45. When the number of participants, and therefore the number of pairs of scores (N), is twelve, the probability of getting this value by chance is 0.13. As this probability is higher than the applicable alpha level (0.05), this value of the correlation coefficient, and therefore the effect (the correlation), is deemed to be not statistically significant.

TABLE 25.5 Ratings of BLS knowledge and performance

BLS KNOWLEDGE	BLS PERFORMANCE
5, 4, 3, 4, 2, 3, 4, 2, 3, 3, 4, 3	4, 3, 3, 3, 1, 2, 2, 4, 3, 2, 4, 2

Multiple regression

Multiple regression
analysis: A multivariate
procedure that assesses
the degree to which scores
for a subset of variables
predict scores for another
variable in the set.

A **multiple regression analysis** is a multivariate procedure that can be used when there are three or more variables and the data are interval or ratio. It assesses the degree to which scores for a subset of these variables predict scores for another variable in the set. The degree of predictability is related to the degree of correlation between the predicted variable and its predictor variables. For example, measures could be made, for a group of participants, of blood cholesterol level, blood sugar level and level of physical activity. The degree to which scores on these variables predict scores on a measure of BMI could be assessed using a multiple regression analysis. Multiple regression, and associated procedures such as logistic regression, where the predicted variable is nominal or categorical, are being used increasingly in health research. An example of a categorical variable in this context would be diabetic/not diabetic. While these procedures are beyond the scope of this chapter, discussion is provided in a number of texts (e.g. Grove 2007; Tabachnick & Fidell 2012).

BODY IMAGE IN CHILDREN

Fernanda Nava, in collaboration with Paul O'Halloran and Jane Pierson, has recently completed a study of body image in children, and its relationship with participation in various types of sports. With regard to body image in children *per se*, one of the aspects that was investigated was desire for muscularity. Boys and girls who participated in the study were asked a number of questions pertaining to muscularity, including whether they would like to have bigger muscles. Children answered the question 'Would you like to have bigger muscles?' by selecting one of the following answers: 'No, not at all', 'No, not much', 'Yes, a little', 'Yes, a lot'. One of the research questions, with regard to muscularity, was about whether there was a relationship between age and desire to be more muscular. As this was a correlational design, and one of the variables (age) was ratio and the other variable (desire for muscularity) was ordinal, there were a number of ways of determining whether the relationship between the two variables was statistically significant. After considering these possibilities (some of which were outlined in the section on correlational designs), it was decided that the best course of action was to treat the four response choices to the question about muscularity as being a set of (ordinal) categories, and to treat age as a categorical variable, with each category corresponding to each of the age groups of the study participants (eight years old, nine years old, ten years old, eleven years old, and twelve/thirteen years old). A two-way chi-square test was then used to determine if there was a relationship (a statistically significant association) between age and desire for muscularity.

RESEARCH IN PRACTICE

Summary

This chapter has discussed a number of fundamental aspects of data analysis in quantitative research, in the context of health practice that is informed by research evidence. It has outlined the nature of statistical significance and its place in making decisions about whether evidence deriving from research studies should be used in practice. It has also described and explained the conduct of a number of statistical tests that are commonly encountered in health research and are used in determining if the outcome of a quantitative research study is statistically significant. These discussions should have given readers a better understanding of the purpose and nature of data analysis in quantitative research.

Practice exercises

1   The (hypothetical) study summarised in Table 25.6 examined the effect of alcohol consumption on video-game playing performance. Each of the participants played the video game under two conditions: sober, and under the influence.

Jane Pierson

TABLE 25.6   Mean number of points scored on the video game and standard deviation (in brackets) when participants were sober/under the influence

	SOBER	UNDER THE INFLUENCE
Number of points	932.50 (18.32)	921.92 (15.13)

(a) Describe the design of this study.

(b) What was measured in this study and what level of measurement was used?

(c) Which statistical test could be used to analyse these data?

2   The (hypothetical) study summarised in Table 25.7 examined the relationship between degree of overweight and blood cholesterol level.

TABLE 25.7   Body mass index (BMI) and blood cholesterol level

BMI	CHOLESTEROL LEVEL (MMOL/L)
30, 28, 25, 26, 32, 31, 29, 26, 27, 28, 29, 30	7.5, 6.5, 6.0, 6.5, 8.5, 7.5, 5.5, 5.5, 6.0, 7.0, 8.5

(a) Describe the design of this study.

(b) What was measured in this study and what level of measurement was used?

(c) What statistic could be used in the analysis of these data?

3   Locate a journal paper online, which reports a study in which ANOVA was used for data analysis.

(a) Describe the design of this study.

(b) What was measured in this study and what level of measurement was used?

(c) For one of the ANOVAs, what was/were the value/values of F? What were the associated degrees of freedom? What was/were the probability or probabilities of obtaining the result(s) by chance?

Notes

1   For an independent groups t-test, the degrees of freedom are equal to the number of participants in the first group plus the number of participants in the second group minus 2. For a related t-test, the degrees of freedom are equal to the number of participants minus 1.

2   There are two types of degrees of freedom associated with a value of F. The first is equal to the number of levels minus 1, and the second is equal to the total number of participants minus the number of levels (for an independent groups ANOVA).

3   For the two-way chi-square, the number of degrees of freedom is equal to the number of rows minus 1 multiplied by the number of columns minus 1.

Further reading

Elliot, A.C. & Woodward, W.A. (2006). *Statistical analysis quick reference and guide book with SPSS examples*. Thousand Oaks, CA: Sage.

Grove, S.K. (2007). *Statistics for health care research: a practical workbook*. Edinburgh: Elsevier Saunders.

Maxwell, S.E. & Delany, H.D. (2004). *Designing experiments and analysing data: a model comparison perspective*, 2nd edn. Mahwah, NJ.: Lawrence Erlbaum Associates.

Salkind, N.J. (2014). *100 questions (and answers) about statistics*. London: Sage.

Tabachnick, B.G. & Fidell, L.S. (2012). *Using multivariate statistics*, 6th edn. Boston: Pearson Education.

Websites

There are a number of websites that provide online calculators that can be used to conduct statistical tests, as well as providing information about these tests. Such websites can be found by typing the name of the test (e.g. t-test) into an internet search engine, and/or the name of the test plus the word 'calculator' into the search engine. Using the calculators to work out the statistics for some of the examples in this chapter, and/or creating a hypothetical data set and using a calculator to do the analysis, can be a good way of gaining further understanding of statistical procedures.

Jane Pierson

26

How to Read and Make Sense of Statistical Data

PAUL O'HALLORAN

Chapter objectives

In this chapter you will learn:

- to identify key issues when interpreting descriptive and inferential statistics
- to describe the differences between statistical and clinical significance
- to describe how clinical significance can be determined
- how to calculate effect size
- how to read results sections of quantitative research papers or mixed methods papers with confidence

Key terms

ANOVA

Clinical significance

Confidence intervals

Degrees of freedom

Descriptive statistics

Effect size

Inferential statistics

p value

Statistical significance

Types I and II statistical error

Introduction

I have been teaching research methods at undergraduate and postgraduate levels for over ten years. One of the biggest challenges students report when reading research papers is interpreting the results sections of quantitative research papers. Indeed, many students comment that they bypass the results section and go straight to the discussion section of a research paper. While you can often get the gist of the results in the opening paragraphs of the discussion, the problem with this approach is that the consumer (student, practitioner or other researcher) of the research article must assume that the researcher has interpreted the results without bias and correctly. Unfortunately, this is not always the case. As readers will discover in this chapter, even researchers can occasionally make errors when interpreting their results. The ability to interpret quantitative results is important even if you choose not to do any of your own research. As a practitioner, you will need to be able to read research papers for information regarding the latest techniques and so on, and be able to make some preliminary distinctions between good and poor research papers.

The main purpose of this chapter is to provide foundation knowledge and skills for you to be able to read and interpret statistical data, whether it be your own that you obtained in a small research project or, more typically, what you are reading in refereed research articles.

Where to begin

Students often comment that when reading a results section of a research article they become overwhelmed by the mass of figures, whether these are in a table, in text, in a graph or some other pictorial representation of the data. One of the first questions students ask is, 'Where do I begin?' One of the best places to begin when reading quantitative data is with the summary or **descriptive statistics**.

Reading and interpreting descriptive statistics

Descriptive statistics include measures of central tendency such as means, median (50th percentile) or mode (most frequently occurring score) (see Chapter 25). However, these figures are difficult to interpret unless we also have some measure of dispersion, such as variance, standard deviation or semi inter-quartile range. These measures of dispersion give the reader an indication of how much variation there is in scores. In other words, they provide an indicator of how representative or reliable the mean or median is. The following is a data set from my own study, which examined the effect of a walking program on mood in persons with type 2 diabetes (O'Halloran 2007).

Interpreting descriptive statistics: an example

Type 2 diabetes and mood study

Background to the study: Physical activity plays an important role in the management of type 2 diabetes, yet people with type 2 diabetes are less active than the general population (Dunstan

Descriptive statistics: These include measures of central tendency such as means, median (50th percentile) or mode (most frequently occurring score), and measures of dispersion (e.g. the standard deviation and the range).

Paul O'Halloran

et al. 2002). One of the challenges when working with people with type 2 diabetes is to have people make long-term changes to their physical activity patterns. It has been suggested that how individuals feel immediately after a bout of physical activity can affect the likelihood of maintaining involvement in the activity (Biddle *et al.* 2000). My study determined whether sessions of walking led to improvements in mood in persons with type 2 diabetes. Specifically, using the Subjective Exercise Experience Scale (SEES: McAuley & Courneya 1994), the mood of twenty-four previously sedentary people with type 2 diabetes was measured before and after twenty- and forty-minute bouts of group walking. The data that relate to the Positive Well-being scale of the SEES are presented in Table 26.1.

TABLE 26.1   Pre- and post-exercise Positive Well-being scores: means, standard deviations and effect sizes

SEES SUBSCALE	PRE-EXERCISE		POST-EXERCISE		
	M	SD	M	SD	d*
Positive Well-being					
20-minute walk	17.7	5.2	21.8	5.1	0.79
40-minute walk	18.4	5.8	22.1	5.4	0.67

*Effect sizes were calculated by subtracting mean scores at the post-exercise assessment from the pre-exercise mean then dividing this by the pooled standard deviation.

The table shows a number of figures in columns under the symbol headings *M, SD* and *d*. Often, one of the first things that students become confused by is the symbols that are used by researchers. Table 26.2 shows some commonly used statistical symbols.

TABLE 26.2   Statistical symbols

NAME	SYMBOL (EXAMPLES)	DEFINITION
Mean	M	The arithmetic mean
Median	MD	The point that cuts the distribution in half
Mode	Mode	The most common value
Variance	s2	Squared average amount of variability around the mean
Standard deviation	sd, s, SD	Average amount of variability around the mean
Effect size	ES, d, r, q, g, w, f, f2	A measure of change or association that is independent of sample size
Correlation coefficients	r	Measures the degree of relationship between two variables

NAME	SYMBOL (EXAMPLES)	DEFINITION
Confidence interval	CI	An expected range in which the population value will be found at a given level of probability
t-test	t	Compares differences between two means
ANOVA	F	Compares differences between three or more means
Regression	R2	The prediction of the relationship between two or more variables
chi-square	x2	Measure of association when categorical data are used

M is one of the symbols that is used for mean, SD is used to represent standard deviation and d for Cohen's (1992) effect size. We will be referring to effect size a little later when we discuss key considerations when interpreting inferential statistics.

From Table 26.1, we can ascertain that the mean for Positive Well-being was $M = 17.7$ before the twenty-minute walk and $M = 21.8$ after the walk. In order to obtain a sense of the meaning of these figures, it is important to have some understanding of the scale on which they were measured. The measures section of the paper (O'Halloran 2007) shows that people rated their moods on the SEES on a 7-point scale (1 = not at all, 7 = very much so) and, since each mood subscale has four items, the minimum score must be 4 and the maximum 28. Thus higher scores are indicative of a more positive mood. A score of around 18 on the Positive Well-being scale before exercise would suggest that people were feeling relatively positive before exercise. That people scored 21.8 after exercise indicated that they were feeling even better after exercise. However, we cannot confidently reach conclusions about data on the basis of descriptive statistics alone. This requires reference to inferential statistics (discussed later). Once these steps have been followed, the next thing to examine is the standard deviation or average amount of variation around the mean.

As can be seen in Table 26.1, the standard deviation for the twenty-minute walk on the Positive Well-being scale was $sd = 5.2$ before exercise and $sd = 5.1$ after exercise. This suggests that scores varied on average about 5 from the means. Given this value relative to the means of 17.7 and 21.8, the standard deviation suggests a relatively small amount of variation between scores and that the mean may be representative of scores at each assessment. Had the standard deviation been around the 15–20 mark rather than 5, these conclusions would have been less certain. Students often ask, 'When should I worry about the size of the standard deviation?' There is no definitive answer, but common sense is often a useful guide (e.g. how large it is relative to the mean, and what this degree of variation indicates given the scale used to measure the variable of interest).

Paul O'Halloran

Confidence intervals

Confidence interval: An
important indicator of the
representativeness of the
mean, particularly with
respect to a population.

Inferential statistics: These
include a variety of
procedures that are
commonly referred to as
'statistical tests'.

A further important indicator of the representativeness of the mean, particularly with respect to a population, is that of **confidence intervals**. Whenever a mean is calculated using a sample, there is always going to be a degree of error. One way of ascertaining the amount of error is to calculate the confidence interval of the mean. Although confidence intervals are actually an **inferential statistic**, they will be discussed here because they provide one of the best indicators of the representativeness of the mean. A common practice for researchers is to calculate the 95 or 99 per cent confidence intervals for reported means (Edwards 2008). The 95 per cent confidence interval, for example, enables us to conclude that we are 95 per cent certain that the true population mean lies between two values.

Returning to the type 2 diabetes and mood study (O'Halloran 2007), if the 95 per cent confidence intervals for the Positive Well-being scale means for the twenty minutes of walking were calculated, it would appear in text as follows: for the Pre-exercise mean ($M = 17.7$, 95% CI 15.6–19.9) and for the Post-exercise mean ($M = 21.8$, 95% CI 19.6–23.9). The way that this would be interpreted is that we are 95 per cent certain that the true population mean of the Positive Well-being scale before exercise for people with type 2 diabetes lies somewhere between 15.6 and 19.9 and after exercise it lies somewhere between 19.6 and 23.9.

The narrower the range in these values, the more representative the mean. Conversely, a wide range in these values suggests that the sample mean does not give a useful guide to the population value. The relatively small range of values reported above suggests that the mean values of 17.7 before exercise and 21.8 after exercise are fairly good representations of the true population value. For further information on confidence intervals and how to calculate and interpret them, see Polgar and Thomas (2013) or Edwards (2008).

Where does that leave us? Making sense of descriptive statistics in the type 2 diabetes and mood study

The case study above examined descriptive statistics relating to a measure of Positive Well-being in persons with type 2 diabetes before and after a twenty-minute session of group walking. Reference to the mean values and standard deviations in the summary table (Table 26.1), in conjunction with an understanding of what the scores represent, suggested that people scored fairly high on Positive Well-being before exercise and even higher after exercise (although we could not yet determine if this was statistically significant). Further, we were able to conclude that variation among the mean scores was small to moderate at both assessment points, and the calculation of confidence intervals enabled us to determine that these mean scores were a reasonable indicator of population values. Our next key question is, are the differences between these mean scores before and after exercise 'real' or did they occur by chance? This determination requires inferential statistics.

STEPS FOR READING/MAKING SENSE OF DESCRIPTIVE STATISTICS

1   Go to the summary table or figure.

2   Examine measures of central tendency (e.g. means, medians).

3   Examine the method section for a description of the measure/questionnaire etc., to understand what the scores represent.

4   Examine measures of dispersion (e.g. variance, standard deviation).

5   Look for confidence intervals.

Reading and interpreting inferential statistics

While descriptive statistics provide a useful starting point for reading and interpreting quantitative statistics, they tell only part of the story. They provide a preliminary overview of what was found in a particular study and might give some clues about the effect of a treatment or intervention or the relevance of associations between factors in health settings. But descriptive statistics alone are not sufficient for reaching valid conclusions about what seem to be meaningful associations or treatment effects. This is because whenever you use a sample to make inferences about what is happening in a population (generally the essence of quantitative research), there is going to be some error involved with issues such as sampling and the measurement of the variable of interest. For example, in the type 2 diabetes and mood study discussed above, although the mean mood scores were based on twenty-four people with type 2 diabetes, the aim is to make inferences relating to the wider population of previously sedentary persons with type 2 diabetes. In other words, we aim to generalise our findings to the wider population of persons with type 2 diabetes. However, there would have been a degree of error involved in activities in the study, such as the measurement of mood. Thus there are two major potential interpretations for the increase in Positive Well-being scores from before the twenty-minute walk (M = 17.1) to after the walk (M = 21.8). One interpretation is that the walk seemed to have some positive influence on mood in these people, the other is that the means differed due to chance. Inferential statistics enable us to determine which of these explanations is more probable or likely to be correct (see Chapter 25).

STOP AND THINK

In what ways are descriptive statistics useful for understanding the outcomes of a study?

What are the most useful descriptive statistics to examine when attempting to obtain the general outcomes of the study? Consult a research paper on a topic of your interest and look for these statistics.

What are some of the potential limitations of descriptive statistics?

Paul O'Halloran

Interpreting outcomes from inferential tests

As discussed in Chapter 25, there are a host of inferential tests such as t-tests, chi-square, ANOVA and so on that can be used to determine the probability of an outcome being due to chance. The appropriateness of these tests will be determined by questions such as the number of groups, type of data, and the studies of particular research question(s) (Polgar & Thomas 2013). However, all inferential tests produce a common value that is crucial in the interpretation of findings, the **p value**. This *p* value is the first thing to examine when reading inferential statistics, because it represents the probability of the 'null hypothesis' being true. That is, the probability of no treatment effect (i.e. no effect of exercise on mood in persons with type 2 diabetes) or no association between two variables (e.g. the consumption of green leafy vegetables and colon cancer). The way that this hypothesis-testing works is that if the probability of there being no treatment effect or no association is low enough, this suggests that there must indeed be a treatment effect or association. While this sounds a little convoluted, mathematically you can only assess the probability of a null effect (e.g. no difference between means or treatment effects), not the probability of a treatment effect being true. If this *p* value is equal to or below a predetermined value (the alpha level, α) set by researchers before the study, we say that the finding is statistically significant. If the *p* value exceeds this predetermined value, we say that the finding is not **statistically significant**. This predetermined alpha level is most typically set at 0.05 or 0.01 (Cowles & Davis 1982). If an alpha level of $\alpha = 0.05$ is set, it means that for something to be considered statistically significant the probability of it being due to chance must be equal to or below 5 in 100. If an alpha level of $\alpha = 0.01$ is set, it means that for something to be considered statistically significant the probability of it being due to chance must be equal to or below 1 in 100.

Interpreting inferential statistics: the type 2 diabetes and mood study

We will examine this in relation to data from the type 2 diabetes and mood study (O'Halloran 2007). To determine whether walking had an effect on mood in these people, a form of **ANOVA** (see Chapter 25) was calculated that enabled the researcher to compare two different levels of a variable or factor (in this case, duration of the walks) across time. This two-way repeated-measures ANOVA is able to examine if there are differences over time (from the pre-exercise assessment of mood to that following exercise), duration (do average means during the twenty-minute walk differ from those in the forty-minute walk?), or between different walk durations (the interaction effect that examines if the pattern of change in mood differs between the twenty- and forty-minute walks). This analysis produced a single significant finding in relation to Positive Well-being. Specifically, there was a significant time effect for Positive Well-being. If you look at the Positive Well-being means in Table 26.1, average scores were higher at the post-exercise assessments than they were prior to exercise for both the twenty-and forty-minute walks. This was reported as follows ($F(1,23) = 25.61$, $p = 0.000$). There are several important pieces of information within these brackets, which are discussed next.

How to make sense of reported inferential statistics: a step-by-step approach

The following example relates to a form of ANOVA, but the principles hold true regardless of whether you are reading statistical output from a t-test, correlation coefficient, chi-square or multiple regression (see Chapter 25). There will always be at least three sets of values: a test statistic (in this case $F = 25.61$), some figures in parentheses known as degrees of freedom (in this case $(1,23)$) and a p value, which is the probability of the null hypothesis being true (in this case $p = 0.000$). The meaning of each of these values and how to interpret them further is outlined below.

Step 1: Look at the p value

The thing that most people will examine first is the p value, which indicates the probability of the null hypothesis being true. While the p was $= 0.000$ in the type 2 diabetes study, it does not indicate that we can be 100 per cent certain that the null hypothesis is false. This can never be the case in inferential statistics. There is always going to be some probability of the null hypothesis being true. What it does suggest is that the probability of the null hypothesis being true in this example was less than 1 in 1000. It is convention to report to two or three decimal places, so it may have been $p = 0.00001$ and then rounded to $p = 0.000$. Therefore in this case, the p value indicates that there was a very low probability of there being no difference between means at the pre-exercise assessment and those at the post-exercise assessment (the 'null hypothesis' being true). In other words, the probability was so low, well below the predetermined level set by the researcher ($\alpha = 0.05$), that the finding would be deemed statistically significant. We would therefore conclude that there must be a difference in means between these time-points. It is worth noting that since most statistical tests are calculated using computer programs, exact probabilities are typically reported. But in some research articles, instead of the statistic been reported as $(F(1,23) = 25.61, p = 0.000)$, you may see $(F(1,23) = 25.61, p < .05)$ or $(F(1,23) = 25.61, p < .01)$. In all cases, this clearly indicates that the result was statistically significant.

What if instead of being $(F(1,23) = 25.61, p = 0.000)$, it was $(F(1,23) = 2.61, p = 0.08)$? This would suggest that the probability of there being no difference between means is now 8 in 100. This is higher than most alpha levels set by researchers, and had this been the case we would have concluded that there was no difference between Positive Well-being means before and after exercise. The finding would have been considered not statistically significant.

Step 2: Examine test values and degrees of freedom

In addition to examining the p value, it is also important to look at the specific value produced by the test such as $F = 25.61$ in the example above or $t = 8.91$ in the case of a t-test or $r = 0.7$ in the case of a correlation coefficient. These values refer to different things in different tests, and it is important to have an understanding of what the test is actually calculating (see Chapter 25). At a basic level, typically the larger the value the stronger the effect, whether that be a treatment effect as reflected by differences in means or an association or correlation between variables such as number of physiotherapy sessions attended and flexibility in a knee joint during rehabilitation. In the example above, an F of 25.61 is large. This can be determined by looking at an F table in most books on quantitative statistics (Schwartz & Polgar 2003).

Degrees of freedom are the values reported in the parentheses or brackets before the test value. In the above example, these degrees of freedom were (1,23). The precise meaning of degrees of freedom will vary across different tests. For some tests, such as Pearsons correlation coefficient, there will be only one value in these brackets (e.g. r (41) = 0.7); for others, such as an ANOVA, there will be two. In all cases, these degrees of freedom refer in some way to the number of scores in a sample that are free to vary. Larger degrees of freedom are typically reflective of larger sample sizes.[1]

Degrees of freedom: Values that represent the number of scores that are free to vary associated with a test statistic. Used to calculate the statistical significance of a test statistic.

STOP AND THINK

- What does the p value mean?
- If a correlation between physical activity and mental health was $r = 0.5$, $p = 0.02$, what would be an appropriate conclusion to make about this finding?
- What impact does sample size have on statistical significance?

How to interpret findings that are statistically significant

So far we have looked at an example of how to read and interpret inferential statistics as they relate to whether a finding is statistically significant or not. But it does not end there. There can be a number of potential explanations for results that are statistically significant. These are outlined below.

The finding was *not* due to chance and it was meaningful

In most cases, this is the ideal scenario for researchers—this type of finding is clearly interpretable. Not only is the finding unlikely to be due to chance but it also has some 'real' meaning. This begs the question of how we determine if a finding has some real meaning. There are several indicators of determining whether a finding may be meaningful as well as statistically significant. One is to examine the **effect size** of a statistic, if reported. Effect size, which can be measured in various ways and depends on the particular statistical test that was undertaken (Cohen 1992), is a measure of the strength of a finding (whether that is a difference between means or relationships between factors) that is independent of sample size. Such a measure is important because the size of a sample plays a substantial role in determining whether a finding is statistically significant or not. For instance, if there

Effect size: A measure of the strength of a finding that is independent of sample size.

are hundreds or thousands of people in a sample, the study has so much power to detect findings that even very minor differences or relationships can be deemed statistically significant.

For example, a study asked a sample of more than 350 students whether they thought it was acceptable for a therapist to tell a client's partner that the client was HIV-positive, even if it meant going against the client's wishes (Collins & Knowles 1995). The researchers asked female (n = 164) and male students (n = 203) to rate this on a 5-point scale from 1 (strongly agree/always) to 5 (strongly disagree/never). Results showed a significant difference ($F(1) = 17.51$, $p < .001$) between the mean for females ($M = 2.71$) and that for males ($M = 2.11$). However, since it seems that both females and males were undecided on this issue and that scores only differed by 0.6 on a 5-point scale, it would be difficult to argue that the results were meaningful. The researchers in this study would have been well advised to calculate an effect size, or a measure of the differences between these means that did not take sample size into account. The appropriate effect size statistic for comparing two means is Cohen's (1992) equation:

$$d = MA - MB\ \sigma$$

With this measure of effect size, one mean is subtracted from the other, divided by the standard deviation (the standard of the comparison group is often used, or the average standard deviation of the two groups). Sample size is not included in this calculation. Once this has been calculated, this value can be compared to criteria that Cohen (1992) developed for interpreting the magnitude of an effect or finding. According to Cohen, a small effect is defined as $d = 0.20$, a medium effect as $d = 0.50$, and a large effect as $d = 0.80$. Examination of the data in Table 26.1 shows that the effects for differences between pre- and post-exercise Positive Well-being means in the twenty-minute ($d = 0.79$) and forty-minute ($d = 0.67$) walks were in the medium to large range. This would be one indicator that, as well as being statistically significant, these results are also likely to be meaningful.

Another very useful indicator of whether statistical findings are meaningful is **clinical significance**, which is the practical or applied value of a finding or sets of findings (Kazdin 2015). As such, there are no precise calculations for determining if something is clinically significant. Rather, according to Kazdin (2015), clinical significance can be gauged by factors such as those below.

Clinical significance: The practical or applied value of a finding or sets of findings.

- Amount of change as a result of an intervention (can be determined by effect size, or if clients or patients are no longer experiencing problems or symptoms). For example, a patient is no longer experiencing the symptoms of depression.

- Subjective evaluations from a client or patient regarding the effects of a factor or intervention. That is, do participants from a study report noticeable differences in how they are feeling or functioning, and are these differences noticed by significant others in the person's life? For example, a patient's wife might comment on his improvement in activity levels and general well-being.

- Social impact. That is, can the information from the study or a new treatment or intervention have a measurable impact on things such as rates of an illness, days missed at work, or days of hospitalisation? For example, evaluating the effect of a stress management program conducted in a workplace setting on rates of absenteeism.

- Comparison. The client or patient is compared with the performance of others such as a normative sample or a patient group. For example, if a physiotherapist developed a new intervention for assisting patients to rehabilitate following a hip replacement, it would be useful to examine not only if there has been a significant improvement in this group's quality of life or some measure of disability but also how these people compare with normative samples on these measures.

The finding was *not* due to chance but it was *not* meaningful

As noted above, findings can occasionally be statistically significant without necessarily being meaningful. That is, the findings are unlikely to be due to chance but they also have little practical significance or meaning. This can occur with particularly large sample sizes.[2] This was illustrated above in the study by Collins and Knowles (1995), where relatively minute mean differences in the responses of males and females were found to be statistically significant. There are also cases where a correlation coefficient can be as low as r = 0.2 yet still be significant if the sample size is large enough. The key, as suggested above, is to give an indicator of the meaningfulness of a result, such as effect size or clinical significance. When reading statistical findings, it is therefore useful to check whether the investigator has provided a measure of effect size or an indicator of clinical significance. Even if they have not, by referring to the factors that are indicators of clinical significance (Kazdin 2015) you can often get a sense of this. For example, applying these clinical significance criteria to findings in Collins and Knowles' study, it would be fair to conclude that while the gender difference in opinions about disclosing information on HIV status is indeed significant there is little practical or applied value in a difference so small.

The finding was due to chance—an error was made

By its nature, statistical testing is probabilistic—there is always going to be some probability that a mistake has been made. We can, for example, mistakenly conclude that something was statistically significant when this was not the case. This is termed a **Type I error**. The maximum probability of making such an error is equal to the alpha level in the study. If the researcher selected an alpha level of 0.05, they will mistakenly conclude that a finding is significant a maximum of 5 times in 100. This is why some researchers adopt a more conservative alpha level, such as 0.01. This means that the probability of a researcher mistakenly concluding that a result is significant will be 1 in 100. You might wonder why researchers do not always go with a more conservative alpha level, such as 0.01. The reason is that the lower the alpha level, the greater the chance of incorrectly concluding a result to be non-significant. This is termed a **Type II error** and is discussed next (see also Chapter 15).

Type I statistical errors: These occur when researchers mistakenly conclude that a finding was statistically significant when it may be a result of chance rather than being a real difference.

Type II statistical errors: These occur when, although there may have been a clinically important effect, the trial did not have a large enough sample size to detect it statistically.

We can summarise this by saying there are two key steps in interpreting findings that are statistically significant.

> **STEPS FOR INTERPRETING FINDINGS THAT ARE STATISTICALLY SIGNIFICANT**
>
> 1   Ask how likely it is that the result was due to chance. In other words, what is the probability that we have made a mistake (i.e. Type I error)? This can be determined by examining the p value. Look for confidence intervals.
>
> 2   Determine if the finding was meaningful. This can be determined in several ways, for example examining factors such as the effect size (Cohen 1992), if reported, and looking at indicators of clinical significance.

How to interpret findings that are not statistically significant

Just as there are several explanations for findings that are statistically significant, there is more than one explanation for findings that are not deemed statistically significant. These are outlined below.

The finding was due to chance and was *not* meaningful

This type of finding is generally clearly interpretable. In the diabetes study discussed earlier, as well as examining the effect of walking on positive mood (Positive Well-being), Psychological Distress was measured before and after the twenty- and forty-minute walks. This information is presented in Table 26.3.

TABLE 26.3   Pre- and post-exercise Psychological Distress scores: means, standard deviations and effect sizes

SEES SUBSCALE	PRE-EXERCISE		POST-EXERCISE		
	M	SD	M	SD	d*
Psychological Distress					
20-minute walk	7.0	4.4	6.1	3.7	−0.22
40-minute walk	7.1	3.7	7.0	4.0	−0.01

*Effect sizes were calculated by subtracting mean scores at the post-exercise assessment from the pre-exercise mean then dividing this by the pooled standard deviation.

Paul O'Halloran

As can be seen in Table 26.3, there is very little difference between pre-exercise and post-exercise means for both the twenty- and forty-minute walks. In contrast to the findings regarding Positive Well-being, there was no significant effect for time for Psychological Distress ($F(1,23) = 0.89$, $p = 0.355$). Reference to the table shows that the effect size was $d = -0.22$ for the twenty-minute walk and $d = -0.01$ for the forty-minute walk. Reference to the criteria supplied by Cohen (1992) suggests the differences between pre- and post-exercise Psychological Distress means were small to very small. By considering these results, you could clearly conclude that the study showed that walking did not seem to influence Psychological Distress.

The finding was due to chance but possibly meaningful

Suppose, however, that the effect sizes for Psychological Distress had been $d = 0.5$ to $d = 0.8$ and above. This finding would have been more difficult to interpret as these effect sizes would be indicators of medium to large differences (Cohen 1992). Had this been the case, the correct interpretation would have been that this finding, while seemingly due to chance, is nevertheless potentially meaningful. This can occur quite often, particularly when sample sizes are relatively small, which reduces the probability of being able to detect a true difference (the test has low power). Therefore it is always worth considering the possibility that non-significant findings could potentially be meaningful. In order to rule this possibility out, it is sensible to examine information such as the effect size for the result and other potential indicators of clinical significance, such as whether participants with a physical condition are no longer troubled by symptoms after a treatment or whether their scores on a measure following a treatment place them within a 'normal range'. Another example where you need to be careful in interpreting a non-significant result is where a correlation appears moderate to large (e.g. $r = 0.5$ or more) yet not significant. This can also occur when the sample size is low. Once you have examined these indicators of clinical significance, you are able to make an interpretation with some confidence one way or another.

The finding was not due to chance—an error was made

As with findings that are statistically significant, it is also possible to make an error when a non-significant result is produced in a study. This is a Type II error, where the researcher mistakenly concludes that there was no difference, no association and so on. This is more likely to occur when sample sizes are low and/or a stringent alpha level has been adopted ($\alpha < 0.01$). For instance, in some studies alpha levels of 0.008 or less can be adopted, particularly when researchers are trying to account for multiple comparisons in their study. Such situations reduce the power of the study, making it more difficult to correctly identify a true difference or relationship. A further useful indicator of whether a Type II error has occurred is if the effect size of the statistic is in the medium to high range (Cohen 1992).

We can summarise this by saying there are two key steps in interpreting findings that are not statistically significant.

**STEPS FOR INTERPRETING FINDINGS THAT ARE
NOT STATISTICALLY SIGNIFICANT**

1   Determine if the finding was meaningful. This can be determined by examining factors such as the effect size (Cohen 1992) and certainly by looking at indicators of clinical significance (Kazdin 2015).

2   Determine if a Type II error may have occurred. Examine the sample size in the study and see if the alpha level set by the researchers was low.

Simple decision rules for making sense of inferential statistics

Before the last twenty years or so, interpreting statistical tests was as simple as examining the probability levels and ensuring that a Type I error had not occurred (Schmidt 1996). If a finding was statistically significant, it was interpreted as meaningful; if not significant, the assumption was made that no effect was present. However, as can be ascertained from the discussion above, there has been a shift to recognising that interpretation of quantitative data cannot rely on the outcome of inferential statistics in isolation (Cohen 1992; Schmidt 1996; Kazdin 2015). Indeed, there are several considerations that need to be taken into account when interpreting the outcome of inferential statistics. These include the size of the effect, potential errors in statistical decision-making, the influence of sample size and alpha levels on the power to detect differences, and indicators of clinical significance. These considerations can lead a consumer of quantitative data to feel somewhat confused about how this can all fit together, particularly how statistical and clinical significance influence our interpretations of data. One way of simplifying this is to create some simple decision rules for combining statistical and clinical significance to reach an overall conclusion regarding a result. These are given in Table 26.4.

Using the information in this table, we would conclude that the findings regarding the effect of Positive Well-being and Psychological Distress in the type 2 diabetes and mood study could both be interpreted clearly. For Positive Well-being, both the twenty- and forty-minute walks resulted in significant improvements on this measure and the size of the effects suggested that these improvements could also be clinically significant. Further, there was consistency between statistical and clinical significance in relation to the effect that walking had on Psychological Distress. In both cases, neither seemed to be significant (p was > 0.05 and the effect sizes were small). On the other hand, in the Colin and Knowles (1995) study, where the difference between males and females with respect to their views on confidentiality of information about HIV status was statistically significant yet seemingly minor in magnitude (unlikely to be clinically significant), we would conclude that results are inconclusive. The recommendation using the decision rules in Table 26.4 would be to suspend judgment about that finding until confirmation with further research.

Paul O'Halloran

TABLE 26.4   Simple decision rules for interpreting inferential statistics

		STATISTICAL SIGNIFICANCE	
		YES	NO
Clinical significance	YES	**Clear** Strong evidence for a treatment effect or finding	**Inconclusive** Suspend judgment There is a need for further research (e.g. with larger samples)
	NO	**Inconclusive** Suspend judgment Suggests findings may not be meaningful- need for further research	**Clear** Strong evidence for lack of a treatment effect or lack of relationship between factors

STOP AND THINK

- What does statistical significance tell us about a particular set of results?
- Consult a research paper of interest and examine how the researchers have interpreted statistically significant results. Does this fit with your interpretation?
- Why is statistical significance alone not enough when interpreting results?
- What does the concept of clinical significance add to our interpretation of results of a study?
- Perform a quick literature search, entering the name of a topic of interest and clinical significance as search terms and examine how the investigators have used this concept to interpret their findings.

Summary

The purpose of this chapter was to provide information to help you read and interpret statistical data. The best place to start is with the summary of a study or descriptive statistics. With descriptive statistics, it is recommended that, as a minimum, it is important to examine the measures of central tendency, such as the mean or median, in conjunction with measures of dispersal such as the standard deviation and confidence intervals if available. This examination is an indicator of how representative the mean or median is of what is happening in the sample and/or population. These descriptive statistics often provide an overall indicator of how data relate to a study's aims or research questions. For example, the descriptive statistics in the investigation of the effect of walking on mood in persons with type 2 diabetes revealed that walking for either twenty or forty minutes may have led to an improvement in Positive Well-being. But before we could draw such conclusions with any confidence, inferential statistics had to be examined to determine the probability that the findings were not due to chance. Through inspection of the *p* values from the statistical test that was used to examine the effect of walking on mood, we were able to conclude that it was very unlikely that the improvements in Positive Well-being were in fact due to chance. However, it was emphasised that statistical significance alone is not adequate to interpret results from statistical tests. It is crucial to consider whether findings have any practical or applied value. That is, the potential clinical significance of the findings must be examined. I have argued that it is only by examining statistical and clinical significance in conjunction that we can reach meaningful conclusions from statistical tests. The discussion concluded with a set of simple decision rules that combine statistical and clinical significance.

Practice exercises

1   When interpreting descriptive statistics, why is it important to examine measures of dispersal as well as the means or medians?

2   Why is it important to examine inferential statistics?

3   What does it mean when a researcher concludes that their findings were statistically significant?

4   What are some of the limitations of relying on statistical significance alone when interpreting statistical data?

5   What conclusions would you reach in interpreting the following sets of results?

   (a) A researcher found that the difference between a new and old treatment for rehabilitation from a hip replacement was significant. Patients who received the new treatment returned to their usual work and leisure activities substantially earlier than the group receiving the old treatment.

   (b) A researcher found that the correlation between sessions of treatment in a health setting and recovery time in 2000 patients was significant ($r(1999) = 0.3$, $p = 0.002$).

   (c) Researchers found that differences in two treatment groups wearing different orthoses in distance walked, as measured by pedometer, were not significant in a sample of sixteen people. They calculated an effect size on the number of steps taken by each group and found that $d = 0.91$.

Notes

1   This is true of statistical tests such as t-tests, correlation coefficients and outputs from an ANOVA such as interaction effects, where participant numbers feature in the calculations of the degrees of freedom etc. However, with some statistical tests such as chi-square, sample sizes are not used to compute the degrees of freedom (see Edwards 2008).

2   This is not to suggest that large sample sizes are a negative. On the contrary, the larger the sample size the better in terms of power and often in terms of generalisability.

Further reading

Edwards, T. (2008). *Research design and statistics: a bio-behavioural approach*. Boston: McGraw-Hill.

Gordon, R.A. (2010). *Applied statistics for the social and health sciences*. London: Routledge.

Grissom, R.J. & Kim, J.J. (2012). *Effect sizes for research: univariate and multivariate applications*. New York: Routledge.

Kazdin, A.E. (ed.) (2015). *Methodological issues and strategies in clinical research*, 4th edn. Washington, DC: American Psychological Association.

Pagano, R.R. (2012). *Understanding statistics in the behavioral sciences*, 10th edn. Belmont, CA: Cengage Learning US.

Terrell, S.R. (2012). *Statistics translated: a step-by-step guide to analyzing and interpreting data*. New York: Guilford Press.

Websites

www.statsoft.com/textbook/esc.html#What_is_"statistical_significance"_(p-level)

> For further explanation of significance testing.

www.sportsci.org/resource/stats/generalize.html#effect

> For discussion of confidence intervals.

www.indiana.edu/~stigtsts/quotsagn.html

> For discussion of limitations of significance testing.

Writing and Appraising Research Reports

PRANEE LIAMPUTTONG, NORA SHIELDS AND ANNEMARIE GALLICHIO

Chapter objectives

In this chapter you will learn:

- how to write up research papers
- about commonalities and differences in writing qualitative and quantitative papers
- suggested structures for writing a research paper
- how to critically appraise qualitative and quantitative published papers

Introduction

> Writing is an integral part of research. How you write about your research topic will shape the way you and others come to understand it (Gabriel 2013, p. 356).

Once we have conducted a good piece of research, what shall we do with our interesting and important findings? We need to put our information down on paper. We need to write about it so that our research findings can be disseminated and other people can read and make use of them, whether for improving current health and welfare practices or as the basis for developing new research projects. We also have an obligation to our participants, to make sure their contributions to our work reach as wide a target audience as possible.

It is essential to be able to critically appraise published materials arising out of research. This will help readers evaluate the evidence that they might need in their evidence-based practice. How do we know if the published material is rigorous and trustworthy enough?

The nature of qualitative research writing

> Writing is an ongoing and socially embedded practice. It is about 'textwork' … or the practice, art, and craft of writing (Marvasti 2008, p. 613).

Qualitative writing is different from quantitative writing. A quantitative report consists of a concise presentation of the methods and results of the study (Neuman 2011; Bryman 2016). Qualitative writing, on the other hand, 'must be a convincing argument systematically presenting data to support the researcher's case and to refute alternative explanations' (Morse 1994b, p. 231).

Unlike quantitative research, which usually presents statistical findings in the form of tables and summaries, qualitative research requires different ways of showing the accessibility and usability of its findings. Therefore, it is important that when composing qualitative research outcomes, the report is written in the language of the readership (Sandelowski & Leeman 2012). For this reason, writing that is based on qualitative research, be it a report, article or book, tends to be longer than quantitative writing. The written report must contain enough detail to tell readers about the research and its findings. There are several reasons for this (Neuman 2011; Gabriel 2013; Liamputtong 2013).

1   Qualitative data are more difficult to condense. Qualitative data contain words, not numbers, and include many quotes and extended case examples.

2   In a qualitative report, detailed descriptions of the research sites and the population under study need to be provided so that readers will have a better understanding of the research setting.

3   Qualitative researchers employ less standardised data collection methods, ways of developing analytical categories and modes of organising evidence. The methods chosen depend on the conditions of the research site and the researchers' preferences. Hence qualitative researchers need to explain what they did, and why, in greater detail.

4   The goals of qualitative studies are to explore new settings and construct new theories. Detailed descriptions of the development of new concepts, their relationships and the interpretations of evidence need to be provided. This adds to the length of the report.

5   The nature of qualitative data gives the writer freedom to use literary devices to maintain the readers' interest and accurately translate a meaning system for the readers. This, again, lengthens the paper.

There are three ways that we can write to present the results of our research (Neuman 2011; Liamputtong 2013). First, the findings are given without comments or interpretations; interpretations can be discussed later in the discussion section. Second, interpretations are used to make some connections between lines of evidence; again, further detail is provided in the discussion section. Finally, the results and discussion of each point may need to go together if an in-depth discussion is required to give meaning to the findings. However, because of the nature of qualitative research, which needs some interpretation to make the findings more meaningful, qualitative writing tends to include discussion throughout (as opposed to the specific 'Discussion' section in quantitative reports). This makes the report's organisational structure more critical for ensuring clarity. Writing a qualitative report therefore requires careful attention to structure and meaning. Writers need to make a special effort to achieve coherence and conciseness (Belgrave *et al.* 2002; Wolcott 2009; Neuman 2011; Liamputtong 2013).

In qualitative reports, the language is not as objective or formal as in quantitative papers. A writer usually uses the first person (I, we) in describing the research processes and in discussing the findings (Gabriel 2013; Bryman 2016). We can witness this style of writing in most qualitative papers in many journals such as *Qualitative Health Research*, *Qualitative Research*, *Sociology of Health and Illness*, *Qualitative Inquiry* and so on. Wolcott (2009) argues that since the researcher's role is an integral part of qualitative study, descriptive accounts need to be made in the first person. This is what Pranee Liamputtong tends to use in her qualitative research reports, whether these are a journal paper, report or book.

Like quantitative reports, qualitative reports also make use of graphic representations, such as pictures and diagrams. Very often, tables are used to describe the major background characteristics of the people under study, but the tables and graphics are used to supplement the discussion, not to replace it (Liamputtong 2013).

One important point we wish to make is that in reporting qualitative findings it is not essential to state the number of people who discuss a particular issue (Hennink *et al.* 2011; Liamputtong 2013). For example, when you write about the perceptions of infant feeding among Australian mothers, you will not say that four women believe breastfeeding is the best option for newborn infants. You will explain in detail about how these mothers, whatever the number, perceive breastfeeding. There may be a range of perceptions, but qualitative researchers do not indicate how many of the women participants have these perceptions. Some researchers who do not have a good understanding of the nature of qualitative research may demand that you do so. But we suggest that you should adhere to the practice of qualitative research when writing up a qualitative research piece.

Pranee Liamputtong, Nora Shields and Annemarie Gallichio

STOP AND THINK

Once upon a time, Pranee wrote an article which stemmed from her qualitative research regarding the mental health issues of ethnic communities living in Melbourne. She was told by her superior that the paper was full of 'flowery language' and that a table should be included. Pranee had used the first person 'I' in the paper, and was told that the first person should not be used in an 'academic' article.

Considering what has been discussed above, what is your opinion about this? Was Pranee correct in the way she wrote her qualitative paper or should she follow the advice given by her superior? What is your reason for your opinion?

The nature of quantitative research writing

Quantitative research writing often reflects the type of research it is describing: it is quite a standardised affair (Gabriel 2013; Bryman 2016). Here you are more likely to include tables of numerical data to describe participant characteristics, or to display your overall findings in graphic form. Quantitative research writing is usually written in the third person (Billig 2013), although many health-related journals are now encouraging authors to write in the first person, particularly when describing what methods they used and how they were applied. This is similar to how authors of qualitative research write their reports. Although there is a basic framework for presenting the results from any quantitative study, the fundamental point to remember is that you are telling a story to your reader. In this regard, quantitative research writing is comparable to qualitative research writing.

A major problem with many published reports on quantitative research (particularly clinical research reports) is that the methods used and the results found are often inadequately described (Zhang & Shaw 2012). This has implications for the readers. For example, if a report of a clinical trial does not tell you that the person employed to assess the participants did not know which group the participants were allocated to, you might not believe the results to the same extent as when the authors explicitly state this information. The reason you may not believe the outcomes is that an assessor who is not blind to group allocation is a potential source of bias to the results. So it is very important that you describe your research methods, providing as much detail as possible.

In a positive move to address poor reporting of clinical trials, various groups have taken the initiative of developing guidelines on how to write about this type of research. For example, the CONSORT Statement (see Chapter 15) is an evidence-based set of recommendations for reporting randomised controlled trials (RCTs) and offers a standard way for authors to prepare the reports of their research findings (Altman *et al.* 2001). Although the statement focuses on RCTs, many of its recommendations are relevant and applicable to all types of quantitative clinical research. The CONSORT group has also published a statement for clinical trials of non-pharmacological treatments (Boutron *et al.* 2008).

It is important when writing a quantitative research report for publication in a health journal to keep in mind who is likely to read your article. Health professionals generally read research reports because they want to be effective clinicians and offer their patients the most up-to-date treatment approaches and management strategies. Most clinicians read journal articles as part of their continued professional development—they are 'research consumers'. It can be easy for them to get lost in the technical jargon and statistical analysis of a research report. Writing about your research in a clear and transparent way helps those who read it to interpret it with greater ease.

You also need to think about why people might read your article. What most readers are interested in is how your work might endorse their approaches to practice or how it suggests ways for them to change their practice. So it is important, when writing a quantitative research report, that you discuss the implications of your statistical analysis for everyday clinical practice. If you want clinicians and health professionals to change their practice as a result of your research, you need to tell them in a simple and straightforward way how your analysis applies to them (see Chapter 25).

STOP AND THINK

What are the similarities between quantitative report writing and qualitative report writing? What are the differences? Think about the following aspects of the report in particular: describing the research design, reporting ethical issues, outlining the method of data analysis and presenting the results.

The structure of research writing: commonality and divergence

There are common structures that make the presentation of research findings clear and easy to follow:

1 title
2 abstract or summary
3 introduction
4 literature review and theory
5 research design and method
6 findings or results
7 discussion and conclusion
8 acknowledgments
9 references

Pranee Liamputtong, Nora Shields and Annemarie Gallichio

Title

The title should capture the essence of your text. Sometimes researchers may use a very interesting title to catch the attention of the audience. The CONSORT Statement recommends including the research design of the study in the title because this can help readers locate literature more quickly and easily.

Abstract or summary

This section is brief but needs to contain essential information about your paper. When readers read this section, they can immediately see what the paper is about, how you carried out the research and what are the main findings of the study. Structured abstracts are best for quantitative research. A structured abstract includes a series of subheadings (e.g. research design, participants, method, results, discussion and keywords), and generally the information included under each heading is standardised. Writing your abstract using a structured format helps readers find the information they need more easily (Hartley *et al.* 1996). In qualitative research, you will include essential parts such as we have presented earlier, but they do not need to be separated by subheadings, though subheadings may be required by particular journals that publish qualitative papers. You need to follow the guidelines of a journal if you wish to write your work for publication.

Introduction

The introduction explains the reasons why you did your research. It indicates the nature, importance and urgency of the research or the gap in knowledge that you are attempting to fill (Bryman 2016). The emphasis here is typically on relevant previous research. It also emphasises the situation and factors that prompted the proposed project. Evidence from a literature review or a systematic review should be used to explain the exact nature and extent of the health issue that has led to the development of your research. This section is important since it demonstrates how much you understand and how familiar you are with the literature. It also allows you to justify the need for your research in a strong and compelling way (see the CONSORT website).

At the end of your introduction you should list the specific aims and objectives of your research. These are the questions you want to answer in your study (Bryman 2016). For qualitative research, you need to provide your research questions or suppositions (Liamputtong 2013). For quantitative research, you should also include your hypotheses. These are more specific than your objectives and can be tested using statistical methods (see the CONSORT website; see also Chapter 2). Often, your objectives and hypotheses will be very similar.

Literature review and/or theory

It is common for a literature review to be included in this section (Bryman 2016). However, with the word limits of a particular journal, some papers may not present this section separately from the Introduction. Additionally, many researchers include in this section the theoretical framework they are using. This is to give readers enough detail about the theory or framework that was applied in the research. It must be noted that this theoretical framework may not be referred to by all researchers, and is more common among papers that make use of the qualitative approach (see Chapter 2).

Research design and method

This section discusses the design of the research and the method you employ. It generally contains subheadings such as participants, method, intervention, outcome measures, procedure, data analysis. For a qualitative piece, you will not include the intervention and outcome measures, but you will have to explain the need for the qualitative approach and give a discussion of rigour and trustworthiness (see Chapter 1). Often, too, you may need to discuss some ontological and epistemological positions of your research (see Chapter 1).

Every research study addresses an issue relevant to a particular population, or people with a particular health issue, concern or condition. The participants' section includes some description of the research participants, for example who they were and how they were selected. A description of the participants usually includes some of their socio-demographic characteristics such as age, sex, education level, employment and diagnosis. These eligibility criteria are particularly important in clinical research because they help readers know who the information will be relevant to or how generalisable the research findings are likely to be. How the participants were recruited (e.g. by referral or self-selection through advertising) should also be described. In qualitative research, you include some socio-demographic characteristics of the participants as indicated above.

The method section must outline the method used in the study and give some explanation of it. We cannot assume that readers will know what the method is, without some explanation. For example, if you use a focus group method for data collection, you must explain what a focus group is, what the method can offer you, and how it is usually conducted (see Chapter 5). Similarly, if you use a survey method, you will have to provide some discussion on what the method can offer and how it is generally used (see Chapter 13).

Some quantitative research studies investigate the effect of a particular intervention or treatment. If your study does, then you should fully describe the intervention that was implemented. Relevant details might include what the intervention is, what it does, the dose applied (intensity, frequency and duration), who administered it (what personnel, what training they had), any specific equipment used and where it took place (contextual factors). It is also important to give details about any control or placebo interventions. For example, if your control group was a usual care group, you need to describe what usual care is.

One of the key features of a quantitative research study is the outcome measures used; they are what determine whether an intervention was effective or, in a comparative study, if there is a difference between the groups of participants (see Chapter 11). A full description of the outcome measures includes information on the psychometric properties of the outcome measure (e.g. validity and reliability) relevant to the study participants, details of how the outcomes were measured, and steps taken to improve reliability (e.g. were multiple measures taken and the average calculated, or were the assessors trained to perform the assessments in a standard way). Most research studies employ several outcome measures, but the most important is the primary outcome measure. All other outcome measures are secondary outcome measures. The sample size calculation is usually based on data relating to the primary outcome measure. It is important to document if the participant and assessor were blind to group allocation, since this removes a potential source of bias. In health research, while it is often possible to employ an assessor who is blinded, it is not always possible to blind the participant or the health professional to the intervention.

In the procedure section you describe what happened during the study in time sequence. In qualitative research, you describe the process of data collection and how you went about doing your research. For example, if you selected a focus group method as your data collection tool, you would need to explain in detail how you actually used it. In quantitative research, you would describe when the outcome measures were assessed, particularly if they were assessed on more than one occasion. Other important aspects of the research design that should be mentioned are randomisation and concealment of group allocation.

The final part of your methods section is the data analysis component. In qualitative research, you need to explain what data analysis method you employed, for example, thematic or content analysis (see Chapter 23). An important thing to remember is that it is not enough for you to say that the data analysis was carried out using thematic data analysis. The readers may not know what this method is. You must explain the nature of the method and how you used it in your study. If you have used computer programs to help analyse the data (see Chapter 24), you have to give some explanation of what the package can do and the way you used it.

In quantitative research, the data analysis section is where you describe the statistical methods used to complete your analysis, and state why you chose those particular methods. You might start by saying how you analysed the participants' demographic data (e.g. calculating means and standard deviations). When comparing groups, you might calculate an estimate of how large the treatment effect was (an effect size and the associated 95 per cent confidence interval). This analysis helps readers interpret the difference in outcome between the groups and the range of uncertainty around the true treatment effect. Many people report the statistical significance of their findings using p-values; these values are the probability that your findings could have occurred by chance. It is always best to report the actual p value (e.g. $p = 0.023$) rather than stating the threshold ($p < 0.05$) (see Chapters 25, 26).

Findings

The results of your research are presented in this section. In qualitative research, the findings are separated into different themes, and verbatim quotations are used to elaborate your explanation of the findings. In quantitative research, the results are often presented as tables and figures (Bryman 2016).

Discussion and conclusion

What you have found in your research is discussed in this section. An important aspect that you should remember is that you need to link your findings to the literature and theory you provided in the introduction (Bryman 2016). Readers would like to see how your study can confirm or contribute to new knowledge in the area or discipline. In the conclusion, researchers often make some recommendations for further research or note the implications for health care practices. This will allow readers to see that your research findings can be used in real life and/or allow others to duplicate or extend your research in the field.

Acknowledgments

It is customary to acknowledge the assistance of others in this section. In particular, you express your gratitude to your research participants, who have given you valuable knowledge so that you could undertake your research. You should also acknowledge funding agencies who have given you money to carry out the research.

References

This section lists all the references you have cited in the text. You need to ensure that they are complete and that the format is consistent throughout.

You may like to read Bryman (2016, pp. 661–87) for writing up qualitative, quantitative and mixed methods research. There are many useful tips in this piece.

QUALITATIVE WRITING

Here is an example from Helen and Pranee's qualitative research. The research is based on the work of Helen's PhD study and was published in *Sexual Health* (see Rawson & Liamputtong 2009). For reasons of length, we present only certain sections of the paper and exclude all references cited. You may wish to read this paper from the journal directly.

Title

'The influence of traditional Vietnamese culture on the utilisation of mainstream health services for sexual health issues by second-generation Vietnamese Australian young women.'

Abstract

This paper discusses the impact traditional Vietnamese culture has on the uptake of mainstream health services for sexual health matters by Vietnamese Australian young women. It is part of a wider qualitative study which explored the factors that shaped the sexual behaviour of Vietnamese Australian young women living in Australia. A grounded theory method was employed, involving in-depth interviews with 15 Vietnamese Australian young women aged 18–25 years who reside in Melbourne. The findings demonstrated that the ethnicity of the general practitioner had a clear impact on the women utilising the health service. They perceived that a Vietnamese doctor would hold the traditional view of sex held by their parents' generation. They reasoned that due to cultural mores, optimum sexual health care could only be achieved with a non-Vietnamese health professional. It is evidenced from the present study that cultural influences can impact on the sexual health of young people from culturally diverse backgrounds and, in Australia's multicultural society, provision of sexual health services must acknowledge the specific needs of ethnically diverse young people.

RESEARCH IN PRACTICE

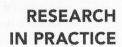

Pranee Liamputtong, Nora Shields and Annemarie Gallichio

Introduction

The sexual and reproductive development and health of young people are important global health concerns, and while its importance is widely acknowledged in contemporary research, research centres primarily on young people's sexual activity, unsafe sexual practices and the potential outcomes of risk-taking behaviour (such as sexually transmitted infections and teenage pregnancies), and sex education. A biomedical perspective underpins this body of work to the exclusion of the relevance of prevailing social factors and processes, thus effectively denying the importance of socially informed enquiry. It has been argued that a comprehensive sexual health strategy, involving medical, social, cultural, gendered and age-specific aspects, is needed to ensure that the global population receives and maintains optimum sexual and reproductive health. As part of a wider study, we sought to help fill this void by exploring the factors which influence the sexual behaviour of young women in Australia with a specific cultural heritage.

In this paper, we discuss how the parental Vietnamese culture influences the way these young women utilised mainstream health services for sexual health matters. Specifically, we examine how the parental Vietnamese culture influenced the young women's choice of general practitioner (GP).

Method

This research adopted a qualitative methodology as this enabled us to examine and learn from the experiences of the young women who are living them. In addition, the exploratory nature of this research into the complex interplay of sexuality, second-generation and gender issues is well suited to a qualitative research design. Grounded theory allowed us to uncover the young women's thoughts, perceptions and feelings, and so ensure that behaviour is understood through the meanings and interpretations they attach to it. Data were gathered by in-depth interviews with 15 second-generation Vietnamese young women living in Melbourne, Australia. An 'interview guide' was utilised and consisted of a list of topics deemed pivotal to the

research question. The inclusion criteria for participation in the study were (1) be a second-generation immigrant, that is, be born or live in Australia, in accordance with national census data; (2) be Vietnamese Australian, that is, have lived in Australia from a young age with one or both parents being born in Vietnam; (3) be aged 18 to 25 years, and (4) be fluent in English.

The 15 interviews were audiotaped, allowing for an uninterrupted flow of discussion, and the tapes were transcribed by the first author and analysed. In keeping with grounded theory method, the tapes were transcribed and analysed at the completion of each interview. Data analysis was informed by grounded theory and involved assessment and interpretation of the commonalities, contradictions and differences of the young women's lived experiences using open, axial and selective coding. To ensure anonymity, the young women are referred to by pseudonyms.

Findings

The analysis process for the wider study resulted in the development of four main categories as shaping the sexual behaviour of Vietnamese Australian young women. The results presented in this section relate to the category 'The impact of sexual and reproductive health services on sexual behaviour', specifically the subcategory we have termed 'Choice of general practitioner', and how accessing health care for sexual health purposes is influenced and impacted by the parental Vietnamese culture. This subcategory consisted of two key elements: 'Parental influence over choice of general practitioner' and 'Ethnicity of general practitioner'. Analysis of the interview data produced significant insights into the young women's preferences regarding optimum sexual health care and factors which would hinder their access to such care.

Parental influence over choice of general practitioner

The young women who lived with their parents viewed them as controlling their choice of GP. They had the same GP as their parents and expressed concern about this situation, feeling that it could create problems if they wanted, or needed, to see the GP about sexual health matters. This concern was generated, and fuelled, by fear and resulted in participants 'changing' their GP for consultations about sex-related issues.

The young women viewed having access to adequate and appropriate health care as important in relation to sexual and reproductive health. While they stated that they 'occasionally' needed to visit their family GP or other family health practitioners, they indicated their reluctance to do so. This reluctance was based on two concerns: first, having the 'same GP as parents' and second, the ethnicity of the GP. Participants voiced the need for 'trust' when talking about sexual health issues. They had a 'fear of being found out'. They used phrases such as 'concerned about people finding out', 'parents might find out' and 'Vietnamese people gossip'. Their preferred site for 'treatment' was a family health clinic, which they viewed as offering the possibility of a confidential and anonymous service.

The generation of fear

The young women's concern about having the same GP as their parents arose from the fear that their parents, or other members of the Vietnamese community, may learn that a visit concerned sexual health matters. Nga indicated her concern:

> It's a bit scary. I'd feel 'Are they [the doctors] going to say something and it gets back to my parents?'

Changing general practitioner for sexual health issues

To avoid the possibility of being 'exposed', the young women indicated that they would change their GP. Those who no longer lived in the parental home stated that they had changed their GP from the one they shared with their parents:

> When I lived at home we all had the same doctor as my parents and that's awkward for certain things. Now I have my own doctor, nothing to do with my family (Lan).

Discussion and conclusion

In the traditional Vietnamese culture, the prescribed conduct of women is rooted in Confucian tenets which enjoin female submission and premarital female chastity.

Young women are deemed to be guardians of the 'traditional moral values', and immense importance is placed on female virginity before marriage and on family honour. Thus the young women perceived that a Vietnamese GP would be upholding this traditional moral code. Their expressions of fear, embarrassment and judgment stemmed from this perception of sexuality within the Vietnamese community. In most Asian cultures, open discussion about sexuality is unusual, even among close friends, since sex is considered a very sensitive and taboo subject and is generally not discussed. During their interviews the young women stressed that within the traditional culture, discussion of sexual issues would be perceived as indicative of engagement in sexual activities. They were only too aware of the cultural expectations and the notion that any premarital sexual expression could compromise their, and their family's, moral reputation within the community. They later discussed the consequences of shame and dishonour for non-adherence to traditional sexual mores. (This will be addressed in a later paper.) For these young women, trust was the underlying component in gaining optimum sexual health care. They believed this to be unachievable with a Vietnamese GP.

The findings indicate that the factors which impact on the sexual behaviour of Vietnamese Australian young women have significant implications for the provision of sexual health services. Cultural taboos can limit young people's access to sexual and reproductive services and information. Thus there is a clear need for health care providers working within a multicultural society such as Australia to acknowledge that cultural context and social environment constitute multifaceted aspects of human behaviour. If the overall morbidity of young Australians is to be addressed through the development and implementation of appropriate strategies then, in addition to having culturally based and appropriate sex education information, the sexual health care services provided must be culturally sensitive.

Pranee Liamputtong, Nora Shields and Annemarie Gallichio

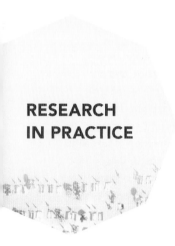

RESEARCH IN PRACTICE

QUANTITATIVE WRITING

Here we provide an example from Nora Shields' quantitative research. The research was published in *Archives of Physical Medicine and Rehabilitation* in 2008. Again, we present only certain sections of the paper and exclude all references. You may wish to read this paper from the journal directly (see Shields *et al.* 2008b).

Title

'Effects of a community-based progressive resistance training program on muscle performance and physical function in adults with Down syndrome: a randomised controlled trial.'

Structured abstract

Objective: Does progressive resistance training improve muscle strength, muscle endurance, and physical function in adults with Down syndrome? *Design*: Single-blind randomised controlled trial. *Participants*: Adults ($N = 20$) with Down syndrome (13 men, 7 women; mean age, 26.8 ± 7.8y) were randomly assigned to either an intervention group ($n = 9$) or a control group ($n = 11$). *Intervention*: The intervention was a supervised, group, progressive resistance training program, using weight machines performed twice a week for 10 weeks. Participants completed 2–3 sets of 10–12 repetitions of each exercise until they reached fatigue. The control group continued with their usual activities. *Main outcome measures*: The outcomes measured by blinded assessors were muscle strength (1-RM), muscle endurance (number of repetitions at 50% of 1-RM) for chest press, and the grocery shelving task. *Results*: The intervention group demonstrated significant improvement in upper-limb muscle endurance compared to the control group (mean difference 16.7 reps, 95% confidence interval, [CI] 7.1–26.2), and a trend towards an improvement in upper-limb muscle strength (mean difference 8.6 kg, 95% CI, –1.3–18.5 kg) and in upper-limb function (mean difference –20.3s, 95% CI, –45.7–5.2s). *Conclusions*: Progressive resistance training is a safe and feasible fitness option that can improve upper-limb muscle endurance in adults with Down syndrome.

Introduction

People with Down syndrome (DS) have reduced muscle strength and muscular endurance compared to their peers without disability. Muscle weakness can impact the ability of people with DS to perform everyday activities. Only three trials have investigated the effects of progressive resistance training in people with DS. Each of these trials found improved muscle strength with training, but none of the trials reported the effects of the programs on muscle endurance or functional activities. These trials were also limited as none employed blinded assessors to collect the data and two studies did not include a control group in their design. As no randomised controlled trial (RCT) has been conducted, it is not known to what extent the reported effects of progressive resistance training in people with DS are due to the strength training intervention rather than due to series effects. The aim of this trial was to determine if a progressive resistance training program for adults with DS can lead to increased muscle strength and endurance, and to improved physical function in this population.

Methods

We conducted an RCT. The trial received ethics approval from the university ethics committee, and all participants and their carers gave written informed consent to take part.

Participants

Adults with DS were included if they were aged 18 years or more, had the ability to follow simple verbal instructions in English, and were well enough to participate in a progressive resistance training program. The exclusion criterion was participation in a strength training program in the six months prior to the start of the study. Adults with DS were randomised using a concealed allocation, block randomisation method to either an intervention group or a control group.

Intervention

Participants in the intervention group completed a 10-week, twice a week progressive resistance training program at a community gymnasium. The program included three exercises for the upper limbs using weight machines (shoulder press, seated chest press, seated row). Participants completed 2–3 sets of 10–12 repetitions of each exercise until they reached fatigue. A 2-minute rest period was given between each set, and the resistance was increased when two sets of 12 repetitions of an exercise could be completed. Participants completed the program as a group, supervised by two accredited fitness trainers. Participants in the control group continued with their typical daily activities.

Outcome measurements

All participants were assessed at baseline and immediately after the intervention period. The outcome measurements were taken by assessors who were blind to group allocation. Maximal muscle force generation was tested by establishing the amount of weight each participant could lift in a single seated chest press (1-RM). Muscle endurance was measured by counting the number of repetitions that could be completed when the weight on the seated chest press was lowered to 50% of 1-RM. Physical function was measured using the grocery shelving task. Participants were asked to carry two grocery bags each containing 10 × 410 g items to a bench two metres away. The participants then stacked the items onto a shelf at shoulder height. Participants completed the task as quickly as possible and the time taken was measured.

Data analysis

Data were analysed using SPSS statistical software to determine if there were any significant baseline demographic differences between the groups. Outcomes were analysed using analysis of covariance on the change scores with the baseline measure of that variable used as the covariate. The mean difference within each group and the mean difference between the groups and the 95% CIs of the mean differences were also calculated. Effect sizes and 95% CIs were also calculated for the change scores.

Results

Twenty adults (13 men, 7 women) with DS took part (see Table 27.1). Participants in the intervention group attended 92.8% of scheduled training sessions. No sessions were missed due to injury. The intervention group had a statistically significant improvement in upper-limb muscle endurance compared to the control group (mean difference in repetitions of the chest press at 50% of 1-RM, 16.7; 95% CI, 7.1–26.2; $p <.01$). There were also trends towards improvement in upper-limb muscle strength (mean difference 1-RM, 8.6 kg; 95% CI, −1.3–18.5 kg; $p = 0.08$) and upper-limb function (mean difference in grocery shelving task, −20.3s; 95% CI, −45.7–5.2s; $p = 0.11$) that favoured the intervention group (Table 27.2).

Discussion and conclusion

The main finding was that upper-limb muscle performance improved in adults with DS after a 10-week progressive resistance exercise program. There was a significant increase in chest press endurance and a trend toward an increase in upper-limb strength as measured by a 1-RM chest press and upper-limb functional activity as measured by a grocery shelving task. The effect sizes observed were moderate to large (0.76–.90), and

TABLE 27.1   Demographic data for intervention and control groups

CHARACTERISTIC	INTERVENTION (N = 9)	CONTROL (N = 11)
Mean age ± SD (y)	25.8 ± 5.4	27.6 ± 9.5
Sex (male/female)	7/2	6/5
Height (cm)	158.8 (7.12)	152.0 (10.0)
Weight (kg)	78.4 (13.5)	61.2 (6.7)
Level of perceived intellectual disability		
Mild	2	2
Moderate or severe	7	9

TABLE 27.2   Mean (SD) score and mean (95% CI) difference between groups for upper-limb outcomes for the intervention group and the control group

OUTCOME	SCORE				DIFFERENCE BETWEEN GROUPS*		
	Baseline (week 0)		Post-intervention (week 10)		Week 10–Week 0? (95% CI)	p-value	Effect size (95% CI)
	Int	Con	Int	Con	Int-Con		
Chest press 1-RM (kg)	35.9 (15.4)	28.0 (10.2)	44.9 (15.2)	31.6 (13.3)	8.6 (-1.3–18.5)	0.08	0.63 (-0.20–1.59)
Chest press endurance (no. of repetitions)	15.0 (4.7)	19.0 (8.1)	25.9 (8.3)	17.5 (9.5)	16.7 (7.1–26.2)	0.00	1.51 (0.46–2.44)
Grocery shelving task (sec)	85.1 (49.1)	122.8 (84.0)	67.5 (33.4)	110.7 (66.4)	-20.3 (-45.7–5.2)	0.11	0.22 (-0.68–1.09)

*Derived from ANCOVA with dependent variable on admission and baseline weight as covariates

Con = control group; Int = intervention group

the changes in upper-limb strength carried over to trends to changes in upper-limb physical function tasks suggests that these results may be clinically significant. The change in upper-limb endurance may be relevant in these adults, whose employment involves manual work of the upper limbs.

The progressive resistance exercise program implemented for this study was feasible for adults with DS. It might be expected that adults with DS have difficulty taking part in or being motivated to continue with a progressive resistance exercise program. The participants were all capable of taking part in the program and experienced benefits from doing so despite their intellectual disability. Compliance with the program was excellent and there were no withdrawals from the study, indicating that a strength training program was an acceptable form of exercise to the participants. Another positive finding was that the training program appeared to be a safe intervention for people with DS. No major adverse events were reported during the program. This finding is consistent with conclusions that strength training appears to be a relatively safe intervention for people with a broad range of health conditions.

The main strength of this trial was that it was an RCT. It adds to an area of research where to date only three previous studies have investigated if strength training programs are beneficial for adults with DS. This trial was limited by the relatively small sample size of 20 participants, which required the effects of the intervention to be large in order to detect any changes as a result of the strength training program.

How to critically appraise qualitative and quantitative published papers

Qualitative papers

It has been suggested that qualitative research is difficult to evaluate or appraise as there are many kinds of qualitative enquiry depending on the epistemology and methodology adopted in the research (Bochner 2000; Dixon-Woods *et al.* 2004; Guba & Lincoln 2005, 2008; Green & Thorogood 2009; Tracy 2010; Mackey 2012; Creswell 2013). We agree with many qualitative researchers in the field. However, we believe that for a student or practitioner who wishes to appraise qualitative research for EBP (evidence-based practice), it is necessary to have some guidelines that they can use. We find the guidelines provided by Mildred Blaxter (1996) a very useful set of criteria for evaluating papers based on qualitative research. The criteria presented in the box below are taken from her suggestions, published by the British Sociology Association (see also Blaxter 1996).

CRITERIA FOR THE EVALUATION OF QUALITATIVE PAPERS

General

- Are the methods of the research appropriate to the nature of the question of the research? That is, what does the research seek to understand? Could a quantitative method have addressed the issue better?
- Is the connection to an existing body of knowledge or theory clear? That is, is there enough reference to the literature? Does the paper cohere with, or critically address, existing theory?

Methods

- Are there clear descriptions of the criteria used for the selection of participants, the data collection and the analysis?
- Is the selection of participants theoretically justified?

Pranee Liamputtong, Nora Shields and Annemarie Gallichio

- Does the sensitivity of the methods match the needs of the research questions? Is there any consideration of the limitations of the methods?
- Has the relationship between field workers and participants been considered?
- Is there evidence about how the research was presented and explained to the participants?
- Was the data collection and record-keeping systematic and appropriate?

Analysis

- Is reference made to accepted procedures for analysis?
- How systematic is the analysis?
- Is there adequate discussion of how themes, concepts and categories were derived from the data?
- Is there adequate discussion of the evidence both for and against the researcher's arguments? In particular, are negative data given? Has there been any search for cases that might refute the conclusions?
- Have measures been taken to test the validity of the findings? That is, have methods such as feeding the findings back to the participants, triangulation or procedures based on grounded theory been used?
- Have any steps been taken to see whether the analysis would be comprehensible to participants? In particular, has the meaning of their accounts been explored with participants?

Presentation

- Is the research clearly contextualised? That is, is relevant information about the social context of the setting and participants provided?
- Are the data presented systematically? That is, are quotations and field notes identified for readers to judge the range of evidence being used?
- Is a clear distinction made between the data and their interpretation? In particular, do the conclusions follow from the data?
- Is enough of the original evidence presented to satisfy the reader of the relationship between the evidence and the conclusions?
- Is the researcher's own position (e.g. role, possible bias and influence on the research) clearly stated?
- Are the results credible and appropriate? That is, do they address the research question? Are they plausible and coherent? Are they important theoretically or practically?

Ethics

- Have ethical issues been adequately considered?

If a qualitative article can provide answers to all or most of these questions in a positive way, it is likely that the paper is of high quality. In critically appraising a paper, readers can look for any gaps by using these questions to judge if the paper is trustworthy or not.

It must be noted that these guidelines are constructed for qualitative papers in general. It is argued that some qualitative enquiry would need some explicit criteria (Green & Thorogood 2009; Tracy 2010; Mackey 2012). Additionally, due to the word limit of some journals, particularly medical journals which allow a limit of only 3000–4000 words, it can be very difficult for the author to include all these criteria. This may lead to difficulties in appraising some qualitative papers. However, writers have developed some guidelines to evaluate qualitative material. We recommend readers to consult the work of Patton (2003), Russell and Gregory (2003), Green and Thorogood (2009), Tracy (2010), Hennink *et al.* (2011), Spencer and Ritchie (2011) and Mackey (2012).

STOP AND THINK

Considering the criteria discussed above and the example of a qualitative research provided in this chapter, what is your opinion of the strength of the paper? Does it present enough evidence that you can use in your work? Can you rely on this research report in your attempt to provide sexual health education for Vietnamese young women?

Quantitative papers

This section of the chapter aims to examine ways to critically appraise published quantitative research papers (Kempe & Nevill 2010). However, before we discuss the critical appraisal process, it is important to address one assumption about the hierarchy of evidence or levels of evidence (see Chapter 1).

Different types of clinical or research questions require different types of evidence which will arise from a variety of study designs—depending on the research question being asked. A methodological distinction is made between quantitative research (which is associated with experimental research and statistical analyses, such as RCTs and cohort studies) and qualitative research (which is associated with naturalistic enquiry such as ethnography and phenomenology). The distinction between these two paradigms is made on the basis of the type of data (numbers or words) and the type of question the research was trying to address. The latter is a very important distinction, as it relates to how we critically appraise the research (see also Chapter 1). Here are two examples to illustrate this.

If we were interested in the experiences of a young person with HIV/AIDS in Australia, it would be inappropriate to conduct an RCT or a cohort study. We would not ask them to complete a survey with predetermined response options. It would be more suitable and more effective to talk to them about their experiences and ask them to tell us their story. So in this example, the best evidence to answer this research question would arise from a qualitative study design.

If we were interested in finding out the number of people between the ages of eighteen and thirty who had found employment in Australia, we could conduct a cross-sectional survey. Again, it would not be appropriate or effective to conduct an RCT, as we cannot randomise people as employed (case) and unemployed (control) and an RCT would not give us the right type of evidence.

Pranee Liamputtong, Nora Shields and Annemarie Gallichio

In summary, different types of research questions require different types of evidence that will arise from different types of research designs. While RCTs provide us with high-quality evidence, it is not always effective or appropriate to use them to answer all the research questions we are interested in.

The box below illustrates how to critically appraise RCTs in a systematic manner. See also the explanatory notes that follow the box.

CRITERIA FOR THE ASSESSMENT OF QUANTITATIVE PAPERS: EVALUATION OF AN RCT

1   Are the results of the study valid?

   A   Screening questions:

      Ai Did the study ask a clearly focused research question?

Consider if the research question is 'focused' in terms of:

- *the population studied*
- *the intervention given*
- *the outcomes considered.*

      Aii Was this a randomised controlled trial (RCT) and was this the appropriate design for the research question?

Consider:

- *Why was this study carried out as an RCT?*
- *Was this the right research study design for the research question being asked?*
- *Is it worth continuing?*

   B   Detailed questions:

      Bi Did the reviewers try to identify the following?

Consider:

- *How were participants allocated to intervention and control groups? Was the process truly random?*
- *Was the method of allocation described? Was a method used to balance the randomisation, e.g. stratification?*
- *How was the randomisation schedule generated and how was a participant allocated to a study group?*
- *Where the groups well balanced? Are any differences between the groups at entry to the trial reported?*
- *Were there differences reported that might have explained any outcome(s) (confounding)?*

      Bii Were the participants, staff and study personnel 'blind' to participants' study group?

Consider:

- *the fact that blinding is not always possible*
- *if every effort was made to achieve blinding*
- *if you think it matters in this study*
- *the fact that we are looking for 'observer bias'.*

    Biii Were all of the participants who entered the trial accounted for at its conclusion?

Consider:

- *if any intervention-group (treatment) participants got a control-group option or vice versa*
- *if all participants were followed up in each study group (was there loss to follow-up)*
- *if all the participants' outcomes were analysed by the groups to which they were originally allocated (intention-to-treat analysis)*
- *what additional information would you like to have seen to make you feel better about this.*

    Biv Were the participants in all groups followed up and data collected in the same way?

Consider:

- *if, for example, they were reviewed at the same time intervals and if they received the same amount of attention from researchers and health workers. Any differences may introduce performance or measurement bias.*

    Bv Did the study have enough participants to minimise the possibility of chance?

Consider:

- *Is there a power calculation? This will estimate how many participants are needed to be reasonably sure of finding something important (if it really exists and for a given level of uncertainty about the final result).*

  C What are the results?

    Ci How are the results presented and what is the main result (the statistical information)?

Consider:

- *if, for example, the results are presented as a proportion of people experiencing an outcome such as 'risk' or as a measurement such as mean or median differences, or as survival curves and hazards*
- *the magnitude of the results and how meaningful they are*
- *how you would sum up the 'bottom-line' result of the trial in one sentence.*

Pranee Liamputtong, Nora Shields and Annemarie Gallichio

Cii How precise are the results (i.e. look for confidence intervals or *p* values)?

Consider:

- *Is the result precise enough to make a decision?*
- *Was a confidence interval reported? Would your decision about the effectiveness of this intervention be the same at the upper confidence limit as the lower confidence limit?*
- *Is a p value reported where confidence intervals are unavailable?*

D Will the results of this study help me in my clinical situation with my patient/ client?

Di Were all the important outcomes considered so the results can be applied to my specific clinical situation for my patient/client?

Consider whether:

- *the people included in the trial could be different from your population in ways that might produce different results*
- *your local setting differs from that of the trial*
- *you can provide the same treatment in your setting.*

Consider outcomes from the point of view of the:

- *individual*
- *policy-maker and professionals*
- *family/carers*
- *wider community.*

Consider:

- *Does any benefit reported outweigh any harm and/or cost? If this information is not reported, can it be filled in from elsewhere?*
- *Should policy or practice change as a result of the evidence contained in this trial?*

Source: Adapted from Solutions for Public Health (2007)

Explanatory notes

The first two questions are screening questions and can be answered quickly. If the answer to both is 'yes', it is worth proceeding with the remaining questions.

- There is a degree of overlap between several of the questions.
- You are asked to record a Yes, No or Can't tell to most of the questions.
- A number of italicised hints are given after each question. These are designed to remind you why the question is important.

Critical appraisal tools for other quantitative study designs

If the published research report you are reviewing uses a different study design, you can find the appropriate critical appraisal questions at the website of the Critical Appraisal Skills Program (CASP) (Public Health Resource Unit 2007; see also Guyatt *et al.* 1993), which also covers other research study designs.

The documents available from CASP are titled as follows:

1 'Case Control Study'

2 'Cohort Study'

3 'Economic Evaluations'

4 'Systematic Review'.

STOP AND THINK

Considering the criteria discussed above and the example of a quantitative research paper provided in this chapter, what is your opinion regarding the strengths of the paper? Does it provide enough evidence that you can use this intervention in your work? Can you rely on this research report to help provide opportunities for exercise among adults with Down syndrome?

Summary

We strongly believe that writing up our research findings is an essential component of the research process if we wish to complete it. Writing about our findings helps to communicate the important issues arising from our research to wider audiences, be they academics, health and welfare professionals or policy-makers. More importantly, what we find in conducting any piece of research may prove useful in improving the health and well-being of many individuals and in the provision of health and welfare services for many people. Our research findings can be used as 'evidence' in health and social care, so it is our moral obligation to write after we have completed our research. How will anyone find this information if we do not write about it? Research dissemination through writing is therefore an important part of the research process. As van Manen (2006, p. 715) says:

> It is in the act of … writing that insights emerge. The [writing] involves textual material that possesses … interpretive significance. It is precisely in the process of writing that the data of the research are gained as well as interpreted and that the fundamental nature of the research question is perceived.

Pranee Liamputtong, Nora Shields and Annemarie Gallichio

It is also important that we know how to critically appraise published material so that we can evaluate its rigour and trustworthiness. This way we can be more confident about the evidence that we will use in our EBP. This chapter has also discussed the way that all readers can appraise both qualitative and quantitative published materials that they think will be useful.

Practice exercises

1   Obtain four articles on any issue relevant to your study, from journals. Two papers must be based on qualitative methods and the other two on quantitative methods. Read and critically examine the format that each paper has adopted. Do you see any commonality or difference between the four papers? Discuss the commonalities and differences.

2   Using the same articles, critically appraise their strength and trustworthiness. Follow the guidelines given in this chapter. What can you say about the rigour and trustworthiness of the articles?

3   You have done a piece of research using one of the methods covered in this book. You have finished your data analysis and now it is time to write up your research findings. Start composing your paper, using the structures provided in this chapter.

Notes

1   This paper is used with permission from CSIRO Publishing. The link to this issue of *Sexual Health* is <www.publish.csiro.au/nid/166/issue/5048.htm>.

2   This paper is used here with permission from Elsevier Science.

Further reading

Belgrave, L.L., Zablotsky, D. & Guadagno, M.A. (2002). How do we talk to each other? Writing qualitative research for quantitative readers. *Qualitative Health Research*, 12(10), 1427–39.

Berg, K. & Latin, R. (2008). *Essentials of research methods in health, physical education, exercise science, and recreation*, 3rd edn. Baltimore: Lippincott Williams & Williams.

Goodall, H.L. (2008). *Writing qualitative inquiry: self, stories, and academic life*. Walnut Creek, CA: Left Coast Press.

Johnstone, M-J. (2004). *Effective writing for health professionals: a practical guide to getting published*. Sydney: Allen & Unwin.

Liamputtong, P. (2013). *Qualitative research methods*, 4th edn. Melbourne: Oxford University Press.

Marvasti, A.B. (2011). Three aspects of writing qualitative research: practice, genre, and audiences. In D. Silverman (ed.), *Qualitative research: issues of theory, method and practice*, 3rd edn. London: Sage, 383–96.

Moore, N. (2006). *How to do research: a practical guide to designing and managing research projects*, 3rd edn. London: Facet.

Neuman, W.L. (2011). *Social research methods: qualitative and quantitative Methods,* 7th edn. Boston: Allyn & Bacon, 542–72).

Sandelowski, M. & Leeman, J. (2012). Writing usable qualitative health research findings. *Qualitative Health Research*, 22(10), 1404–13.

Tracy, S.J. (2010). Qualitative quality: eight 'big tents' criteria for excellent qualitative research. *Qualitative Inquiry*, 16(10), 837–51.

Wolcott, H.F. (2009). *Writing up qualitative research*, 3rd edn. Thousand Oaks, CA: Sage.

Websites

www.consort-statement.org

> The CONSORT website. This website provides a current definitive version of the CONSORT statement and up-to-date information on extensions, a library of examples of good reporting and useful resources related to the statement.

http://cnx.org/content/m14576/latest

> This webpage contains vivid discussions on writing up qualitative theses. It gives some ideas about what the author calls the haziness of writing a qualitative dissertation that readers may find useful.

http://research.avondale.edu.au/cgi/viewcontent.cgi?article=1038&context=edu_papers

> The website contains information about a framework for assessing the quality of qualitative research.

www.phru.nhs.uk/pages/PHD/CASP.htm

> This website belongs to the Solutions for Public Health (2007). It has information about the critical appraisal skills program and information about the quality in qualitative evaluation. It discusses a framework for evidence.

www.equator-network.org/

> This is the EQUATOR Network website, the resource centre for good reporting of health research studies. It is a great resource for health researchers.

GLOSSARY

Allocation bias
A type of selection bias that occurs when the process of allocating participants to groups leads to differences in the baseline characteristics of those groups.

Allocation concealment
The randomised allocation sequence being concealed from investigators who are involved in recruiting participants.

Alternating treatment design
Two or three treatments of interest are provided in rapid succession and in an alternating format, within a session, in a session-by-session format or in a day-by-day format. The results are graphed together to clearly show the difference in rate and stability of learning in each treatment condition.

Analysis of narratives
The type of data analysis where themes are derived from the stories to demonstrate commonalities and dissimilar experiences.

Analysis of variance (ANOVA)
One of the most commonly used analyses in quantitative data analysis procedures. An ANOVA is used to compare the means of three or more sets of scores to determine if there are statistically significant differences between them.

Analytical cross-sectional study
A study which involves taking a 'snapshot' or cross-section of the population at a particular point in time. It aims to address questions about associations between exposures and outcomes.

Analytical epidemiological studies
Are designed to test hypotheses about associations between an exposure of interest and a particular health outcome. Thus they aim to identify or describe cause-and-effect relationships or associations between exposure and outcome factors.

Anonymity
Refers to a person being unknown to the researcher and hence to anyone else. Further, if the person took part in a public health survey their confidentiality was maintained.

Ascertainment bias
Occurs when the results or conclusions of the trial are distorted by the knowledge of which intervention each participant is receiving.

Assessment
The process of gathering quantitative data in general, also referred to as evaluation.

Assessment bias
Occurs if an investigator's assessment of a participant lacks objectivity. Subjective outcome measures are prone to exaggerate the effect of the intervention.

Axial coding
The step in coding that requires moving towards a greater level of abstraction from the data. The task at this level of coding will be to further evaluate the codes to determine what needs to be reassembled or reorganised. This may involve processes such as breaking codes into smaller categories or collapsing more than one code into a single category.

Bias
A concept used in randomised controlled trials and other positivist research designs. Researchers may unknowingly influence or bias the outcome of a study. Such bias can distort the results or conclusions away from the truth, the result being a poor-quality trial that underestimates, or more likely overestimates, the benefits of an intervention. There are five main types of

bias: selection, allocation, assessment, ascertainment and stopping rule biases.

Blinding
A technique used in randomised controlled trials to prevent assessors, participants or data analysis staff knowing which group a participant is in after s/he has been allocated.

Boolean operator
A term that determines the relationship between two or more search words in searching through electronic databases. There are three basic terms: 'and', 'or' and 'not'. These three terms can be linked to expand or condense the search.

Bracketing or epoché
The fundamental concept underpinning phenomenological reduction. The aim is to suspend all judgments and prior ideas about the phenomenon 'in order to enter the unique world of the individual whose experience is the focus of the research' (Carpenter & Suto 2008, p. 67). The concept of bracketing is characteristic of descriptive phenomenology.

CAQDAS (computer-assisted qualitative data analysis software)
A specifically designed program (there are many versions) that can take over a substantial amount of the manual labour involved with analysing the data. CAQDAS offers a highly efficient data management system for storing, coding, organising, sorting and retrieving data.

Case study in qualitative research
The study of a particular issue which is examined through one or more cases within a bounded system such as a setting or context.

Case-control study
A study that compares a group of people who have the outcome factor of interest (cases) with a group of people who do

not (controls). Investigators look back through time to identify exposures in the two groups. The two groups are then compared using measures of association, most commonly the odds ratio.

Chi-square test
A test of statistical significance, used when the level of measurement is nominal and the data therefore consist of frequency counts for categories. There is the one-way chi-square test, which is sometimes called the goodness of fit test, and the two-way chi-square test. The latter, which is commonly encountered in health research, is used when there are two variables and determines if the relationship (association) between the two variables is statistically significant.

Citation bias
Occurs where articles that have statistically significant findings are cited more often than others.

Clinical audit
A process that provides a systematic framework for establishing care standards based on best evidence. It is a practical way to compare day-to-day practice with best evidence care standards and it can identify areas of care that require improvement.

Clinical data-mining
Provides practice-based evidence, i.e. evidence or information derived from practice. Such evidence underscores the importance of experiential knowledge in clinical decision-making and its contribution to establishing broad-based best practice models.

Clinical practice guidelines
'Systematically developed statements which assist the health professional and the patient to make decisions about what is the appropriate health care in specific circumstances' (Field & Lohr 1990, p. 38).

Clinical significance

The practical or applied value of a finding or set of findings. Clinical significance can be gauged by factors such as amount of change as a result of an intervention, subjective evaluations from a client or patient regarding the effects of a factor or intervention, and social impact of the intervention.

Clinical trial

A trial that is conducted to determine if an intervention is effective, i.e. whether it is beneficial to patients. A clinical trial can be used to investigate the efficacy of interventions.

Code

'A word or short phrase that symbolically assigns a summative, salient essence-capturing and/or evocative attribute for a portion of language-based or visual data' (Saldaña 2009, p. 3).

Coding

Part of the data analysis process where codes are applied to segments, or chunks, of data. It is central to qualitative research and is typically the starting point for most forms of qualitative analysis. Coding is the first step that allows researchers to move beyond tangible data to make analytical interpretations.

Cohort study

A study that follows, over time, a group (cohort) of people who have been exposed to a possible risk factor for a health outcome, and another group who have not been exposed. The incidence of the outcome in the exposed group is then compared to the incidence of the outcome in the group that is not exposed. This enables the relationship between the exposure and the outcome to be assessed.

Collaborative participatory research

A term that highlights the importance of collaboration and participation. This model recognises that the researcher has certain technical expertise, and that community leaders and community members have knowledge of their community needs and perspectives. The approach involves a transfer of knowledge, including knowledge of how to undertake research with community organisations.

Community

Can refer to any group of people living in geographic proximity or sharing an interest, a history or a cultural affinity.

Concurrent design

With this design, the questions that the researchers ask would tend to be framed from the start and they could consider using multiple reference points where intact but separate data sets are collected concurrently.

Confidence interval

An important indicator of the representativeness of the mean, particularly with respect to a population. One way of ascertaining the amount of error in statistical analysis is to calculate the confidence interval of the mean. The narrower the range in these values, the more representative the mean.

Confidentiality

Aims to conceal the true identity of people who participate in the research. Revealing their true identities could lead to danger and other negative consequences for these people. It is extremely important with some vulnerable groups, particularly those who are marginalised and stigmatised in the society.

Confounder

An extraneous factor that distorts (or confounds) the true effect of an intervention.

Confounding effect

Distortion of the true effect of an intervention by extraneous unwanted factors.

Consolidated Standards of Reporting Trials (CONSORT) Statement
Guidelines that aim to ensure accurate and complete reporting of the design, conduct, analysis and generalisability of trials, thus ensuring the highest possible standards are met when clinical trials are published.

Constant comparative analysis
An analytical technique used in grounded theory, during which information obtained from data collection is constantly compared with the emerging categories and concepts.

Constructivism
An epistemology that dominates the qualitative approach, also referred to as interpretivism. It suggests that 'reality' is socially constructed. Constructivist researchers reject the ideal of a single truth. They believe that there are multiple truths, which are individually constructed. Reality is seen as being shaped by social factors such as class, gender, race, ethnicity, culture and age. To constructivist researchers, reality is not firmly rooted in nature, but is a product of our own making.

Content analysis
A form of data analysis used by both qualitative and quantitative researchers that involves identifying codes before searching for their occurrence in the data. It is a deductive method, in contrast to the inductive method of thematic analysis.

Convenience sampling
This technique allows researchers to find individuals who are conveniently available and willing to participate in a study. Convenience sampling is crucial when it is difficult to find individuals who meet some specified criteria such as age, gender, ethnicity or social class. It is a form of a non-probability sampling technique.

Correlation coefficient
Used to summarise the degree of relationship (correlation) between variables. In the case of bivariate correlation, these variables correspond to two sets of measures (scores) for one group of participants.

Critical appraisal
The systematic examination of a research study to assess its strengths, weaknesses and trustworthiness, as well as its value and relevance in different contexts.

Cross-sectional study
A study that involves the measurement of exposure and outcome simultaneously within the population of interest. Cross-sectional studies are often described as providing a snapshot of the frequency and characteristics of a health state in a population at a particular point in time. They are also referred to as prevalence studies.

Cross-sectional survey
It is used where the primary purpose is descriptive. A cross-sectional survey gives a profile of the sample at one point in time. It cannot make inferences about past or future and relies largely on descriptive and correlational analyses. It can tell us what proportion of a sample or population reports certain symptoms, diseases or characteristics, and whether these are more prevalent among certain sections of the population.

Culture
The knowledge people use to generate and interpret social behaviour.

Data analysis
The way that researchers make sense of their data. In qualitative research it means looking for patterns of ideas or themes, whereas in quantitative research data are

analysed by counting various response alternatives.

Data display
An 'organised, compressed assembly of information that permits conclusion drawing' (Miles & Huberman 1994, p. 11).

Data extraction
The process by which information that will help answer the review question, such as data on study characteristics and findings, is obtained from the studies included in the systematic review.

Data-mining
The process of extracting and analysing data to uncover hidden patterns and useful information. It is used commonly in retail, marketing and fraud detection. In social work research and practice, it is a form of research most often done by practitioners themselves, rather than by external researchers.

Data reduction
Occurs when raw data are transcribed and transformed into summaries, initial codes and preliminary themes. Data reduction forms the preliminary phase of analysis.

Data saturation (theoretical saturation)
Data saturation occurs during the final stage of analysis, when no new categories or concepts can be derived from the data and any further data collected will fit within already developed categories.

Data synthesis
Summarising and collating the findings of the individual studies included in the systematic review. It can include descriptive analysis or more formal quantitative analysis such as meta-analysis.

Degrees of freedom
Value(s) associated with a test statistic that represent the number of scores that are free to vary. These values are used in determining the statistical significance of a test statistic.

Deontological ethics
An approach to ethics which holds that acts are inherently good or evil, regardless of their consequences.

Descriptive coding (open coding)
Often, the first level or step in coding in qualitative data analysis, in which the central aim is to sort and organise the data so that further analysis can take place. In grounded theory, this is referred to as open coding. This initial phase of coding stays close to the data themselves.

Descriptive epidemiology
Focuses on describing health states and events and their distribution. It describes morbidity and mortality within the population using person, place and time variables. Descriptive studies are often carried out using pre-existing population health data. There are two common types of descriptive epidemiological studies: cross-sectional studies and longitudinal studies.

Descriptive phenomenology
An approach to studying 'things as they appear' in order to arrive at a rigorous and unbiased understanding of the essential human consciousness and experience. Descriptive phenomenology develops detailed concrete descriptions of experience.

Descriptive statistics
Include measures of central tendency such as the mean (average), median (50th percentile) or mode (most frequently

occurring score), and measures of dispersion (e.g. the standard deviation and the range).

Descriptive test
Describes the difference between individuals within a group.

Discourses
Provide 'historically variable ways of specifying knowledge and truth—what is possible to speak of at any given moment' (Ramazanoğlu 1993, p. 19). In other words, discourses are not simply systems of signs, but systems of practices, and these systems or discourses bring objects into existence as they are spoken. In Chapter 6, discourse means 'communication of thought by words; talk; conversation' rather than its specific meaning in the social sciences.

Discriminative test
Distinguishes between individuals with and without a characteristic or trait.

Ecological study
An epidemiological study in which the unit of analysis is groups or aggregates rather than individuals. For instance, an ecological study may look at the association between rates of smoking and lung mortality in different countries. A limitation of ecological studies is that we cannot infer that associations observed at the aggregate level exist at the individual level—this is known as the ecological fallacy.

Effectiveness/efficacy
A measure used to determine whether the treatment or intervention has an intended or expected outcome. In medicine, however, it refers to the ability of a treatment or intervention to reproduce a desired outcome under ideal circumstances.

Effect size
Effect size, which can be measured in various ways and depends on the particular statistical test used, is a measure of the strength of a finding (whether that is difference between means or relationships between factors) that is independent of sample size.

Electronic databases
Electronic databases include general medical databases, discipline-specific databases and other speciality databases. They catalogue published health-related literature including journal articles, textbooks and reports.

Emic
An insider's perspective. It is a perspective conducted in a person's own culture, such as an intensive care nurse conducting research within an intensive care ward.

Empathic neutrality
This occurs in an interview whereby the researcher can validate the interviewee while remaining neutral to the content of what is being said.

Epidemiology
The study of the distribution and determinants of health states in populations. Epidemiology can provide the answers to questions asked in the health sector such as: How much disease is there? Who gets it? Where are most people affected? When did they have it? What happens over time?

Epistemology
Is concerned with the nature and scope (limitations) of knowledge. It addresses the questions: What is knowledge? How is knowledge acquired? What do people know? How do we know what we know? Why do we know what we know?

Essence

The essential structure of a phenomenon that would reflect the experience of people in general rather than that of individuals. The essence is derived through a rigorous analytic process during which the researcher brackets out their habitual ways of perceiving the phenomenon.

Ethical principles

There are four principles that researchers must adhere to in their research: *respecting autonomy*—the person making an informed decision about being involved; *beneficence*—the obligation to provide benefits, not to the participant necessarily, but certainly to the public good; *non-maleficence*—avoiding bad intention or the causation of harm or discomfort disproportionate to the benefits of the research; and *justice*—the concept that benefits, risks and costs are equitably distributed.

Ethnography

A research method that focuses on the scientific study of the lived culture of groups of people, used to discover and describe individual social and cultural groups. Crucial features include the use of participant observation in the fieldwork, along with other qualitative methods such as in-depth interviewing, focus groups and unobtrusive methods.

Ethno-nursing

The use of ethnography as a method for research in nursing allows nursing to be studied within the natural setting of local or indigenous communities and viewed within the context in which it occurs, as well as studying areas that have not been previously explored. It can be used to document, describe and explain nursing phenomena in relation to care, health, illness prevention and illness or injury recovery by nurses, clients and nursing or health institutions. It can provide in-depth data and detailed accounts of nursing phenomena or experiences, in a holistic view not gained through other research methods.

Etic

An outsider's perspective. In ethnographic studies conducted from the etic perspective, the researcher has no knowledge of or experience in the culture they are studying.

Evaluative tests

These are designed to measure change over time and are often called outcome measures. To accurately measure the amount of change, evaluative tools need to collect data at interval or ratio levels.

Evidence

Evidence, in the context of evidence-based practice, is what results from a systematic review and appraisal of all available literature relevant to a carefully designed question and protocol. It is information that can be used to support and guide practices, programs and policies in health and social care in order to enhance the health and well-being of individuals, families and communities.

Evidence-based practice

The use of best research evidence, along with clinical expertise, available resources and the patient's preferences, to determine the optimal management options in a specific situation.

Evidence-based practice in health care

A process that requires the practitioner to find empirical evidence about the effectiveness or efficacy of different treatment options and then determine the relevance of that evidence to a particular client's situation. The information is carefully considered in light of the available resources and the clinician's expertise, in order to determine the selected treatment plan for the client. EBP emphasises the importance of practice being based on, and supported by, sound empirical research, with the preferred gold standard being the conduct of randomised controlled trials.

Explanatory trial

A trial that is highly controlled and hence has reduced the number of variables that can affect the final outcome. It has more ability to explain what variable caused the result detected. However, because of the tight controls, the results of an explanatory trial may not be able to be generalised to everyday practice.

Exposure

A potential risk or protective factor for a health state. The exposure may represent an actual exposure (e.g. environmental pollution), a behaviour (e.g. physical inactivity, cigarette smoking) or an individual attribute (e.g. age) (Oleckno 2002). Exposure is often referred to as a study factor or independent variable.

External validity

The extent to which the findings from a study relate to patients or clients in the real world, i.e. how much the results can be applied to the wider population. This relates to the generalisability of a study's findings.

Fieldwork

A period of data collection commonly employed in the ethnographic method. Fieldwork may take a year or longer. The researcher usually stays in the community being studied throughout the period.

Focus groups

A data collection method based on group discussion. Typically, there is a moderator who acts as leader of the group and a notetaker who records field notes of the discussion. The participants (usually between eight and ten) express their views by interacting in a group discussion of the issues.

Focused coding

A step that follows descriptive or open coding. This is when researchers begin working with the codes in order to start making sense of the data. This may involve synthesising the codes and determining relationships between various events or phenomena.

Focused ethnography

Concentrates on a single problem in a particular setting. Rather than attempting to portray an entire cultural system, focused ethnography draws on the cultural ethos of a microcosm to study selected aspects of everyday life. It gives emphasis to particular behaviours in specific settings and allows researchers to work within time and scope limitations by narrowing the focus and providing objectives that are more manageable. Focused ethnography is also known as specific, particularistic or mini-ethnography.

Funnel format survey

In this model, the questions move from a broad focus to more specific content, from non-sensitive questions to more sensitive questions, and from more impersonal to more personal. In an inverted funnel format survey, questions move from more specific to more general, from more sensitive to less sensitive, and from personal to impersonal.

Generalisability

To ensure the findings of a clinical trial are generalisable, practitioners need to assess whether the participants, interventions and protocols employed in the trial are similar to their practice.

Grounded theory

A qualitative research method that uses a systematic set of procedures to collect and analyse data with the aim of developing an inductively derived theory that is 'grounded' in the data.

Hermeneutics

A theory of the process of interpretation. Hermeneutics is used in qualitative research to examine the way people develop interpretations of their life in relation to their life experiences.

Human research ethics committee

A group of people that includes researchers, health and social care professionals, a lawyer, lay members, and someone with a pastoral role in the community. There must also be a balance of men and women, and a balance of people who are regularly present and those who are co-opted for specialist expertise.

Inclusion/exclusion criteria

The rules set *a priori* (before the review is completed) that determine which studies are selected for inclusion in the systematic review and which are to be omitted.

In-depth interviewing

A method of qualitative data collection. The interview does not used fixed questions, though it can be guided by a set of broad questions. It aims to engage interviewees in conversation to elicit their understandings and interpretations. Within this method, it is assumed that people have particular and essential knowledge about the social world that is obtainable through verbal messages.

Indigenous people

The original inhabitants of countries that have been colonised by other cultural groups. Indigenous peoples are often marginalised from the mainstream political and social systems of these countries, and are widely recognised to be disadvantaged across a range of social, political and health indicators.

Inferential statistics

Include a variety of procedures that are commonly referred to as statistical tests.

Informed consent

A process that precedes the data collection. The people to be involved in the research process are informed of the aims and methods of the research and asked for their consent to participate. It shows that people from whom data was collected understood the research, and agreed to participate based on that understanding.

Institutional ethnography

Developed with the aim of discovering or exposing the chains of coordination and control in a social system or among settings of everyday life. Institutional ethnography is not empirically focused on 'experience' or 'culture' but on social organisation. It is concerned with exploring and describing social and institutional forces that shape, limit and otherwise organise people's everyday worlds.

Intention-to-treat analysis

A concept used in randomised controlled trials. It should be conducted as the primary analysis. With this type of analysis, outcome measures are obtained regardless of compliance with the trial protocol, and data from all participants are analysed according to allocation, even if the participants had adverse events or unexpected outcomes.

Intentionality

The assumption that the life-world 'is not an objective environment or a subjective consciousness or a set of beliefs; rather, [it] is what we

perceive and experience it to be'
(Finlay 1999, p. 302).

Internal validity
The truthfulness of the findings of a
study based on the methods used in that
study, i.e. are the methods used valid
and reliable, and is there little chance of
confounders or bias?

Interpretive or hermeneutic phenomenology
Focuses on describing the meanings
attributed by individuals' 'being in the
world and how these meanings influence
the choices that they make' (Lopez & Willis
2004, p. 729). Researchers working in this
tradition would encourage participants to
describe interactions, relations with others,
physical experiences and so on in order to
place the lived experience in the context of
daily life.

Interval data
These have the property of a rank order,
and distances or intervals between the
units of measurement are equal. Interval
data meet the criteria for measurement
because it is possible to define the
distance between values and therefore
identify how much one individual or group
differs from another.

Interview transcript
The written record of an interview that
has been transcribed from the verbal
conversation. It is used for in-depth data
analysis in qualitative research.

Inverted funnel format survey
See Funnel format survey.

Key informant
An individual who is able to provide in-
depth information to an ethnographer.
It is a concept that is used more often
in ethnographic research than in other
qualitative methods.

Knowledge
'An accepted body of facts or ideas that
is acquired through the use of the senses
or reason' (Grinnell *et al.* 2011a, p. 9). It is
recognised that knowledge can also be
acquired through research methods.

Knowledge acquisition
Takes the position that the most efficient
way of 'knowing something' is through
research findings, which have been gathered
through the use of research methods.

Life-world
'The world of experience as it lived'
(Finlay 1999, p. 301), 'our sense of lived life'
(Rapport 2005, p. 131).

Likert scale
Is used to measure subjective variables
such as attitudes. The researcher
generates a number of statements (e.g.
attitudes) and wishes to measure the
extent to which participants agree or
disagree with the statements.

Line of argument
In meta-ethnography, the studies can be
tied to one another by noting just how one
study informs and goes beyond another.
The guiding question is what can be
said about the whole, based on selective
studies of the part.

Literature review
A written presentation resulting from
reviewing literature. It provides a critical
analysis of what is known and what is
not known, and lays the groundwork for
research which would lead to evidence-
based practice in health care.

Longitudinal cohort survey
A type of survey in which the primary
purpose is to track changes over time.
Longitudinal surveys administer the same
set of questions to individuals on repeated
occasions, and seek to understand how

individuals or groups change over time. They could be undertaken to monitor changes in health or some other variable over time, or to measure outcomes of certain interventions or treatments.

Longitudinal studies
These are useful to identify new cases (incidence) of a health state in a defined population and time-period. They follow a group of people over time to identify new cases (incidence) of a health state in a defined population and period.

MANOVA
See Multivariate analysis of variance.

Measurement
This term is used in a number of different contexts, including where the instrument or tool meets the requirements for being a measure, i.e. it is capable of measuring the magnitude of the attribute under evaluation using a calibrated scale. Measurement involves the process of description and quantification. It means recording physical or behavioural characteristics by assigning a value to aspects such as the quality, quantity, frequency or degree of those attributes.

Measurement errors
Occur when researchers do not measure accurately or when they measure a different variable from the one intended. Measurement errors can be either systematic or random, depending on whether they have a constant pattern.

Memos
Memos are documented accounts of the researcher's thoughts, ideas and reflections about the research process. Memos provide an audit trail of the researcher's analytical decision-making and logistical details about research activities.

Meta-analysis
A statistical technique that combines the results of similar studies into a single result that provides an estimate of the overall effect.

Meta-data analysis
Analysis of processed data from selected qualitative research studies.

Meta-ethnography
An approach that enables a rigorous procedure for deriving substantive interpretations about any set of ethnographic or interpretive studies.

Meta-method analysis
The study of research methods to determine the way qualitative methods are interpreted and implemented. Underlying methodological assumptions and trends and their meaning for the research finding are studied.

Metaphor
Used in narrative enquiry to enhance the meaning of stories by making an analogy with something familiar, or emphasising the meaning of experience that might be difficult to understand or convey in any other way.

Meta research
Critical analysis and synthesis, resulting in a deepened interpretive understanding and development of new or modified theory, thus creating a qualitative knowledge base for evidence-based care.

Meta-study
A systematic interpretive research approach that involves a tripartite analysis of data, method and theory, and finally a metasynthesis of an existing body of qualitative research and creative interpretation of the primary research to produce new and expanded understandings.

Metasummary

Aggregation of reports of primary qualitative studies containing findings in the form of topical or thematic summaries or surveys of data, which are not interpretive syntheses of data.

Metasynthesis

A generic term that represents qualitative review approaches on previous qualitative studies in a field of interest.

Meta-theory

Part of a meta-study. Determines the link between the theoretical perspective that frames each primary study and the methods, findings and conclusions of the research.

Method

The strategies and techniques that researchers use to acquire knowledge and collect data.

Methodology

'A specific philosophical and ethical approach to developing knowledge; a theory of how research should, or ought, to proceed given the nature of the issue it seeks to address' (Hammell 2006, p. 167).

Mixed format survey

This is particularly relevant for longer surveys covering a number of domains. Here, the questions are organised in sections or domains and particular formats are applied within domains.

Mixed methods

A research design that combines research methods from qualitative and quantitative research approaches within a single research study.

Moderator

A key person in focus groups method, who may or may not be the researcher. A moderator leads and guides group discussions; in some contexts 'facilitator' is the preferred term.

Morbidity

The state of a person's health, i.e. illness, disability, chronic disease and so forth.

Mortality

Death.

Multiple baseline design

When it is unlikely that treated behaviours will return to baseline levels after withdrawal of the treatment, multiple baseline designs are frequently the design of choice. In this design, the effects of treatment are replicated in several participants or in different target behaviours. The design also allows for replication in different treatment conditions within a single participant so that the relative effectiveness of one treatment over another can be investigated.

Multiple probe design

In some situations, the multiple probe design offers a cost-effective alternative to the multiple baseline design. Not all probes are taken in every session; rather, some are taken on a predetermined and less frequent schedule or once a requisite skill is obtained.

Multiple realities

The same objects or situations can mean different things to different people, and 'people and the worlds they occupy are inextricably intertwined' (Carpenter & Suto 2008, p. 66).

Multiple regression analysis

A multivariate procedure that can be used when there are three or more variables and the level of measurement is interval or ratio. It assesses the degree to which scores for a subset of these variables predict scores for another variable in the set.

Multivariate analysis of variance (MANOVA)

Used when there are two or more dependent variables (measures), each of which is measured on an interval or ratio scale, and where the set of scores for each is reasonably normally distributed. A MANOVA can be applied to designs where there are one or more independent variables, each with two or more levels.

Narrative analysis

An approach to the analysis of data generated mainly from a narrative enquiry approach, which can also used to analyse other qualitative data. Within this method, a story is created by imposing order on narrative data.

Narrative enquiry

A research method that focuses on the structure and nature of the narratives, or stories, produced.

Narrative review

Illustrates how ideas, conceptual frameworks and methodologies have become established within a specific health issue. Researchers critique existing research by evaluating, scrutinising and integrating it and place it within the context of their research.

Netnography

Collecting data on, and conveying, cultural institutions and experiences online.

Nominal data

Occur where objects or people are assigned to named categories according to some criterion, such as male/female.

Non-probability sampling

In this method, the probability of a potential research participant being selected is not known in advance. This sampling method does not provide representative samples for the populations from which they are drawn, so the findings cannot be generalised to a larger group of people. However, these methods are useful for research questions, particularly for qualitative research, that do not need to involve large populations.

Observation

The process of collecting data by looking rather than listening.

Observational epidemiological study

This type of study does not seek to intervene or change people's exposure status. Rather, the aim is to collect information about people's exposure and health outcomes as these naturally occur within the population. Observational studies can be considered as either descriptive or analytical.

Ontology

The study of the nature of being, existence or reality in general. It is concerned with understanding the kinds of things that construct the world. It asks whether or not there is a single objective reality in this world.

Open coding

See Descriptive coding.

Ordinal data

Result when observations are rank-ordered and values are assigned sequentially to reflect the logical ordering of categories. Common examples are Likert scales, which rank responses from low to high.

Outcome

In epidemiology, it refers to the health state that is under investigation and of interest. The outcome of interest is often referred to as the dependent variable. Other authors use the term 'disease'. In epidemiology, however, not all outcomes are diseases and in fact some outcomes may be desirable or favourable health states. It would be unfortunate and inappropriate to label these outcomes as disease.

Outcome measure

A term used in reference to the evaluative test used to measure the effect of the intervention (*see* Evaluative tests). Outcome measures should be both valid and reliable.

p value

All inferential tests produce a common value, the *p* value, that is critical in the interpretation of findings. This *p* value is one thing to examine when reading inferential statistics, because it represents the probability of the null hypothesis being true.

Participant observation

A particular method of collecting data, employed in ethnography. The researcher lives in the community under study, observes people's daily activities, participates in their everyday life, learns how they view the world and witnesses first-hand how they behave.

Participatory action research

A method in which research and action are joined in order to plan, implement and monitor change. The informants become co-researchers and hence have their voices heard in all aspects of the research. The researcher becomes a participant in the initiatives and uses their research knowledge and expertise to assist the informants in self-research.

Patient-reported outcome

An outcome where the patient, rather than the clinician, reports on the impact of a disease or intervention on the status of their health. When evaluating the effect of an intervention on a patient, the patient's perspective on whether that intervention is effective is most important.

Phenomenological reduction

The goal is to search for all possible meanings, to describe rather than explain, to gain rich, thick information that represents the essential nature of the individuals' experiences and that 'communicates the sense and logic of the phenomenon to others' (Todres 2005, p. 110) in a new way.

Phenomenology

A methodological approach that has a strong and dynamic philosophical and epistemological foundation that seeks to understand, describe and interpret human behaviour and the meaning individuals make of their experiences. Phenomenologists study people's understandings and interpretations of their experiences in their own terms, emphasising these as explanations for their actions.

Photovoice

This method rejects traditional paradigms of power and the production of knowledge within the research relationship. It allows people to record and reflect the concerns and needs of their community by taking photographs. It also promotes critical discussion about important issues through dialogue about the photographs. Using a camera to record their concerns and needs allows individuals who rarely have contact with those who make decisions over their lives to make their voices heard.

Physiotherapy Evidence Database (PEDro)

For the profession of physiotherapy, a relatively large body of relevant research evidence is available and has been collected, appraised and made available.

PICO concept or logic grid

A useful process to start a systematic review. PICO stands for Population, Intervention or indicator, Comparator or control, and Outcome.

Plot

A forestructure of narrative indicating how people think in recounting stories and revealing the meaning and significance of various story elements. Plot also indicates how people extract understanding from past events to make sense of present circumstances.

Population

In statistical research, the group or cases from which the sample in a research project is selected. The term is used in epidemiology to refer to all the people who live in a defined area or country.

Population-based health data

'Ongoing systems that collect and register all cases of a particular disease or class of diseases as they develop in a defined population' (Oleckno 2002, p. 349) or in a specific population group, e.g. women, children or indigenous people.

Population health data

A number of sources of population health data are freely available both internationally and nationally. Common sources of population health data that are routinely collected include census data and disease registries (e.g. births, deaths, cancer and infectious diseases). The collection of registry data is a national responsibility and often these data are provided to both the United Nations and the World Health Organization. Other sources of data include regular surveys such as the National Health Survey and hospital records.

Positionality

Is related to the 'position' from which a person 'chooses' to speak. The research question or aim is developed from this 'position' and to some extent it lends credibility and authority to the study. In addressing issues of positionality, researchers need to make a full explanation of their experience and knowledge of the research topic and their relationship with the participants.

Positivism

An approach to research derived from a belief that social science research methods should be scientific in the same way as the physical sciences such as physics or chemistry. Positivism views reality as being independent of our experiences of it, and being accessible through careful thinking, and observing and recording of our experiences. Qualitative researchers reject the arguments of positivism, pointing out that meanings and interpretations cannot be measured like physical objects.

Postmodern ethnography

Postmodern ethnography still requires the traditional methodological commitment to observation found in realist ethnography. But the use of key informants is required as the basis for detailed description and structural analysis of the social world, and the use of cases, particularly conflicts where individual interests seem opposed to social forces. It also requires an embedded sense of what it is like to live in the social world so described; the approaches used most commonly are life history. Ethnographers use these techniques in combination to provide greater ethnographic richness, as well as to improve the reliability of both data and interpretation.

Practice-based research

It has the following essential attributes: it is inductive (concepts derived from practice wisdom); it makes use of non-experimental or quasi-experimental designs; it seeks descriptive or correlational knowledge; it may be either retrospective or prospective; it may be quantitative or qualitative but tends to rely on instruments tailored to the needs of social practice rather than external standardised research instruments; it is collaborative in nature; and practice requirements tend to outweigh research considerations.

Pragmatic trial

One in which the investigators attempt to mimic common practice, thereby endeavouring as much as possible to make the results generalisable to everyday practice. Pragmatic trials have become more common over the past decade or so in an effort to make clinical trials more meaningful to clinicians and the public.

Pragmatism

A paradigm that has been promoted as an attractive philosophy within methodological pluralism. It argues that reality exists not only as natural and physical realities, but also as psychological and social realities, which include subjective experience and thought, language and culture. Knowledge is both constructed and based on the reality of the world in which we live and which we experience. Therefore researchers should employ a combination of methods that works best for answering their research questions.

Predictive test

It aims to assess individuals in terms of their likely future outcomes, e.g. hospital admission scores on the Functional Independence Measure were used to predict length of stay and discharge scores.

PRISMA statement

The PRISMA statement (Preferred Reporting Items for Systematic Reviews and Meta-Analyses) is an evidence-based set of twenty-seven items for reporting in systematic reviews and meta-analyses.

Probability sampling method

The method that requires that the probability of a participant being selected is known in advance. This method is important in quantitative research where, in most cases, the intent is to generalise the findings for the sample to the population from which the sample was taken. The four most common methods for drawing random samples are simple random sampling, systematic random sampling, stratified random sampling and cluster random sampling.

Project agreement or memorandum of understanding

It is drawn up to clarify the roles, responsibilities and expectations of the researcher and the community partners around particular issues such as ownership of data, outcomes and publications. While MOUs are seldom legally binding, this process is important for the collaborating partners to develop an understanding of each other's values and expectations.

Publication bias

Occurs when a trial is published or not published because of the direction of its findings. Studies that have a positive result are more likely to be published; trials finding no difference between groups are, on average, less likely or will take longer to be published.

Purposive sampling

Purposive sampling looks for cases that will be able to provide rich or in-depth information about the issue being examined in the research. It does not look for cases that will provide a representative sample, as in random sampling techniques in quantitative research.

Q² or Q squared

The combination of quantitative and qualitative approaches in a research study. It is the concept used in mixed methods research design.

Qualitative data analysis

An ongoing, cyclical process that occurs from the very beginning of the research.

Qualitative research

Research strategies that emphasise words rather than numbers in the process of data collection and analysis. The focus of qualitative research is on the generation of theories.

Qualitative research synthesis

It is both an interpretive product, i.e. the synthesis itself, and the methods and techniques used to create that product.

Quality assessment

An evaluation of the methodological quality of a particular study or studies. In systematic reviews, the quality assessment process can guide the interpretation of the review findings and help determine the strength of inferences we can make from the results. In clinical trials, a high-quality assessment rating is an indication that a study is not likely to be prone to confounders or bias, and is more likely to accurately reflect the effect of the intervention.

Quantitative research

Research strategies that place their emphasis on numbers in the process of data collection and analysis. The focus of the quantitative approach is on the testing of theories.

Questionnaire

A specific type of written survey made up of a structured series of questions. Questionnaires usually have highly standardised response options so that data can be easily analysed and compared across individuals or groups.

Randomisation

A mechanism where participants are randomly allocated an intervention, e.g. the active test intervention versus a placebo or a sham intervention. It is a powerful tool that ensures the study groups are as similar as possible except for the intervention being studied.

Randomised controlled trial

A clinical trial where participants are randomly assigned to groups in order to receive different interventions. This randomisation removes many of the effects that may bias the true result. It is currently considered the gold standard for evaluating the efficacy of an intervention, as it removes many of the effects that may bias the true result. Randomised controlled trials can either be explanatory or pragmatic.

Ratio data

These have the same properties as interval data, and have an empirical rather than an arbitrary zero. This is the highest level of measurement, and data from ratio scales have the greatest statistical utility because of their mathematical properties.

Reciprocal translation

In meta-ethnography, the studies can be combined such that one study can be presented in terms of another. They are then directly comparable as reciprocal and analogous translations.

Reflexivity

An essential strategy that makes explicit the deep-seated views and judgments that affect the research topic, including a full assessment of the influence of the researcher's background, assumptions, perceptions, values, beliefs and interests on the research process.

Refutational

In meta-ethnography, the studies can be set against one another such that the grounds for one study's refutation of another become visible. The accounts stand in relative opposition to each other and are essentially refutational or oppositional.

Reliability

The extent to which a measurement instrument is dependable, stable and consistent when repeated under identical conditions. 'Reliability' refers to the ability of the scale to provide consistent, stable information across time and across respondents. For instance, if someone completes the scale today and again in two days' time, do you get essentially the same responses?

Research

A planned activity that results in the construction of new knowledge which can be used to provide answers to some health problems or as evidence for health care practice.

Research-based practice

Has the following characteristics: it is deductive (concepts derived from theory); it seeks causal knowledge therefore it gives priority to experimental, randomised control group designs; it is prospective; and it relies on standardised, quantitative research instruments. While it is collaborative, research requirements tend in the main to outweigh practice considerations.

Research design

Refers to the type of research enquiry as well as an outline of the study.

Research ethics

Contemporary research ethics is understood as finding the balance between the risks and benefits associated with a research project. Risks relating to issues such as confidentiality, anonymity, discomfort from the procedures and so forth are set against the benefits not just to the participants but to the public at large. Decisions about research proposals are usually made by ethics committees. *See Human Research Ethics Committee.*

Research participant

A person who agrees to take part in the study on equal terms.

Research problem

An area of concern about which little is known, and which needs to be answered in order to improve health care practice. Often, it determines the complexity of the research project.

Research process

A planned activity that researchers use to construct their research project. It must be choreographed according to the research questions that they intend to examine.

Research proposal

A formal written document which provides full details of the research that researchers intend to conduct.

Research question

Questions that researchers intend to answer by conducting their proposed research.

Rigour

Rigorous qualitative research is trustworthy and can be relied upon by other researchers. In qualitative research, 'rigour' is preferred to 'validity' and 'reliability', terms used by quantitative researchers, because rigour indicates the different methodology involved in research that focuses on meanings and interpretations.

Risk of bias
The degree to which a study has employed measures to minimise bias.

Sample size
In a randomised controlled trial, this must be determined before the start of the trial. It should be large enough to be able to detect if the intervention being evaluated leads to a clinically worthwhile effect.

Search strategy
The process by which the potential literature to be included in the systematic review is identified.

Secondary data analysis
An analysis of data collected for purposes other than for a specific piece of research. Often, the data are taken from existing research results from other researchers.

Selection bias
Arises if the investigators systematically manipulate enrolment into the trial.

Selective coding
A level of analysis beyond axial coding, whereby a central or core theme is identified using the previous levels of analysis. At this point, researchers can begin formulating propositions by drawing conclusions, making causal connections and developing theoretical constructs.

Semi-structured interview
A technique that is often referred to as an 'in-depth interview' but that more accurately refers to an interview where the researchers have prepared some pre-interview questions (theme lists) and used them to elicit information, but at the same time allow the participants to elaborate on their responses.

Sensitive topics
May arise in research that involves the private sphere of an individual. Sensitive research includes studies that are intimate,

discreditable or incriminating, and may cause emotional upset or pose some physical and emotional risk to the participants.

Sequential design
A research design when one data set follows another and extends or explores the findings from the first set.
For example, a qualitative study is undertaken to explore a particular issue or phenomenon; researchers could create hypotheses from these results which they could then test using a survey or experimental design.

Single-subject experimental design
An experimental research method that focuses on a single individual and their response to treatment/s over time. Several terms have been used interchangeably for SSEDs: single-case designs or single-case experimental designs; single-subject designs; interrupted time series designs; N of 1; small N designs.

Snowball sampling
Sampling that relies on existing participants to identify acquaintances who fit the inclusion criteria of a study in order to increase the size of the sample, particularly when a population is difficult to locate.

Standardised scale
It provides a scientific form of health assessment that is particularly useful for measuring subjective constructs such as pain, mood and level of symptoms. Standardised scales are made up of a series of self-report questions, ratings or items that measure a specific concept, and response categories are in the same format and can be summed or aggregated in some weighted form.

Statistical significance
Whether or not an outcome is statistically significant can be established by using a statistical test to decide whether the

outcome is likely to be due to chance or to be real. If the probability of obtaining the effect by chance is low, then it is concluded that the effect is real, i.e. it is statistically significant.

Steering committee or advisory group
Researchers using CPR often establish a steering committee or advisory group to provide advice and guidance on all matters pertaining to the community with whom and for whom the research is being conducted.

Stopping rule bias
A concept relevant to randomised controlled trials. It can occur if a trial is stopped inappropriately.

Surrogate outcome measure
An outcome that is measured from a source that is not directly from the patient; for example, a blood test or an x-ray measurement, which is used because it may have a relationship with change in the patient's health.

Survey
A descriptive research method where respondents are asked a series of questions in a standard manner so that responses can be easily quantified and analysed statistically. This enables the researcher to describe the characteristics of the sample being studied and to make generalisations to the larger population of interest.

Survey to test intervention effects
A survey in which the primary question is whether a particular intervention or experiment produces change in outcomes. It takes measures before and after a treatment or intervention to determine whether the intervention is associated with hypothesised improvement.

Symbolic interactionism
A theoretical perspective that explains human behaviour and human interaction through the use of symbolic communication and shared meanings. People interact with others and objects based on the meaning those things have for the individual.

Systematic review
A comprehensive identification and synthesis of the available literature on a specified topic. Systematic reviews are different from narrative reviews in that they provide an objective or scientific summary of the literature rather than a subjective opinion-based summary. In a systematic review, literature is treated as data.

Thematic analysis
The identification of themes through a careful reading and rereading of the data. The method is inductive, building up concepts and theories from the data, compared with the deductive method of content analysis.

Theme
A grouping of data emerging from the research, to which the researcher gives a name.

Theoretical assumptions
Hypothetical statements that explain, or are used to predict, certain phenomena. Theoretical models are diagrammatic explanations of hypothetical relationships. They are used to guide what is to be measured. If the intention is to improve participation, then participation must be carefully defined and measured. If the intention is to investigate relationships between constructs within the model, e.g. the relationship between impairments of body function and participation, then both elements must be evaluated. Careful consideration of the theoretical assumptions under investigation (in practice and research) is an essential component of all test selection.

Theoretical sampling
The procedure for collecting data in order to generate theory. The researcher adopts an iterative process of concurrently collecting, analysing and coding data to determine the type of data that should be collected next, so as to develop the emerging theory.

Theoretical sensitivity
The researcher's ability to have insight into the nuances inherent within the data based on previous knowledge and experiences relevant to the area. Sources of theoretical sensitivity may be the literature and personal and professional experience.

Theory-builders in CAQDAS
CAQDAS programs offer different facilities such as conceptual mapping to help researchers examine relationships between codes and categories from text. Often, these facilities are referred to as 'theory-builders'. Importantly, this capacity does not mean that the program can build theory on its own. Rather, the CAQDAS will have various in-built tools that help researchers to make comparisons and develop some theoretical ideas.

Thick description
Descriptions based on qualitative research, typically ethnography, where ample detail and background information are provided so that people's actions can be understood in the context of the experiences and patterns of meaning that influence them.

Transformative paradigm
The transformative paradigm emphasises that all research should address issues of social justice and be for the betterment of the human race. In addition, within the research design any issues of power imbalance between the researcher and the researched must be addressed.

Triangulation
The use of multiple methods, researchers, data sources or theories in a research project. It recognises the value of different methods of data collection and/or different methods of analysis in teasing out answers to complex questions regarding health-related behaviours.

t-test
It is used to compare two means with each other, to establish if there is a statistically significant difference between them. There are several versions of the t-test. These include the one-sample t-test, which is used to compare a mean for a single set of scores with another mean, and two-sample t-tests, which are used when there are two sets of scores, the means of which are to be compared with each other.

Type I statistical error
It occurs when the researchers mistakenly conclude that a finding was statistically significant when it may actually have been the result of chance rather than a real difference. Testing multiple non-prespecified hypotheses inflates the Type I statistical error rate, resulting in spurious and often implausible findings.

Type II statistical error
It occurs when the investigators conclude that there is no significant different between the groups (i.e. that the intervention being studied is not effective); there may have been a clinically important effect but the trial did not have a sufficiently large sample size to detect it statistically. This is more likely to occur when sample sizes are low.

Unobtrusive method
A method that does not require direct contact with the informants. It makes use of data that have been published

or are available in libraries, the press or other media. Indirect and unobtrusive observation, where the informants have no knowledge about the research, is also employed.

Utilitarian

An ethical issue based on the assumption that it is possible to predict the likely consequences of an action (in this case research) and the likely benefit it will have for the greatest number of people.

Validity

The extent to which an instrument measures what it is intended to measure. 'Validity' refers to the degree to which the scale measures what it is supposed to measure (content and construct validity). For instance, does it have a good correlation with another gold standard measure?

Variable

An attribute that varies between individuals, objects, qualities and properties. It may refer to health issues, for example respiratory rate and blood pressure, or characteristics of people, such as male and female, occupations such as farmers, medical practitioners and nurses, or concepts such as anxiety, coping strategy, stigma and discrimination, which

can be measured directly using scales and questionnaires

Verbal rating scale

It is commonly used where a question is asked and a range of verbal response categories is provided. Participants circle the response that most closely represents their view.

Virtue ethics

A situation where judgments are made about a person (*qua* researcher) by their demonstrated moral character.

Visual analogue scale

Allows respondents to rate items on a continuous line between two end points. Typically, participants are asked to mark a position on the line that goes from 0 to 10 or from 0 to 100.

Vulnerable people

Individuals who are marginalised and discriminated against in society because of their social positions, based on class, ethnicity, gender, age, illness, disability or sexual preferences. Often, they are difficult to reach and require special consideration when they are involved in research. The term is also used to refer to people who are difficult to access in societies.

REFERENCES

Aagaard, H. & Hall, E.O.C. (2008). Mothers' experiences of having a preterm infant in the neonatal care unit: a meta-synthesis. *Journal of Pediatric Nursing*, 23(3), 26–36.

Aamodt, A. (1982). Examining ethnography for nurse researchers. *Western Journal of Nursing Research*, 4(2), 209–21.

ABS (2006a). *National health survey: summary of results, Australia 2004–05*. Cat. No. 4364.0. Canberra: Australian Bureau of Statistics. <www.ausstats.abs.gov.au/ausstats/subscriber.nsf/0/3 B1917236618A042CA25711F00185526/$File/43640_2004-05.pdf>.

ABS (2006b). *2004–05 National Health Survey: user's guide—electronic publication*. Cat. No. 4363.0.55.001. Canberra: Australian Bureau of Statistics.

ABS (2007). *1986, 1996 and 2006 Census of population and housing, customised tables*. Canberra: Australian Bureau of Statistics.

ABS (2009a). Births. Canberra: Australian Bureau of Statistics. <www.abs.gov.au/AUSSTATS/abs@. nsf/DSSbyCollectionid/C25FB9875049D14ACA256BD000281108?opendocument>.

ABS (2009b). 2007–08 *National Health Survey: Summary of results, Australia*. ABS Cat. No. 4364.0. Reissue. Canberra: Australian Bureau of Statistics. www.abs.gov.au/AUSSTATS/abs@.nsf/mf/4364.0.

ABS (2011a). *Gender indicators, Australia July 2011*. Cat. No. 4125.0. Canberra: Australian Bureau of Statistics. <www.abs.gov.au>.

ABS (2011b). *Census dictionary*. Cat. No. 2901.0 – Marital status. www.abs.gov.au/ausstats/abs@.nsf/ Lookup/2901.0Chapter40402011.

Acocella, I. (2012). The focus groups in social research: advantages and disadvantages. *Quality and Quantity*, 46(4), 1125–36.

Adams, S. (2015). Identifying research questions. In N.A. Schmidt & J.M. Brown (eds), *Evidence-based practice for nurses: appraisal and application of research*, 3rd edn. Burlington, MA: Jones & Bartlett Learning, 70–93.

Ahern, K.J. (1999). Ten tips for reflexive bracketing. *Qualitative Health Research*, 9, 407–11.

AIHW (2009). *National Hospital Morbidity Data Collection*. Canberra: Australian Institute of Health and Welfare. <www.aihw.gov.au/hospitals/nhm_database.cfm>.

AIHW (2015a). *Aboriginal and Torres Strait Islander health performance framework 2014 report: detailed analyses*. Cat. No. IHW 167. Canberra: Australian Institute of Health and Welfare.

AIHW (2015b). *The health and welfare of Australia's Aboriginal and Torres Strait Islander peoples 2015*. Cat. No. IHW 147. Canberra: Australian Institute of Health and Welfare.

AIHW (2015c). *Cervical screening in Australia 2012–2013*. Cancer series no. 93. Cat. No. CAN 91. Canberra: Australian Institute of Health and Welfare. <http://www.aihw.gov.au/publication-detail/?id=60129550871>.

AIHW (2015d). GRIM (General Record of Incidence of Mortality) books. Canberra: Australian Institute of Health and Welfare. <http://www.aihw.gov.au/deaths/grim-books/>.

AIHW (n.d.). Data online 2009.Canberra: Australian Institute of Health and Welfare. <www.aihw.gov. au/dataonline.cfm>.

Al-Abbad, H. & Simon, J.V. (2013). The effectiveness of extracorporeal shock wave therapy on chronic achilles tendinopathy: a systematic review. *Foot & Ankle International*, 34(1), 33–41.

Alexopoulos, G.S., Abrams, R.C., Young, R.C. & Shamoian, C.A. (1988). Cornell scale for depression in dementia. *Biological Psychiatry*, 23, 271–84.

Altheide, D.L. & Johnson, J.M. (2011). Reflections on interpretive adequacy in qualitative research. In N.K. Denzin & Y.S. Lincoln (eds), *The Sage handbook of qualitative research*, 4th edn. Thousand Oaks, CA: Sage, 581–94.

Altman, D.G. (1980). Statistics and ethics in research. III. How large a sample? *British Medical Journal*, 281, 1336–8.

Altman, D.G., Schulz, K.F., Moher, D., Egger, M., Davidoff, F., Elbourne, D. *et al.* (2001). The revised CONSORT statement for reporting randomized trials: explanation and elaboration. *Annals of Internal Medicine*, 134(8), 663–94.

Alvesson, M. & Sandberg, J. (2013). *Constructing research questions: doing interesting research*. London: Sage.

American Academy of Orthopaedic Surgeons (2014). *Management of anterior cruciate ligament injuries: evidence-based clinical practice guideline*. Rosemont, IL: American Academy of Orthopaedic Surgeons.

American Association for the Advancement of Science & Mead, M. (1968). *Science and the concept of race*. New York: Columbia University Press.

American Educational Research Association, A.P.A. & National Council on Measurement in Education (2014). *Standards for educational and psychological testing*. Washington DC: American Educational Research Association.

Anastas, J. (2005). Observation. In R. Grinnell & Y. Unrau (eds), *Social work research and evaluation: quantitative and qualitative approaches*. New York: Oxford University Press, 213–30.

Anderson, K. (2012). The teaching and practice of health promotion in nursing: the missed opportunities. Unpublished PhD thesis. School of Public Health, La Trobe University, Bendigo.

Andrew, S., Salamonson, Y., Everrett, B., Halcomb, E.J. & Davidson, P.M. (2011). Beyond the ceiling effect: using a mixed methods approach to measure patient satisfaction. *International Journal of Multiple Research Approaches*, 5(1), 52–63.

Anfara, V.A. & Mertz, N.T. (2014). *Theoretical frameworks in qualitative research*, 2nd edn. Los Angeles: Sage.

Angell, B. (2011). The occupational experiences of mothers caring for a young person with first episode psychosis: a narrative study. Unpublished honours thesis. La Trobe University, Melbourne.

Angen, M.J. (2000). Evaluating interpretive inquiry: reviewing the validity debate and opening the dialogue. *Qualitative Health Research*, 10(3), 378–95.

Annells, M. (1996). Grounded theory method: philosophical perspectives, paradigm of inquiry, and postmodernism. *Qualitative Health Research*, 6(3), 379–93.

Annells, M. (1997a). Grounded theory method, part I: Within the five moments of qualitative research. *Nursing Inquiry*, 4, 120–9.

Annells, M. (1997b). Grounded theory method, part II: Options for users of the method. *Nursing Inquiry*, 4, 176–80.

Annells, M. (2005). A qualitative quandary: alternative representation and meta-synthesis. *Journal of Clinical Nursing*, 14, 535–6.

Anusasananun, B., Pothiban, L., Kasemkitwatana, S., Soivong, P. & Trakultivakorn, H. (2013). Coping behaviors and predicting factors among breast cancer survivors during each phase of cancer survivorship. *Pacific Rim International Journal of Nursing Research*, 17(2), 148–66.

Aoun, S.M. & Kristjanson, L.J. (2005). Evidence in palliative care research: how should it be gathered? *Medical Journal of Australia*, 183(5), 264–6.

Ardern, C.L., Webster, K.E., Taylor, N.F. & Feller, J.A. (2011). Return to sport following anterior cruciate ligament reconstruction surgery: a systematic review and meta-analysis of the state of play. *British Journal of Sports Medicine*, 45, 596–606.

Argyris, C. & Schon, D. (1974). *Theory and practice: increasing professional effectiveness*. San Francisco: Jossey-Bass.

Arndt, M., Murchie, F., Schembri, A. & Davidson, P. (2009). 'Others had similar problems and you were not alone': evaluation of an open group mutual aid model in cardiac rehabilitation. *Journal of Cardiovascular Nursing*, 24(4), 328–35.

Arroll, B., Robb, G. & Sutich, E. (2003). *The diagnosis and management of soft tissue knee injuries: internal derangements. Best practice evidence-based guideline*. New Zealand Guidelines Group.

Asadoorian, J., Hearson, B., Satyanarayana, S. & Ursel, J. (2010). Evidence based practice in dental hygiene: exploring the enhancers and barriers across disciplines. *Canadian Journal of Dental Hygiene*, 44(6), 271–6.

Atkinson, R. (2007). The life story interview as a bridge in narrative inquiry. In D.J. Clandinin (ed.), *Handbook of narrative inquiry: mapping a methodology*. Thousand Oaks, CA: Sage.

Audet, J. & d'Amboise, G. (2001). The multi-site study: an innovative research methodology. *The Qualitative Report* (2). <www.nova.edu/ssss/QR/QR6-2/index.html>.

Audrey, S. (2011). Qualitative research in evidence-based medicine: improving decision-making and participation in randomized controlled trials of cancer treatment. *Palliative Medicine*, 25(8), 758–65.

Auslander, G., Dobrof, J. & Epstein, I. (2001). Comparing social work's role in renal dialysis in Israel and the United States: a practice-based research potential of available clinical information. *Social Work in Health Care*, 33(3/4), 129–51.

Austin, P.C., Mamdani, M.M., Juurlink, D.N. & Hux, J.E. (2006). Testing multiple statistical hypotheses resulted in spurious associations: a study of astrological signs and health. *Journal of Clinical Epidemiology*, 59(9), 964–9.

Australian Centre for Evidence Based Aged Care (2009). *Strengthening care outcomes for residents with evidence (SCORE) summary report May 2009*. <www.health.vic.gov.au/agedcare/downloads/score/score_summary_report_may_09.pdf>.

Australian Council on Healthcare Standards (2004). *ACHS News*, 12, 4.

Australian Nursing and Midwifery Federation (2014). *National practice standards for nurses in general practice*. Melbourne: Australian Nursing and Midwifery Federation, Federal Office.

Aveyard, H. (2014). *Doing a literature review in health and social care*, 3rd edn. Maidenhead: Open University Press.

Avis, M. (2003). Do we need methodological theory to do qualitative research? *Qualitative Health Research*, 13(7), 995–1004.

Babbie, E. (2014). *The basics of social research*, 6th edn. Belmont, CA: Wadsworth.

Babbie, E. (2016). *The practice of social research*, 14th edn. Boston, MA: Cengage Learning.

Bailey, A. (2008). Let's tell you a story: use of vignettes in focus group discussions on HIV/AIDS among migrant and mobile men in Goa, India. In P. Liamputtong (ed.), *Doing cross-cultural research: ethical and methodological perspectives*. Dordrecht: Springer, 253–64.

Bailey, D. & Kerlin, L. (2015). Can health trainers make a difference with difficult-to-engage clients? A multisite case study. *Health Promotion Practice*, 16(5), 756–64.

Baillie, L. (1995). Ethnography and nursing research: a critical appraisal. *Nurse Researcher*, 3(2), 5–21.

Baluch, B. & Davies, P. (2008). Poverty dynamics and life trajectories in rural Bangladesh. *International Journal of Multiple Research Approaches*, 2(2), 176–90.

Bamberg, M. (2007). *Narrative: state of the art*. Amsterdam: John Benjamins.

Barbour, R. (2008). *Introducing qualitative research: a student's guide to the craft of doing qualitative research*. London: Sage.

Barbour, R. (2014). *Introducing qualitative research: a student's guide*, 2nd edn. London: Sage.

Barclay, R., Ripat, J. & Mayo, N. (2015). Factors describing community ambulation after stroke: a mixed-methods study. *Clinical Rehabilitation*, 29(5), 509–21.

Barnett-Page, E. & Thomas, J. (2009). Methods for the synthesis of qualitative research: a critical review. *BMC Medical Research Methodology*, 9(59). Doi:10.1186/1471-2288-9-59.

Barratt, R. (1991). *Culture and conduct: an excursion in anthropology*, 2nd edn. Belmont, CA: Wadsworth.

Barroso, J., Gollop, C.J., Sandelowski, M., Meynell, J., Pearce, P.F. & Collonis, L.J. (2003). The challenges of searching for and retrieving qualitative studies. *Western Journal of Nursing Research*, 25(2), 153–78.

Barter-Godfrey, S.H. & Taket, A.R. (2007). Understanding women's breast screening behaviour: a study carried out in South East London, with women aged 50–64 years. *Health Education Journal*, 66(4), 335–46.

Bateson, G. & Mead, M. (1942). *Balinese character: a photographic analysis*. New York: New York Academy of Sciences.

Bateson, G. (1973). *Steps towards an ecology of mind*. London: Paladin.

Baum, F. (2015). *The new public health*, 4th edn. Melbourne: Oxford University Press.

Bauman, Z. (2005). Afterthought: on writing: on writing sociology. In N.K. Denzin & Y.S. Lincoln (eds), *The Sage handbook of qualitative research*. Thousand Oaks, CA: Sage, 1089–98.

Bazeley, P. (2007). *Qualitative data analysis with NVivo*, 3rd edn. London: Sage.

Bazeley, P. (2012). Regulating qualitative coding using QDAS. *Sociological Methodology*, 42(1), 77–8.

Bazeley, P. (2013). *Qualitative data analysis: practical strategies*. Thousand Oaks, CA: Sage.

Bazeley, P. & Jackson, K. (2013). *Qualitative data analysis with NVivo*, 2nd edn. London: Sage.

Beadle-Brown, J., Mansell, J. & Kozma, A. (2007). De-institutionalization in intellectual disabilities. *Current Opinion in Psychiatry*, 20, 437–42.

Beauchamp, T.L. & Childress, J.F. (2001). *Principles of biomedical ethics*, 5th edn. Oxford: Oxford University Press.

Beck, C.T. (2002a). Mothering multiples: a meta-synthesis of qualitative research. *American Journal of Maternal Child Nursing*, 27(4), 214–21.

Beck, C.T. (2002b). Postpartum depression: a metasynthesis. *Qualitative Health Research*, 12(4), 453–72.

Beck, C.T. (2009). Metasynthesis: a goldmine for evidence-based practice. *AORN Journal*, 90(5), 701–10.

Beck, C.T. (2011). A meta-ethnography of traumatic childbirth and its aftermath: amplifying causal looping. *Qualitative Health Research*, 21(3), 301–11.

Beck, C.T. (ed.) (2013). *Routledge international handbook of qualitative nursing research*. New York: Routledge.

Becker, P. (1993). Common pitfalls of published grounded theory research. *Qualitative Health Research*, 3(2), 254–60.

Beckerman, H., Roebroeck, M.E., Lankhorst, G.J., Becher, J.G., Bezemer, P.D. & Verbeek, A.L.M. (2001). Smallest real difference: a link between reproducibility and responsiveness. *Quality of Life Research*, 10, 571–8.

Beckett, K. (2013). Professional wellbeing and caring: exploring a complex relationship. *British Journal of Nursing*, 22(19), 1118–24.

Begg, C., Cho, M., Eastwood, S., Horton, R., Moher, D., Olkin, I. *et al.* (1996). Improving the quality of reporting of randomized controlled trials: the CONSORT statement. *Journal of the American Medical Association*, 276, 637–9.

Belgrave, L.L., Zablotsky, D. & Guadagno, M.A. (2002). How do we talk to each other? Writing qualitative research for quantitative readers. *Qualitative Health Research*, 12(10), 1427–39.

Bench, S. & Day, T. (2010). The user experience of critical care discharge: a meta-synthesis of qualitative research. *International Journal of Nursing Studies*, 47, 487–99.

Benjaminse, A., Gokeler, A. & van der Schans, C.P. (2006). Clinical diagnosis of an anterior cruciate ligament rupture: a meta-analysis. *Journal of Orthopaedic & Sports Physical Therapy*, 36(5), 267–88.

Benning, A., Ghaleb, M., Suokas, A., Dixon-Woods, M., Dawson, J., Barber, N. *et al.* (2011). Large-scale organisational intervention to improve patient safety in four UK hospitals: mixed method evaluation. *British Medical Journal*, 342, d195.

Beretvas, S. & Chung, H. (2008). A review of meta-analyses of single-subject experimental designs: methodological issues and practice. *Evidence-based Communication Assessment and Intervention*, 2(3), 129–41.

Bettelheim, B. (1943). Individual and mass behavior in extreme situations. *Journal of Abnormal and Social Psychology*, 38, 417–52.

Bhagwanjee, S., Muckart, D.J., Jeena, P.M. & Moodley, P. (1997a). Does HIV status influence the outcome of patients admitted to a surgical intensive care unit? A prospective double blind study. *British Medical Journal*, 314, 1077–81.

Bhangwanjee, S., Muckart, D.J., Jeena, P.M. & Moodley, P. (1997b). Letter: Why we did not seek informed consent before testing patients for HIV. *British Medical Journal*, 314, 1081–84.

Biddle, S.J.H., Fox, K.R., Boutcher, S.H. & Faulkner, G.E. (2000). The way forward for physical activity and the promotion of psychological well-being. In S.J.H. Biddle, K.R. Fox & S. H. Boutcher (eds), *Physical activity and psychological well-being*. New York: Routledge, 154–68.

Biesta, G. (2010). Pragmatism and the philosophical foundations of mixed methods research. In A. Tashakkori and C. Teddlie (eds), *The Sage handbook of mixed methods in social and behavioural research*. Thousand Oaks, CA: Sage, 95–117.

Billig, M. (2013). *Learn to write badly: how to succeed in the social sciences*. Cambridge: Cambridge University Press.

Bingham, S.A., Day, N.E., Luben, R. *et al.* (2003). Dietary fibre in food and protection against colorectal cancer in the European Prospective Investigation into Cancer and Nutrition (EPIC): an observational study. *Lancet*, 361, 1496–501.

Birks, M. & Mills, J. (2012). *Grounded theory: a practical guide*. London: Sage.

Birks, M., Chapman, Y. & Francis, K. (2008). Memoing in qualitative research: probing data and processes. *Journal of Research in Nursing*, 13(1), 68–75.

Bland, J.M. & Altman, D.G. (1986). Statistical methods for assessing agreement between two methods of clinical measurement. *The Lancet*, 1(8476), 307–10.

Blaxter, M. (1996). Criteria for the evaluation of qualitative research papers. *Medical Sociology News*, 22(1), 68–71.

Bloom, J.R., Stewart, S.L., Johnston, M., Banks, P. & Fobair, P. (2001). Sources of support and the physical and mental well-being of young women with breast cancer. *Social Science & Medicine*, 53(11), 1513–24.

Blumer, H. (1969). *Symbolic interactionism: perspective and method*. Englewood Cliffs, NJ: Prentice-Hall.

Blumer, H. (1969/1986). *Symbolic interactionism: perspective and method*. Berkeley, CA: University of California Press.

Bochner, A. (2000). Criteria against ourselves. *Qualitative Inquiry*, 6(2), 266–72.

Bochner, A. & Riggs, N. (2014). Practicing narrative inquiry. In P. Leavy (ed.), *The Oxford handbook of qualitative research*. Oxford: Oxford University Press.

Bogdan, R.C. & Biklen, S.K. (2007). *Qualitative research for education: an introduction to theory and methods*, 5th edn. Boston, MA: Pearson.

Bond, T.G. & Fox, C. (2007). *Applying the Rasch model: fundamental measurement in the human sciences*, 2nd edn. New Jersey: Lawrence Erlbaum.

Bondas, T. (2013). Finland and Sweden: qualitative research from nursing to caring. In C.T. Beck (ed.), *Routledge international handbook of qualitative nursing research*. New York: Routledge, 527–45.

Bondas, T. & Hall, E. (2007a). Challenges in the approaches to metasynthesis research. *Qualitative Health Research*, 17, 113–21.

Bondas, T. & Hall, E. (2007b). A decade of metasynthesis research: a meta-method study. *International Journal of Qualitative Studies on Health and Wellbeing*, 2(2), 101–13.

Booth, A., Carroll, D., Ilott, I., Low, L.L. & Cooper, K. (2013). Desperately seeking dissonance: identifying the disconfirming case in qualitative evidence synthesis. *Qualitative Health Research*, 23(1), 126–41.

Booth, A., Papaioannou, D. & Sutton, A. (2012). *Systematic approaches to a successful literature review*. London: Sage.

Booth, T. (1999). Doing research with lonely people. *British Journal of Learning Disabilities*, 26(1), 132–4.

Bourgois, P.I. (1995). *In search of respect: selling crack in El Barrio*. Cambridge: Cambridge University Press.

Bourgois, P.I. & Schonberg, J. (2009). *Righteous dopefiend*. Berkeley, CA: University of California Press.

Boutron, I., Guittet, L., Estellat, C., Moher, D., Hróbjartsson, A. & Ravaud, P. (2007). Reporting methods of blinding in randomized trials assessing nonpharmacological treatments. *PLoS Medicine*, 4(2), e61.

Boutron, I., Moher, D., Altman, D., Schulz, K. & Ravaud, P. (2008). Methods and processes of the CONSORT Group: example of an extension for trials assessing nonpharmacologic treatments. *Annals of Internal Medicine*, 148, W60–W66.

Bowling, A. (2005). *Measuring health: a review of quality of life measurement scales*, 3rd edn. Maidenhead, UK: Open University Press.

Boychuk-Duchscher, J.E. & Morgan, D. (2004). Grounded theory: reflections on the emergence vs. forcing debate. *Journal of Advanced Nursing*, 48, 605–12.

Boydell, N., Fergie, G., McDaid, L. & Hilton, S. (2014). Avoiding pitfalls and realising opportunities: reflecting on issues of sampling and recruitment for online focus groups. *International Journal of Qualitative Methods*, 13, 206–23.

Braun, V. & Clarke, V. (2006). Using thematic analysis in psychology. *Qualitative Research in Psychology*, 3, 77–101.

Braun, V. & Clarke, V. (2013). *Successful qualitative research: a practical guide for beginners*. London: Sage.

Bray, J., Lee, L., Smith, S. & Yorks, L. (eds) (2000). *Collaborative inquiry in practice: action, reflection and making meaning*. Thousand Oaks, CA: Sage.

Brinkmann, S. & Kvale, S. (2014). *InterViews: learning the craft of qualitative research interviewing*, 3rd edn. Sage: London.

Britten, N., Campbell, R., Pope, C., Donovan, J. & Morgan, M. (2002). Using meta-ethnography to synthesise qualitative research: a worked example. *Journal of Health Service Research & Policy*, 7(4), 209–15.

Brotherton, J.M.L., Fridman, M., May, C.L., Chappell, G., Saville, A.M. & Gertig, D.M. (2011). Early effect of the HPV vaccination programme on cervical abnormalities in Victoria, Australia: an ecological study. *The Lancet*, 377(9783), 2085–9.

Bruce, C., Parker, A. & Renfrew, L. (2006). 'Helping or something': perceptions of students with aphasia and tutors in further education. *International Journal of Language & Communication Disorders*, 41(2), 137–54.

Brusco, T., Taylor, N., Watts, J. & Shields, N. (2014). Economic evaluation of adult rehabilitation: a systematic review and meta-analysis of randomized controlled trials in a variety of settings. *Archives of Physical Medicine and Rehabilitation*, 95, 94–116.

Bryman, A. (2007). Barriers to integrating qualitative and quantitative research. *Journal of Mixed Methods Research*, 1(1), 8–22.

Bryman, A. (2016). *Social research methods*, 5th edn. Oxford: Oxford University Press.

Bryman, A., Becker, S. & Sempik, J. (2008). Quality criteria for quantitative, qualitative and mixed methods research: a view from social policy. *International Journal of Social Research Methodology*, 11(4), 261–76.

Bull, M.J. (2014). Strategies for sustaining self used by family caregivers for older adults with dementia. *Journal of Holistic Nursing*, 32(2), 127–35.

Bulmer, M. (ed.) (1982). *Social research ethics*. London: Macmillan.

Bussing, R., Koro-Ljungberg, M., Gagnon, J.C., Mason, D.M., Ellison, A., Noguchi, K., Garvan, C.W. & Albarracin, D. (2014). Feasibility of school-based ADHD interventions: a mixed-methods study of perceptions of adolescents and adults. *Journal of Attention Disorders*. Doi:10.1177/1087054713515747.

Buston, K. (1997). NUD*IST in action: its use and its usefulness in a study of chronic illness in young people. *Sociological Research Online*, 2(3). <www.socresonline.org.uk/socresonline/2/3/6.html>.

Butera-Prinzi, F. & Perlesz, A. (2004). Children's experience of living with a parent with a head injury. *Brain Injury*, 18(1), 83–101.

Byham-Gray, L.D., Gilbride, J.A., Dixon, B. & Stage, F.K. (2005). Evidence-based practice: what are dieticians' perceptions, attitudes, and knowledge? *Journal of the American Dietetic Association*, October, 1574–81.

Byrne, M. (2001). Ethnography as a qualitative research method. *AORN Journal*, 74(1), 82–4.

Cabrall, A. (2012). *Why use NVivo for your literature review?* https://anujacabraal.wordpress.com/2012/08/01/why-use-nvivo-for-your-literature-review/

Callahan, C.M., Sachs, G.A., LaMantia, M.A., Unroe, K.T., Arling, G. & Boustani, M.A. (2014). Redesigning systems of care for older adults with Alzheimer's disease. *Health Affairs*, 33(4), 626–32.

Campbell, R., Pound, P., Pope, C., Britten, N., Pill, R., Morgan, M. *et al.* (2003). Evaluating meta-ethnography: a synthesis of qualitative research on lay experiences of diabetes and diabetes care. *Social Science & Medicine*, 56, 671–84.

Cao, Y., Davidson, P.M. & Digiacomo, M. (2009a). Cardiovascular disease in China: an urgent need to enhance the nursing role to improve health outcomes. *Journal of clinical nursing*, 18(5), 687–93.

Cao, Y., DiGiacomo, M., Du, H.Y. & Davidson, P.M. (2009b). Chinese nurses' perceptions of heart health issues facing women in China: a focus group study. *Journal of Cardiovascular Nursing*, 24(6), E2–E29.

Caplan B. & Reidy, K. (1996). Staff–patient–family conflicts in rehabilitation: sources and solutions. *Topics in Spinal Cord Injury Rehabilitation*, 2, 21–33.

Caracelli, V.J. & Riggin, L.J.C. (1994). Mixed-method evaluation: developing quality criteria through concept mapping. *Evaluation Practice*, 15, 139–52.

Carding, P. & Hillman, R. (2001). More randomised controlled studies in speech and language therapy. *British Medical Journal*, 323, 645–6.

Carlsen, B. & Glenton, C. (2011). What about N? A methodological study of sample-size reporting in focus group studies. *BMC Medical Research Methodology*, 11(1), 26.

Carpenter, C. (1994). The experience of spinal cord injury: the individual's perspective: implications for rehabilitation practice. *Physical Therapy*, 74(7), 614–29.

Carpenter, C. (2013). Phenomenology in rehabilitation research. In P. Liamputtong (ed.), *Research methods in health: foundations for evidence-based practices*, 2nd edn. Melbourne: Oxford University Press, 115–31.

Carpenter, C. & Hammell, K. (2000). Evaluating qualitative research. In K.W. Hammell, C. Carpenter & I. Dyck (eds), *Using qualitative research: a practical introduction for occupational and physical therapists*. Edinburgh: Churchill Livingstone, 107–19.

Carpenter, C. & Suto, M. (2008). *Qualitative research for occupational and physical therapists: a practical guide*. Oxford: Wiley-Blackwell.

Carr, W. & Kemmis, S. (1986). *Becoming critical: education, knowledge, and action research*. Philadelphia, PA: Falmer Press.

Carroll, C. (2010). 'It's not everyday that parents get a chance to talk like this': exploring parents' perceptions and expectations of speech-language pathology services for children with intellectual disability. *International Journal of Speech-Language Pathology*, 12(4), 352–61.

CASP (2013). *Qualitative checklist*. Critical Appraisal Skills Programme. http://media.wix.com/ugd/dd ed87_29c5b002d99342f788c6ac670e49f274.pdf.

Catterall, M. & MacLaren, P. (1997). Focus group data and qualitative analysis programs: coding the moving picture as well as snapshots. *Sociological Research Online*, 2(1). <www.socresonline.org.uk/2/1/6.html>.

Celik, H., Abma, T.A., Klinge, I. & Widdershoven, G.A.M. (2012). Process evaluation of a diversity training program: the value of a mixed method strategy. *Evaluation and Program Planning*, 35(1), 54–65.

Centre for Reviews and Dissemination (2009). *Report No 4: Undertaking systematic reviews of research on effectiveness*. University of York. <www.york.ac.uk/inst/crd/index.htm>.

Chalmers, T.C., Celano, P., Sacks, H.S. & Smith, H. Jr (1983). Bias in treatment assignment in controlled clinical trials. *New England Journal of Medicine*, 309(22), 1358–61.

Chan, A.-W., Hróbjartsson, A., Haahr, M.T., Gøtzsche, P.C. & Altman, D.G. (2004). Empirical evidence for selective reporting of outcomes in randomized trials: comparison of protocols to published articles. *Journal of the American Medical Association*, 291(20), 2457–65.

Charles, P., Giraudeau, B., Dechartres, A., Baron, G. & Ravaud, P. (2009). Reporting of sample size calculation in randomised controlled trials: review. *British Medical Journal*, 338, b1732. doi: 10.1136/bmj.b1732.

Charmaz, K. (2000). Grounded theory: objectivist and constructivist methods. In N.K. Denzin & Y.S. Lincoln (eds), *Handbook of qualitative research*, 2nd edn. Thousand Oaks, CA: Sage, 509–35.

Charmaz, K. (2002). Stories and silences: disclosures and self in chronic illness. *Qualitative Inquiry*, 8(3), 302–28.

Charmaz, K. (2006). *Constructing grounded theory: a practical guide through qualitative analysis*. London: Sage.

Charmaz, K. (2009). Shifting the grounds: constructivist grounded theory methods. In J.M. Morse, P.N. Stern, J. Corbin, B. Bowers, K. Charmaz & A.E. Clarke (eds), *Developing grounded theory: the second generation*. Walnut Creek, CA: Left Coast Press.

Charmaz, K. (2011). Grounded theory methods in social justice research. In N.K. Denzin & Y.S. Lincoln (eds), *The Sage handbook of qualitative research*, 4th edn. Thousand Oaks, CA: Sage, 359–80.

Charmaz, K. (2014). *Constructing grounded theory*, 2nd edn. London: Sage.

Charon, R. (2012). At the membranes of care: stories in narrative medicine. *Academic Medicine*, 87(3), 342.

Cheek, J., Onslow, M. & Cream, A. (2004). Beyond the divide: comparing and contrasting aspects of qualitative and quantitative research approaches. *Advances in Speech-Language Pathology*, 63, 147–52.

Chen, Z. (2013). *Constipation management: evidence summaries*. Joanna Briggs Institute.

Chenitz, W.C. & Swanson, J.M. (1986). *From practice to grounded theory: qualitative research in nursing*. California: Addison-Wesley.

Chester, R., Costa, M.L., Shepstone, L., Cooper, A. & Donell, S.T. (2008). Eccentric calf muscle training compared with therapeutic ultrasound for chronic Achilles tendon pain: a pilot study. *Manual Therapy*, 13(6), 484–91.

Chevalier, J.M. and Buckles, D.J. (2013). *Participatory action research: theory and methods for engaged inquiry*. London: Routledge.

Chirgwin, S. & D'Antoine, H. (2016). The health of indigenous people. In P. Liamputtong (ed.), *Public health: local and global perspectives*. Cambridge: Cambridge University Press, 313–29.

Cho, J. & Trent, C. (2014). Evaluating qualitative research. In P. Leavy (ed.), *The Oxford handbook of qualitative research*. Oxford: Oxford University Press, 677ff.

Chow, A. (2010). Optimizing the use of video-tapes of clinical sessions: the data-mining approach for scale construction in theory-building for bereaved persons in Hong Kong. *Social Work and Health Care*, 49(9), 832–55.

Christiansen, O.B., Mathiesen, O. & Lauritsen, J.G. (1992). Study of the birthweight of parents experiencing unexplained recurrent miscarriages. *British Journal of Obstetrics and Gynaecology*, 99(5), 408–11.

Chronister, J.A., Lynch, R.T., Chan, F., Rosenthal, D. & da Silva Cardoso, E. (2008). The evidence-based practice movement in healthcare: implications for rehabilitation. *Journal of Rehabilitation*, 74(2), 6–15.

Cisneros Puebla, C.A. (2003). Computer-assisted qualitative analysis. *Sociologías*, (9), 288-313.

Clandinin, J.D. (ed.) (2007). *Handbook of narrative inquiry: mapping the methodology*. Thousand Oaks, CA: Sage.

Clandinin, J. (2013). *Engaging in narrative inquiry*. Walnut Creek, CA: Left Coast Press.

Clark, V. & Braun, V. (2013). Teaching thematic analysis. *The Psychologist*, 26, 120–3.

Coa, K.I., Smith, K.C., Klassen, A.C., Thorpe, R.J. & Caulfield, L.E. (2015). Exploring important influences on the healthfulness of prostate cancer survivors' diets. *Qualitative Health Research*, 25(6), 857–70.

Coates, V. (2004). Qualitative research: a source of evidence to inform nursing practice? *Journal of Diabetes Nursing*, 8(9), 329–34.

Cochrane, A.L. (1979). 1931–1971: a critical review, with particular reference to the medical profession. In *Medicines for the year 2000*. London: Office of Health Economics, 1–11.

Coenen, M., Stamm, T.A., Stucki, G. & Cieza, A. (2012). Individual interviews and focus groups in patients with rheumatoid arthritis: a comparison of two qualitative methods. *Quality of Life Research*, 21(2), 359–70.

Coffin, J., Drysdale, M., Hermeston, W., Sherwood, J. & Edwards, T. (2008). Ways forward in Indigenous health. In S.-T. Liaw & S. Kilpatrick (eds), *A textbook of Australian rural health*. Canberra: Australian Rural Health Education Network, 141–52.

Cohen, J. (1977). *Statistical power analysis for the behavioural sciences*. New York: Academic Press.

Cohen, J. (1992). A power primer. *Psychological Bulletin*, 112, 155–9.

Cohen, L. & Manion, L. (2000). *Research methods in education*, 2nd edn. New York: Routledge.

Cohen, S., Gottlieb, B. & Underwood, L. (2000). Social relationships and health. In S. Cohen, L. Underwood & B. Gottlieb (eds), *Social support measurement and intervention*. New York: Oxford University Press, 3–28.

Colaizzi, P.F. (1978). Psychological research as the phenomenologist views it. In R.S. Valle & M. King (eds), *Existential phenomenological alternatives for psychology*. New York: Oxford University Press, 48–71.

Collins, J. & Fauser, B. (2005). Balancing the strengths of systematic and narrative reviews. *Human Reproduction Update*, 11, 103–4.

Collins, K., Onwuegbuzie, T. & Jaio, Q. (2007). A mixed-methods investigation of mixed methods in sampling designs in social and health science research. *Journal of Mixed Methods Research*, 1(3), 267–94.

Collins, K.M.T., Onwuegbuzie, A.J. & Johnson, R.B. (2012). Securing a place at the table: a review and extension of legitimation criteria for the conduct of mixed research. *American Behavioral Scientist*, 56(6), 849–65.

Collins, N. & Knowles, A.D. (1995). Adolescents' attitudes towards confidentiality between the school counsellor and the adolescent client. *Australian Psychologist*, 30(3), 179–82.

Commonwealth of Australia, Department of the Prime Minister and Cabinet (2016). *Closing the gap. Prime Minister's Report 2016*. Canberra.

Condero, A. (2004). When family reunification works: data-mining foster care records. *Families in Society*, 85(4), 571–80.

Cook, D., Mulrow, C. & Haynes, R.B. (1997). Systematic reviews: synthesis of best evidence for clinical decisions. *Annals of Internal Medicine*, 126, 376–80.

Cooke, A., Smith, D. & Booth, A. (2012). Beyond PICO: the SPIDER tool for qualitative evidence synthesis. *Qualitative Health Research*, 22(10), 1435–43.

Cooper, H. (2010). *Research synthesis and meta-analysis: a step-by-step approach*, 4th edn. Thousand Oaks, CA: Sage.

Cooper, K., Smith, B.H. & Hancock, E. (2009). Patients' perceptions of self-management of chronic low back pain: evidence for enhancing patient education and support. *Physiotherapy*, 95, 43–50.

Corbin, J. (2009). Taking an analytic journey. In J.M. Morse, P.N. Stern, J. Corbin, B. Bowers, K. Charmaz & A.E. Clarke (eds), *Developing grounded theory: the second generation*. Walnut Creek, CA: Left Coast Press, 35–53.

Corbin, J. & Strauss, A. (2008). *Basics of qualitative research: techniques and procedures for developing grounded theory*, 3rd edn. Thousand Oaks, CA: Sage.

Corbin, J. & Strauss, A. (2015). *Basics of qualitative research: techniques and procedures for developing grounded theory*, 4th edn. Thousand Oaks, CA: Sage.

Corti, L. & Thompson, P. (2004). Secondary analysis of archived data. In C. Seale, G. Gobo, J.F. Gubrium & D. Silverman (eds), *Qualitative research practice*. London: Sage, 327–43.

Cotchett, M.P., Landorf, K.B., Munteanu, S.E. & Raspovic, A.M. (2011). Consensus for dry needling for plantar heel pain (plantar fasciitis): a modified Delphi study. *Acupuncture in Medicine*, 29(3), 193–202.

Council for Aboriginal Reconciliation (1994). *Addressing disadvantage: a greater awareness of the causes of Indigenous Australians' disadvantage*. Canberra: Australian Government Publishing Service.

Coupland, H., Ritchie, J. & Maher, L. (2004). *Within reach: a participatory needs assessment of young injecting drug users in south western Sydney*. Sydney: UNSW Publishing and Printing Service.

Couzos, S., Nicholson, A.K., Hunt, J.M., Davey, M.E., May, J.K., Bennet, P.T., Westphal, D.W. & Thomas, D. (2015). Talking about the smokes: a large-scale, community-based participatory research project. *Medical Journal of Australia*, 202(10), S13–19.

Covey, S.R. (2004). The 8th habit: from effectiveness to greatness. New York: Free Press.

Cowles, M. & Davis, D. (1982). On the origins of the .05 level of statistical significance. *American Psychologist*, 37, 553–8.

Coyne, I.T. (1997). Sampling in qualitative research. Purposeful and theoretical sampling: merging or clear boundaries? *Journal of Advanced Nursing*, 26, 623–30.

Craig, J.V. & Smyth, R.L. (2012). *The evidence-based practice manual for nurses*, 3rd edn. Edinburgh: Churchill Livingstone.

Crapanzano, V. (1980). *Tuhami: portrait of a Moroccan*. Chicago: University of Chicago Press.

Creswell, J.W. (2003). *Research design: qualitative, quantitative, and mixed methods approaches*, 2nd edn. London: Sage.

Creswell, J.W. (2007). *Qualitative inquiry and research design: choosing among five approaches*, 2nd edn. Thousand Oaks, CA: Sage.

Creswell, J.W. (2013). *Qualitative inquiry and research design: choosing among five approaches*, 3rd edn. Thousand Oaks, CA: Sage.

Creswell, J.W. (2014). *Research design: qualitative, quantitative and mixed methods approaches*, 4th edn. Thousand Oaks, CA: Sage.

Creswell, J.W. (2015). *A concise introduction to mixed methods research*. Thousand Oaks, CA: Sage.

Creswell, J.W. & Plano Clark, V.L. (2011). *Designing and conducting mixed methods research*, 2nd edn. Thousand Oaks, CA: Sage.

Creswell, J.W. & Plano Clark, V.L. (2014). The mixed methods approach. In R.M. Grinnell Jr & Y.A. Unrau (eds), *Social work research and evaluation: foundations of evidence-based practice*, 10th edn. New York: Oxford University Press, 99–110.

Creswell, J.W., Fetters, M.D. & Ivankova, N.V. (2004). Designing a mixed methods study in primary care. *Annals of Family Medicine*, 2, 7–12.

Crowther, M. & Cook, D. (2007). Trials and tribulations of systematic reviews and meta-analyses. *Hematology*, 2007, 493–7.

Cumming, S., Fitzpatrick, E., McAuliffe, D., McKain, S., Martin, C. & Tonge, A. (2007). Raising the Titanic: rescuing social work documentation from the sea of ethical risk. *Australian Social Work*, 60(2), 239–57.

Curry, L. & Nunez-Smith, M. (2015). *Mixed methods in health sciences research*. Thousand Oaks, CA: Sage.

Curtin, M. & Fossey, E. (2007). Appraising the trustworthiness of qualitative studies: guidelines for occupational therapists. *Australian Occupational Therapy Journal*, 54, 88–94.

Cusick, A., Vasquez, M., Knowles, L. & Wallen, M. (2005). Effect of rater training on reliability of Melbourne Assessment of Unilateral Upper Limb Function scores. *Development Medicine & Child Neurology*, 47(1), 39–45.

Cussen, A., Howie, L. & Imms, C. (2012). Looking to the future: adolescents with cerebral palsy talk about their aspirations—a narrative study. *Disability and Rehabilitation*, 34(24), 2103–10.

Cutcliffe, J.R. (2000). Methodological issues in grounded theory. *Journal of Advanced Nursing*, 31(6), 1476–84.

Cutcliffe, J. & Ramcharan, P. (2002). Leveling the playing field? Exploring the merits of the ethics-as-process approach for judging qualitative research proposals. *Qualitative Health Research*, 12, 1000–10.

D'Arcy Hart, P. (1999). A change in scientific approach: from alternation to randomised allocation in clinical trials in the 1940s. *British Medical Journal*, 319, 572–3.

Dalley, J. & Sim, J. (2001). Nurses' perceptions of physiotherapists as rehabilitation team members. *Clinical Rehabilitation*, 15, 380–9.

Daly, K.J. (2007). *Qualitative methods for family studies and human development*. Thousand Oaks, CA: Sage.

Daly, J., Jackson, D. & Nay, R. (2014). Visionary leadership for a 'greying' health care system. In R. Nay, S. Garratt & D. Fetherstonhaugh (eds), *Older people: issues and innovations in care*, 4th edn. Elsevier: Sydney, 489–501.

Daly, J., Willis, K., Small, R., Green, J., Welch, N., Kealy, M. & Hughes, E. (2007). A hierarchy of evidence for assessing qualitative health research. *Journal of Clinical Epidemiology*, 60, 43–9.

Dam, K. & Hall, E.O.C. (2016). Navigating in an unpredictable daily life: a metasynthesis on children's experiences living with a parent with severe mental illness. Unpublished paper submitted to *Scandinavian Journal of Caring Sciences*.

Dattilio, F. (2006). Case-based research in family therapy. *Australian and New Zealand Journal of Family Therapy*, 27(4), 208–13.

David, R. & Whitehouse, J. (1998). Modelling the consultation process in a secondary referral unit for children. *International Journal of Language & Communication Disorders*, 33(Suppl.), 532–7.

Davidson, M. (2002). The interpretation of diagnostic tests: a primer for physiotherapists. *Australian Journal of Physiotherapy*, 48(3), 227–32.

Davidson, P.M., Daly, J., Meleis, A. & Douglas, M. (2003). Globalisation as we enter the 21st century: reflections and directions for nursing education, science, research and clinical practice. *Contemporary Nurse*, 15(3), 162–74.

Davison, C., Davey-Smith, G. & Frankel, S. (1991). Lay epidemiology and the prevention paradox: the implication of coronary candidacy for health education. *Sociology of Health and Illness*, 13(1), 1–19.

Davison, C., Davey-Smith, G. & Frankel, S. (1992). The limits of lifestyle: re-assessing 'fatalism' in the popular culture of illness prevention. *Social Science & Medicine*, 34, 675–85.

De Bie, R. (2001). Critical appraisal of prognostic studies: an introduction. *Physiotherapy Theory & Practice*, 17, 161–71.

de Koning, K. & Martin, M. (1996). *Participatory research in health: issues and experiences*. London: Zed Books.

de Laine, M. (1997). *Ethnography: theory and applications in health research*. Sydney: McLennan & Petty.

de Laine, M. (2000). *Fieldwork, participation and practice: ethics and dilemmas in qualitative research*. London: Sage.

De Matteo, C., Law, M., Russell, D., Pollock, N., Rosenbaum, P.L. & Walter, C.B. (1991). *QUEST: quality of upper extremity skills test manual*. Hamilton, ON: McMaster University.

de Vaus, D.A. (2007). *Social surveys 2: survey instruments and data sources*, vol. 2. London: Sage.

de Visser, R., Badcock, P.L., Rissel, C., Richters, J., Smith, A.M.A., Grulich, A. & Simpson, J.M. (2014). Safer sex and condom use: findings from the Second Australian Study of Health and Relationships. *Sexual Health*, 11, 495–504.

de Visser, R.O., Smith, A.M.A., Rissel, C., Richters, J. & Grulich, A.E. (2003). Sex in Australia: safer sex and condom use among a representative sample of adults. *Australian and New Zealand Journal of Public Health*, 27(2), 223–9.

De Vries, R., DeBruin, D.A. & Goodgame, A. (2004). Ethics review of social, behavioural and economic research: where should we go from here? *Ethics and Behavior*, 14(4), 351–68.

DeFina, A. & Georgakopoulou, A. (eds) (2015). *The handbook of narrative analysis*. Chichester, UK: Wiley Blackwell.

Del Mar, C., Glasziou, P. & Mayer, D. (2004). Teaching evidence based medicine. *British Medical Journal*, 329, 989–90.

Dellinger, A.B. & Leech, N.L. (2007). Toward a unified validation framework in mixed methods research. *Journal of Mixed Methods Research*, 1(4), 309–32.

Denny, E., Culley, L., Papadopoulos, I. & Apenteng, P. (2011). From womanhood to endometriosis: findings from focus groups with women from different ethnic groups. *Diversity in Health and Care*, 8(3), 167–80.

Denzin, N.K. (1982). On the ethics of disguised observation: an exchange between Norman K. Denzin and Kai T. Erikson. In M. Bulmer (ed.), *Social research ethics*. London: Macmillan, 139–51.

Denzin, N.K. (2008). The new paradigm dialogs and qualitative inquiry. *International Journal of Qualitative Studies in Education*, 21(4), 315–25.

Denzin, N.K. (2009). The elephant in the living room: or extending the conversation about the politics of evidence. *Qualitative Research*, 9(2), 139–60.

Denzin, N.K. (2010). Moments, mixed methods and paradigm dialogs. *Qualitative Inquiry*, 16, 419–27.

Denzin, N.K. (2011). The politics of evidence. In Denzin, N.K. and Lincoln, Y.S. (eds), *The Sage handbook of qualitative research*, 4th edn. Thousand Oaks, CA: Sage, 645–57.

Denzin, N.K. & Lincoln, Y.S. (2005). Methods of collecting and analysing empirical materials. In N.K. Denzin & Y.S. Lincoln (eds), *The Sage handbook of qualitative research*. Thousand Oaks, CA: Sage, 641–9.

Denzin, N.K. & Lincoln, Y.S. (2008). Introduction: the discipline and practice of qualitative research. In N.K. Denzin & Y.S. Lincoln (eds), *Strategies of qualitative inquiry*, 3rd edn. Thousand Oaks, CA: Sage, 1–43.

Denzin, N.K. & Lincoln, Y.S. (2011). Introduction: the discipline and practice of qualitative research. In N.K. Denzin & Y.S. Lincoln (eds), *The Sage handbook of qualitative research*, 4th edn. Thousand Oaks, CA: Sage, 1–19.

Department of Health (2001). *The expert patient: a new approach to chronic disease management in the twenty-first century*. London: Department of Health.

Department of Health (2005a). *Research governance framework for health and social care*. London: Department of Health. <www.dh.gov.uk/en/Publicationsandstatistics/Publications/PublicationsPolicyAndGuidance/DH_4008777>.

Department of Health (2005b). *Creating a patient-led NHS: delivering the NHS Improvement Plan*. London: Department of Health.

Department of Veterans' Affairs (2007). *Constipation: a quality of life issue for veteran patients*. Therapeutic brief. <www.veteransmates.net.au/VeteransMATES/documents/module_materials/M10_TherBrief.pdf> and <www.va.gov/oig/54/reports/VAOIG-06-03145-23.pdf>.

DeVault, M. & McCoy, L. (2002). Institutional ethnography: using interviews to investigate ruling relations. In J. Gubrium & J. Holstein (eds), *Handbook of interview research: context and method*. Thousand Oaks, CA: Sage.

Dew, K. (2007). A health researcher's guide to qualitative methodologies. *Australian and New Zealand Journal of Public Health*, 31(5), 433–7.

Dey, I. (1999). *Grounding grounded theory: guidelines for qualitative inquiry.* San Diego: Academic Press.

Dickson-Swift, V., James, E.L., Kippen, S. & Liamputtong, P. (2007). Doing sensitive research: what challenges do qualitative researchers face? *Qualitative Research*, 7(3), 327–53.

Dickson-Swift, V., James, E. & Liamputtong, P. (2008a). *Undertaking sensitive research in the health and social sciences: managing boundaries, emotions and risks.* Cambridge: Cambridge University Press.

Dickson-Swift, V., James, E.L., Kippen, S. & Liamputtong, P. (2008b). Risk to researchers in qualitative research on sensitive topics: issues and strategies. *Qualitative Health Research*, 18(1), 133–44.

DiGiacomo, M., Delaney, P., Abbott, P., Davidson, P.M., Delaney, J. & Vincent, F. (2013). 'Doing the hard yards': carer and provider focus group perspectives of accessing Aboriginal childhood disability services. *BMC Health Services Research*, 13(1), 326.

Dillman, D.A., Smyth, J.D. & Christian, L.M. (2014). *Internet, phone, mail, and mixed-mode surveys: the tailored design method*, 4th edn. Hoboken, NJ: John Wiley.

Dingwall, R. & McDonnell, M.B. (2015). *The Sage handbook of research management.* London: Sage.

Disler, R., Spiliopoulos, N., Inglis, S., Currow, N. & Davidson, P.M. (2015). Attitudes to cognitive impairment and testing in patients with chronic obstructive pulmonary disease: focus group study. *American Journal of Respiratory Critical Care Medicine*, 191, A5291.

Dixon-Woods, M., Shaw, R.L., Agarwal, S. & Smith, J.A. (2004). The problem of appraising qualitative research. *Quality and Safety in Health Care*, 13, 223–5.

Dixon-Woods, M., Agarwal, S., Jones, D., Young, B. & Sutton, A. (2005). Synthesising qualitative and quantitative evidence. *Journal of Health Services Research and Policy*, 10, 45–53.

Dixon-Woods, M., Bonas, S., Booth, A., Jones, D.R., Miller, T.A., Shaw, R.L. *et al.* (2006a). How can systematic qualitative reviews incorporate qualitative research? A critical perspective. *Qualitative Research*, 6, 27–44.

Dixon-Woods, M., Cavers, D., Agarwal, S., Annandale, E., Arthur, A., Harvey, J., Hsu, R., Katbamna, S., Olsen, R., Smith, L., Riley, R. & Sutton, A.J. (2006b). Conducting a critical interpretive synthesis of the literature on access to healthcare by vulnerable groups. *BMC Medical Research Methodology*, 6, 35. <www.biomedcentral.com/1471-2288/6/35>.

Dixon-Woods, M., Booth, A. & Sutton, A. (2007a). Synthesizing qualitative research: a review of published reports. *Qualitative Research*, 7(3), 375–422.

Dixon-Woods, M., Sutton, A., Shaw, R., Miller, T., Smith, J., Young, B., Bonas, S., Booth, A. & Jones, D. (2007b). Appraising qualitative research for inclusion in systematic reviews: a quantitative and qualitative comparison of three methods. *Journal of Health Service & Research Policy*, 12(1), 42–7.

Dobrof, J., Ebenstein, H., Dodd, S.-J. & Epstein, I. (2006). Caregivers and professionals partnership caregiver resource center: assessing a hospital support program for family caregivers. *Journal of Palliative Medicine*, 9(1), 196–205.

Doll, R. (1998). Controlled trials: the 1948 watershed. *British Medical Journal*, 317, 1217–20.

Doll, R., Peto, R., Boreham, J. & Sutherland, I. (2005). Mortality from cancer in relation to smoking: 50 years observations on British doctors. *British Journal of Cancer*, 92(3), 426–9.

Dominelli, L. & Holloway, M. (2008). Ethics and governance in social work research in the UK. *British Journal of Social Work*, 38(5), 1009–28.

Donovan, J., Mills, N., Smith, M., Brindle, L., Jacoby, A., Peters, T., Frankel, S., Neal, D. & Hamdy, F. (2002). Improving design and conduct of randomised trials by embedding them in qualitative research: ProtecT (prostate testing for cancer and treatment) study. *British Medical Journal*, 325, 766–70.

Dougherty, J. (2015). Collecting evidence. In N.A. Schmidt & J.M. Brown (eds), *Evidence-based practice for nurses: appraisal and application of research*, 3rd edn. Burlington, MA: Jones & Bartlett Learning, 262–93.

Douglas, J.D. (1976). *Investigative social research*. Beverly Hills, CA: Sage.

Dowling, M. (2007). From Husserl to van Manen: a review of different phenomenological approaches. *International Journal of Nursing Studies*, 44(1), 131–42.

Drageset, S., Lindstrøm, T.C., Giske, T. & Underlid, K. (2012). 'The support I need': women's experiences of social support after having received breast cancer diagnosis and awaiting surgery. *Cancer Nursing*, 35(6), E39–E47.

Drayton-Brooks, S. & White, N. (2004). Health promoting behaviors among African American women with faith-based support. *Association of Black Nursing Faculty (ABNF) Journal*, 15(5), 84–90.

Duggleby, W., Hicks, D., Nekolaichuk, C., Holtslander, L., Williams, A., Chambers, T. & Eby, J. (2012). Hope, older adults, and chronic illness: a metasynthesis of qualitative research. *Journal of Advanced Nursing*, 68(6), 1211–23.

Duley, L. & Farrell, B. (2002). *Clinical trials*. London: BMJ Books.

Dumrongthanapakorn, P. & Liamputtong, P. (2015). Social support coping means: the lived experiences of northeastern Thai women with breast cancer. *Health Promotion International*. Doi: 10.1093/heapro/dav023.

Dunning, H., Williams, A., Abonyi, S. & Crooks, V. (2008). A mixed method approach to quality of life research: a case study approach. *Social Indicators Research*, 85, 145–58.

Dunstan, D.W., Zimmet, P.Z., Welborn, T.A., de Courten, M.P., Cameron, A.J., Sicret, R.A. *et al.* (2002). The rising prevalence of diabetes mellitus and impaired glucose tolerance: the Australian Diabetes, Obesity and Lifestyle study. *Diabetes Care*, 25, 829–34.

Dyer, K. & das Nair, R. (2012). Why don't healthcare professionals talk about sex? A systematic review of recent qualitative studies conducted in the United Kingdom. *Journal of Sex Medicine*, published online 31/7/12. <http://onlinelibrary.wiley.com/doi/10.1111/j.1743-6109.2012.02856.x/pdf>.

Dykes, F. & Flacking, R. (eds) (2016). *Ethnographic research in maternal and child health*. Abingdon: Routledge.

Dysart, A.M. & Tomlin, G.S. (2002). Factors related to evidence-based practice among US occupational therapy clinicians. *American Journal of Occupational Therapy*, 56(3), 275–84.

Edmonds, W.A. & Kennedy, T.D. (eds) (2012). *An applied reference guide to research designs: quantitative, qualitative, and mixed methods*. Thousand Oaks, CA: Sage.

Edwards, T. (2008). *Research design and statistics: a bio-behavioural approach*. Boston, MA: McGraw-Hill.

Edwards, S.J.L., Ashcroft, R. & Kirchin, S.T. (2004). Research ethics committees: differences and moral judgements. *Bioethics*, 18(5), 407–27.

Egger, M., Jüni, P., Bartlett, C., Holenstein, F. & Sterne, J. (2003). How important are comprehensive literature searches and the assessment of trial quality in systematic reviews? Empirical study. *Health Technology Assessment*, 7, 1.

Ell, K., Nishimoto, R., Mediansky, L., Mantell, J. & Hamovitch, M. (1992). Social relations, social support and survival among patients with cancer. *Journal of Psychosomatic Research*, 36(6), 531–41.

Ellen, R.F. (1984). *Ethnographic research: a guide to general conduct*. London: Academic Press.

Elliot, A.C. & Woodward, W.A. (2006). *Statistical analysis quick reference and guide book with SPSS examples*. Thousand Oaks, CA: Sage.

Elo, S. & Kyngäs, H. (2008). The qualitative content analysis process. *Journal of Advanced Nursing*, 62(1), 107–15.

Embretson, S.E. & Hershberger, S.L. (1999). *The new rules of measurement: what every psychologist and educator should know*. Mahwah, NJ: Lawrence Erlbaum.

Endacott, R. (2008). Clinical research 6: writing and research. *International Emergency Nursing*, 16(3), 211–14.

Engel, U. (2015). *Improving survey methods: Lessons from recent research*. Routledge: London.

Engström, Å. & Söderberg, S. (2004). The experiences of partners of critically ill persons in an intensive care unit. *Intensive & Critical Care Nursing*, 20(5), 299–308.

Ennals, P. & Fossey, E. (2009). Using the OPHI-II to support recovery for people with mental illness. *Occupational Therapy in Mental Health*, 25, 13.

Epstein, I. (2001). Using available clinical information in practice-based research: mining for silver while dreaming of gold. *Social Work in Health Care*, 33(3/4), 15–32.

Epstein, I., Zilberfein, F. & Snyder, S. (1997). Using available information in practice-based outcomes research: a case study of psycho-social risk factors and liver transplant outcomes. In E.J. Mullen & J.L. Magnabosco (eds), *Outcomes in the human services: cross-cutting issues and methods*. Washington, DC: NASW Press, 224–33.

Eri, S.T., Bondas, T., Gross, M., Janssen, P. & Green, J.A. (2015). A balancing act in an unknown territory: a metasynthesis on first-time mothers' experiences in early labour. *Midwifery*. Doi. org/10.1016/j-midw.2014.11.007.

Erickson, S. & Serry, T.A. (2016). Comparing alternate learning pathways within a problem-based learning speech-language pathology curriculum. *International Journal of Speech-Language Pathology*, 18(1), 97–107.

Erikson, F. (2011). A history of qualitative inquiry in social and educational research. In N.K. Denzin & Y.S. Lincoln (eds), *The Sage handbook of qualitative research*, 4th edn. Thousand Oaks: Sage, 43–59.

Erikson, K.T. (1967). A comment on disguised observation in sociology. *Social Problems*, 14, 366–73.

Estabrooks, C.A., Field, P.A. & Morse, J.M. (1994). Aggregating qualitative findings: an approach to theory development. *Qualitative Health Research*, 4(4), 503–11.

Esterberg, K.G. (2002). *Qualitative methods in social research*. Boston, MA: McGraw-Hill.

Evans, D. (2003). Hierarchy of evidence: a framework for ranking evidence evaluating healthcare interventions. *Journal of Clinical Nursing*, 12, 77–84.

Evans-Pritchard, E.E. (1937). *Witchcraft, oracles, and magic among the Azande*. Oxford: Clarendon Press.

Evans-Pritchard, E.E. (1951). *Social anthropology*. London: Cohen & West.

Fahy, K. (2008). Evidence-based midwifery and power/knowledge. *Women and Birth*, 21, 1–2.

Fawcett, A.J.L. (2007). *Principles of assessment and outcome measurement for occupational therapists and physiotherapists: theory, skills and application*. <http://library.latrobe.edu.au/record=b2264691~S5>.

Fawcett, B. & Pockett, R. (2015). *Turning ideas into research: theory, design and practice.* London: Sage.

Fegran, L., Hall, E.O.C., Uhrenfeldt, L., Aagaard, H. & Ludvigsen, M.S. (2014). Adolescents' and young adults' transition experiences when transferring from paediatric to adult care: a qualitative metasynthesis. *International Journal of Nursing Studies*, 51, 123–35. Doi:10.1016/j.ijnurstu.2013.02.001.

Feilzer, M.V. (2010). Doing mixed methods research pragmatically: implications for the rediscovery of pragmatism as a research paradigm. *Journal of Mixed Methods Research*, 4(1), 6–16.

Feldman, S. & Howie, L. (2009). Looking back, looking forward: reflections on using a life history review tool with older people. *Journal of Applied Gerontology*, 28(5), 621–37.

Ferguson, F.C., Brownless, M. & Webster, V. (2008). A Delphi study investigating consensus among expert physiotherapists in relation to the management of low back pain. *Musculoskeletal Care*, 6(4), 197–210.

Fergusson, D., Aaron, S.D., Guyatt, G. & Hebert, P. (2002). Post-randomisation exclusions: the intention to treat principle and excluding patients from analysis. *British Medical Journal*, 325, 652–4.

Fernandes, A.F., Cruz, A., Moreira, C., Santos, M.C. & Silva, T. (2014). Social support provided to women undergoing breast cancer treatment: a study review. *Advances in Breast Cancer Research*, 3(2), 47–53.

Field, K. & Murphy, D.J. (2015). Perinatal outcomes in a subsequent pregnancy among women who have experienced recurrent miscarriage: a retrospective cohort study. *Human Reproduction*, 30(5), 1239–45.

Field, M.J. & Lohr, K.N. (1990). *Clinical practice guidelines: directions for a new program.* Institute of Medicine, Washington, DC: National Academy Press.

Fielding, N. & Lee, R.M. (1998). *Computer analysis and qualitative research.* London: Sage.

Figert, A. & Kuehnert, P. (1997). Reframing knowledge about the AIDS epidemic: academic and community-based interventions. In P. Nyden, A. Figert, M. Shibley & D. Burrows (eds), *Building community: social science in action.* Thousand Oaks, CA: Pine Forge Press, 154–60.

Finfgeld, D.L. (2003). Metasynthesis: the state of the art-so far. *Qualitative Health Research*, 13(7), 893–904.

Finfgeld-Connett, D. (2010). Generalizability and transferability of meta-synthesis research findings. *Journal of Advanced Nursing*, 66(2), 246–54.

Finfgeld-Connett, D. (2014). Metasynthesis findings: potential versus reality. *Qualitative Health Research*, 24(11), 1581–91.

Finlay, L. (1999). Applying phenomenology in research: problems, principles and practice. *British Journal of Occupational Therapy*, 62(7), 299–306.

Finlay, L. (2009). Exploring lived experience: principles and practice of phenomenological research. *International Journal of Therapy and Rehabilitation*, 16(9), 474–81.

Fisher, A.G. & Fisher, A.G. (1993). The assessment of IADL motor skills: an application of many-faceted Rasch analysis. *American Journal of Occupational Therapy*, 47(4), 319–29.

Fleck, C. & Muller, A. (1997). Bruno Bettelheim and the concentration camps. *Journal of the History of Behavioural Sciences*, 33(1), 1–37.

Flemming, K. (2009). Synthesis of quantitative and qualitative research: an example using critical interpretive synthesis. *Journal of Advanced Nursing*, 66(1), 201–17.

Flemming, K. (2010). The use of morphine to treat cancer-related pain: a synthesis of quantitative and qualitative research. *Journal of Pain and Symptom Management*, 39(1), 139–54.

Flick, U. (2006). *An introduction to qualitative research*, 3rd edn. Newbury Park, CA: Sage.

Flick, U., Garms-Homolová, V., Herrmann, W.J., Kuck, J. & Röhnsch, G. (2012). 'I can't prescribe something just because someone asks for it ...': using mixed methods in the framework of triangulation. *Journal of Mixed Methods Research*, 6(2), 97–110.

Floersch, J. (2000). Reading the case record: the oral and written narratives of social workers. *Social Service Review*, 74(2), 169–91.

Floersch, J. (2004). A method for investigating practitioner use of theory in practice. *Qualitative Social Work*, 3(2), 161–77.

Flyvbjerg, B. (2011). Case study. In N.K. Denzin and Y.S. Lincoln (eds), *The Sage handbook of qualitative research*, 4th edn. Thousand Oaks, CA: Sage, 301–16.

Fontana, A. & Prokos, A.H. (2007). *The interview: from formal to postmodern*. Walnut Creek, CA: Left Coast Press.

Fook, J. (ed.) (1996). *The reflective researcher: social workers' theories of practice research*. Sydney: Allen & Unwin.

Fook, J. & Gardner, F. (2007). *Practising critical reflection: a resource handbook*. Maidenhead, UK: Open University Press.

Fook, J., Collington, V., Ross, V., Ruch, G. & West, L. (2015). *Researching critical reflection: multidisciplinary perspectives*. Abington: Routledge.

Fossey, E., Harvey, C., McDermott, F. & Davidson, L. (2002). Understanding and evaluating qualitative research. *Australian and New Zealand Journal of Psychiatry*, 36(6), 717–32.

Foster, A., Worrall, L., Rose, M.L. & O'Halloran (2014). Turning back the tide: putting acute aphasia management back on the agenda through evidence-based practice. *Aphasiology*, 27(4), 420–43.

Fox, F.E., Morris, M. & Rumsey, N. (2007). Doing synchronous online focus groups with young people: methodological reflections. *Qualitative Health Research*, 17(4), 539–47.

France, E.F., Ring, N., Thomas, R., Noyes, J., Maxwell, M. & Jepson, R. (2014). A methodological systematic review of what's wrong with meta-ethnography reporting. *BMC Medical Research Methodology*, 14, 119. Doi: 10.1186/1471-2288-14-119.

Frank, A. (2000). The standpoint of the storyteller. *Qualitative Health Research*, 10, 354–65.

Frank, A. (2010). *Letting stories breathe: a socio-narratology*. Chicago: University of Chicago Press.

Franklin, R., Allison, D. & Gorman, B. (eds) (1996). *Design and analysis of single-case research*. New Jersey: Lawrence Erlbaum.

Franz, A., Worrell, M. & Vögele, C. (2013). Integrating mixed method data in psychological research: combining Q methodology and questionnaires in a study investigating cultural and psychological influences on adolescent sexual behavior. *Journal of Mixed Methods Research*, 7(4), 370–89.

Franzel, B., Schwiegershausen, M., Heusser, P. & Berger, B. (2013). Individualized medicine from the perspectives of patients using complementary therapies: a metaethnography approach. *BMC Complementary & Alternative Medicine*, 13, 124. Doi: 10.1186/1472-6882-13-124.

Freire, P. (1972). *Pedagogy of the oppressed*. London: Sheed & Ward.

Freud, S. (1974). *The standard edition of the complete psychological works of Sigmund Freud*. <http://freud.org.uk/furfaq.htm>.

Freudenthal, S., Ahlberg, B.M., Mtweve, S., Nyindo, P., Poggensee, G. & Krantz, I. (2006). School-based prevention of schistosomiasis: initiating a participatory action research project in northern Tanzania. *Acta Tropica*, 100, 79–87.

Friedman, L.M., Furberg, C.D. & DeMets, D.L. (1998). *Fundamentals of clinical trials*. New York: Springer.

Frizziero, A., Trainito, S., Oliva, F., Nicoli Aldini, N., Masiero, S. & Maffulli, N. (2014). The role of eccentric exercise in sport injuries rehabilitation. *British Medical Bulletin*, 110(1), 47–75.

Gabler, N., Duan, W., Vohra, S. & Kravitz, R. (2011). N-of-1 trials in the medical literature: a systematic literature review. *Medical Care*, 49(8), 761–8.

Gabriel, M. (2013). Research: writing through, writing up. In M. Walter (ed.), *Social research methods*, 3rd edn. Melbourne: Oxford University Press, 355–80.

Gaiser, T.J. (2008). Online focus groups. In N. Fielding, R.M. Lee & G. Blank (eds), *The Sage handbook of online research methods*. London: Sage, 290–307.

Gamberini, L. & Spagnolli, A. (2003). Display techniques and methods for cross-medial data analysis. *PsychNology Journal* 1(2), 131–40. <www.psychnology.org/File/PSYCHNOLOGY_JOURNAL_1_2_GAMBERINI.pdf>.

Gapp, R., Harwood, I., Stewart, H. & Woods, P. (2013). Viewing computer-assisted qualitative data analysis (CAQDAS) through Leximancer. In Proceedings of the 27th ANZAM Conference, Hobart, Australia, 4–6 December 2013. http://eprints.soton.ac.uk/356871/.

García-Horta, J.B. & Guerra-Ramos, M.T. (2009). The use of CAQDAS in educational research: some advantages, limitations and potential risks. *International Journal of Research & Method in Education*, 32(2), 151–65.

Geertz, C. (1973). *The interpretation of cultures: selected essays*. New York: Basic Books.

Geertz, C. (1995). *After the fact*. Cambridge, MA: Harvard University Press.

Genat, W. (2006). *Aboriginal health workers: primary health care at the margins*. Perth: University of Western Australia Press.

Gergen, K.J. & Gergen, M. (1988). Narrative and the self as relationship. In L. Berkowitz (ed.), *Advances in experimental social psychology*. San Diego: Academic Press.

Gergen, K.J. & Gergen, M. (2011). Narrative tensions: perilous and productive. *Narrative Inquiry*, 21, 374–81.

Gergen, M.M. & Gergen, K.J. (2006). Narratives in action. *Narrative Inquiry*, 16, 112–21.

Germov, J. (ed.) (2014). *Second opinion: an introduction to health sociology*, 5th edn. Melbourne: Oxford University Press.

Gholizadeh, L. (2009). *The discrepancy between perceived and estimated absolute risks of coronary heart disease in Middle Eastern women: implications for cardiac rehabilitation*. Unpublished PhD thesis, University of Western Sydney, Sydney.

Gibbons, J.D. (1993). *Nonparametric statistics: an introduction*. Newbury Park, CA.: Sage.

Gibbs, G.R. (2002). *Qualitative data analysis: explorations with NVivo*. Buckingham, UK: Open University.

Gibbs, G.R. (2008). *Analyzing qualitative data*. London: Sage.

Gibbs, L. & Gambrill, E. (2002). Evidence-based practice: counterarguments to objections. *Research on Social Work Practice*, 12(3), 452–76.

Gibson, B. (2012). Editorial. Beyond methods: the promise of qualitative inquiry for physical therapy. *Physical Therapy Reviews*, 17(6), 357–9.

Gibson, B.E. & Martin, D.K. (2003). Qualitative research and evidence-based physiotherapy practice. *Physiotherapy*, 89(6), 350–8.

Gilles, M.T., Dickinson, J.E., Cain, A., Turner, K.A., McGuckin, R., Loh, R. *et al.* (2007). Perinatal HIV transmission and pregnancy outcomes in indigenous women in Western Australia. *Australian and New Zealand Journal of Obstetrics and Gynaecology*, 47, 362–7.

Gillett, K., O'Neill, B. & Bloomfield, J.G. (2016). Factors influencing the development of end-of-life communication skills: a focus group study of nursing and medical students. *Nurse Education Today*, 36, 395–400.

Giorgi, A.P. (1997). The theory, practice, and evaluation of the phenomenological method as a qualitative research procedure, *Journal of Phenomenological Psychology*, 28(2), 235–60.

Giorgi, A.P. & Giorgi, B.M. (2003). The descriptive phenomenological psychological method. In P.M. Camic, J.E. Rhodes & L. Yardley (eds), *Qualitative research in psychology: expanding perspectives in methodology and design*. Washington, DC: American Psychological Association, 243–71.

Glaser, B.G. (1978). *Theoretical sensitivity: advances in the methodology of grounded theory*. Mill Valley, CA: Sociology Press.

Glaser, B.G. (1992). *Emergence vs forcing: basics of grounded theory analysis*. Mill Valley, CA: Sociology Press.

Glaser, B.G. (ed.) (1996). *Gerund grounded theory: the basic social process dissertation*. Mill Valley, CA: Sociology Press.

Glaser, B.G. (1998). *Doing grounded theory: issues and discussions*. Mill Valley, CA: Sociology Press.

Glaser, B.G. (2001). *The grounded theory perspective: conceptualization contrasted with description*. Mill Valley, CA: Sociology Press.

Glaser, B.G. (2002a). Conceptualisation: on theory and theorizing using grounded theory [electronic version]. *International Journal of Qualitative Methods*, 1, 1–31. <www.ualberta.ca/~iiqm/backissues/1_2Final/pdf/glaser.pdf>.

Glaser, B.G. (2002b). Constructivist grounded theory? [electronic version]. *Forum: Qualitative Social Research*, 3. <http://nbn-resolving.de/urn:nbn:de:0114-fqs0203125>.

Glaser, B.G. (2003). *The grounded theory perspective II: Description's remodelling of grounded theory*. Mill Valley, CA: Sociology Press.

Glaser, B.G. (2004). Naturalistic inquiry and grounded theory [electronic version]. *Forum: Qualitative Social Research*, 5. <http://nbn-resolving.de/urn:nbn:de:0114-fqs040170>.

Glaser, B.G. & Holton, J. (2004). Remodeling grounded theory [electronic version]. *Forum: Qualitative Social Research*, 5. <www.qualitative-research.net/fqs-texte/2-04/2-04glaser-e.pdf>.

Glaser, B.G. & Strauss, A. (1967). *The discovery of grounded theory: strategies for qualitative research*. New York: Aldine.

Glass, G.V., McGraw, B. & Smith, M.L. (1981). *Meta-analysis in social research*. Beverly Hills, CA: Sage.

Goethals, S., Dierckx de Casterlé, B. & Gastmans, C. (2012). Nurses' decision-making in cases of physical restraint: a synthesis of qualitative evidence. *Journal of Advanced Nursing*, 68(6), 1198–210.

Goffman, I. (1969). *Where the action is: three essays*. London: Allen Lane.

Goleman, D. (2006). *Social intelligence: the new science of human relationships*. New York: Bantam Books.

Gomersall, T., Madill, A. & Summers, L.K.M. (2011). A metasynthesis of the self-management of type 2 diabetes. *Qualitative Health Research*, 2(6), 853–71.

Gomm, R. (2004). *Social research methodology: a critical introduction*. London: Palgrave Macmillan.

Goodfellow, J. (1997). Narrative inquiry: musings, methodology and merits. In J. Higgs (ed.), *Qualitative research: discourse on methodologies*. Sydney: Hampden Press, 61–74.

Gordis, L. (2009). *Epidemiology*, 4th edn. Edinburgh: Elsevier Saunders.

Gough, D., Thomas, J. & Oliver, S. (2012). Clarifying differences between review designs and methods. *Systematic Reviews*, 1, 28. Doi: 10.1186/2046-4053-1-28.

Goulding, C. (2002). *Grounded theory: a practical guide for management, business and market researchers*. London: Sage.

Grady, C. (2001). Money for research participation: does it jeopardize informed consent? *American Journal of Bioethics*, 1(2), 40–4.

Graham, M. (2015). Is being childless detrimental to a woman's health and well-being across her life course? *Women's Health Issues*, 25(2), 176–84.

Grant, S., Aitchison, T., Henderson, E., Christie, J., Zare, S., McMurray, J. & Dargie, H. (1999). A comparison of the reproducibility and the sensitivity to change of visual analogue scales, Borg scales, and Likert scales in normal subjects during submaximal exercise. *Chest*, 116, 1208–17.

Graves, J. (2007). Factors influencing indirect speech and language therapy interventions for adults with learning disabilities: the perceptions of carers and therapists. *International Journal of Language and Communication Disorders*, 42(suppl. 1), 103–21.

Grbich, C. (2007). *Qualitative data analysis: an introduction*. London: Sage.

Grbich, C. (2013). *Qualitative data analysis: an introduction*, 2nd edn. London: Sage.

Greaves, S., Imms, C., Dodd, K. & Krumlinde-Sundholm, L. (2013). Development of the Mini-Assisting Hand Assessment: evidence for content and internal scale validity. *Developmental Medicine and Child Neurology*, 55(11), 1030–7.

Green, A., DiGiacomo, M., Luckett, T., Abbott, P., Davidson, P.M., Delaney, J. & Delaney, P. (2014). Cross-sector collaborations in Aboriginal and Torres Strait Islander childhood disability: a systematic integrative review and theory-based synthesis. *International Journal for Equity in Health*, 13(1), 1–16.

Green, J. & Thorogood, N. (2009). *Qualitative methods for health research*, 2nd edn. London: Sage.

Greene, J.C. (2007). *Mixed methods in social inquiry*. San Francisco: Jossey-Bass.

Greenfield, B.H. (2006). The meaning of caring in five experienced physical therapists. *Physiotherapy Theory and Practice*, 22, 175–87.

Greenfield, B.H. & Jensen, G.M. (2012). Phenomenology: a powerful tool for patient-centered rehabilitation. *Physical Therapy Reviews*, 17(6), 417–24.

Greenfield, B.H., Anderson, A., Cox, B. & Tanner, M.C. (2008). Meaning of caring to 7 novice physical therapists during their first year of clinical practice. *Physical Therapy*, 88(10), 1154–66.

Greenhalgh, T. (1997). How to read a paper: papers that summarise other papers (systematic reviews and meta-analyses). *British Medical Journal*, 315, 672–5.

Greenhalgh, T. (2006). *How to read a paper: the basics of evidenced based medicine*, 2nd edn. Malden, MA: Blackwell Publishing/BMJ Books.

Greenhalgh, T. (2014). *How to read a paper: the basics of evidence based medicine*, 5th edn. Chichester, West Sussex: Johns Wiley & Sons/BMJ Books.

Greenhalgh, T. & Peacock, R. (2005). Effectiveness and efficiency of search methods in systematic reviews of complex evidence: audit of primary sources. *British Medical Journal*, 331, 1064–5.

Griffiths, F.E., Boardman, F.K., Chondros, P., Dowrick, C.F., Densley, K., Hegarty, K.L. & Gunn, J. (2015). The effect of strategies of personal resilience on depression recovery in an Australian cohort: a mixed methods study. *Health*, 19(1), 86–106.

Grinnell, R.M. & Unrau, Y.A. (eds) (2008). Preface. *Social work research and evaluation: foundations of evidence-based practice*, 8th edn. New York: Oxford University Press.

Grinnell, R.M. Jr, Unrau, Y.A. & Williams, M. (2011a). Introduction. In R.M. Grinnell & Y.A. Unrau (eds), *Social work research and evaluation: foundations of evidence-based practice*, 8th edn. New York: Oxford University Press, 1–16.

Grinnell, R.M. Jr, Williams, M. & Unrau, Y.A. (2011b). Research problems and questions. In R.M. Grinnell & Y.A. Unrau (eds), *Social work research and evaluation: foundations of evidence-based practice*, 9th edn. New York: Oxford University Press, 19–31.

Grinnell, R.M., Williams, M. & Unrau, Y.A. (2011c). The quantitative research approach. In R.M. Grinnell & Y.A. Unrau (eds), *Social work research and evaluation: foundations of evidence-based practice*, 9th edn. New York: Oxford University Press, 32–51.

Grinnell, R.M. Jr, Unrau, Y.A. & Williams, M. (2014a). Introduction. In R.M. Grinnell & Y.A. Unrau (eds), *Social work research and evaluation: foundations of evidence-based practice*, 10th edn. New York: Oxford University Press, 1–29.

Grinnell, R.M., Williams, M. & Unrau, Y.A. (2014b). The quantitative approach. In R.M. Grinnell & Y.A. Unrau (eds), *Social work research and evaluation: foundations of evidence-based practice*, 10th edn. New York: Oxford University Press, 58–77.

Grønkjær, M., Curtis, T., de Crespigny, C. & Delmar, C. (2011). Analysing group interaction in focus group research: impact on content and the role of the moderator. *Qualitative Studies*, 2(1), 16–30.

Grove, S.K. (2007). *Statistics for health care research: a practical workbook*. Edinburgh: Elsevier Saunders.

Grove, S.K., Burns, N. & Gray, J.R. (2013). *The practice of nursing research: appraisal, synthesis, and generation of evidence*, 7th edn. St Louis, MO: Elsevier.

Grypdonck, M.H.F. (2006). Qualitative health research in the era of evidence-based practice. *Qualitative Health Research*, 16(10), 1371–85.

Guba, E.G. & Lincoln, Y.S. (1994). Competing paradigms in qualitative research. In N.K. Denzin & Y.S. Lincoln (eds), *Handbook of qualitative research*. Thousand Oaks, CA: Sage, 105–17.

Guba, E.G. & Lincoln, Y.S. (2005). Paradigmatic controversies, contradictions and emerging confluences. In N.K. Denzin & Y.S. Lincoln (eds), *The Sage handbook of qualitative research*. Thousand Oaks, CA: Sage, 191–215.

Guba, E.G. & Lincoln, Y.S. (2008). Paradigmatic controversies, contradictions, and emerging confluences. In N.K. Denzin & Y.S. Lincoln (eds), *The landscape of qualitative research*, 3rd edn. Thousand Oaks, CA: Sage, 255–86.

Gubrium, J.F. & Holstein, J.A. (1997). *The new language of qualitative method*. New York: Oxford University Press.

Gubrium, J.F., Holstein, J.A., Marvasti, A.B. & McKinney, K.D. (2012). *The Sage handbook of interview research: the complexity of the craft*, 2nd edn. London: Sage.

Guest, G., Bunce, A. & Johnson, L. (2006). How many interviews are enough? An experiment with data saturation and variability. *Field Methods*, 18(1), 59–82.

Guest, G., MacQueen, K.M. & Namey, E.E. (2012). *Applied thematic analysis*. Thousand Oaks, CA: Sage.

Guillemin, M. & Drew, S. (2010). Questions of process in participant-generated visual methodologies. *Visual Studies*, 25(2), 175–88.

Guillemin, M. & Gillam, L. (2004). Ethics, reflexivity and 'ethically important moments' in research. *Qualitative Inquiry*, 10(2), 261–81.

Guillemin, M. (2004). Understanding illness: using drawings as research method. *Qualitative Health Research*, 14(2), 272–89.

Guyatt, G.H., Oxman, A.D., Kunz, R., Vist, G.E., Falck-Ytter, Y. & Schünemann, H.J. (2008a). GRADE: What is 'quality of evidence' and why is it important to clinicians? *British Medical Journal*, 336, 995–8.

Guyatt, G.H., Oxman, A.D., Kunz, R., Jaeschke, R., Helfand, M., Liberati, A., Vist, G.E. & Schünemann, H.J. (2008b). Incorporating considerations of resources use into grading recommendations. *British Medical Journal*, 336, 1170–3.

Guyatt, G.H., Oxman, A.D., Kunz, R., Falck-Ytter, Y., Vist, G.E., Liberati, A. & Schünemann, H.J. (2008c). GRADE: going from evidence to recommendations. *British Medical Journal*, 336, 1049–51.

Guyatt, G.H., Oxman, A.D., Vist, G.E., Kunz, R., Falck-Ytter, Y., Alonso-Coello, P. & Schünemann, H.J. (2008d). GRADE: an emerging consensus on rating quality of evidence and strength of recommendations. *British Medical Journal*, 336, 924–6.

Guyatt, G.H., Sackett, D. & Cook, D.J. (1993). Users' guides to the medical literature. II. How to use an article about therapy or prevention: A. Are the results of the study valid? *Journal of the American Medical Association*, 270(21), 2598–601.

Haahr, M.T. & Hróbjartsson, A. (2006). Who is blinded in randomized clinical trials? A study of 200 trials and a survey of authors. *Clinical Trials*, 3(4), 360–5.

Habets, B. & van Cingel, R.E. (2015). Eccentric exercise training in chronic mid-portion Achilles tendinopathy: a systematic review on different protocols. *Scandinavian Journal of Medicine & Science in Sports*, 25(1), 3–15.

Haesler, E., Bauer, M. & Nay, R. (2007). Staff–family relationships in the care of older people: a report on a systematic review. *Research in Nursing & Health*, 30(4), 385–98.

Haesler, E., Bauer, M. & Nay, R. (2010). Factors associated with constructive nursing staff–family relationships in the care of older adults in the institutional setting: an update to a systematic review. *International Journal of Evidence-Based Healthcare*, 8(2), 45–74.

Hagey, R.S. (1997). Editorial. The use and abuse of participatory action research. *Chronic Diseases in Canada*, 18(1), 1–4.

Hajiro, T. & Nishimura, K. (2002). Minimal clinically significant difference in health status: the thorny path of health status measures? *European Respiratory Journal*, 19, 390–1.

Halcomb, E.J., Gholizadeh, L., DiGiacomo, M., Phillips, J. & Davidson, P.M. (2007). Literature review: considerations in undertaking focus group research with culturally and linguistically diverse groups. *Journal of Clinical Nursing*, 16(6), 1000–11.

Hall, W.A. & Callery, P. (2001). Enhancing the rigor of grounded theory: incorporating the reflexivity and relationality. *Qualitative Health Research*, 11(2), 257–72.

Hammell, K.W. (2006). *Perspectives on disability and rehabilitation: contesting assumptions; challenging practice*. Edinburgh: Churchill Livingstone/Elsevier.

Hammell, K.W. & Carpenter, C. (2000). Introduction to qualitative research in occupational therapy and physical therapy. In K.W. Hammell, C. Carpenter & I. Dyck (eds), *Using qualitative research: a practical introduction for occupational and physical therapists*. Edinburgh: Churchill Livingstone, 1–12.

Hammell, K.W. & Carpenter, C. (2004). *Qualitative research in evidence-based rehabilitation*. Edinburgh: Churchill Livingstone.

Hammersley, M. (1996). The relationship between qualitative and quantitative research: paradigm loyalty versus methodological eclecticism. In J.T.E. Richardson (ed.), *Handbook of research methods for psychology and the social sciences*. Leicester: BPS Books, 159–74.

Hammersley, M. (2005). Close encounters of a political kind: the threat from the evidence-based policy-making and practice movement. *Qualitative Researcher*, 1, 2–4.

Hammersley, M. (2008). The issue of quality in qualitative research. *International Journal of Research & Method in Education*, 30(3), 287–305.

Hammersley, M. & Atkinson, P. (1995). *Ethnography: principles in practice*, 2nd edn. London: Routledge & Kegan Paul.

Hammersley, M. & Atkinson, P. (2007). *Ethnography: principles in practice*, 3rd edn. Milton Park, Abingdon, UK: Routledge.

Hanna, S., Russell, D., Bartlett, D., Kertoy, M., Rosenbaum, P. & Swinton, M. (2005). *Clinical measurement guidelines for service providers*. <http://canchild.icreate3.esolutionsgroup.ca/en/canchildresources/resources/ClinicalMeasurement.pdf>.

Hannes, K. & Lockwood, C. (2011). Pragmatism as the philosophical foundation for the Joanna Briggs meta-aggregative approach to qualitative evidence synthesis. *Journal of Advanced Nursing*, 67(7), 1632–42.

Hannes, K. & Macaitis, K. (2012). A move to more systematic and transparent approaches in qualitative evidence synthesis: update on a review of published papers. *Qualitative Research*, 12(4), 402–42.

Hannes, K., Lockwood, C. & Pearson, A. (2010). A comparative analysis of three online appraisal instruments' ability to assess validity in qualitative research. *Qualitative Health Research*, 20(12), 1736–43.

Harper, P.J. (2007). Writing research proposals: five rules. *HIV Nursing*, 8(2), 15–17.

Hart, E. & Bond, M. (1995). *Action research for health and social care: a guide to practice*. Buckingham, UK: Open University Press.

Hartley, J., Sydes, M. & Blurton, A. (1996). Obtaining information accurately and quickly: are structured abstracts more efficient? *Journal of Information Science*, 22, 349–56.

Hartsock, N. (1987). The feminist standpoint: developing the ground for a specifically feminist historical materialism. In S. Harding (ed.), *Feminism and methodology*. Bloomington, IN: Indiana University Press, 157–80.

Hauck, Y., Nguyen, T., Frayne, J., Garefalakis, M. & Rock, D. (2015). Sexual and reproductive health trends among women with enduring mental illness: a survey of Western Australian community mental health services. *Health Care for Women International*, 36(4), 499–510.

Havill, N.L., Leeman, J., Shaw-Kokot, J., Knafl, K., Crandell, J. & Sandelowski, M. (2014). Managing large-volume literature searches in research synthesis studies. *Nursing Outlook*, 62(2), 112–18.

Havstam, C., Laakso, K., Lohmander, A. & Ringsberg, K.C. (2011). Taking charge of communication: adults' descriptions of growing up with a cleft-related speech impairment. *Cleft Palate–Craniofacial Journal*, 48(6), 717–26.

Hawker, S., Payne, S., Kerr, C., Hardey, M. & Powell, J. (2002). Appraising the evidence: reviewing disparate data systematically. *Qualitative Health Research*, 12(9), 1284–99.

Heaton, J. (1998). Secondary analysis of qualitative data. *Social Research Update* (22). Online journal. <http://www.soc.surrey.ac.uk/sru/SRU22.html>.

Heaton, J. (2004). *Re-working qualitative data*. London: Sage.

Heaton, J. (2008). Secondary analysis of qualitative data: an overview. *Historical Social Research*, 3, 33–45.

Heinemann, A.W., Linacre, J.M., Wright, B.D. & Hamilton, B.B. (1994). Prediction of rehabilitation outcomes with disability measures. *Archives of Physical Medicine and* Rehabilitation, 75, 133–43.

Hennink, M., Hutter, I. & Bailey, A. (2011). *Qualitative research methods*. London: Sage.

Henry, J., Dunbar, T., Arnott, A., Scrimgeour, M., Matthews, S., Murakami-Gold, L., et al. (2002a). *Indigenous research reform agenda: Changing institutions*, vol. 3. Casuarina, NT: Cooperative Research Centre for Aboriginal and Tropical Health.

Henry, J., Dunbar, T., Arnott, A., Scrimgeour, M., Matthews, S., Murakami-Gold, L., et al. (2002b). *Indigenous research reform agenda: Rethinking methodologies*. Casuarina, NT: Cooperative Research Centre for Aboriginal and Tropical Health.

Herbert, R., Jamtvedt, G., Birger Hagen, K. & Mead, J. (2011). *Practical evidence-based physiotherapy*, 2nd edn. Edinburgh: Elsevier.

Hersh, D. (2003). 'Weaning' clients from aphasia therapy: speech pathologists' strategies for discharge. *Aphasiology*, 17(11), 1007–29.

Hesse-Biber, S.N. (2014). *The practice of qualitative research*, 3rd edn. Thousand Oaks, CA: Sage.

Hesse-Biber, S.N. & Leavy, P. (2011). *The practice of qualitative research*, 2nd edn. Thousand Oaks, CA: Sage.

Hewitt, A., Howie, L. & Feldman, S. (2010). Retirement: what will you do? A narrative inquiry of occupation-based planning for retirement: implications for practice. *Australian Occupational Therapy Journal*, 57(1), 8–16.

Hewitt, C., Hahn, S., Torgerson, D.J., Watson, J. & Bland, J.M. (2005). Adequacy and reporting of allocation concealment: review of recent trials published in four general medical journals. *British Medical Journal*, 330, 1057–8.

Heyvaert, M., Hannes, K., Maes, B. & Onghena, P. (2013). Critical appraisal of mixed methods studies. *Journal of Mixed Methods Research*, 7(4), 302–27.

Higginbottom, G. & Liamputtong, P. (2015). Diverse ethno-cultural groups and the use of participatory research. In G. Higginbottom & P. Liamputtong (eds), *Participatory qualitative research methodologies in health*. London: Sage, 161–82.

Higgins, J.P.T. & Green, S. (2008). *Cochrane handbook for systematic reviews of interventions. Version 5.0.1* [updated September 2008]. <www.cochrane-handbook.org>.

Higgins, J.P.T. & Green, S. (2011). *Cochrane handbook for systematic reviews of interventions. Version 5.1.0* [updated March 2011]. <www.cochrane-handbook.org>.

Hill, E.L., Graham, M.L. & Shelley, J.M. (2010). Hysterectomy trends in Australia—between 2000/01 and 2004/05. *Australian and New Zealand Journal of Obstetrics and Gynaecology*, 50(2), 153–8.

Hillier, L., Mitchell, K.J. & Ybarra, M.L. (2012). The internet as a safety net: findings from a series of online focus groups with LGB and non-LGB young people in the United States. *Journal of LGBT Youth*, 9(3), 225–46.

Hirschi, T. (1969). *Causes of delinquency*. Berkeley, CA: University of California Press.

Hobart, J. & Cano, S. (2009). Improving the evaluation of therapeutic interventions in multiple sclerosis: the role of new psychometric methods. *Health Technology Assessment*, 13(12), 1–200.

Hochschild, A. (1990). *The second shift: working parents and the revolution of the home*. New York: Viking.

Hochschild, A. (2003). *The commercialization of intimate life: notes from home and work*. Berkeley, CA: University of California Press.

Hoffman, T., Bennett, S. & Del Mar, C. (2010). *Evidence-based practice across the health professions*. Sydney: Churchill Livingstone.

Hoffman, T., Bennett, S. & Del Mar, C. (2013). *Evidence-based practice across the health professions*, 2nd edn. Sydney: Churchill Livingstone.

Holland, K.D. & Holahan, C.K. (2003). The relation of social support and coping to positive adaptation to breast cancer. *Psychology & Health*, 18(1), 15–29.

Hollis, S. & Campbell, F. (1999). What is meant by intention to treat analysis? Survey of published randomised controlled trials. *British Medical Journal*, 319, 670–4.

Holloway, I. & Wheeler, S. (2002). *Qualitative research in nursing*, 2nd edn. Oxford: Blackwell Science.

Holloway, I. & Wheeler, S. (2013). *Qualitative research in nursing and healthcare*, 3rd edn. Somerset: Wiley.

Holmefur, M. (2009). *The Assisting Hand Assessment: continued development, psychometrics and longitudinal use*. PhD dissertation, Karolinska Institutet, Stockholm.

Holmefur, M. & Krumlinde-Sundholm, L. (2015). Psychometric properties of a revised version of the Assisting Hand Assessment (Kids-AHA 5.0). *Developmental Medicine & Child Neurology*. Doi: 10.1111/dmcn.12939.

Holton, J.A. (2007). The coding process and its challenges. In A. Bryant & K. Charmaz (eds), *The Sage handbook of grounded theory*. London: Sage, 265–89.

Hopkins, T., Clegg, J. & Stackhouse, J. (2015). Young offenders' perspectives on their literacy and communication skills. *International Journal of Language & Communication Disorders*. Doi: 10.1111/1460-6984.12188.

Hopkinson, J.B. & Richardson, A. (2015). A mixed-methods qualitative research study to develop a complex intervention for weight loss and anorexia in advanced cancer: the family approach to weight and eating. *Palliative Medicine*, 29(2), 164–76.

Horner, R.D. & Baer, D.M. (1978). Multiple-probe technique: a variation of the multiple baseline. *Journal of Applied Behavior Analysis*, 11(1), 189–96.

Houser, J. (2015). *Nursing research: reading, using, and creating evidence*, 3rd edn. Sudbury, MA: Jones & Bartlett Learning.

Howie, L., Coulter, M. & Feldman, S. (2004). Crafting the self: narratives of occupational identity. *American Journal of Occupational Therapy*, 58(4), 446–54.

Hróbjartsson, A. & Boutron, I. (2011). Blinding in randomized clinical trials: imposed impartiality. *Clinical Pharmacology and Therapeutics*, 90(5), 732–6.

Hróbjartsson, A. & Gøtzsche, P.C. (2010). Placebo interventions for all clinical conditions. *Cochrane Database of Systematic Reviews*, Issue 1, Art. No. CD003974. Doi: 10.1002/14651858.CD003974. pub3.

Hróbjartsson, A., Gøtzsche, P. & Gluud, C. (1998). The controlled clinical trial turns 100 years: Fibiger's trial of serum treatment of diphtheria. *British Medical Journal*, 317, 1243–5.

Hudson, A.L., Nyamathi, A., Greengold, B., Koniak-Griffin, A.S.D., Khalilifard, F. & Getzoff. D. (2010). Health-seeking challenges among homeless youth. *Nursing Research*, 59(3), 212–18.

Hughes, C. (1992). 'Ethnography': what's in a word—process? product? promise? *Qualitative Health Research*, 2(4), 439–50.

Hughes, P.C., Taylor, N.F. & Green, R.A. (2008). Most clinical tests cannot accurately diagnose rotator cuff pathology: a systematic review. *Australian Journal of Physiotherapy*, 54, 159–70.

Humphery, K. (2001). Dirty questions: Indigenous health and 'western research'. *Australian and New Zealand Journal of Public Health*, 25(3), 197–202.

Humphreys, L. (1975). *Tearoom trade: impersonal sex in public places*. New York: Aldine.

Iacono, T. (2006). Ethical challenges and complexities of including people with intellectual disability as participants in research. *Journal of Intellectual and Developmental Disability*, 31(3), 173–9.

Iles, R. & Davidson, M. (2006). Evidence based practice: a survey of physiotherapists' current practice. *Physiotherapy Research International*, 11(2), 93–103.

International Committee of Medical Journal Editors (2012). *Uniform requirements for manuscripts submitted to biomedical journals: writing and editing for biomedical publication. III. J. Obligation to register clinical trials*. <www.icmje.org/#clin_trials>.

Ioannidis, J.P.A. (1998). Effect of the statistical significance of results on the time to completion and publication of randomized efficacy trial. *Journal of the American Medical Association*, 279(4), 281–6.

Israel, M. (2015). *Research ethics and integrity for social scientists: beyond regulatory compliance*, 2nd edn. London: Sage.

Israel, B.A., Eng, E., Schulz, A.J. & Parker, E.A. (eds) (2005). *Methods in community-based participatory research for health*. San Francisco: Jossey-Bass.

Israel, B.A., Eng, E., Schultz, A.J. & Parker, E.A. (eds) (2012). *Methods for community-based participatory research for health*, 2nd edn. San Francisco: Jossey-Bass.

Ittenbach, R. & Lawhead, W. (1996). Historical and philosophical foundation of single-case research. In R. Franklin, D. Allison & B. Gorman (eds), *Design and analysis of single-case research*. New Jersey: Lawrence Erlbaum, 13–39.

Jacelon, C.S. & O'Dell, K.K. (2005). Analyzing qualitative data. *Urologic Nursing*, 25(3), 217.

Jack, S.M. (2006). Utility of qualitative research findings in evidence-based public health practice. *Public Health Nursing*, 23(3), 277–83.

Jadad, A.R. (1998). *Randomised controlled trials: a user's guide*. London: BMJ Books.

Jadad, A.R., Moore, R.A., Carroll, D., Jenkinson, C., Reynolds, D.J.M., Gavaghan, D.J. *et al.* (1996). Assessing the quality of reports of randomized clinical trials: is blinding necessary? *Controlled Clinical Trials*, 17, 1–12.

Jamieson, L.M., Paradies, Y.C., Eades, S., Chong, A., Maple-Brown, L., Morris, P., Bailie, R., Cass, A., Roberts-Thomson, K. & Brown, A. (2012). Ten principles relevant to health research among Indigenous Australian populations. *Medical Journal of Australia*, 197(1), 16–18.

Jamtvedt, G., Young, J.M., Kristoffersen, D.T., O'Brien, M.A. & Oxman, A.D. (2006). Audit and feedback: effects on professional practice and health care outcomes. *Cochrane Database of Systematic Reviews. Issue 2.* <www.cochrane.org/reviews/en/ab000259.html>.

Janssen, S.L. & Stube, J.E. (2014). Older adults' perceptions of physical activity: a qualitative study. *Occupational Therapy International,* 21, 53–62.

Jeffrey, J.E. & Foster, N.E. (2012). A qualitative investigation of physical therapists' experiences and feelings managing patients with non-specific low back pain. *Physical Therapy*, 92(2), 266–78.

Jenkinson, C. & McGee, H. (1998). *Health status measurement: a brief but critical introduction.* Oxford: Radcliffe Medical Press.

Jensen, L.A. & Allen, M.N. (1996). Meta-synthesis of qualitative findings. *Qualitative Health Research*, 6(4), 553–60.

Joanna Briggs Institute (2008a). *Management of constipation in older adults.* Best practice information sheet 12(7). Adelaide: Joanna Briggs Institute.

Joanna Briggs Institute (2008b). *JBI QARI critical appraisal checklist for interpretive and critical research.* <www.joannabriggs.edu.au/documents/jbireviewmanual_cip11449.pdf>.

Joanna Briggs Institute (2008c). *Reviewers' manual: the synthesis of qualitative research findings.* Adelaide: Joanna Briggs Institute.

Johansson, M., Rubertsson, C., Rådestad, I. & Hildingsson, I. (2012). Childbirth: an emotionally demanding experience for fathers. *Sexual and Reproductive Healthcare*, 3, 11–20.

John, A. (2012). Stress among mothers of children with intellectual disabilities in urban India: role of gender and maternal coping. *Journal of Applied Research in Intellectual Disabilities*, 25(4), 372–82.

Johnson, B. (2008). Editorial. Living with tensions: the dialectic approach. *Journal of Mixed Methods Research*, 2(3), 203–7.

Johnson, B. & Turner, L.A. (2003). Data collection strategies in mixed methods research. In A. Tashakkori & C. Teddlie (eds), *Handbook of mixed methods in social and behavioral research.* London: Sage, 297–319.

Johnson, J.M. & Rowlands, T. (2012). The interpersonal dynamics of in-depth interviewing. In J.F. Gubrium & J.A. Holstein (eds), *Handbook of interview research: the complexity of the craft.* Thousand Oaks, CA: Sage, 99–113.

Johnson, M. & Hengstberger-Sims, C. (2014). Introducing the research process. In S. Jirojwong, M. Johnson & A. Welch (eds), *Research methods in nursing and midwifery: pathways to evidence-based practice*, 2nd edn. Melbourne: Oxford University Press, 34–63.

Johnson, R. & Onwuegbuzie, T. (2006). Mixed methods research: a research paradigm whose time has come. *Educational Researcher*, 33(7), 14–26.

Johnson, R. & Waterfield, J. (2004). Making words count: the value of qualitative research. *Physiotherapy Research International*, 9(3), 121–31.

Johnson, L.M., Randall, M., Reddihough, D., Oke, L.E., Byrt, T.A. & Bach, T.M. (1994). Development of a clinical assessment of quality of movement for unilateral upper limb function. *Developmental Medicine & Child Neurology*, 36, 965–73.

Jones, K. (2013). Doing a literature review in health. In M. Saks & J. Allsop (eds), *Researching health: qualitative, quantitative and mixed methods*, 2nd edn. London: Sage, 42–63.

Jones, M.L. (2004). Application of systematic review methods to qualitative research: practical isues. *Journal of Advanced Nursing*, 48(3), 271–8.

Jones, P. (1987). The untreatable family. *Child Abuse and Neglect*, 11, 409–20.

Jones, F., Rodger, S., Ziviani, J. & Boyd, R. (2012). Application of a hermeneutic phenomenologically orientated approach to qualitative study. *International Journal of Theory and Practice*, 19(7), 370–8.

Jorgensen, D.L. (1989). *Participant observation: a methodology for human studies*. Newbury Park, CA: Sage.

Josselson, R. (2006). Narrative research and the challenge of accumulating knowledge. *Narrative Inquiry*, 16, 4–10.

Josselson, R. (2007). The ethical attitude in narrative research: principles and practicalities. In J.D. Clandinin (ed.), *Handbook of narrative inquiry: mapping the methodology*. Thousand Oaks, CA: Sage, 537–66.

Josselson, R. (2011). Narrative research: constructing, deconstructing and reconstructing story. In F. Wertz, K. Charmaz, L. McMullen, R. Josselson, R. Anderson & E. McSpadden (eds), *Five ways of doing qualitative analysis*. New York: Guildford Press, 224–42.

Jüni, P., Altman, D.G. & Egger, M. (2001). Systematic reviews in health care: assessing the quality of controlled clinical trials. *British Medical Journal*, 323, 42–6.

Kaida, A., Gray, G., Bastos, F.I., Andia, I., Maier, M., McIntyre, J. *et al.* (2008). The relationship between HAART use and sexual activity among HIV-positive women of reproductive age in Brazil, South Africa and Uganda. *AIDS Care*, 20(1), 21–5.

Kale, R. (1997). Letter. Failing to seek patients' consent to research is always wrong. *British Medical Journal*, 314, 1081–4.

Kaplan, S.A., Ruddock, C., Golub, M., Davis, J., Foley Sr, R., Devia, C. *et al.* (2009). Stirring up the mud: using a community-based participatory approach to address health disparities through a faith-based initiative. *Journal of Health Care for the Poor and Underserved*, 20(4), 1111–23.

Kaptchuk, T.J. & Miller, F.G. (2015). Placebo effects in medicine. *New England Journal of Medicine*, 373(1), 8–9.

Kavitha, R. & Jayan, C. (2014). Role of social support on cancer distress among breast cancer patients. *Guru Journal of Behavioral and Social Sciences*, 2(1), 247–51.

Kazdin, A.E. (2003). Clinical significance: measuring whether interventions make a difference. In A.E. Kazdin (ed.), *Methodological issues and strategies in clinical research*, 3rd edn. Washington, DC: American Psychological Association, 547–68.

Kazdin, A.E. (2011). Single-case research designs: methods for clinical and applied settings, 2nd edn. New York: Oxford University Press.

Kazdin, A.E. (ed.) (2015). *Methodological issues and strategies in clinical research*, 4th edn. Washington, DC: American Psychological Association.

Kearney, M.H. (1998a). Ready-to-wear: discovering grounded formal theory. *Research in Nursing and Health*, 21,179–86.

Kearney, M.H. (1998b). Truthful self-nurturing: a grounded formal theory of women's addiction recovery. *Qualitative Health Research*, 8, 495–512.

Kearney, M.H. (2001a). Levels and applications of qualitative research evidence. *Research in Nursing & Health*, 24, 145–53.

Kearney, M.H. (2001b). New directions in grounded formal theory. In R. Schreiber & P.N. Stern (eds), *Using grounded theory in nursing*. New York: Springer, 227–46.

Kearney, R. & Costa, M.L. (2010). Insertional achilles tendinopathy management: a systematic review. *Foot and Ankle International*, 31(8), 689–94.

Keech, A., Gebski, V. & Pike, R. (eds) (2007). *Interpreting and reporting clinical trials: a guide to the CONSORT statement and the principles of randomised controlled trials*. Sydney: MJA Books.

Keene, J. (2001). *Clients with complex needs: inter-professional practice*. Oxford: Blackwell Science.

Kellehear, A. (1993). *The unobtrusive researcher: a guide to methods*. Sydney: Allen & Unwin.

Keller, C., Fleury, J., Perez, A., Ainsworth, B. & Vaughan, L. (2008). Using visual methods to uncover context. *Qualitative Health Research*, 18(3), 428–36.

Kelly, M. (2012). Research questions and proposals. In C. Seale (ed.), *Researching society and culture*, 3rd edn. London: Sage, 97–117.

Kelly, S.E. (2010). Qualitative interviewing techniques and styles. In I. Bourgeault, R. Dingwell & R. De Vries (eds), *The Sage handbook of qualitative methods in health research*. London: Sage, 307–26.

Kelly, T. & Howie, L. (2007). Working with stories in nursing research: procedures used in narrative analysis. *International Journal of Mental Health Nursing*, 16, 136–44.

Kelly, J., Saggers, S., Taylor, K., Pearce, G., Massey, P., Bull, J., Odo, T., Thomas, J., Billycan, R., Judd, J., Reilly, S. & Ahboo, S. (2012). 'Makes you proud to be black eh?': reflections on meaningful indigenous research participation. *International Journal of Equity in Health*, 11, 40. Doi: 10.1186/1475-9276-11-40.

Kempe, A. & Nevill, A. (2010). *HBS108 Health Information and Data Topic 9 content*. Deakin University, HBS108 Health Information and Data curriculum.

Kenaszchuk, C., Conn, L.G., Dainty, K., McCarthy, C., Reeves, S. & Zwarenstein, M. (2012). Consensus on interprofessional collaboration in hospitals: statistical agreement of ratings from ethnographic fieldwork and measurement scales. *Journal of Evaluation in Clinical Practice*, 18(1), 93–9.

Kent, G. (1996). Shared understandings for informed consent: the relevance of psychological research on the provision of information. *Social Science and Medicine*, 43(10), 1517–23.

Khanlou, N. & Peter, E. (2004). Participatory action research: considerations for ethical review. *Social Science and Medicine*, 60(10), 2333–40.

Kidd, P.S. & Parshall, M.B. (2000). Getting the focus and the group: enhancing analytical rigor in focus group research. *Qualitative Health Research*, 10(3), 293–308.

Kielhofner, G. (2002). *A model of human occupation: theory and application*, 3rd edn. Baltimore: Lippincott, Williams & Wilkins.

Kielhofner, G. (ed.) (2008). *Model of human occupation*, 4th edn. Baltimore: Lippincott, Williams & Wilkins.

Kielhofner, G., Mallinson, T., Crawford, C., Nowak, M., Rigby, M., Henry, A. & Walens, A. (2004). *A user's manual for the Occupational Performance History Interview (Version 2.1), OPHI-II*. Chicago: Model of Human Occupation Clearing House, Department of Occupational Therapy, College of Applied Health Sciences, University of Illinois.

Kielhofner, G., Borell, L., Holzmueller, R., Jonsson, H., Josephsson, S., Keponen, R. *et al.* (2008). Crafting an occupational life. In G. Kielhofner (ed.), *Model of human occupation*, 4th edn. Baltimore: Lippincott, Williams & Wilkins, 110–25.

Kim, S. & Yoon, G. (2015). An innovation-driven culture in local government: do senior managers' transformational leadership and the climate for creativity matter? *Public Personnel Management*, 44(2), 147–68.

King, N. & Horrocks, C. (2010). *Interviews in qualitative research*. London: Sage.

Kingma, J.J., de Knikker, R., Wittink, H.M. & Takken, T. (2007). Eccentric overload training in patients with chronic Achilles tendinopathy: a systematic review. *British Journal of Sports Medicine*, 41(6), e3.

Kirkevold, M. (1997). Integrative nursing research: an important strategy to further development of nursing science and nursing practice. *Journal of Advanced Nursing*, 25, 977–84.

Kirkham, S. (2003). The politics of belonging and intercultural health care. *Western Journal of Nursing Research*, 25(7), 762–80.

Kitzinger, J. (1995). Qualitative research: introducing focus groups. *British Medical Journal*, 311(7000), 299–302.

Klauda, S.L. & Wigfield, A. (2012). Relations of perceived parent and friend support for recreational reading with children's reading motivations. *Journal of Literacy Research*, 44(1), 3–44.

Kleinman, A. (1988). *The illness narratives*. New York: Basic Books.

Kline, T.J.B. (2005). *Psychological testing: a practical approach to design and application*. Thousand Oaks, CA: Sage.

Klingels, K., De Cock, P., Desloovere, K., Huenaerts, C., Molenaers, G., Van Nuland, I. *et al.* (2008). Comparison of the Melbourne Assessment of Unilateral Upper Limb Function and the Quality of Upper Extremity Skills Test in hemiplegic CP. *Development Medicine & Child Neurology*, 50(12), 904–9.

Knight, L.V. & Mattick, K. (2006). 'When I first came here, I thought medicine was black and white': making sense of medical students' ways of knowing. *Social Science and Medicine*, 63, 1084–96.

Koch, T. & Kralik, D. (2001). Chronic illness: reflections on a community-based action research programme. *Journal of Advanced Nursing*, 36(1), 23–31.

Koch, T., Selim, P. & Kralik, D. (2002). Enhancing lives through the development of a community-based participatory action research programme. *Journal of Clinical Nursing*, 11, 109–17.

König, T. (2004). *Routinizing frame analysis through the use of CAQDAS*. Paper presented at the biannual RC-33 meeting, Amsterdam, 17–20 August 2004.

Kozinets, R.V. (2002). The field behind the screen: using netnography for marketing research in online communities. *Journal of Marketing Research*, 39, 61–72.

Kozinets, R.V. (2015). *Netnography: redefined*, 2nd edn. London: Sage.

Krueger, R. A. (1997). *Analyzing and reporting focus group results*. London: Sage.

Krueger, R.A. (1998). *Focus group kit: analyzing and reporting focus group results*, 6th edn. Thousand Oaks, CA: Sage.

Krueger, R.A. & Casey, M.A. (2009). *Focus groups: a practical guide for applied research*. Thousand Oaks, CA: Sage.

Krumlinde-Sundholm, L. & Eliasson, A. (2003). Development of the Assisting Hand Assessment: A Rasch-built measure intended for children with unilateral upper limb impairments. *Scandinavian Journal of Occupational Therapy*, 10(1), 16–26.

Kummerer, S.E., Lopez-Reyna, N.A. & Hughes, M.T. (2007). Mexican immigrant mothers' perceptions of their children's communication disabilities, emergent literacy development, and speech-language therapy program. *American Journal of Speech-Language Pathology*, 16(3), 271–82.

Kvale, S. (2007). *Doing interviews*. London: Sage.

La Pelle, N. (2004). Simplifying qualitative data analysis using general purpose software tools. *Field Methods*, 16(1), 85–108.

Lacey, E.A. (1998). Social and medical research: is there a difference? *Social Sciences in Health*, 4(4), 211–17.

Lai Fong Chiu (2002). *Straight talking: communicating breast screening information in primary care*. Leeds, UK: Nuffield Institute for Health.

Laine, C., Horton, R., DeAngelis, C.D., Drazen, J.M., Frizelle, F.A., Godlee, F. *et al.* (2007). Clinical trial registration: looking back and moving ahead. *New England Journal of Medicine*, 356(26), 2734–6.

Lalayants, M., Epstein, I., Auslander, G.K., Chi Ho Chan, W., Fouche, C., Giles, R., Joubert, L., Rosenne, H. & Vertigan, A. (2012). Clinical data-mining: learning from practice in international settings. *International Social Work*, 56(6), 775–97.

Lam, J. (2012). *Falls in older persons: an exploration of factors impacting on the decision to participate in an exercise program amongst recent fallers*. Unpublished Master's thesis. School of Public Health, La Trobe University, Melbourne.

Lam, P. & Beaulieu, M. (2004). Experiences of families in the neurological ICU: a bedside phenomenon. *Journal of Neuroscience Nursing*, 36(3), 142–55.

Landmark, B.T., Strandmark, M. & Wahl, A. (2002). Breast cancer and experiences of social support: in-depth interviews of 10 women with newly diagnosed breast cancer. *Scandinavian Journal of Caring Sciences*, 16(3), 216–23.

Landorf, K.B. & Burns, J. (2009). Health outcome assessment. In B. Yates (ed.), *Merriman's assessment of the lower limb*. Edinburgh: Elsevier/Churchill Livingstone, 35–51.

Landorf, K.B., Keenan, A.-M. & Herbert, R.D. (2006). Effectiveness of foot orthoses to treat plantar fasciitis: a randomized trial. *Archives of Internal Medicine*, 166(12), 1305–10.

Landorf, K.B., Radford, J.A., Keenan, A.-M. & Redmond, A.C. (2005). Effectiveness of low-dye taping for the short-term management of plantar fasciitis. *Journal of the American Podiatric Medical Association*, 95(6), 525–30.

Lang, T.A. & Secic, M. (1997). *How to report medical statistics in medicine*. Philadelphia, PA: American College of Physicians.

Larkin, P.M., Begley, C.M. & Devane, D. (2014). Breaking from binaries: using a sequential mixed methods design. *Nurse Researcher*, 21(4), 8–12.

Last, J.M., Abramson, J.H., Friedman, G.D., Porta, M., Spasoff, R.A. & Thuriaux, M. (eds), (1995). *A dictionary of epidemiology*, 3rd edn. New York: Oxford University Press.

Laugharne, C. (1995). Ethnography: research method or philosophy? *Nurse Researcher*, 3(2), 45–54.

Law, M. (2004). *Outcome measures rating form guidelines*. <www.canchild.ca/en/canchildresources/resources/measguid.pdf>.

Laycock, A. with Walker, D., Harrison, N. & Brands, J. (2011). *Researching Indigenous health: a practical guide for researchers*. Melbourne: Lowitja Institute.

Leblanc, M.C., Kowalczuk, M., Andruszkiewicz, N., Simunovic, N., Farrokhyar, F., Turnbull, T.L. *et al.* (2015). Diagnostic accuracy of physical examination for anterior knee instability: a systematic review. *Knee Surgery Sports Traumatology Arthroscopy Journal*, 23(10), 2805–13.

Lee, P. (2005). The process of gatekeeping in health care research. *Nursing Times*, 101(32), 36–8.

Lee, P. (2016). Assessing the health of populations: epidemiology in public health. In P. Liamputtong (ed.), *Public health: local and global perspectives*. Cambridge: Cambridge University Press, 188–212.

Lee, C. & Gramotnev, H. (2006). Predictors and outcomes of early motherhood in the Australian longitudinal study on women's health. *Psychology, Health and Medicine*, 11(1), 29–47.

Lee, R. & Fielding, N.G. (1991). Computing for qualitative research: options, problems and potential. In N.G. Fielding & R.M. Lee (eds), *Using computers in qualitative research*. London: Sage, 1–13.

Lee, R.M. & Renzetti, C.M. (1993). The problems of researching sensitive topics: introduction. In C.M. Renzetti & R.M. Lee (eds), *Researching sensitive topics*. London: Sage, 3–13.

Lee, H., Tamminen, K.A., Clark, A.M., Slater, L., Spence, J.C. & Holt, N.L. (2015). A meta-study of qualitative research examining determinants of children's independent active free play. *International Journal of Behavioural Nutrition and Physical Activity*, 12, 5. Doi: 10.1186/s12966-015-0165-9.

Leech, N.L., Dellinger, A.B., Brannagan, K.B. & Tanaka, H. (2010). Evaluating mixed research studies: a mixed methods approach. *Journal of Mixed Methods Research*, 4(1), 17–31.

Leech, N.L., Onwuegbuzie, A.J. & Combs, J.P. (2011). Writing publishable mixed research articles: guidelines for emerging scholars in the health sciences and beyond. *International Journal of Multiple Research Approaches*, 5(1), 7–24.

Leeman, J., Sandelowski, M., Havill, N.L. & Knafl, K. (2015). Parent-to-child transition in managing cystic fibrosis: a research synthesis. *Journal of Family Theory & Review*, 7, 167–83.

Leininger, M.M. (1979). *Transcultural nursing*. New York: MASSON International Nursing Publications.

Leininger, M.M. (1985). *Qualitative research methods in nursing*. Orlando, FL: Grune & Stratton.

Leininger, M.M. (1994). *Nursing and anthropology: two worlds to blend*. Columbus, OH: Greyden Press.

Lenton, S., Dietze, P., Olsen, A., Wiggins, N., McDonald, D. & Fowler, C. (2014). Working together: expanding the availability of naloxone for peer administration to prevent opioid overdose deaths in the Australian Capital Territory and beyond. *Drug and Alcohol Review*, 34 (4), 404–11.

Levack, W.M.M. (2012). The role of qualitative metasynthesis in evidence-based physical therapy. *Physical Therapy Reviews*, 17(6), 390–7.

Levy, R.I. (1988). *Tahitians: mind and experience in the Society Islands* (Midway reprint edn). Chicago: University of Chicago Press.

Lewin, K. (1946/1988). Action research and minority problems. In Deakin University (ed.), *The action research reader*. Melbourne: Deakin University. Originally published in 1946, 41–6.

Lewins, A. & Silver, C. (2007). *Using software in qualitative research: a step-by-step guide*. Los Angeles: Sage.

Liamputtong, P. (2007). *Researching the vulnerable: a guide to sensitive research methods.* London: Sage.

Liamputtong, P. (2010). *Performing qualitative cross-cultural research.* Cambridge: Cambridge University Press.

Liamputtong, P. (2011). *Focus group methodology: principles and practice.* London: Sage.

Liamputtong, P. (2013). *Qualitative research methods*, 4th edn. Melbourne: Oxford University Press.

Liamputtong, P. (2016). Qualitative research methodology and evidence-based practice in public health. In P. Liamputtong (ed.), *Public health: local and global perspectives.* Melbourne: Cambridge University Press, 171–87.

Liamputtong, P. & Haritavorn, N. (2016). To tell or not to tell: disclosure and women living with HIV/AIDS in Thailand. *Health Promotion International*, 31(1), 23–32. Doi:10.1093/heapro/dau057.

Liamputtong, P. & Rumbold, J. (2008). Knowing differently: setting the scene. In P. Liamputtong & J. Rumbold (eds), *Knowing differently: art-based and collaborative research.* New York: Nova Science Publishers, 1–23.

Liamputtong, P. & Suwanhong, D. (2015). Breast cancer diagnosis: biographical disruption, emotional experiences and strategic management in Thai women with breast cancer. *Sociology of Health & Illness*, 37(7), 1086–1101.

Liamputtong, P., Haritavorn, N. & Kiatying-Angsulee, N. (2009). HIV and AIDS, stigma and AIDS support groups: perspectives from women living with HIV and AIDS in central Thailand. *Social Science and Medicine*, special issue on Women, Mothers and HIV Care in Resource-Poor Settings, 69(6), 862–8.

Liamputtong, P., Haritavorn, N. & Kiatying-Angsulee, N. (2012). Living positively: the experiences of Thai women in central Thailand. *Qualitative Health Research*, 22(4), 441–51.

Lincoln, Y.S. & Guba, E.G. (1985). *Naturalistic inquiry.* Beverly Hills, CA: Sage.

Lincoln, Y.S. & Guba, E.G. (1989). *Fourth generation evaluation.* Newbury Park, CA: Sage.

Lincoln, Y.S., Lynham, S.A. & Guba, E.G. (2011). Paradigmatic controversies, contradictions, and emerging confluences, revisited. In N.K. Denzin & Y.S. Lincoln (eds), *The Sage handbook of qualitative research*, 4th edn. Thousand Oaks, CA: Sage, 97–128.

Locke, L.F., Spirduso, W. & Silverman, S.J. (2013). *Proposals that work: a guide for planning dissertations and grant proposals*, 6th edn. Thousand Oaks, CA: Sage.

Logemann, J.A. (2004). Evidence-based practice. *Advances in Speech-Language Pathology*, 6(2), 134–5.

Long, C.L. & Hollin, C.R. (1997). The scientist-practitioner model in clinical psychology: a critique. *Clinical Psychology and Psychotherapy*, 4(2), 75–83.

Long, C.O. (2015). Other sources of evidence. In N.A. Schmidt & J.M. Brown (eds), *Evidence-based practice for nurses: appraisal and application of research*, 3rd edn. Burlington, MA: Jones & Bartlett Learning, 320–40.

Long-Sutehall, T., Sque, M. & Addington-Hall, J. (2010). Secondary analysis of qualitative data: a valuable method for exploring sensitive issues with an elusive population. *Journal of Research in Nursing*, 16(4), 335–44.

Lopez, K.A. & Willis, D.G. (2004). Descriptive versus interpretive phenomenology: the contributions to nursing knowledge. *Qualitative Health Research*, 14(5), 726–35.

Low, J. (2007). Unstructured interviews and health research. In M. Saks & J. Allsop (eds), *Researching health: qualitative, quantitative and mixed methods.* London: Sage, 74–91.

Low, J. (2013). Unstructured interviews and health research. In M. Saks & J. Allsop (eds), *Researching health: qualitative, quantitative and mixed methods*, 2nd edn. London: Sage, Ch. 5.

Ludvigsen, M.S., Hall, E.O.C., Fegran, L., Aagaard, H. & Uhrenfeldt, L. (2016). Using Sandelowski and Barroso's metasynthesis method in advancing qualitative evidence. *Qualitative Health Research*, 26(3), 320–9.

Ludvigsen, M.S., Meyer, G., Hall, E., Fegran, L., Aagaard, H. & Uhrenfeldt, L. (2013). Development of clinically meaningful complex interventions: the contribution of qualitative research. *Pflege*, 26(3), 207–14.

Lueboonthavatchai, P. (2007). Prevalence and psychosocial factors of anxiety and depression in breast cancer patients. *Journal of the Medical Association of Thailand*, 90(10), 2164–74.

Lunde, Å., Heggen, K. & Strand, R. (2013). Knowledge and power: exploring unproductive interplay between quantitative and qualitative researchers. *Journal of Mixed Methods Research*, 7(2), 197–210.

Lundgren, I., Begley, C., Gross, M.M. & Bondas, T. (2012). 'Groping through the fog': a metasynthesis of women's experiences on VBAC (vaginal birth after caesarean section). *BMC Pregnancy and Childbirth*, 12, 85. Doi: 10.1186/1471-2393-12-85.

Lynoe, N., Sandlund, M. & Jacobsson, L. (1999). Research ethics committees: a comparative study of assessment of ethical dilemmas. *Scandinavian Journal of Psychiatry*, 2, 152–9.

MacKenzie, A. (1992). Learning from experience in the community: an ethnographic study of district nurse students. *Journal of Advanced Nursing*, 17, 682–91.

Mackey, M.C. (2012). Evaluation of qualitative research. In P.L. Munhall (ed.), *Nursing research: a qualitative perspective*, 5th edn. Sudbury, MA: Jones & Bartlett, 517–31.

MacMillan, K. & Koenig, T. (2004). The wow factor: preconceptions and expectations for data analysis software in qualitative research. *Social Science Computer Review*, 22(2), 179–86.

Magnussen, R.A., Dunn, W.R. & Thomson, A.B. (2009). Non-operative treatment of midportion Achilles tendinopathy: a systematic review. *Clinical Journal of Sport Medicine*, 19(1), 54–64.

Maher, L., Tran, T., Sargent, P., Tran, M.G. & Musson, R. (2002). Participatory action research with PLWHA in Vietnam. In *Proceedings of the XIV International AIDS Conference*, Barcelona, 7–12 July, 14.

Major, C.H. & Savin-Baden, M. (2010). *An introduction to qualitative research synthesis*. London: Routledge.

Malinowski, B. (1922/1961). *Argonauts of the western Pacific: an account of native enterprise and adventure in the archipelagoes of Melanesian New Guinea*. New York: E.P. Dutton.

Malinowski, B. (1932). *The sexual life of savages in north-western Melanesia: an ethnographic account of courtship, marriage and family life among the natives of the Trobriand islands, British New Guinea*, 3rd edn. London: Routledge & Kegan Paul.

Malliaras, P., Barton, C.J., Reeves, N.D. & Langberg, H. (2013). Achilles and patellar tendinopathy loading programmes: a systematic review comparing clinical outcomes and identifying potential mechanisms for effectiveness. *Sports Medicine*, 43(4), 267–86.

Malpass, A., Shaw, A., Sharp, D., Walter, F., Feder, G., Ridd, M. & Kessler, D. (2009). 'Medication career' or 'moral career'? The two sides of managing anti-depressants: a meta-ethnography of patients' experience of antidepressants. *Social Science & Medicine*, 68(1),154–68.

Malterud, K. (2001). Qualitative research: standards, challenges, and guidelines. *Lancet*, 358(9280), 483–8.

Mani-Babu, S., Morrissey, D., Waugh, C., Screen, H. & Barton, C. (2015). The effectiveness of extracorporeal shock wave therapy in lower limb tendinopathy: a systematic review. *American Journal of Sports Medicine*, 43(3), 752–61.

Mansell, J. & Beadle-Brown, J. (2004). Person-centred planning or person-centred action? A response to the commentators. *Journal of Applied Research in Intellectual Disabilities*, 17, 31–5.

Mantzoukas, S. (2008). Facilitating research students in formulating qualitative research questions. *Nursing Education Today*, 28, 371–7.

Mantzoukas, S. (2009). The research evidence published in high impact nursing journals between 2000 and 2006: a quantitative content analysis. *International Journal of Nursing Studies*, 46(4), 479–89.

Manuel, J., Fang, L., Bellamy, J.L. & Bledsoe, S.E. (2011). Evaluating evidence. In R.M. Grinnell & Y.A. Unrau (eds), *Social work research and evaluation: foundations of evidence-based practice*, 9th edn. New York: Oxford University Press, 145–59.

Manuel, J., Fang, L., Bellamy, J.L. & Bledsoe, S.E. (2014). Evaluating existing evidence. In R.M. Grinnell & Y.A. Unrau (eds), *Social work research and evaluation: foundations of evidence-based practice*, 10th edn. New York: Oxford University Press, 185–98.

Marcus, G.E. & Fischer, M.M.J. (1999). *Anthropology as cultural critique: an experimental moment in the human sciences*, 2nd edn. Chicago: University of Chicago Press.

Markham, C. & Dean, T. (2006). Parents' and professionals' perceptions of quality of life in children with speech and language difficulty. *International Journal of Language & Communication Disorders*, 41(2), 189–212.

Marková, I. (2012). *Dialogue in focus groups*. London: Equinox Books.

Marshall, J., Goldbart, J. & Phillips, J. (2007). Parents' and speech and language therapists' explanatory models of language development, language delay and intervention. *International Journal of Language & Communication Disorders*, 42(5), 533–55.

Martin, G.M. (2015). Obesity in question: understandings of body shape, self and normalcy among children in Malta. *Sociology of Health & Illness*, 37(2), 212–26.

Martone, M. (2001). Decisionmaking issues in the rehabilitation process. *Hastings Center Report*, 31, 36–41.

Marvasti, A. (2008). Writing and presenting social research. In P. Alasuutari, L. Bickman & J. Brannen (eds), *The Sage handbook of social research methods*. London: Sage, 602–16.

Marvasti, A.B. (2004). *Qualitative research in sociology*. London: Sage.

Mason, J. (2002). *Qualitative researching*, 2nd edn. London: Sage.

Massey, O.T. (2011). A proposed model for the analysis and interpretation of focus groups in evaluation research. *Evaluation and Program Planning*, 34(1), 21–8.

Matthews, J.N.S. (2006). *An introduction to randomized controlled clinical trials*. Boca Raton, FL: Chapman & Hall/CRC.

Matthews, S., Scrimgeour, M., Dunbar, T., Arnott, A., Chamberlain, A., Murakami-Gold, L. & Henry, J. (2002). *Indigenous research reform agenda: Promoting the use of health research*. Links Monograph Series 4. Darwin: Cooperative Research Centre for Aboriginal Health.

Matyas, T.A. & Greenwood, K.M. (1990). Visual analysis of single-case time series: effects of variability, serial dependence, and magnitude of intervention effects. *Journal of Applied Behavioral Analysis*, 23, 333–9.

Mauk, K.L. (2015). Qualitative designs: using words to provide evidence. In N.A. Schmidt & J.M. Brown (eds), *Evidence-based practice for nurses: appraisal and application of research*, 3rd edn. Burlington, MA: Jones & Bartlett Learning, 228–61.

Maxwell, S.E. & Delaney, H.D. (2004). *Designing experiments and analysing data: a model comparison perspective*, 2nd edn. Mahwah, NJ.: Lawrence Erlbaum.

Mayer, F., Hirschmuller, A., Muller, S., Schuberth, M. & Baur, H. (2007). Effects of short-term treatment strategies over 4 weeks in Achilles tendinopathy. *British Journal of Sports Medicine*, 41(7), e6.

Mayo, K., Tsey, K. & Empowerment Research Team (2009). *Research dancing: reflections on the relationships between university-based researchers and community-based researchers at Gurriny Yealamucka Health Services Aboriginal Corporation, Yarabah*. Casuarina, NT: Cooperative Research Centre for Aboriginal Health.

Mays, N., Pope, C. & Popay, J. (2005). Systematically reviewing qualitative and quantitative evidence to inform management and policy-making in the health field. *Journal of Health Services Research & Policy*, 10(suppl. 1), 6–20.

Mbekenga, C.K., Christensson, K., Lugina, H. & Olsson, P. (2011). Joy, struggle and support: postpartum experiences of first-time mothers in a Tanzanian suburb. *Women and Birth*, 24(1), 24–31.

McAuley, E. & Courneya, K.S. (1994). The subjective exercise experiences scale (SEES): development and preliminary validation. *Journal of Sport and Exercise Psychology*, 16, 163–77.

McBrien, B. (2008). Evidence-based care: enhancing the rigour of a qualitative study. *British Journal of Nursing*, 17(20), 1286–9.

McCann, T.V. & Clark, E. (2003a). Grounded theory in nursing research, Part 1: methodology. *Nurse Researcher*, 11(2), 7–18.

McCann, T.V. & Clark, E. (2003b). Grounded theory in nursing research, Part 2: critique. *Nurse Researcher*, 11(2), 19–28.

McConnell-Henry, T., Chapmen, Y. & Francis, K. (2009). Husserl and Heidegger: exploring the disparity. *International Journal of Nursing Practice*, 15, 7–15.

McCormick, J., Rodney, P. & Varcoe, C. (2003). Reinterpretations across studies: an approach to meta-analysis. *Qualitative Health Research*, 13(7), 933–44.

McCurdy, D.W., Spradley, J.P. & Shandy, D.J. (2005). *The cultural experience: ethnography in complex society*, 2nd edn. Long Grove, IL.: Waveland Press.

McDonald, E., Carroll, A., Albiston, D. & Epstein, I. (2005). Social relationships in early psychosis: clinical data-mining for practice-based evidence. *Journal of Social Work Research and Evaluation*, 6(2), 155–66.

McDonald, K. (1999). *Struggles for subjectivity: identity, action and experience*. Cambridge: Cambridge University Press.

McDonald, M., Townsend, A., Cox, S.M., Paterson, N.D. & Lafreniere, D. (2008). Trust in health research relationships: accounts of human subjects. *Journal of Empirical Research on Human Research Ethics*, 3(4), 35–47.

McDowell, I. (2006). *Measuring health: a guide to rating scales and questionnaires*. New York: Oxford University Press.

McDowell, I. & Newell, C. (1996). *Measuring health: a guide to rating scales and questionnaires*. New York: Oxford University Press.

McKiernan, M. & McCarthy, G. (2010). Family members' lived experience in the intensive care unit: a phemenological study. *Intensive & Critical Care Nursing*, 26(5), 254–61.

McLauchlan, G. & Handoll, H.H.G. (2011). Interventions for treating acute and chronic Achilles tendinitis. *Cochrane Database of Systematic Reviews*, Art. No. CD000232. Doi: 10.1002/14651858. CD000232.

McMillan, A.M., Landorf, K.B., Gilheany, M.F., Bird, A.R., Morrow, A.D. & Menz, H.B. (2012). Ultrasound guided corticosteroid injection for plantar fasciitis: randomised controlled trial. *British Medical Journal*, 344, e3260.

McPherson, K., Herbert, A., Judge, A., Clarke, A., Bridgman, S., Maresh, M. *et al.* (2005). Psychosexual health 5 years after hysterectomy: population-based comparison with endometrial ablation for dysfunctional uterine bleeding. *Health Expectations*, 8, 234–43.

McPherson, K.M. & Kayes, N.M. (2012). Qualitative research: its practical contribution to physiotherapy. *Physical Therapy Reviews*, 17(6), 382–9.

McReynolds, L. & Kearns, K. (1984). *Single-subject experimental designs in communicative disorders*. Baltimore, MA: University Park Press.

Mead, M. (1942). *Growing up in New Guinea: a study of adolescence and sex in primitive societies*. Harmondsworth: Penguin.

Mead, M. (1944). *The American character*. Harmondsworth: Penguin.

Mead, M. (1949). *Male and female: a study of the sexes in a changing world*. New York: W. Morrow.

Mead, M. (1951). *The school in American culture*. Cambridge, MA: Harvard University Press.

Mead, M. (1956). *New lives for old: cultural transformation—Manus, 1928–1953*. London: Gollancz.

Mead, M. (1961). *Coming of age in Samoa: a psychological study of primitive youth for western civilization*. New York: W. Morrow.

Mead, M. (1965). *And keep your powder dry: an anthropologist looks at America (new expanded edn)*. New York: Morrow.

Mead, M. (1968). *The mountain Arapesh*. Garden City, NY: Natural History Press.

Mead, M. (1977). *Sex and temperament in three primitive societies*. London: Routledge & Kegan Paul.

Mead, M. & American Museum of Natural History (1970). *Culture and commitment: a study of the generation gap*. London: Bodley Head.

Mead, M. & Baldwin, J. (1971). *A rap on race*. Philadelphia, PA: Lippincott.

Mead, M. & Heyman, K. (1965). *Family*. New York: Macmillan.

Mead, M. & Macgregor, F.M.C. (1951). *Growth and culture: a photographic study of Balinese childhood*. New York: Putnam.

Mead, M. & Wolfenstein, M. (1955). *Childhood in contemporary cultures*. Chicago: University of Chicago Press.

Meadows-Oliver, M. (2009). Does qualitative research have a place in evidence-based nursing practice? *Journal of Pediatric Health Care*, 23(5), 352–4.

Melia, K.M. (1996). Rediscovering Glaser. *Qualitative Health Research*, 6(3), 368–78.

Meltzer, P.J., Abbott, P. & Spradling, P. (2002). Teaching gerontology using the Self-Discovery Tapestry: an innovative instrument. *Gerontology & Geriatrics Education*, 23(2), 49–63.

Menz, H.B., Munteanu, S.E., Landorf, K.B. *et al.* (2007). Radiographic classification of osteoarthritis in commonly affected joints of the foot. *Osteoarthr Cartil*, 15,1333–8.

Merighi, J., Ryan, M., Renouf, N. & Healy, B. (2005). Reassessing a theory of professional expertise: a cross-national investigation of expert mental health social workers. *British Journal of Social Work*, 35, 709–25.

Merrill, M.L., Taylor, N.L., Martin, A.J., Maxim, L.A., D'Ambrosio, R., Gabriel, R.M., Wendt, S.J., Mannix, D. & Wells, M.E. (2012). A mixed-method exploration of functioning in Safe Schools/Healthy Students partnerships. *Evaluation and Program Planning*, 35(2), 280–6.

Mertens, D. (2010). Philosophy in mixed methods teaching: the transformative paradigm as illustration. *International Journal of Multiple Research Approaches*, 4, 9–18.

Mileham, P. (2015). Finding sources of evidence. In N.A. Schmidt & J.M. Brown (eds), *Evidence-based practice for nurses: appraisal and application of research*, 3rd edn. Burlington, MA: Jones & Bartlett Learning, 94–131.

Miles, M.B. & Huberman, A.M. (1994). *Qualitative data analysis: a methods sourcebook*, 2nd edn. Los Angeles, CA: Sage.

Miles, M.B., Huberman, A.M. & Saldana, J. (2013). *Qualitative data analysis: a methods sourcebook*, 3rd edn. Los Angeles: Sage.

Milgram, S. (1974). *Obedience and authority: an experimental view*. New York: Harper Collins.

Miller, W.L. & Crabtree, B.F. (2005). Clinical research. In N.K. Denzin & Y.S. Lincoln (eds), *The Sage handbook of qualitative research*, 2nd edn. Thousand Oaks, CA: Sage, 605–39.

Minichiello, V., Aroni, R. & Hays, T. (2008). *In-depth interviewing*, 3rd edn. Sydney: Pearson Prentice Hall.

Minichiello, V., Sullivan, G., Greenwood, K. & Axford, R. (eds) (2004). *Handbook of research methods for nursing and health science*, 2nd edn. Sydney: Pearson Education Australia.

Minkler, M. & Wallestein, N. (2008). *Community-based participatory research for health: from process to outcomes*, 2nd edn. San Francisco: Jossey-Bass.

Mirabito, D. (2001). Mining treatment termination data in an adolescent mental health service: a quantitative study. *Social Work in Health Care*, 33(3/4), 71–90.

Mishler, E.G. (1999). *Storylines: craftartists' narratives of identity*. Cambridge, MA: Harvard University Press.

Moher, D. & Tricco, A. (2008). Issues related to the conduct of systematic reviews: a focus on the nutrition field. *American Journal of Clinical Nutrition*, 88, 1191–9.

Moher, D., Dulberg, C.S. & Wells, G.A. (1994). Statistical power, sample size, and their reporting in randomized controlled trials. *Journal of the American Medical Association*, 272(2), 121–4.

Moher, D., Hopewell, S., Schulz, K.F., Montori, V., Gøtzsche, P.C., Devereaux, P.J., Elbourne, D., Egger, M. & Altman, D.G. (2010). CONSORT 2010 explanation and elaboration: updated guidelines for reporting parallel group randomised trials. *Journal of Clinical Epidemiology*, 63(8), e1–e37.

Moher, D., Schulz, K.F., Altman, D.G. for the CONSORT Group (2012). *The CONSORT statement: revised recommendations for improving the quality of reports of parallel-group randomized trials*. <http://www.consort-statement.org>.

Mokkink, L.B., Terwee, C.B., Patrick, D.L., Alonso, J., Stratford, P.W., Knola, D.L. *et al.* (2010a). International consensus on taxonomy, terminology, and definitions of measurement properties for health-related patient-reported outcomes: results of the COSMIN study. *Journal of Clinical Epidemiology*, 63(7), 737–45.

Mokkink, L.B., Terwee, C.B., Patrick, D.L., Alonso, J., Stratford, P.W., Knola, D.L. & de Vet, H.C.W. (2010b). *TheCOSMIN checklist manual.* <www.cosmin.nl/images/upload/File/COSMIN%20 checklist%20manual%20v6.pdf>.

Moran, G., Fongay, P., Kurtz, A., Bolton, A. & Brook, C. (1991). A controlled study of the psychoanalytic treatment of brittle diabetes. *Journal of the American Academy of Child and Adolescent Psychiatry*, 30(6), 926–35.

Morgan, D. (2007). Paradigms lost and pragmatism regained: methodological implications of combining qualitative and quantitative methods. *Journal of Mixed Methods Research*, 1(Jan.), 48–76.

Morgan, D.L. (1993). Qualitative content analysis: a guide to paths not taken. *Qualitative Health Research*, 3, 112–21.

Morgan, D.L. (1997). *The focus group guidebook.* Thousand Oaks, CA: Sage.

Morgan, D.L. (1998a). *Focus group kit vol. 1: focus group guidebook.* Thousand Oaks, CA: Sage.

Morgan, D.L. (1998b). *Focus group kit vol. 2: planning focus groups.* Thousand Oaks, CA: Sage.

Morgan, D.L. (1998c). *The focus group guidebook.* Thousand Oaks, CA: Sage.

Morgan, D. & Morgan, R. (2009). *Single-case research methods for the behavioural and health sciences.* Los Angeles: Sage.

Morikawa, M., Okada, T., Ando, M., Aleksic, B., Kunimoto, S., Nakamura, Y. *et al.* (2015). Relationship between social support during pregnancy and postpartum depressive state: a prospective cohort study. *Scientific Reports*, 5, 105–20.

Morrell, C. & Harvey, G. (2003). *The clinical audit handbook.* London: Elsevier Science.

Morris, A. (2015). *A practical introduction to in-depth interviewing.* London: Sage.

Morse, J.M. (1994a). Designing funded qualitative research. In N.K. Denzin & Y.S. Lincoln (eds), *Handbook of qualitative research.* Thousand Oaks, CA: Sage, 220–35.

Morse, J.M. (1994b). *Critical issues in qualitative research methods.* Thousand Oaks, CA: Sage.

Morse, J.M. (1998). What's wrong with random selection? *Qualitative Health Research*, 8(6), 733–5.

Morse J.M. (2000). Editorial. Determining sample size. *Qualitative Health Research*, 10(1), 3–5.

Morse, J.M. (2007). Strategies of intraproject sampling. In P.L. Munhall (ed.), *Nursing research: a qualitative perspective*, 4th edn. Sudbury, MA: Jones & Bartlett, 529–39.

Morse, J.M. & Richards, L. (2002). *Read me first for a user's guide to qualitative methods.* Thousand Oaks, CA: Sage.

Morse, J.M., Barrett, M., Mayan, M., Olson, K. & Spiers, J. (2002). Verification strategies for establishing reliability and validity in qualitative research. *International Journal of Qualitative Methods*, 1(2), Art. 2. <www.ualberta.ca/~iiqm/backissues/1_2Final/pdf/morseetal.pdf>.

Moses, J.W. & Knutsen, T.L. (2007). *Ways of knowing: competing methodologies in social and political research.* Basingstoke: Palgrave Macmillan.

Moustakas, C. (1994). *Phenomenological research methods.* Thousand Oaks, CA: Sage.

Muecke, M. (1994). On the evaluation of ethnographies. In J. Morse (ed.), *Critical issues in qualitative research methods.* Thousand Oaks, CA: Sage, 187–209.

Mullen, E.J., Bellamy, J.L. & Bledsoe, S.E. (2011). Evidence-based practice. In R.M. Grinnell & Y.A. Unrau (eds), *Social work research and evaluation: foundations of evidence-based practice*, 9th edn. New York: Oxford University Press, 160–77.

Mullen, E.J., Bellamy, J.L. & Bledsoe, S.E. (2014). Evidence-based practice. In R.M. Grinnell & Y.A. Unrau (eds), *Social work research and evaluation: foundations of evidence-based practice*, 10th edn. New York: Oxford University Press, 200–17.

Munteanu, S.E., Zammit, G.V., Menz, H.B., Landorf, K.B., Handley, C.J., Elzarka, A. & DeLuca, J. (2011). Effectiveness of intra-articular hyaluronan (Synvisc, hylan G-F 20) for the treatment of first metatarsophalangeal joint osteoarthritis: a randomised placebo-controlled trial. *Annals of the Rheumatic Diseases*, 70(10), 1838–41.

Murphy, A. & McDonald, J. (2004). Power, status and marginalisation: rural social workers and evidence-based practice in multidisciplinary teams. *Australian Social Work*, 57(2), 127–36.

Mykhalovskiy, E. & McCoy, L. (2002). Troubling ruling discourses of health: using institutional ethnography in community-based research. *Critical Public Health*, 12(1), 17–37.

Nair, M., Kurinczuk, J.J., Brocklehurst, P., Sellers, S., Lewis, G. & Knight, M (2015). Factors associated with maternal death from direct pregnancy complications: a UK national case-control study. *British Journal of Obstetrics and Gynaecology*, 122, 653–62.

Natalier, K. (2013). Research design. In M. Walter (ed.), *Social research methods*, 3rd edn. Melbourne: Oxford University Press, pp. 25-49.

Nathan, P. & Gorman, J. (eds) (2002). *A guide to treatments that work*, 2nd edn. Oxford: Oxford University Press.

Nathan, P., Gorman, J. & Salkind, N. (1999). *Treating mental health disorders: a guide to what works*. New York: Oxford University Press.

National Aboriginal and Torres Strait Islander Health Council (2003). *National strategic framework for Aboriginal and Torres Strait Islander health 2003–2013: framework for action by governments*. Canberra: NATSIHC.

National Aboriginal Health Strategy Working Party (1989). *A national Aboriginal health strategy*. Canberra: Australian Government Publishing Service.

Nay, R. (1993). Benevolent oppression: lived experiences of nursing home life. Unpublished PhD thesis, University of New South Wales, Sydney.

Nay, R. & Fetherstonhaugh, D. (2007). Evidence-based practice: limitations and successful implementation. *Annals of the New York Academy of Science*, 1114, 456–63.

Nay, R. & Fetherstonhaugh, D. (2012). What is pain? A phenomenological approach to understanding. *International Journal of Older People Nursing*, 7, 233–9.

Nettleton, J. & Reilly, O. (1998). Facilitating effective learning during clinical placement. *International Journal of Language & Communication Disorders*, 33(suppl.), 250–4.

Neuman, W.L. (2006). *Social research methods: qualitative and quantitative approaches*, 6th edn. Boston, MA: Pearson/Allyn & Bacon.

Neuman, W.L. (2011). *Social research methods: qualitative and quantitative approaches*, 7th edn. Boston, MA: Allyn & Bacon.

Neutens, J.J. (2014). *Research techniques for the health sciences*, 5th edn. Boston, MA: Pearson.

Neville, C. & Byrne, G. (2014). Depression and suicide in older people. In R. Nay, S. Garratt & D. Fetherstonhaugh (eds), *Interdisciplinary care of older people: issues and innovations*, 4th edn. Australia: Elsevier, 267–84.

Newell, D.J. (1992). Intention-to-treat analysis: implications for quantitative and qualitative research. *International Journal of Epidemiology*, 21, 837–41.

References

NHMRC (1999a). *A guide to the development, implementation and evaluation of clinical practice guidelines*. Canberra: National Health and Medical Research Council.

NHMRC (1999b). *National statement on research involving humans*. Canberra: National Health and Medical Research Council.

NHMRC (2003). *Values and ethics: guidelines for ethical conduct in Aboriginal and Torres Strait Islander health research*. Canberra: National Health and Medical Research Council.

NHMRC (2005). *Keeping research on track: a guide for Aboriginal and Torres Strait Islander peoples about health research ethics*. Canberra: National Health and Medical Research Council.

NHMRC (2007). *National statement on ethical conduct in human research*. Canberra: National Health and Medical Research Council.

Nicholls, D. (2012). Postmodernism and physiotherapy research. *Physical Therapy Reviews*, 17(6), 360–8.

Nieminen, P., Rucker, G., Miettunen, J., Carpenter, J. & Schumacher, M. (2007). Statistically significant papers in psychiatry were cited more often than others. *Journal of Clinical Epidemiology*, 60(9), 939–46.

Nilsson, D. (2001). Psycho-social problems faced by 'frequent flyers' in a paediatric diabetes unit. *Social Work in Health Care*, 33(3/4), 53–69.

Noblit, G.W. & Hare, R.D. (1988). *Meta-ethnography: synthesizing qualitative studies*. Newbury Park, CA: Sage.

NOP World (2005). International survey on breast cancer. Offprint of study tables provided on request from ann.taket@deakin.edu.au.

Norris, W.M., Wenrich, M.D., Nielsen, E.L., Treece, P.D., Jackson, J.C. & Curtis, J.R. (2005). Communication about end-of-life care between language-discordant patients and clinicians: insights from medical interpreters. *Journal of Palliative Medicine*, 8(5), 1016–24.

Northam, E., Anderson, P., Adler, R., Werther, G. & Warne, G. (1996). Psychosocial and family functioning in children with insulin-dependent diabetes at diagnosis and one year later. *Journal of Pediatric Psychology*, 21(5), 699–717.

Northam, E., Anderson, P., Werther, G., Adler, R. & Andrewes, D. (1995). Neuropsychological complications of insulin dependent diabetes in children. *Child Neuropsychology*, 1(1), 74–87.

Northcutt, N. & McCoy, D. (2004). *Interactive qualitative analysis: a systems method for qualitative research*. London: Sage.

NVIVO (2016). *The #1 software for qualitative data analysis*. <http://www.qsrinternational.com/product>.

Nyden, P. & Wiewel, W. (1992). Collaborative research: harnessing the tensions between researcher and practitioner. *American Sociologist*, 23(4), 43–55.

O'Cathain, A., Murphy, E. & Nicholl, J. (2007). Why, and how, mixed methods research is undertaken in health services research in England: a mixed methods study. *BMC Health Services Research*, 7.

O'Cathain, A., Murphy, E. & Nicholl, J. (2008). The quality of mixed methods studies in health services research. *Journal of Health Services Research & Policy*, 13(2), 92–8.

O'Halloran, P.D. (2007). Mood changes in weeks 2 and 6 of a graduated group walking program in previously sedentary persons with type 2 diabetes. *Australian Journal of Primary Health*, 13, 68–73.

O'Leary, P., Easton, S.D. & Gould, N. (2015). The effect of child sexual abuse on men: toward a male sensitive measure. *Journal of Interpersonal Violence*. Doi:10.1177/0886260515586362.

O'Reilly, K. (2005). *Ethnographic methods*. London: Routledge.

O'Reilly, K. (2012). *Ethnographic methods*, 2nd edn. London: Routledge.

O'Reilly, M. & Kiyimba, N. (2015). *Advanced qualitative research: a guide to using theory.* London: Sage.

Oakley, A. (2009). Interviewing women: a contradiction in terms. In N. Fielding (ed.), *Interviewing II*, vol. 1. London: Routledge, 93–115.

OCEBM Levels of Evidence Working Group (2011). *The Oxford 2011 levels of evidence*. Oxford Centre for Evidence-Based Medicine. <www.cebm.net/index.aspx?o=5653>.

Odgaard-Jensen, J., Vist, G.E., Timmer, A., Kunz, R., Akl, E.A., Schünemann, H., Briel, M., Nordmann, A.J., Pregno, S. & Oxman, A.D. (2011). Randomisation to protect against selection bias in healthcare trials. *Cochrane Database of Systematic Reviews*, Issue 4, Art. No. MR000012. Doi: 10.1002/14651858.MR000012.pub3.

Oetzel, J.G., Simpson, M., Berryman, K. & Reddy, R. (2015). Differences in ideal communication behaviours during end-of-life care for Māori carers/patients and palliative care workers. *Palliative Medicine*. Doi: 0269216315583619.

Oleckno, W.A. (2002). *Essential epidemiology: principles and applications*. Long Grove, IL: Waveland Press.

Olsen, K., Young, R.A. & Schultz, I.Z. (eds) (2016). *Handbook of qualitative health research for evidence-based practice*. Dordrecht: Springer.

Onwuegbuzie, A.J. & Johnson, R.B. (2006). The validity in mixed research. *Research in the Schools*, 13(1), 48–63.

Onwuegbuzie, A., Bustamante, R. & Nelson, J. (2010). Mixed research as a tool for developing quantitative instruments. *Journal of Mixed Methods Research*, 4(1), 56–78.

Onwuegbuzie, A.J., Dickinson, W.B., Leech, N.L. & Zoran, A.G. (2009). A qualitative framework for collecting and analyzing data in focus group research. *International Journal of Qualitative Methods*, 8(3), 1–21.

Orbach, S. (1984). *Fat is a feminist issue*. London: Hamlyn.

Orbach, S. (2009). *Bodies*. London: Picador.

Osterlind, S.J. (2006). *Modern measurement: theory, principles, and applications of mental appraisal*. New Jersey: Pearson Education/Merrill Prentice Hall.

Pace, R., Pluye, P., Bartlett, G., Macaulay, A.C., Salsberg, J., Jagosh, J. & Seller, R. (2012). Testing the reliability and efficiency of the pilot Mixed Methods Appraisal Tool (MMAT) for systematic mixed studies review. *International Journal of Nursing Studies*, 49, 47–53.

Packer, M. (2011). *The science of qualitative research*. Cambridge: Cambridge University Press.

Padgett, D.K. (2008). *Qualitative methods in social work research*, 2nd edn. Los Angeles: Sage.

Padgett, D.K. (2012). *Qualitative and mixed methods in public health*. Thousand Oaks, CA: Sage.

Palisano, R.J., Rosenbaum, P.L., Bartlett, D. & Livingston, M.H. (2008). Content validity of the expanded and revised gross motor function classification system. *Developmental Medicine & Child Neurology*, 50, 744–50.

Papaioannou, D., Sutton, A., Carroll, C., Booth, A. & Wong, R. (2009). Literature searching for social science systematic reviews: considerations of a range of search techniques. *Health Information and Libraries Journal*, 27, 114–22.

Papastavrou, E. & Andreou, P. (2012). Exploring sensitive nursing issues through focus group approaches. *Health Science Journal*, 6(2), 185–200.

Parfrey, P. & Ravani, P. (2009). On framing the research question and choosing the appropriate research design. *Methods in Molecular Biology*, 473, 1–17.

Parker, R., Vannest, K. & Brown, L. (2009). The improvement rate difference for single-case research. *Exceptional Children*, 75(2), 135–50.

Parker, R., Vannest, K., Davis, J. & Sauber, S. (2011). Combining nonoverlap and trend for single-case research: Tau-U. *Behavior Therapy*, 42, 284–99.

Paterson, B.L. (2007). Coming out as ill: understanding self-disclosure in chronic illness from a meta-synthesis of qualitative research. In C. Webb & B. Roe (eds), *Reviewing research evidence for nursing practice: systematic reviews*. Oxford: Blackwell, 73–111.

Paterson, B.L. (2013). Metasynthesis. In C.T. Beck (ed.), *Routledge international handbook of qualitative research*. New York: Routledge, 331–46.

Paterson, B.L., Thorne, S.E., Canam, C. & Jillings, C. (2001). *Meta-study of qualitative health research: a practical guide to meta-analysis and meta-synthesis*. Thousand Oaks, CA: Sage.

Paterson, H. & Carpenter, C. (2015). Using different methods to communicate: how adults with severe acquired communication difficulties make decisions about the communication methods they use and how they experience them. *Disability & Rehabilitation*, 37(17), 1522–30.

Patton, M. (2002). *Qualitative research and evaluation methods*, 3rd edn. Thousand Oaks, CA: Sage.

Patton, M.Q. (2003). *Qualitative evaluation checklist*. <www.wmich.edu/evalctr/archive_checklists/qec.pdf>.

Patton, M.Q. (2016). *Qualitative research and evaluation methods*, 4th edn. Thousand Oaks, CA: Sage.

Peat, J.K. (2001). *Health science research: a handbook of quantitative methods*. Sydney: Allen & Unwin.

PEDro (2009). *PEDro rating scale*. Sydney: Centre for Evidence-based Physiotherapy. <www.pedro.org.au>.

Pellatt, G.C. (2007). Patients, doctors, and therapists perceptions of professional roles in spinal cord injury rehabilitation: do they agree? *Journal of Interprofessional Care*, 21(2), 165–77.

Pelto, P.J. & Pelto, G.H. (1978). *Anthropological research: the structure of inquiry*, 2nd edn. Cambridge: Cambridge University Press.

Perlesz, A., Furlong, M. & McLachlan, D. (1992). Family work and acquired brain injury. *Australian and New Zealand Journal of Family Therapy*, 13(3), 145–53.

Perlesz, A., Furlong, M. & the 'D' family (1996). A systemic therapy unravelled: in through the out door. In C. Flaskas & A. Perlesz (eds), *The therapeutic relationship in systemic therapy*. London: Karnac Books, 142–57.

Perlesz, A., Kinsella, G. & Crowe, S. (2000). Psychological distress and family satisfaction following traumatic brain injury: injured individuals and their primary, secondary and tertiary carers. *Journal of Head Injury Rehabilitation*, 15(3), 909–29.

Perry, A., Morris, M., Unsworth, C., Duckett, S., Skeat, J., Dodd, K., Taylor, N. & Riley, K. (2004). Therapy outcome measures for allied health practitioners in Australia: the AusTOMs. *International Journal for Quality in Health Care*, 16(4), 285–91.

Peters, R.M. (2015). What is evidence-based practice? In N.A. Schmidt & J.M. Brown (eds), *Evidence-based practice for nurses: appraisal and application of research*, 3rd edn. Burlington, MA: Jones & Bartlett Learning, 174–97.

Pfeffer, N. (2004). Screening for breast cancer: candidacy and compliance. *Social Science and Medicine*, 58, 151–60.

Phillips, D. (1973). *Abandoning method*. San Francisco: Jossey-Bass.

Piantadosi, S. (2005). *Clinical trials: a methodologic perspective*. New York: Wiley Interscience.

Picot, J., Jones, J., Colquitt, J.L., Gospodarevskaya, E., Loveman, E., Baxter, L. *et al.* (2009). The clinical effectiveness and cost-effectiveness of bariatric (weight loss) surgery for obesity: a systematic review and economic evaluation. *Health Technology Assessment*, 13(41). <www.hta.ac.uk/fullmono/mon1341.pdf>.

Piedra, L.M., Byoun, S.J., Guardini, L. & Cintrón, V. (2012). Improving the parental self-agency of depressed Latino immigrant mothers: piloted intervention results. *Children and Youth Services Review*, 34(1), 126–35.

Pilling, S. & Slattery, J. (2004). Management competencies: intrinsic or acquired? What competencies are required to move into speech pathology management and beyond? *Australian Health Review*, 27(1), 84–92.

Pinnegar, S. & Daynes, G.J. (2007). Locating narrative inquiry historically: thematics in the turn to narrative. In J.D. Clandinin (ed.), *Handbook of narrative inquiry: mapping the methodology*. Thousand Oaks, CA: Sage, 3–34.

Piper, M.C. & Darrah, J. (1994). *Motor assessment of the developing infant*. Philadelphia, PA: W.B. Saunders.

Plakas, S., Taket, A., Cant, B., Fouka, G. & Vardaki, Z. (2014). The meaning and importance of vigilant attendance for the relatives of intensive care unit patients. *Nursing in Critical Care*, 19(5), 243–54.

Plath, D. (2006). Evidence based practice: current issues and future directions. *Australian Social Work*, 59(1), 56–72.

Plath, D. & Gibbons, J. (2010). Discoveries on a data-mining expedition: single session social work in hospitals. *Social Work in Health Care*, 49(8), 703–17.

Pluye, P., Gagnon, M.P., Griffiths, F. & Johnson-Lafleur, J. (2009). A scoring system for appraising mixed methods research, and concomitantly appraising qualitative, quantitative and mixed methods primary studies in mixed studies reviews. *International Journal of Nursing Studies*, 46(4), 529–46.

Pockett, R., Walker, E. & Dave, K. (2010). 'Last orders': dying in a hospital setting. *Australian Social Work*, 63(3), 250–65.

Pocock, S.J. (ed.) (1983). *Clinical trials: a practical approach*. Chichester: John Wiley & Sons.

Polgar, S. & Thomas, S.A. (2013). *Introduction to research in health sciences*, 6th edn. Edinburgh: Churchill Livingstone.

Polit, D.F. & Beck, C.T. (2011). *Nursing research: principles and methods*, 9th edn. Philadelphia, PA: Lippincott Williams & Wilkins.

Polit, D.F. & Beck, C.T. (2014). *Essentials of nursing research: appraising evidence for nursing practice*. Philadelphia, PA: Lippincott Williams & Wilkins.

Polkinghorne, D. (2005). Narrative configuration in qualitative analysis. In A. Hatch & R. Wisniewski (eds), *Life history and narrative: qualitative study series 1, vol. 8*. London: RoutledgeFalmer, 5–24.

Polkinghorne, D.E. (1995). Narrative configuration in qualitative analysis. *International Journal of Qualitative Studies in Education*, 8(1), 5–23.

Poolman, R.W., Struijs, P.A.A., Krips, R., Sierevelt, I.N., Marti, R.K., Farrokhyar, F. & Bhandari, M. (2007). Reporting of outcomes in orthopaedic randomized trials: does blinding of outcome assessors matter? *Journal of Bone and Joint Surgery (American)*, 89(3), 550–8.

Portney, L. & Watkins, M. (2009). *Foundations of clinical research: applications to practice*, 3rd edn. New Jersey: Prentice Hall Health.

Portney, L.G. & Watkins, M.P. (2000). *Foundations of clinical research: applications to practice*, 2nd edn. Upper Saddle River, NJ: Prentice Hall Health.

Praestegaard, J. & Gard, G. (2013). Ethical issues in physiotherapy: reflected from the perspective of physiotherapists in private practice. *Physiotherapy Theory and Practice*, 29(2), 96–112.

Prasad, K.R.S. & Reddy, K.T.V. (2004). Auditing the audit cycle: an open-ended evaluation. *Clinical Governance: An International Journal*, 9(2), 110–14.

Priest, N., Mackean, T., Waters, E., Davis, E. & Riggs, E. (2009). Indigenous child health research: a critical analysis of Australian studies. *Australian and New Zealand Journal of Public Health*, 33(1), 55–63.

Procter, R., Carmichael, R. & Laterza, V. (2008). Co-interpretation of usage data: a mixed methods approach to evaluation of online environments. *International Journal of Multiple Research Approaches*, 2(1), 44–56.

Proschan, M.A. & Waclawiw, M.A. (2000). Practical guidelines for multiplicity adjustment in clinical trials. *Controlled Clinical Trials*, 21, 527–39.

Pryse, Y., McDaniel, A. & Schafer, J. (2014). Psychometric analysis of two new scales: the evidence-based practice nursing leadership and work environment scales. *Worldviews on Evidence-Based Nursing*, 11(4), 240–7.

Public Health Resource Unit (2007). *Critical appraisal skills program*. <www.phru.nhs.uk/pages/PHD/CASP.htm>.

Punch, K.F. (2016). *Developing effective research proposals*, 3rd edn. London: Sage.

Pyett, P. & VicHealth Koori Health Research and Community Development Unit (2002). Towards reconciliation in Indigenous health research: the responsibilities of the non-Indigenous researcher. *Contemporary Nurse*, 14(1), 56–65.

Pyett, P., Waples-Crowe, P. & van der Sterren, A. (2008). Challenging our own practices in Indigenous health promotion and research. *Health Promotion Journal of Australia*, 19(3), 179–83.

Pyett, P., Waples-Crowe, P. & van der Sterren, A. (2009). Engaging with Aboriginal communities in an urban context: some practical suggestions for public health researchers. *Australian and New Zealand Journal of Public Health*, 33(1), 51–4.

Quintanilha, M., Mayan, M.J., Thompson, J., Bell, R.C. & Team, E.S. (2015). Different approaches to cross-lingual focus groups: lessons from a cross-cultural community-based participatory research project in the ENRICH study. *International Journal of Qualitative Methods*, 14(5). Doi: 1609406915621419.

Radcliffe-Brown, A.R. (1922/1964). *The Andaman Islanders*. New York: Free Press of Glencoe.

Radcliffe-Brown, A.R. (1931). *The social organization of Australian tribes*. Melbourne: Macmillan.

Rademaker, L.L., Grace, E.J. & Curda, S.K. (2012). Using computer-assisted qualitative data analysis software (CAQDAS) to re-examine traditionally analyzed data: expanding our understanding of the data and of ourselves as scholars. *Qualitative Report*, 17(22), 1.

Radford, J.A., Landorf, K.B., Buchbinder, R. & Cook, C. (2006). Effectiveness of low-dye taping for the short-term treatment of plantar heel pain: a randomised trial. *BMC Musculoskeletal Disorders*, 7, 64.

Raffel, K.K., Lee, M.Y., Dougherty, C.V. & Greene, G.J. (2013). Making it work: administrator views on sustaining evidence-based mental health interventions. *Administration in Social Work*, 37, 494–510.

Råholm, M.-B. (2010). Abductive reasoning and the formation of scientific knowledge within nursing research. *Nursing Philosophy*, 11, 260–70.

Raines, J.C. (2011). Evaluating qualitative research studies. In R.M. Grinnell & Y.A. Unrau (eds), *Social work research and evaluation: foundations of evidence-based practice*, 9th edn. New York: Oxford University Press, 488–503.

Ramazanoğlu, C. (ed.) (1993). *Up against Foucault: explorations of some tensions between Foucault and feminism*. London: Routledge.

Ramcharan, P. (2006). Ethical challenges and complexities of including vulnerable people in research: some pre-theoretical considerations. *Journal of Intellectual and Developmental Disability*, 31(3), 183–5.

Ramsden, I. (1990). Cultural safety. *New Zealand Nursing Journal*, 83(11), 18–19.

Randall, M. (2009). *Modification and psychometric evaluation of the Melbourne Assessment of unilateral upper limb function*. Unpublished PhD thesis. La Trobe University, Melbourne.

Randall, M., Johnson, L. & Reddihough, D. (1999). *The Melbourne Assessment of unilateral upper limb function: test administration manual*. Melbourne: Royal Children's Hospital.

Randall, M.J., Imms, C. & Carey, L. (2008). Establishing validity of a Modified Melbourne Assessment for children ages 2 to 4 years. *American Journal of Occupational Therapy*, 62(4), 373–83.

Randall, M.J., Imms, C. & Carey, L. (2012). Further evidence of validity of the Modified Melbourne Assessment for neurologically impaired children aged 2 to 4 years. *Developmental Medicine and Child Neurology*, 54, 424–8.

Rapley, T. (2007). *Doing conversation, discourse and document analysis*. London: Sage.

Rapport, F. (2005). Hermeneutic phenomenology: the science of interpretation of texts. In I. Holloway (ed.), *Qualitative research in health care*. Oxford: Blackwell, 125–46.

Rapport, N. & Overing, J. (2000). *Social and cultural anthropology: the key concepts*. Routledge: London.

Rasmussen, S., Christensen, M., Mathiesen, I. & Simonson, O. (2008). Shockwave therapy for chronic Achilles tendinopathy: a double-blind, randomized clinical trial of efficacy. *Acta Orthopaedica*, 79(2), 249–56.

Rauscher, L. & Greenfield, B.H. (2009). Advancements in contemporary physical therapy research: use of mixed methods designs. *Physical Therapy*, 89(1), 91–100.

Rawson, H. & Liamputtong, P. (2009). Influence of traditional Vietnamese culture on the utilisation of mainstream health services for sexual health issues by second-generation Vietnamese Australian young women. *Sexual Health*, 6, 75–81.

Read, C. & Bateson, D. (2009). Marrying research, clinical practice and cervical screening in Australian Aboriginal women in western New South Wales, Australia. *Rural and Remote Health*, 9(1117). <www.rrh.org.au>.

Redmond, L. & Suddick, K. (2012). The lived experience of freezing in people with Parkinson's: an interpretive phenomenological approach. *International Journal of Therapy and Rehabilitation*, 19(3), 169–77.

Registered Nurses' Association of Ontario (2005). *Prevention of constipation in the older adult population*. Ontario: RNAO.

Registered Nurses' Association of Ontario (2011). *Prevention of constipation in the older adult population. Guideline supplement.* Ontario: RNAO.

Reid, B., Sinclair, M., Barr, O., Dobbs, F. & Crealey, G. (2009). A meta-synthesis of pregnant women's decision-making processes with regard to antenatal screening for Down syndrome. *Social Science & Medicine*, 69, 1561–73.

Reid, W.J. (1994). *Qualitative research in social work.* New York: Columbia University Press.

Reilly, S. (2004). The move to evidence-based practice in speech pathology. In S. Reilly, J. Douglas & J. Oates (eds), *Evidence-based practice in speech pathology.* London: Whurr, 3–17.

Richardson, L. (2003). Writing: a method of inquiry. In N.K. Denzin & Y.S. Lincoln (eds), *Collecting and interpreting qualitative materials research*, 2nd edn. Thousand Oaks, CA: Sage, 499–501.

Richters, J., Badcock, P.B., Simpson, J.M., Shellard, D., Rissel, C., de Visser, R.O., Grulich, A.E. & Smith, A.M.A. (2014). Design and methods of the Second Australian Study of Health and Relationships. *Sexual Health*, 11, 383–96.

Richters, J., Grulich, A.E., De Visser, R.O., Smith, A.M.A. & Rissel, C. (2003). Sex in Australia: contraceptive practices among a representative sample of women. *Australian and New Zealand Journal of Public Health*, 27(2), 210–16.

Ridley, D. (2012). *The literature review: a step-by-step guide for students*, 2nd edn. London: Sage.

Riessman, C.K. (2008). *Narrative methods for the human sciences.* Los Angeles: Sage.

Ring, N., Malcolm, C., Wkye, S., MacGillivary, S., Dixon, D., Hoskins, G. *et al.* (2007). Promoting the use of personal asthma action plans: a systematic review. *Primary Care Respiratory Journal*, 16(5), 271–83.

Ritchie, J. & Lewis, J.E. (2005). *Qualitative research practice: a guide for social science students and researchers.* London: Sage.

Ritchie, J., Spencer, L. & O'Connor, W. (2003). Carrying out qualitative analysis. In J. Ritchie & J. Lewis (eds), *Qualitative research practice: a guide for social science students and researchers.* London: Sage.

Ritzer, G. (1990). Metatheorizing in sociology. *Sociological Forum*, 5, 3–15.

Robertson, M. & Boyle, J. (1984). Ethnography: contributions to nursing research. *Journal of Advanced Nursing*, 9(1), 43–9.

Rogers, G. & Bouey, E. (2005). Participant observation. In R. Grinnell & Y. Unrau (eds), *Social work research and evaluation: quantitative and qualitative approaches.* New York: Oxford University Press, 232–44.

Rogers, W.A. (2004). Evidence based medicine and justice: a framework for looking at the impact of EBM upon vulnerable or disadvantaged groups. *Journal of Medical Ethics*, 30(2), 141–5.

Roland, M. & Torgerson, D. (1998a). Understanding controlled trials: what outcomes should be measured? *British Medical Journal*, 317, 1075–80.

Roland, M. & Torgerson, D. (1998b). Understanding controlled trials: what are pragmatic trials? *British Medical Journal*, 316, 285.

Rollans, M., Schmied, V., Kemp, L. & Meade, T. (2013). 'Digging over that old ground': an Australian perspective of women's experience of psychosocial assessment and depression screening in pregnancy and following birth. *BMC Women's Health*, 13, 18.

Rolls, L. & Relf, M. (2006). Bracketing interviews: addressing methodological challenges in qualitative interviewing in bereavement and palliative care. *Mortality*, 11(3), 286–305.

Romanello, M. & Knight-Abowitz, K. (2000). The 'ethic of care' in physical therapy practice and education: challenges and opportunities. *Journal of Physical Therapy Education*, 14(5), 20–5.

Rompe, J.D., Nafe, B., Furia, J.P. & Maffulli, N. (2007). Eccentric loading, shock-wave treatment, or a wait-and-see policy for tendinopathy of the main body of tendo achillis: a randomized controlled trial. *American Journal of Sports Medicine*, 35(3), 374–83.

Rompe, J.D., Furia, J. & Maffulli, N. (2008). Eccentric loading compared with shock wave treatment for chronic insertional achilles tendinopathy: a randomized, controlled trial. *Journal of Bone and Joint Surgery*, 90(1), 52–61.

Rompe, J.D., Furia, J. & Maffulli, N. (2009). Eccentric loading versus eccentric loading plus shock-wave treatment for midportion achilles tendinopathy: a randomized controlled trial. *American Journal of Sports Medicine*, 37(3), 463–70.

Rorty, R. (1989). *Contingency, irony and solidarity*. Cambridge: Cambridge University Press.

Rosaldo, M. (1980). *Knowledge and passion: Ilongot notions of self and social life*. Cambridge: Cambridge University Press.

Rose, M. & Douglas, J. (2006). A comparison of verbal and gesture treatments for a word production deficit resulting from acquired apraxia of speech. *Aphasiology*, 20(12), 1186–209.

Rose, M. & Sussmilch, G. (2008). The effects of semantic and gesture treatments on verb retrieval and verb use in aphasia. *Aphasiology*, 22(7), 691–706.

Rose, M., Douglas, J. & Matyas, T. (2002). The comparative effectiveness of gesture and verbal treatments for a specific phonologic naming impairment. *Aphasiology*, 15(10/11), 977–90.

Rosenberger, W.F. & Lachin, J.M. (2002). *Randomization in clinical trials: theory and practice*. New York: Wiley Interscience.

Ross, L., Lundstrøm, L.H., Petersen, M.A., Johnsen, A.T., Watt, T. & Groenvold, M. (2012). Using method triangulation to validate a new instrument (CPWQ-com) assessing cancer patients' satisfaction with communication. *Cancer Epidemiology*, 36(1), 29–35.

Rossman, G.B. & Rallis, S.F. (2012). *Learning in the field: an introduction to qualitative research*, 3rd edn. Thousand Oaks, CA: Sage.

Rowe, P. & Carpenter, C. (2011). The recent experiences and challenges of military physiotherapists deployed to Afghanistan: a qualitative study. *Physiotherapy Canada*, 63(4), 453–63.

Royal College of Nursing Research Society (2005). *Informed consent in health and social care: RCN guidance for nurses*. London: RCN.

Rubin, A. & Parrish, D. (2007). Views of evidence-based practice among faculty in Master of Social Work programs: a national survey. *Research on Social Work Practice*, 17(1), 110–22.

Rubin, H.J. & Rubin, I.S. (2012). *Qualitative interviewing: the art of hearing data*, 3rd edn. Thousand Oaks, CA: Sage.

Ruel, E.E., Wagner, W.E. & Gillespie, B.J. (2015). *The practice of survey research: theory and applications*. London: Sage.

Russell, C.L. & Gregory, D. (2003). Evaluation of qualitative research studies. *Evidence-Based Nursing*, 6(2), 36–40.

Ryan, G.W. (2004). Using a word processor to tag and retrieve blocks of text. *Field Methods*, 16(1), 109–30.

Ryan, G.W. & Bernard, H.R. (2003). Techniques to identify themes. *Field Methods*, 15(1), 85–109.

Ryan, F., Coughlan, M. & Cronin, P. (2007). Step-by-step guide to critiquing research. Part 2. Qualitative research. *British Journal of Nursing*, 16(12), 738–44.

Ryan, F., Coughlan, M. & Cronin, P. (2009). Interviewing in qualitative research: the one-to-one interview. *International Journal of Therapy and Rehabilitation*, 16(6), 309–14.

Ryan, M. & Sheehan, R. (2009). Research articles in *Australian Social Work* from 1998–2007: a content analysis. *Australian Social Work*, 62(4), 525–42.

Sackett, D.L., Richardson, W.S., Rosenberg, W. & Haynes, R.B. (1997). *Evidence-based medicine: how to practice and teach EBM*. London: Churchill Livingstone.

Sackett, D.L., Rosenburg, W.M., Gray Muir, J.A., Haynes, R.B. & Richardson, W.S. (1996). Evidence-based medicine: what it is and what it isn't. *British Medical Journal*, 312, 71–2.

Sackett, D.L., Straus, S., Richardson, W., Rosenberg, W. & Haynes, R. (2000). *Evidence-based medicine: how to practice and teach EBM*, 2nd edn. Edinburgh: Churchill Livingstone.

Sajatovic, M. & Ramirez, L.F. (2012). *Rating scales in mental health*, 3rd edn. Baltimore, MD: Johns Hopkins University Press.

Saldaña, J. (2009). *Coding in qualitative data analysis*. Thousand Oaks, CA: Sage.

Sale, J.E.M. & Brazil, K. (2004). A strategy to identify critical appraisal criteria for primary mixed-method studies. *Quality and Quantity*, 38(4), 351–65.

Sale, J.E.M., Lohfeld, L.H. & Brazil, K. (2002). Revisiting the quantitative–qualitative debate: implications for mixed-methods research. *Quality and Quantity*, 36(1), 43–53.

Salkind, N.J. (2014). *100 questions (and answers) about statistics*. London: Sage.

Salmond, S.W. (2012). Qualitative metasynthesis. In C. Holly, S.W. Salmond & M.K. Saimbert (eds), *Comprehensive systematic review for advanced nursing practice*. New York: Springer, 209–36.

Sandberg, J. & Alvesson, M. (2011). Ways of constructing research questions: gap spotting or problematization? *Organization*, 18(1), 23–44.

Sandelowski, M. (2000). Focus on research methods combining qualitative and quantitative sampling, data collection, and analysis techniques. *Research in Nursing & Health*, 23, 246–55.

Sandelowski, M. (2001). Real qualitative researchers do not count: the use of numbers in qualitative research. *Research in Nursing & Health*, 24, 230–40.

Sandelowski, M. (2004). Using qualitative research. *Qualitative Health Research*, 14(10), 1366–86.

Sandelowski, M. (2006) 'Meta-jeopardy': tThe crisis of representation in qualitative metasynthesis. *Nursing Outlook*, 54, 10–16.

Sandelowski, M. (2007). From meta-synthesis to method: Appraising the qualitative research synthesis report. In C. Webb & B. Roe (eds), *Reviewing research evidence for nursing practice*. Oxford: Blackwell Publishing, 88–111.

Sandelowski, M. (2014). Unmixing mixed-methods research. *Research in Nursing & Health*, 37, 3–8.

Sandelowski, M. (2015). A matter of taste: evaluating the quality of qualitative research. *Nursing Inquiry*, 22(2), 86–94.

Sandelowski, M. & Barroso, J. (2003). Classifying the findings in qualitative studies. *Qualitative Health Research*, 13(7), 905–23.

Sandelowski, M. & Barroso, J. (2007). *Handbook for synthesizing qualitative research*. New York: Springer.

Sandelowski, M. & Leeman, J. (2012). Writing usable qualitative health research findings. *Qualitative Health Research*, 22(10), 1404–13.

Sandelowski, M., Barroso, J. & Voils, C. (2007). Using qualitative metasummary to synthesize qualitative and quantitative descriptive findings. *Research in Nursing & Health*, 30(1), 99–111.

Sandelowski, M., Docherty, S. & Emden, C. (1997). Qualitative metasynthesis: issues and techniques. *Research in Nursing & Health*, 20, 365–71.

Sandelowski, M., Voils, C.I., Leeman, J. & Crandell, J.L. (2012). Mapping the mixed methods–mixed research synthesis terrain. *Journal of Mixed Methods Research*, 6(4), 317–31.

Sarantakos, S. (2005). *Social research*, 3rd edn. New York: Palgrave Macmillan.

Satyendra, L. & Byl, N. (2006). Effectiveness of physical therapy for Achilles tendinopathy: an evidence-based review of eccentric exercises. *Isokinetics and Exercise Science*, 14(1), 71–80.

Savage, J. (2000). Ethnography and health care. *British Medical Journal*, 321, 1400–2.

Savage, J. (2006). Ethnographic evidence. *Journal of Research in Nursing*, 11(5), 383–93.

Savin-Baden, M. & Niekerk, L.V. (2007). Narrative inquiry: theory and practice. *Journal of Geography in Higher Education*, 31(3), 459–72.

Scally, G. & Donaldson, L.J. (1998). The NHS's 50th anniversary: clinical governance and the drive for quality improvement in the new NHS in England. *British Medical Journal*, 317, 61–5.

Schachter, C.L., Stalker, C.A., Teram, E., Lasiuk, G.C. & Danilkewich, A. (2009). *Handbook on sensitive practice for health care practitioner: lessons from adult survivors of childhood sexual abuse.* Ottawa: Public Health Agency of Canada. <www.phac-aspc.gc.ca/publications-eng.php>.

Schade, D.S., Drumm, D.A., Duckworth, W.C. & Eaton, R.P. (1985). The etiology of incapacitating brittle diabetes. *Diabetes Care*, 1, 12–20.

Schmidt, F.L. (1996). Statistical significance testing and cumulative knowledge in psychology: implications for the training of researchers. *Psychological Methods*, 1, 115–29.

Schmidt, N.A. & Brown, J.M. (2015a). What is evidence-based practice? In N.A. Schmidt & J.M. Brown (eds), *Evidence-based practice for nurses: appraisal and application of research*, 3rd edn. Burlington, MA: Jones & Bartlett Learning, 3–41.

Schmidt, N.A. & Brown, J.M. (eds) (2015b). *Evidence-based practice for nurses: appraisal and application of research*, 3rd edn. Burlington, MA: Jones & Bartlett Learning.

Schneider, S.J., Kerwin, J., Frechtling, J. & Vivari, B.A. (2002). Characteristics of the discussion in online and face-to-face focus groups. *Social Science Computer Review*, 20(1), 31–42.

Scholten, R.J.P.M., Opstelten, W., van der Plas, C.G., Bijl, D., Deville, W.L.J.M. & Bouter, L.M. (2003). Accuracy of physical diagnostic tests for assessing ruptures of the anterior cruciate ligament: a meta-analysis. *Journal of Family Practice*, 52(9), 689–94.

Schon, D. (1983). *The reflective practitioner.* New York: Basic Books.

Schreiber, R.S. & Stern, P.N. (eds) (2001). *Using grounded theory in nursing.* New York: Springer.

Schreiber, R., Crooks, D. & Stern, P.N. (1997). Qualitative meta-analysis. In J.M. Morse (ed.), *Qualitative nursing research: a contemporary dialogue.* London: Sage, 311–27.

Schünemann, H.J., Oxman, A.D., Glasziou, P., Jaeschke, R., Vist, G.E., Williams Jr, J.W., Kunz, R., Craig, J., Montori, V.M., Bossuyt, P. & Guyatt, G.H. (2008). Grading quality of evidence and strength of recommendations for diagnostic tests and strategies. *British Medical Journal*, 36, 1106–10.

Schulz, K.F. (1995). Subverting randomization in controlled trials. *Journal of the American Medical Association*, 274(18), 1456–8.

Schulz, K.F. (1996). Randomised trials, human nature, and reporting guidelines. *Lancet*, 348, 596–8.

Schulz, K.F. & Grimes, D.A. (2002a). Allocation concealment in randomised trials: defending against deciphering. *Lancet*, 359, 614–18.

Schulz, K.F. & Grimes, D.A. (2002b). Blinding in randomised trials: hiding who got what. *Lancet*, 359, 696–700.

Schulz, K.F. & Grimes, D.A. (2002c). Sample size slippages in randomized trials: exclusions and the lost and wayward. *Lancet*, 359, 781–5.

Schulz, K., Altman, D., Moher, D. & CONSORT Group (2010). CONSORT 2010 statement: updated guidelines for reporting parallel group randomised trials. *BMC Medicine*, 8(1), 18.

Schulz, K.F., Chalmers, I., Hayes, R.J. & Altman, D.G. (1995). Empirical evidence of bias: dimensions of methodological quality associated with estimates of treatment effects in controlled trials. *Journal of the American Medical Association*, 273(5), 408–12.

Schutt, R.K. (2014). Sampling. In R.M. Grinnell & Y.A. Unrau (eds), *Social work research and evaluation: foundations of evidence-based practice*, 10th edn. New York: Oxford University Press, 290–312.

Schwandt, T. (1997). *Qualitative inquiry: a dictionary of terms*. Thousand Oaks, CA: Sage.

Schwartz, D. & Lellouch, J. (2009). Explanatory and pragmatic attitudes in therapeutical trials. *Journal of Clinical Epidemiology*, 62(5), 499–505.

Schwartz, H. & Jacobs, J. (1979). *Qualitative sociology*. New York: Free Press.

Schwartz, M. & Polgar, S. (2003). *Statistics for evidence-based health care*. Melbourne: Tertiary Press.

Scott, G. & Garner, R. (2013). *Doing qualitative research: designs, methods, and techniques*. Upper Saddle River, NJ: Pearson Education.

Scott, K. & McSherry, R. (2008). Evidence-based nursing: clarifying the concepts for nursing in practice. *Journal of Clinical Nursing*, 18, 1085–95.

Scurlock-Evans, L., Upton, P. & Upton, D. (2014). Evidence-based practice in physiotherapy: a systematic review of barriers, enablers and interventions. *Physiotherapy*, 100, 208–19.

Seale, C. (2012a). Validity, reliability and the quality of research. In C. Seale (ed.), *Researching society and culture*, 3rd edn. London: Sage, 528–43.

Seale, C. (2012b). Sampling. In C. Seale (ed.), *Researching society and culture*, 3rd edn. London: Sage, 134–52.

Seale, C.F. (2005). Using computers to analyse qualitative data. In D. Silverman (ed.), *Doing qualitative research: a practical handbook*, 2nd edn. London: Sage, 188–208.

Sedgwick, P. (2015). Randomised controlled trials: understanding confounding. *British Medical Journal*, 351, h5119. Doi: http://dx.doi.org/10.1136/bmj.h5119.

Sedgwick, P. & Hooper, C. (2015). Placebos and sham treatments. *British Medical Journal*, 351, h3755. Doi: http://dx.doi.org/10.1136/bmj.h3755.

Seeley, J., Biraro, S., Shafer, L.A., Nasirumbi, P., Foster, S., Whitworth, J. & Grosskurth, H. (2008). Using in-depth qualitative data to enhance our understanding of quantitative results regarding the impact of HIV and AIDS on households in rural Uganda. *Social Science and Medicine*, 67(10), 1434–46.

Serry, T. (2010). *Supplementary reading support for young low-progress readers at school: integrating perspectives about experiences and practices from service providers and parents in an Australian context*. Unpublished PhD thesis. La Trobe University, Melbourne.

Serry, T., Liamputtong, P. & Rose, M. (under review). Perspectives about the role of oral language as a function of learning to read: views from primary school educators. *Language, Speech and Hearing Services in Schools*.

Serry, T., Rose, M. & Liamputtong, P. (2014). Reading recovery teachers discuss reading recovery: a qualitative investigation. *Australian Journal of Learning Difficulties*, 19(1), 61–73.

Shagi, S., Vallely, A., Kasindi, S., Chiduo, B., Desmond, N., Soteli, S. *et al.* (2008). A model for community representation and participation in HIV prevention trials among women who engage in transactional sex in Africa. *AIDS Care*, 20(9), 1039–49.

Shamseer, L., Moher, D., Clarke, M., Ghersi, D., Liberati, A., Petticrew, M., Shekelle, P. & Stewart, L. (2014). Preferred reporting items for systematic review and meta-analysis protocols (PRISMA-P) 2015: elaboration and explanation. *British Medical Journal*, 349, 7647.

Shapiro, D. (2002). Renewing the scientist-practitioner model. *Psychologist*, 15, 232–4.

Shaw, I. & Gould, N. (2001). *Qualitative research in social work*. London: Sage.

Shaw, J.A. & Connelly, D.M. (2012). Phenomenology and physiotherapy: meaning in research and practice. *Physical Therapy Reviews*, 17(6), 398–408.

Shaw, R.L. (2011). Identifying and synthesizing literature. In D. Harper & A.R. Thompson (eds), *Qualitative research methods in mental health and psychotherapy*. Chicago: Wiley-Blackwell, 9–22.

Shea, K.G. & Carey, J.L. (2015). Management of anterior cruciate ligament injuries: evidence-based guidelines. *Journal of the American Academy of Orthopaedic Surgeons*, 23(5), e1-5. Doi:10.5435/JAAOS-D-15-00094.

Sherwood, G.D. (1999). Meta-synthesis: merging qualitative studies to develop nursing knowledge. *International Journal for Human Caring*, 3, 37–42.

Shields, N., Synnot, A. & Barr, M. (2012). Barriers and facilitators to physical activity in children with disabilities: a systematic review. *British Journal of Sports Medicine*, 46, 989–97.

Shields, N., Taylor, N.F. & Dodd, K.J. (2008a). A systematic review comparing the self-concept of children with spina bifida to children with typical development. *Developmental Medicine and Child Neurology*, 50, 733–43.

Shields, N., Taylor, N. & Dodd, K.J. (2008b). Effects of a community-based progressive resistance strength training program on muscle performance and physical function in adults with Down syndrome: a randomized controlled trial. *Archives of Physical Medicine and Rehabilitation*, 89, 1215–20.

Shishehgar, S., Gholizadeh, L., DiGiacomo, M. & Davidson, P.M. (2015). The impact of migration on the health status of Iranians: an integrative literature review. *BMC International Health and Human Rights*, 15(1), 1.

Shore, B. (1982). *Sala'ilua, a Samoan mystery*. New York: Columbia University Press.

Shostak, M. (1983). *Nisa: the life and words of a !Kung woman* (1st Vintage Books edn). New York: Vintage Books.

Shugg, J. & Liamputtong, P. (2002). Being female: the portrayal of women's health in print media. *Health Care for Women International*, 23(6–7), 715–28.

Siegel, S. & Castellan, N.J. (1988). *Nonparametric statistics for the behavioural sciences*, 2nd edn. New York: McGraw-Hill.

Sillitoe, P., Dixon, P. & Barr, J. (2005). Indigenous knowledge inquiries: a methodologies manual for development. Rugby: ITDG Publishing.

Silverman, D. (2010). *Doing qualitative research: a practical handbook*, 3rd edn. London: Sage.

Simonds, J.F. (1977). Psychiatric status of diabetic youth matched with a control group. *Diabetes*, 26(10), 921–5.

Sinha, S., Curtis, K., Jayakody, A., Viner, R. & Roberts, H. (2007). 'People make assumptions about our communities': sexual health amongst teenagers from black and minority ethnic backgrounds in East London. *Ethnicity & Health*, 12(5), 423–41.

Skeat, J. (2013). Using grounded theory in health research. In P. Liamputtong (ed.), *Research methods in health: foundations for evidence-based practice*, 2nd edn. Melbourne: Oxford University Press, 99–114.

Slingsby, B.T. (2006). Professional approaches to stroke treatment in Japan: a relationship-centred model. *Journal of Evaluation in Clinical Practice*, 12(2), 218–26.

Smith, A.M.A., Rissel, C., Richters, J., Grulich, A.E. & De Visser, R.O. (2003). Sex in Australia: the rationale and methods of the Australian Study of Health and Relationships. *Australian and New Zealand Journal of Public Health*, 27(2), 106–17.

Smith, B. (2007). The state of the art in narrative inquiry. *Narrative Inquiry*, 17, 391–8.

Smith, D.E. (1987). *The everyday world as problematic: a feminist sociology*. Boston, MA: Northeastern University Press.

Smith, E. (2008). *Using secondary data in educational and social research*. Maidenhead, UK: McGraw-Hill/Open University Press.

Smith, J.A. (1995). Semi-structured and qualitative analysis. In J.A. Smith, R. Harre & L. Van Langenhove (eds), *Rethinking methods in psychology*. London: Sage, 9–25.

Smith, L.T. (1999). *Decolonizing methodologies: research and Indigenous peoples*. Dunedin, NZ: University of Otago Press.

Smith, J., Osman, C. & Goding, M. (1994). Reclaiming the emotional aspects of the therapist–family system. *Australian and New Zealand Journal of Family Therapy*, 11(3), 139–46.

Smith, L.K., Draper, E.S., Manktelow, B.N., Dorling, J.S. & Field, D.J. (2007). Socioeconomic inequalities in very preterm birth rates. *Archives of Disease in Childhood—Fetal and Neonatal Edition*, 92, F11–14.

Solomon, D.H., Simel, D.L., Bates, D.W., Katz, J.N. & Schaffer, J.L. (2001). The rational clinical examination. Does this patient have a torn meniscus or ligament of the knee? Value of the physical examination. *Journal of the American Medical Association*, 286(13), 1610–20.

Solomons, N.M. & Spross, J.A. (2011). Evidence-based practice barriers and facilitators from a continuous quality improvement perspective: an integrative review. *Journal of Nursing Management*, 19(1), 109–20.

Song, M. & Kong, E.-H. (2015). Older adults' definitions of health: a metasynthesis. *International Journal of Nursing Studies*, 52, 1097–106.

Spector-Mersel, G. (2010). Narrative research: time for a paradigm. *Narrative Inquiry*, 20, 204–24.

Spencer, L. & Ritchie, J. (2011). In pursuit of quality. In D. Harper & A.R. Thompson (eds), *Qualitative research methods in mental health and psychotherapy: a guide for students and practitioners*. Chichester, UK: Wiley-Blackwell, 227–42.

Spicer, N. (2012). Combining qualitative and quantitative methods. In C. Seale (ed.), *Researching society and culture*, 3rd edn. London: Sage, 479–93.

Spink, M.J., Menz, H.B., Fotoohabadi, M.R., Wee, E., Landorf, K.B., Hill, K.D. & Lord, S.R. (2011). Effectiveness of a multifaceted podiatry intervention to prevent falls in community-dwelling older people with disabling foot pain: randomised controlled trial. *British Medical Journal*, 342, d3411.

Sprung, B.R., Janotha, B.L. & Steckel, A.J. (2011). The lived experience of breast cancer patients and couple distress. *Journal of American Academy of Nurse Practitioners*, 23(11), 619–27.

Stacey, J. (1988). Can there be a feminist ethnography? *Women's Studies Forum*, 11(1), 21–7.

Stalker, K. (1998). Some ethical and methodological issues in research with people with learning disabilities. *Disability and Society*, 13(1), 5–19.

Stanley, L. & Temple, B. (1995). Doing the business? Evaluating software packages to aid the analysis of qualitative data sets. *Studies in Qualitative Methodology*, 5, 169–97.

Stanley, M. & Cheek, J. (2003). Grounded theory: exploiting the potential for occupational therapy. *British Journal of Occupational Therapy*, 66(4), 143–50.

Stapleton, E. (2008). *The occupation of caring in later life for an adult child with a mental illness: a narrative study*. Unpublished honours thesis. La Trobe University, Melbourne.

Stern, P.N. (1994). Eroding grounded theory. In J. Morse (ed.), *Critical issues in qualitative research methods*. Thousand Oaks, CA: Sage, 212–23.

Stover, C.M. (2012). The use of online synchronous focus groups in a sample of lesbian, gay, and bisexual college students. *Computers Informatics Nursing*, 30(8), 395–9.

Strathern, M. (ed.) (2000). *Audit cultures: anthropological studies in accountability, ethics and the academy*. London: Routledge.

Straus, S.E., Richardson, W.S., Glasziou, P. & Haynes, R.B. (2005). *Evidence-based medicine: how to practice and teach EBM*. Edinburgh: Churchill Livingstone.

Strauss, A. (1987). *Qualitative analysis for social scientists*. Cambridge: Cambridge University Press.

Strauss, A. & Corbin, J. (1990). *Basics of qualitative research: grounded theory procedures and techniques*. Newbury Park, CA: Sage.

Strauss, A. & Corbin, J. (1998). *Basics of qualitative research: grounded theory procedures and techniques*, 2nd edn. Newbury Park, CA: Sage.

Streiner, D.L, Norman, G.R. & Cairney, J. (2014). *Health measurement scales: a practical guide to their development and use*, 5th edn. Oxford: Oxford University Press.

Streubert, H. & Carpenter, D.R. (2011). *Qualitative research in nursing: advancing the humanistic imperative*, 5th edn. Philadelphia, PA: Lippincott Williams & Wilkins.

Stringer, E. & Genat, W. (2004). *Action research in health*. New Jersey: Pearson.

Stringer, E.T. (1999). *Action research*, 2nd edn. Thousand Oaks, CA: Sage.

Suddick, K.M. & De Souza, L. (2006). Therapists' experiences and perceptions of teamwork in neurological rehabilitation: reasoning behind the team approach, structure and composition of the team and teamworking process. *Physiotherapy Research International*, 11(2), 72–83.

Sue, V.M. & Ritter, L.A. (2012). *Conducting online surveys*, 2nd edn. Thousand Oaks, CA: Sage.

Sulaiman, N., Aroni, R., Thien, F., Schnatter, R., Simpson, P. & Del Colle, E. (2011). Written asthma action plans (WAAPS) in Melbourne general practices: a sequential mixed methods study. *Primary Care Respiratory Journal*, 20(2), 161–9.

Sumsion, T. & Law, M. (2006). A review of evidence on the conceptual elements informing client-centred practice. *Canadian Journal of Occupational Therapy*, 73(3), 153–62.

Suttles, Gerald D. (1968). *The social order of the slum: ethnicity and territory in the inner city*. Chicago: University of Chicago Press.

Suwankhong, D. & Liamputtong, P. (2015). Cultural insiders and research fieldwork: case examples from cross-cultural research with Thai people. *International Journal of Qualitative Methods*. Doi: 10.1177/1609406915621404.

Suwankhong, D. & Liamputtong, P. (2016). Social support among women with breast cancer in southern Thailand. *Journal of Nursing Scholarship*, 48(1), 39-47.

Szklo, M. & Nieto, F.J. (2007). *Epidemiology: beyond the basics*, 2nd edn. Boston, MA: Jones & Bartlett.

Tabachnick, B.G. & Fidell, L.S. (2012). *Using multivariate statistics*, 6th edn. Boston, MA: Pearson Education.

Tashakkori, A. & Creswell, J.W. (2007). Editorial. The new era of mixed methods. *Journal of Mixed Methods Research*, 1(1), 3–7.

Tashakkori, A. & Teddlie, C. (2010). *The Sage handbook of mixed methods in social and behavioural research*, 2nd edn. Thousand Oaks, CA: Sage.

Tate, R., Perdices, M., McDonald, S. & Togher, L. (2011). *Single-case reporting guidelines in behavioural interventions (SCRIBE)*. Sydney: University of Sydney.

Tate, R.L., Perdices, M., Rosenkoetter, U., Wakin, D., Godbee, K., Togher, L. & McDonald, S. (2013). Revision of a method quality rating scale for single-case experimental designs and n-of-1 trials: the 15-item risk of bas in N-of-1 trials (RoBiNT) scale. *Neuropsychological Rehabilitation*, 23(5), 619–38.

Tate, R., Perdices, M., Rosenkeotter, U., Shadfish, W., Vohra, S., Barlow, D. *et al.* (2016). The single-case reporting guidelines in behavioural interventions (SCRIBE) 2015 statement. *Archives of Scientific Psychology*, 4, 1–9.

Tattersall, R.B. (1985). Brittle diabetes. *British Medical Journal*, 291, 555–6.

Taylor, M.C. (2005). Interviewing. In I. Holloway (ed.), *Qualitative research in health care*. Maidenhead, UK: Open University Press, 39–55.

Taylor, S.J. & Bogdan, R. (1998). *Introduction to qualitative research methods*. New York: John Wiley & Sons.

Teddlie, C. & Tashakkori, A. (2009). *Foundations of mixed methods research: integrating quantitative and qualitative approaches in the social and behavioral sciences*. Thousand Oaks, CA: Sage.

Teddlie, C. & Tashakkori, A. (2011). Mixed methods research: contemporary issues in an emerging field. In N.K. Denzin & Y.S. Lincoln (eds), *The Sage handbook of qualitative research*, 4th edn. Thousand Oaks, CA: Sage, 285–99.

Teddlie, C. & Tashakkori, A. (eds) (2003). *Handbook of mixed methods in social and behavioral research*. Thousand Oaks, CA: Sage.

Teddlie, C. & Yu, F. (2007). Mixed method sampling: A typology with examples. *Journal of Mixed Methods Research*, 1(1), 77–100.

Tedlock, B. (2005). The observation of participation and the emergence of public ethnography. In N.K. Denzin & Y.S. Lincoln (eds), *The Sage handbook of qualitative research*. Thousand Oaks, CA: Sage, 467–78.

Tensen, B.L. (2010). *Research strategies for the digital age*, 3rd edn. Boston, MA: Wadsworth.

Terwee, C.B., Bot, A.D.M., de Boer, M.R., van der Windt, D.A.W.M., Knol, D.L., Dekker, J. *et al.* (2007). Quality criteria were proposed for measurement properties of health status questionnaires. *Journal of Clinical Epidemiology*, 60, 34–42.

Thomas, J. & Harden, A. (2008). Methods for the thematic synthesis of qualitative research in systematic reviews. *BMC Medical Research Methodology*, 8, 56. <www.biomedcentral.com/1471-2288/8/45>.

Thompson, C. & Learmonth, M. (2002). How can we develop an evidence-based culture? In J. Craig & R. Smyth (eds), *The evidence-based practice manual for nurses*. Edinburgh: Churchill Livingstone, 211–36.

Thornberg, R. (2012). Informed grounded theory. *Scandinavian Journal of Educational Research*, 56(3), 243–59.

Thorne, S. (1994). Secondary analysis in qualitative research: issues and implications. In J.M. Morse (ed.), *Critical issues in qualitative research methods*. London: Sage, 263–79.

Thorne, S. (1998). Ethical and representational issues in qualitative secondary analysis. *Qualitative Health Research*, 8(4), 547–55.

Thorne, S. (2000). Data analysis in qualitative research. *Evidence Based Nursing*, 3(3), 68–70.

Thorne, S. (2009). The role of qualitative research within an evidence-based context: can metasynthesis be the answer? *International Journal of Nursing Studies*, 46(4), 569–75.

Thorne, S., Jensen, L., Kearney, M.H., Noblit, G. & Sandelowski, M. (2004). Qualitative metasynthesis: reflections on methodological orientation and ideological agenda. *Qualitative Health Research*, 14(10), 1342–65.

Thorne, S.E., Joachim, G., Paterson, B. & Canam, C. (2002). Influence of the research frame on qualitatively derived health science knowledge. *International Journal of Qualitative Methods*, 1, 1. <www.ualberta.ca/~iiqm/backissues/1_1Final/html/thorneeng.html>.

Thurston, W., Cove, L. & Meadows, L. (2008). Methodological congruence in complex and collaborative mixed method studies. *International Journal of Multiple Research Approaches*, 2(1), 2–14.

Tobin, G.A. & Begley, C.M. (2004). Methodological rigour within a qualitative framework. *Journal of Advanced Nursing*, 48(4), 388–96.

Todres, I. (2005). Clarifying the life-world: descriptive phenomenology. In I. Holloway (ed.), *Qualitative research in health care*. Oxford: Blackwell, 104–24.

Toepoel, V. (2015). *Doing surveys online*. London: Sage.

Tollich, M. (2015). *Qualitative ethics in practice*. London: Sage.

Tong, A., Sainsbury, P. & Craig, J. (2007). Consolidated criteria for reporting qualitative research (COREQ): a 32-item checklist for interviews and focus groups. *International Journal for Quality in Health Care*, 19(6), 349–57.

Torgerson, D.J. & Roberts, C. (1999). Understanding controlled trials: randomisation methods: concealment. *British Medical Journal*, 319, 375–6.

Torgerson, D.J. & Torgerson, C.J. (2008). *Designing randomised trials in health education and the social sciences: an introduction*. Basingstoke, UK: Palgrave Macmillan.

Torrance, H. (2008). Building confidence in qualitative research: engaging the demands of policy. *Qualitative Inquiry*, 14(4), 507–27.

Torrance, H. (2011). Qualitative research, science, and government: evidence, criteria, policy, and politics. In N.K. Denzin & Y.S. Lincoln (eds), *The Sage handbook of qualitative research*, 4th edn. Thousand Oaks, CA: Sage, 569–80.

Tourangeau, R., Conrad, F.G. & Couper, M. (2013). *The science of web surveys*. Oxford: Oxford University Press.

Tracy, S.J. (2010). Qualitative quality: eight 'big tents' criteria for excellent qualitative research. *Qualitative Inquiry*, 16(10), 837–51.

Travers, K. (1996). The social organization of nutritional inequities. *Social Science and Medicine*, 43, 543–53.

Trulsson, U. & Klingberg, G. (2003). Living with a child with a severe orofacial handicap: experience from the perspectives of parents. *European Journal of Oral Science*, 111(1), 19–25.

Tsang, E.Y.L., Liamputtong, P. & Pierson, J. (2003). The views of older Chinese people in Melbourne about their quality of life. *Ageing and Society*, 24, 51–74.

Tufford, L. & Newman, P. (2010). Bracketing in qualitative research. *Qualitative Social Work*, 11(1), 80–96.

Turner, D. (2016). *Systematic and literature reviews with CAQDAS or QDA software*. <https://www.youtube.com/watch?v=nkDEOumv6wQ>.

Turner, V.W. (1968). *Schism and continuity in an African society: a study of Ndembu village life*. Manchester: Manchester University Press, on behalf of the Institute for Social Research, University of Zambia.

Uchino, B.N. (2006). Social support and health: a review of psychological processes potentially underlying links to disease outcomes. *Journal of Behavioral Medicine*, 29(4), 377–87.

Uhrenfeldt, L., Aagaard, H., Hall, E.O.C., Fegran, L., Spliid Ludvigsen, M. & Meyer, G. (2013). A qualitative meta-synthesis of patients' experiences of intra- and inter-hospital transitions. *Journal of Advanced Nursing*, 69(8), 1678–90.

Ukrainetz, T.A. & Frequez, E.F. (2003). 'What isn't language?' A qualitative study of the role of the school speech-language pathologist. *Language, Speech, and Hearing Services in Schools*, 34(4), 284–98.

Upton, D. & Upton, P. (2006). Knowledge and use of evidence-based practice by allied health and health science professionals in the United Kingdom. *Journal of Allied Health*, 35(3), 127–33.

Upton, P., Scurlock-Evans, L., Stephens, D. & Upton, D. (2012). The adoption and implementation of evidence-based practice (EBP) among allied health professions. *International Journal of Therapy and Rehabilitation*, 19(9), 497–503.

Vaismoradi, M., Wang, I.-L., Turunen, H. & Bondas, T. (2016). Older people's experiences of caring in nursing homes: a metasynthesis. *International Nursing Review*, 63(1), 111–21.

Vallely, A., Shagi, C., Kasindi, S., Desmond, N., Lees, S., Chiduo, B. *et al.* (2007). The benefits of participatory methodologies to develop effective community dialogue in the context of a microbicide trial feasibility study in Mwanza, Tanzania. *BMC Public Health*, 7, 133.

van Berckelaer, A., DiRocco, D., Ferguson, M., Gray, P., Marcus, N. & Day, S. (2012). Building a patient-centered medical home: obtaining the patient's voice. *Journal of the American Board of Family Medicine*, 25(2), 192–8.

van de Water, A., Shields, N. & Taylor, N. (2011). Systematic review on outcomes in patients with fracture of proximal humerus. *Journal of Shoulder and Elbow Surgery*, 20, 333–43.

van Eck, C.F., van den Bekerom, M.P., Fu, F.H., Poolman, R.W. & Kerkhoffs, G.M. (2013). Methods to diagnose acute anterior cruciate ligament rupture: a meta-analysis of physical examinations with and without anaesthesia. *Knee Surgery Sports Traumatology Arthroscopy Journal*, 21(8), 1895–1903.

van Manen, M. (2006). Writing qualitatively, or the demands of writing. *Qualitative Health Research*, 16(5), 713–22.

van Usen, C. & Pumberger, B. (2007). Effectiveness of eccentric exercises in the management of chronic Achilles tendinosis. *Internet Journal of Allied Health Sciences and Practice*, 5(2), 1–14.

Vandall-Walker, V. & Clark, A.M. (2011). It starts with access: a grounded theory of family members working to get through critical illness. *Journal of Family Nursing*, 17(2), 148–81.

VDHHS (2015). *Victorian health information surveillance system*. Victorian Department of Health and Human Services. <https://www2.health.vic.gov.au/public-health/population-health-systems/health-status-of-victorians#>.

Velicer, W.F., Prochaska, J.O., Fava, J.L., Norman, G.J. & Redding, C.A. (1998). Smoking cessation and stress management: applications of the transtheoretical model of behavior change. *Homeostasis*, 38, 216–33.

Verhaeghe, S.T.L., Defloor, T., Van Zuuren, F.J., Duijnstee, M.S.H. & Grypdonck, M.H.F. (2005). The needs and experiences of family members of adult patients in an intensive care unit: a review of the literature. *Journal of Clinical Nursing*, 14(4), 501–9.

Vlayen, J., Aertgeerts, B., Hannes, K., Sermeus, W. & Ramaekers, D. (2005). A systematic review of appraisal tools for clinical practice guidelines: multiple similarities and one common deficit. *International Journal for Quality in Health Care*, 17(3), 235–42.

Wacjman, J. & Martin, B. (2002). Narratives of identity in modern management: the corrosion of gender difference? *Sociology*, 36(4), 985–1002. <http://soc.sagepub.com/cgi/content/abstract/36/4/985>.

Wadsworth, Y. (2010). *Building in research and evaluation: human inquiry for living systems* [electronic resource]. Sydney: Allen & Unwin.

Wagner, K.D., Davidson, P.J., Pollini, R.A., Strathdee, S.A., Washburn, R. & Palinkas, L.A. (2012). Reconciling incongruous qualitative and quantitative findings in mixed methods research: exemplars from research with drug-using populations. *International Journal of Drug Policy*, 23(1), 54–61.

Walker, D.-M. (2013). The internet as a medium for health services research. Part 2. *Nurse Researcher*, 20(5), 33–7.

Wallis, J.A. & Taylor, N.F. (2011). Pre-operative interventions (non-surgical and non-pharmacological) for patients with hip or knee osteoarthritis awaiting joint replacement surgery: a systematic review and meta-analysis. *Osteoarthritis and Cartilage*, 19(12), 1381–95.

Walsh, D. & Devane, D. (2012). A metasynthesis of midwife-led care. *Qualitative Health Research*, 22(7), 897–910.

Walsh, D. & Downe, S. (2006). Appraising the quality of qualitative research. *Midwifery*, 22, 108–19.

Waltz, C.F., Strickland, O.L. & Lenz, E.R. (2010). *Measurement in nursing and health research*, 4th edn. New York: Springer.

Wand, A. & Eades, S. (2008). Navigating the process of developing a health research project in Aboriginal health. *Medical Journal of Australia*, 188(10), 584–6.

Wang, D. & Bakhai, A. (2006). *Clinical trials: a practical guide to design, analysis, and reporting*. London: Remedica.

Wang, R., Lagakos, S.W., Ware, J.H., Hunter, D.J. & Drazen, J.M. (2007). Statistics in medicine: reporting of subgroup analyses in clinical trials. *New England Journal of Medicine*, 357(21), 2189–94.

Waples-Crowe, P. & Pyett, P. (2005). *The making of a great relationship: a review of a healthy partnership between mainstream and Indigenous organisations*. Melbourne: Victorian Aboriginal Community Controlled Health Organisation.

Ward, L., Treharne, G.J. & Stebbings, S. (2011). The suitability of yoga as a potential therapeutic intervention for rheumatoid arthritis: a focus group approach. *Musculoskeletal Care*, 9(4), 211–21.

Ware, J.E., Kosinski, M. & Keller, S.D. (1994). *SF-36 physical and mental health summary scales: a user's manual*. Boston, MA: Health Institute, New England Medical Center.

Warr, D. & Pyett, P. (1999). Difficult relations: sex work, love and intimacy. *Sociology of Health & Illness*, 21(3), 290–309.

Waterman, H. (1998). Embracing ambiguities and valuing ourselves: issues of validity in action research. *Journal of Advanced Nursing*, 28(1), 101–5.

Waters, M. (director) (2004). *Mean girls* [film]. USA: Paramount Pictures.

Weaver, A. & Atkinson, P. (1995). *Microcomputing and qualitative data analysis*. Aldershot, UK: Avebury.

Weaver, L.J. & Kaiser, B.N. (2015). Developing and testing locally derived mental health scales: examples from North India and Haiti. *Field Methods*, 27(2), 115–30.

Weitzman, E.A. & Miles, M.B. (1995). Choosing software for qualitative data analysis: an overview. *Field Methods*, 7, 1–5.

Weng, Y., Kuo, K.N., Yang, C., Lo, H., Chen, C. & Chiu, Y. (2013). Implementation of evidence-based practice across medical, nursing, pharmacological and allied healthcare professionals: a questionnaire survey in nationwide hospital settings. *Implementation Science*, 8, 112. <http://www.implementationscience.com/content/8/1/112>.

Wertz, F., Charmaz, K., McMullen, L., Josselson, R., Anderson, R. & McSpadden, E. (eds) (2011). *Five ways of doing qualitative analysis*. New York: Guildford Press.

White, A.H. (2015). Using samples to provide evidence. In N.A. Schmidt & J.M. Brown (eds), *Evidence-based practice for nurses: appraisal and application of research*, 3rd edn. Burlington, MA: Jones & Bartlett Learning, 294–319.

White, M. & Epston, D. (1990). *Narrative means to therapeutic ends*. New York: W.W. Norton.

White, S. (2001). Auto-ethnography as reflexive inquiry: the research act as self-surveillance. In I. Shaw & N. Gould (eds), *Qualitative research in social work*. Newbury Park, CA: Sage, 100–15.

Whiting, P., Rutjes, A., Reitsma, J., Bossuyt, P. & Kleijnen, J. (2003). The development of QUADAS: a tool for the quality assessment of studies of diagnostic accuracy included in systematic reviews. *BMC Medical Research Methodology*, 3, 25.

Whittemore, R. & Knafl, K. (2005). The integrative review: updated methodology. *Journal of Advanced Nursing*, 52(5), 546–53.

Whittemore, R., Chao, A., Jang, M., Minges, K. & Park, C. (2014). Methods for knowledge synthesis: an overview. *Heart & Lung*, 43, 453–61.

WHO (2001). *International classification of functioning, disability and health: short version.* Geneva: World Health Organization.

WHO (2012a). *International clinical trials registry platform.* Geneva, World Health Organization. <www.who.int/ictrp/en>.

WHO (2012b). *World Health Organization research policy.* <http://www.who.int/phi/implementation/research/en/>.

WHO, Health and Welfare Canada & Canadian Public Health Association (1986). *Ottawa charter for health promotion.* Ottawa: World Health Organization.

Wiegerinck, J.I., Kerkhoffs, G.M., van Sterkenburg, M.N., Sierevelt, I.N. & van Dijk, C.N. (2013). Treatment for insertional Achilles tendinopathy: a systematic review. Knee Surgery Sports Traumatology Arthroscopy Journal, 21(6), 1345–55.

Wikberg, A. & Bondas, T. (2010). A patient perspective in research on intercultural caring in maternity care: a meta-ethnography. *International Journal of Qualitative Studies on Health and Well-being*, 5(1), 46–8. <www.ijqhw.net/index.php/qhw/rt/printerFriendly/4648/5377>.

Wikberg, A. & Eriksson, K. (2008). Intercultural caring: an abductive model. *Scandinavian Journal of Caring Science*, 22(3), 485–96.

Wiles, R., Heath, S. & Crow, G. (2005). *Methods briefing 2: informed consent and the research process (ESRC Research Methods Programme).* <www.esrc.ac.uk/methods>.

Wilkinson, S.A., Hinchliffe, F., Hough, J. & Chang, A. (2012). Baseline evidence-based practice use, knowledge, and attitudes of allied health professionals. *Journal of Allied Health*, 41(4), 177–84.

Williams, M., Unrau, Y.A., Grinnell, R.M. & Epstein, I. (2011). The qualitative research approach. In R.M. Grinnell & Y.A. Unrau (eds), *Social work research and evaluation: foundations of evidence-based practice*, 9th edn. New York: Oxford University Press, 52–67.

Williams, M., Unrau, Y.A., Grinnell, R.M. & Epstein, I. (2014). The qualitative approach. In R.M. Grinnell & Y.A. Unrau (eds), *Social work research and evaluation: foundations of evidence-based practice*, 10th edn. New York: Oxford University Press, 78–96.

Williamson, K. (2008). Where information is paramount: a mixed methods, multidisciplinary investigation of Australian on-line investor. *Information Research* 13(4). <http://informationr.net/ir/13-4/paper365.html>.

Willis, J.W. (2007). *Foundations of qualitative research: interpretive and critical approaches.* Thousand Oaks, CA: Sage.

Willis, J. & Saunders, M. (2007). Research in a post-colonial world. In M. Pitts & A. Smith (eds), *Researching the margins: strategies for ethical and rigorous research with marginalised communities.* Basingstoke, UK: Palgrave Macmillan, 96–113.

Willis, K., Green, J., Daly, J., Williamson, L. & Bandyopadhyay, M. (2009). Perils and possibilities: achieving best evidence from focus groups in public health research. *Australian and New Zealand Journal of Public Health*, 33(2), 131–6.

Willke, R.J., Burke, L.B. & Erickson, P. (2004). Measuring treatment impact: a review of patient-reported outcomes and other efficacy endpoints in approved product labels. *Controlled Clinical Trials*, 25(6), 535–52.

Wilson, H.S. & Hutchinson, S.A. (1996). Methodological mistakes in grounded theory. *Nursing Research*, 45(2), 122–4.

Winbolt, M., Nay, R. & Fetherstonhaugh, D. (2009). Taking a TEAM (Translating Evidence into Aged care Methods) approach to practice change. In R. Nay & S. Garrett (eds), *Older people: issues and innovations in care*. Sydney: Elsevier Australia, 442–55.

Winkelman, W. & Halifax, N. (2007). Power is only skin deep: an institutional ethnography of nurse-driven outpatient psoriasis treatment in the era of clinic websites. *Journal of Medical Systems*, 31(2), 131–9.

Wolcott, H. (1990). Making a study 'more ethnographic'. *Journal of Contemporary Ethnography*, 19(1), 44–72.

Wolcott, H.F. (2009). *Writing up qualitative research*, 3rd edn. Thousand Oaks, CA: Sage.

Women's Health Australia (2005). The Australian longitudinal study on women's health: the first decade. <www.alswh.org.au/images/content/pdf/achievement_reports/achievements-overview.pdf>.

Wood, L., Egger, M., Gluud, L.L., Schulz, K.F., Jüni, P., Altman, D.G. *et al.* (2008). Empirical evidence of bias in treatment effect estimates in controlled trials with different interventions and outcomes: meta-epidemiological study. *British Medical Journal*, 336, 601–5.

Woodley, B.L., Newsham-West, R.J. & Baxter, G.D. (2007). Chronic tendinopathy: effectiveness of eccentric exercise. *British Journal of Sports Medicine*, 41(4), 188–98; discussion 199.

Woods, M., Paulus, T., Atkins, D.P. & Macklin, R. (2015). Advancing qualitative research using qualitative data analysis software (QDAS)? Reviewing potential versus practice in published studies using ATLAS.ti and NVivo, 1994–2013. *Social Science Computer Review*, 0894439315596311.

World Medical Association (2013). *The World Medical Association Declaration of Helsinki: ethical principles for medical research involving human subjects*. Seoul: Department of Health.

Wright Mills, C. (1967). *The sociological imagination*. London: Oxford University Press.

Wuest, J. (2007). Grounded theory: the method. In P.L. Munhall (ed.), *Nursing research: a qualitative perspective*. Sudbury, MA: Jones & Bartlett, 239–71.

Yoo, G.J., Levine, E.G., Aviv, C., Ewing, C. & Au, A. (2010). Older women, breast cancer, and social support. *Support Care Cancer*, 18(12), 1521–30.

Young, A., Gomersall, T. & Bowne, A. (2012). Trial participants'experiences of early enhanced speech and language therapy after stroke compared with employed visitor support: a qualitative study nested within a randomized controlled trial. *Clinical Rehabilitation*, 27(2), 174–82.

Zhang, Y. & Shaw, J.D. (2012). Publishing in AMJ. Part 5. Crafting the methods and results. *Academy of Management Journal*, 55, 8–12.

Zhao S (1991). Metatheory, metamethod, meta-data-analysis: what, why, and how? *Sociological Perspectives*, 34(3), 377–90.

Zierold, K.M., Sears, C.G. & Brock, G.N. (2015). Exposure-reducing behaviors among residents living near a coal ash storage site. *Health Education & Behavior*. Doi:10.1177/1090198115610573.

Zimmer, L. (2006). Qualitative meta-synthesis: a question of dialoguing with texts. *Journal of Advanced Nursing*, 53, 311–18.

Zuzelo, P.R. (2012). Evidence-based nursing and qualitative research: a partnership imperative for real-world practice. In P.L. Munhall (ed.), *Nursing research: a qualitative perspective*, 4th edn. Sudbury, MA: Jones & Bartlett, 481–500.

Zwarenstein, M. & Treweek, S. (2009). What kind of randomized trials do we need? *Journal of Clinical Epidemiology*, 62(5), 461–3.

NOTES

NOTES

NOTES

NOTES

NOTES

NOTES

NOTES